Advances in Biomedical Science

Advances in Biomedical Science

Editor: Skylar Patton

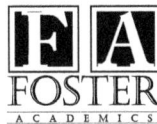

FA FOSTER
ACADEMICS

www.fosteracademics.com

www.fosteracademics.com

FA
FOSTER
ACADEMICS

Cataloging-in-Publication Data

Advances in biomedical science / edited by Skylar Patton.
    p. cm.
Includes bibliographical references and index.
ISBN 978-1-63242-898-1
1. Medical sciences. 2. Medicine. 3. Biomedical engineering. I. Patton, Skylar.
R130 .A38 2020
610--dc23

Foster Academics,
118-35 Queens Blvd., Suite 400,
Forest Hills, NY 11375, USA

ISBN 978-1-63242-898-1 (Hardback)

Contents

Preface

Biomedical sciences refer to a group of applied sciences that apply aspects of natural science for use in healthcare and public health. These applied sciences include medical microbiology, biomedical engineering, clinical virology and clinical epidemiology, among others. These sciences are focused on the study of human health and disease, as well as areas such as human physiology, human nutrition and pharmacology. Laboratory diagnosis is an important aspect of biomedical science. The specializations in biomedical science fall within the array of life sciences, physiological science, and medical physics or bioengineering. Advances in biomedical science have been possible due to an integration of biomedical technologies, biomedical engineering, bioengineering, biotechnology and biomedical informatics. This book aims to shed light on some of the unexplored aspects of biomedical science and the recent researches in this field. It includes some of the vital pieces of work being conducted across the world, on various topics related to this discipline. It is appropriate for students seeking detailed information in this area as well as for experts.

The researches compiled throughout the book are authentic and of high quality, combining several disciplines and from very diverse regions from around the world. Drawing on the contributions of many researchers from diverse countries, the book's objective is to provide the readers with the latest achievements in the area of research. This book will surely be a source of knowledge to all interested and researching the field.

In the end, I would like to express my deep sense of gratitude to all the authors for meeting the set deadlines in completing and submitting their research chapters. I would also like to thank the publisher for the support offered to us throughout the course of the book. Finally, I extend my sincere thanks to my family for being a constant source of inspiration and encouragement.

Editor

CRISPR/Cas9: the Jedi against the dark empire of diseases

Sehrish Khan[1], Muhammad Shahid Mahmood[1], Sajjad ur Rahman[1], Hassan Zafar[1], Sultan Habibullah[2], Zulqarnain khan[2] and Aftab Ahmad[3*]

Abstract

Advances in Clustered Regularly Interspaced Short Palindromic Repeats/CRISPR associated system (CRISPR/Cas9) has dramatically reshaped our ability to edit genomes. The scientific community is using CRISPR/Cas9 for various biotechnological and medical purposes. One of its most important uses is developing potential therapeutic strategies against diseases. CRISPR/Cas9 based approaches have been increasingly applied to the treatment of human diseases like cancer, genetic, immunological and neurological disorders and viral diseases. These strategies using CRISPR/Cas9 are not only therapy oriented but can also be used for disease modeling as well, which in turn can lead to the improved understanding of mechanisms of various infectious and genetic diseases. In addition, CRISPR/Cas9 system can also be used as programmable antibiotics to kill the bacteria sequence specifically and therefore can bypass multidrug resistance. Furthermore, CRISPR/Cas9 based gene drive may also hold the potential to limit the spread of vector borne diseases. This bacterial and archaeal adaptive immune system might be a therapeutic answer to previous incurable diseases, of course rigorous testing is required to corroborate these claims. In this review, we provide an insight about the recent developments using CRISPR/Cas9 against various diseases with respect to disease modeling and treatment, and what future perspectives should be noted while using this technology.

Keywords: CRISPR/Cas9, Disease modeling, Genetic diseases

Background

The potential and versatility of the field of genome engineering are remarkable in the sense of how scientists can utilize it for numerous benefits of mankind. The field has a wide range of applications in therapeutic medicine and biomedical research. The most pivotal aspect of genome engineering is certainly gene therapy, which can provide novelty to the way infectious diseases and genetic disorders are treated. To provide a cure through gene therapy, it is fundamental to study the gene functions and gene regulations through disease models that are in vivo and ex vivo. Another aspect of gene therapy is the way the genome is modified using different approaches, and how this modification could result in either a cure or a harmful mutation.

The genome whether in eukaryotes, prokaryotes or archea is a fascinating plethora of genes with endless protein products and possibilities. The vastness of proteins encoded by genes can be comprehended by a paradigm that twenty thousand proteins can be encoded by genes accumulated in only a meter of linear DNA in the genome [1]. In addition, this DNA also contains non-coding genes too. So, an estimate of the vastness of genes in the genome is tangibly comprehensible. In genetics, data from various studies of the past decade has elaborated the importance of variants and disease. Scientists have apprehended about the pivotal role that genome editing could play in the cure or prevention of infectious diseases. In the field of genome engineering, the term CRISPR/Cas9 has gained much fame in the previous few years. Many research papers are being written and published regarding exceptional experimentation using the technique: also claims of how this innovative, but simple method will prove to be the therapeutic answer to previous incurablediseases. Much testing is being done to confirm the claim of being the divine cure to diseases; in this review, we highlight the advancements that have been made using CRISPR/Cas9 in relation to cancer, genetic diseases, neurological, immunological disorders and viral infections.

* Correspondence: aftab.ahmad@uaf.edu.pk
[3]Department of Biochemistry/U.S.-Pakistan Center for Advanced Studies in Agriculture and Food Security (USPCAS-AFS), University of Agriculture Faisalabad (UAF), Faisalabad 38040, Pakistan
Full list of author information is available at the end of the article

Primordial genome editing to CRISPR/Cas9: The journey

The journey of genetic modification through the past few decades has been remarkable and fascinating. First and foremost, the classical experimentation of Capechhi must be reminisced. He was the first modifier of genes in mammalian cells through his revolutionary research termed, "heteroduplex induced mutagenesis" [2]. In concise, he made possible genetic modification in cells, which potentially paved the way for future genomic modification research. However, modification of the genomes has come a long way since the revolutionary discovery by Capecchi, Many improvements have been indoctrinated into methodologies that have uplifted the technology of genomic modification to a higher level. For many years the field of genetic engineering was based only on simple homologous recombination of DNA, and there was a seemingly limited application of the field due to the requisite of more complex targeting and construct selection.

The consequent development of homologous combination of DNA based upon phages (bacterial viruses) simplified the engineering of much larger DNA fragments, and also made possible the production of target vectors [3]. The headway towards more accomplished gene modification got better when it was demonstrated that double-stranded breaks (DSB) could be induced in mammalian chromosomes [4]. It was further proved that the use of the meganuclease, 'I-SceI' could induce double-stranded breaks increasing the probability to get targeted homologous recombination events [5]. These meganucleases can be cogitated as modified forms of naturally occurring restriction enzymes having extended DNA recognition sequences (14–40 bp) [6]. The engineering of meganucleases is an arduous challenge because the DNA recognition and cleavage function of these enzymes are interwined in a single domain [7].

Further facilitation of genome editing was provided by the use of zinc finger nucleases (ZFNs). These ZFNs have two independent regions: a recognition domain of zinc fingers which identify the target triplet nucleotides in the DNA, while the second region, which is a non-specific nuclease called FokI generates the double stranded breaks (DSB) Since the nuclease has to dimerize to remain active, the ZFNs have to be used in pairs [8]. The ZFNs are small like MNs, but the designing of the recognition domain of ZFNs is more straightforward than MNs. More studies indicated about the potentiality of the use of ZF domains as an effective nuclease system; a target sequence of about 9 bp or 18 bp can be modified using ZFNs in a precise manner [9, 10].

Another genome editing tool is Transcription activator-like effector nucleases (TALENs). These have two independent parts. The first part consists of transcription activator-like factors (TALEs); these proteins were first discovered in the plant pathogen bacteria *Xanthomonas* [11]. During the TALEs infection of plants, these TALEs are transported into the plant cells and bind to DNA sequences resulting in modulation of the expression of the plant genes [11, 12]. These TALEs can be fused to a FokI nuclease domain, which in turn can create DSB in the targeted DNA. The designing of TALENs is simpler than ZFNs, while longer recognition sites enhances its specificity and make it less prone to off-target mutations [13].

Another technology is RNA interference (RNAi), which has also been used to some extent for gene expression modification. But, this technique has certain limitations. The effects of RNAi are generally non-specific, temporary and the technique is restricted to the knocking down of only transcribed genes [14]. These chimeric nucleases ZFNs, TALENs, and meganucleases possess powerful attributes to perform site-specific genome modifications, activation/inactivation of genes, sequence deletion, andrearrangement of the chromosomes [15]. However, an even more efficient genome modification tool was soon to be put to use to modify genomes.

CRISPR/Cas9 miraculous genetic tool

In 2012, the field of genome engineering had one of the most important discoveries ever. Surprisingly, it involved the adaptive immune system of a Gram-positive bacteria *Streptococcus pyogenes*. The adaptive prokaryotic immune system CRISPR/Cas is present in 90% of archea and around 50% of bacteria [16]. The immune system is somewhat analogous to mammalian systems in remembrance of the foreign DNA; a sort of record is kept of prior exposures to phages and plasmids. A recurrent exposure results in a rapid and robust immune response to the invading foreign DNA. The genetic locus of the CRISPR/Cas systems is called "CRISPR array"; the locus contains a base pair range of ~ 20–50 (bp) separated by variable short DNA sequences termed as "Spacers". These spacers are preceded by a leader sequence rich in AT. The sequence of DNA in the invading microbe possesses a sequence identical to the spacers, this foreign sequence is termed as "Protospacer" [17].

The mechanism of immunity generally involves three important phases: adaptation, expression (biogenesis of crRNA) and interference [18]. The first phase, which involves the injection of foreign DNA into the host, the adaption system selects protospacers from the foreign DNA and includes them into the CRISPR locus (array) towards the leader end. During the expression (crRNA biogenesis) phase, there is transcription at the CRISPR locus normally as a single pre-crRNA, which subsequently proceeds into a mature crRNA containing a single spacer. The final phase is the interference in which the crRNA guides the Cas nucleases to precisely-identify and cleave the foreign nucleic acid [19]. A comparison of CRISPR/Cas9, ZFNs, meganucleases, TALENs and RNAi is given in Table 1.

Table 1 Comparison of CRISPR/Cas9, ZFNs, TALENs, meganucleases and RNAi

	CRISPR/Cas9	ZFNs	TALENs	Meganucleases	RNAi
Target site	19–22 bp	18–36 bp	24–40 bp	14–40 bp	Target site should be located 50–100 nt from ATG
Retargeting possibility	Easily retargeted without any complexity	Yes, but requires complex molecular cloning	Yes, but requires protein engineering	Yes, by protein engineering	Yes
Nuclease	Cas9	FokI	FokI	I-SceI	Dicer and Argonaute proteins
Recognition mechanism	RNA-DNA	Protein-DNA	Protein-DNA	Protein-DNA	RNA
Targeting restrictions	Protospacer adjacent motif (PAM) must be present	Non-G-rich sequences are difficult to target	T in the start and A at the end	Novel sequences are difficult to target	Only targets mRNA
Efficiency	High	High	High	High	High
Limitations	Off targets	Both expensive and time consuming to construct	Takes long to construct	Limited versatility in targeting	Off targets
Cytotoxicity	Low	Low	Variable to high	Low	Variable to high
Multiplexing ease	High	Low	Low	Low	High
Cost	Low	High	Moderate	Low	Low

Classification of the CRISPR/Cas system

The diversity of the CRISPR/Cas system is an essential component keeping in mind the wide range of foreign genetic elements that have to be confronted by it. Moreover, there are major differences in the repeated sequences of the CRISPR loci; it also applies to the Cas sequences and overall architecture of the Cas operon [18]. To overcome this ambiguity and to provide a clearer picture of the CRISPR/Cas system, it has been classified into six main types and two main classes shown in Fig 1. Type I-III is better understood, whereas types IV-VI have been identified recently. In the type I system the Cas-3 nuclease-helicase is involved, the type II system has the nuclease Cas9, while the type III systems possess the least understood Cas10. Type IV system possesses an uncharacterized protein Csf1. Type V systems contain either Cpf1, C2c1or C2c3, which are very much similar to Cas9. Type V1 contains a large protein C2c2. Class 1 system comprises of type I, III and IV and the class 2 system comprises of II, V and VI [19].

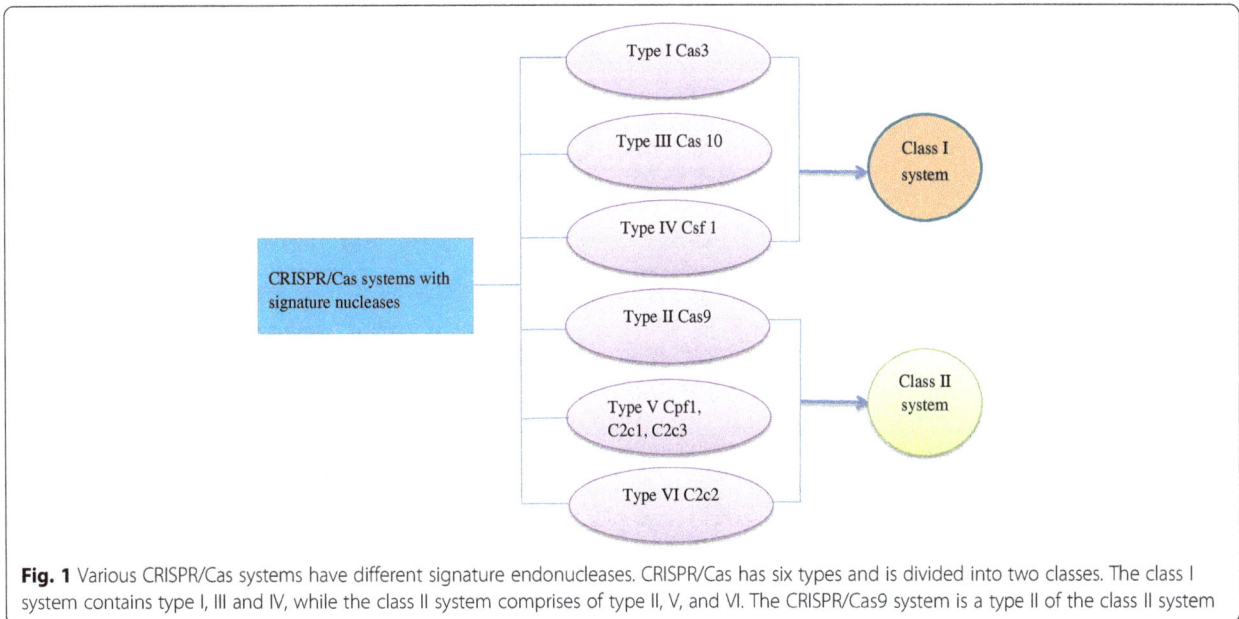

Fig. 1 Various CRISPR/Cas systems have different signature endonucleases. CRISPR/Cas has six types and is divided into two classes. The class I system contains type I, III and IV, while the class II system comprises of type II, V, and VI. The CRISPR/Cas9 system is a type II of the class II system

CRISPR/Cas9 in genome editing

The potential of CRISPR/Cas9 was exploited in mammalian cells for the first time in 2013, the mechanism of action is similar to the prokaryotes with the single guide RNA (sgRNA) derived from the crRNA and trans-acting CRISPR RNA [20]. The CRISPR/Cas9 domains consist of sgRNA, and Cas9 nuclease that has RuyC and HNH as two catalytic active domains [21]. In response to Protospacer adjacent motif (PAM) present on the other strand, the sgRNA directs Cas9 through base pairing to the target site resulting in DSBs generated by Cas9. If homologous sequences are available these DSBs are repaired by homologous directed repair, the absence of homologous sequences will result in non-homologous end joining (NHEJ). The type of joining is pivotal as HDR results in an accurate gene correction while NHEJ may produce insertions/deletion mutations, shown in Figs. 2 and 3.

The reprogrammable property of Cas9 is incredible; it can be reprogrammed through inactivation of either or both HNH or RuvC into nickase Cas9 and dead Cas9 (dCas9). The dCas9 is catalytically inactive, but still shows a promising platform for targeting DNA through RNA guidance [22]. The CRISPR technology for gene regulation is termed as CRISPR interference (CRISPRi for gene repression) or CRISPR activation (CRISPRa for activation). Both use dCas9 fused with transcriptional repressors and activators [23]. In bacteria, dCas9 alone with sgRNA can efficiently silence gene expression [24]. However, only moderate silencing takes place in mammalian cells when dCas9 is used alone [24, 25] The fusing of dCas9 to the repressive KRAB (Krupel associated box) domain of Kox-1 exhibits strong gene silencing [25]. The effective targets sites of CRISPRi include proximal promoters, enhancers and coding region downstream from the transcription site of a gene [25]. The fusion of dCas9 with a transcription activator VP64 can result in the activation of a reporter gene [26, 27].

The CRISPR/Cas9 has many benefits in comparison to TALENs, ZFNs, RNAi and meganucleases. Firstly, in order to target a new DNA sequence the only requirement is a sgRNA, this is much simple and easy as compared to the synthesis of a cumbersome guiding protein for TALENS, ZFNs, RNAi and meganucleases. Furthermore, multiple sgRNAs can be used in the case of CRISPR/Cas9 to target different genomic loci simultaneously this is termed as "multiplexing" [28].

Methods of delivery of CRISPR/Cas9

Both viral and non-viral delivery methods are being used for the delivery of CRISPR/Cas9 components into cell lines and animal models. Viral vectors such as self-inactivating lentivirus, adenovirus and adeno-associated virus (AAV) are potential delivery vehicles for CRISPR/Cas9. For non-viral delivery potential cargoes include plasmid DNA, Cas9/gRNA ribonuleoprotein complexes and donor nucleic acid templates [29]. However, for non-viral delivery various methods such as electroporation, induced osmocytosis, hydrodynamic delivery and lipid-mediated transfection can be used [30].

CRISPR/Cas9 resources

Hundreds of online methods are available for CRISPR/Cas9 gene editing, construct designing with double stranded breaks, single stranded breaks, functional knockouts, plasmid with active gene expression, repress gene expression, tagging protein, finding target sequences and many others. A large number of resources have been developed which are being used for application in genome engineering, for identification of CRISPR target site and for selection of gRNA. Multiple online resources are available

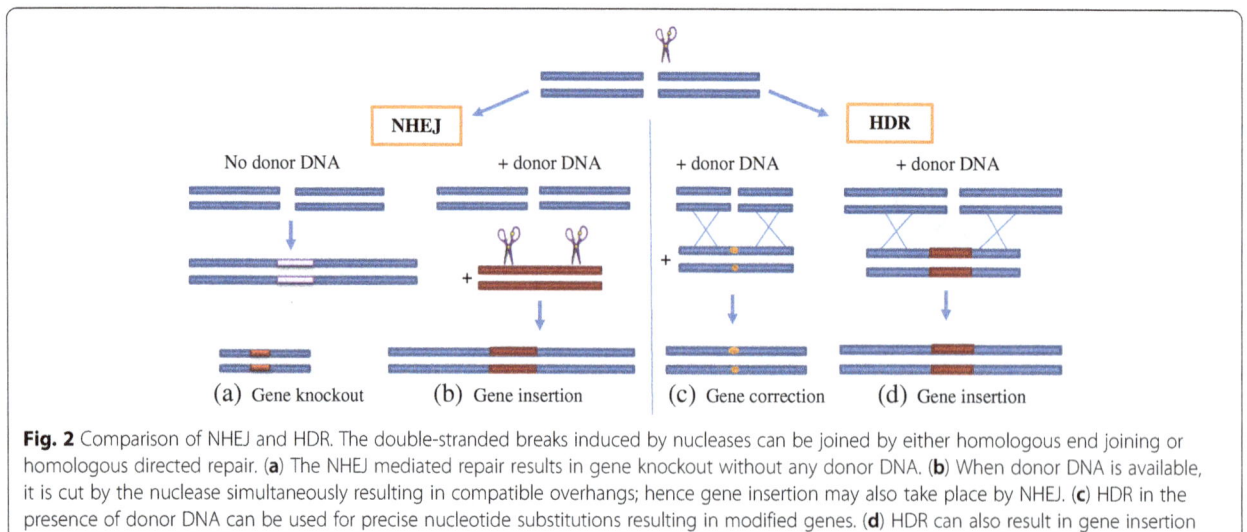

Fig. 2 Comparison of NHEJ and HDR. The double-stranded breaks induced by nucleases can be joined by either homologous end joining or homologous directed repair. (**a**) The NHEJ mediated repair results in gene knockout without any donor DNA. (**b**) When donor DNA is available, it is cut by the nuclease simultaneously resulting in compatible overhangs; hence gene insertion may also take place by NHEJ. (**c**) HDR in the presence of donor DNA can be used for precise nucleotide substitutions resulting in modified genes. (**d**) HDR can also result in gene insertion

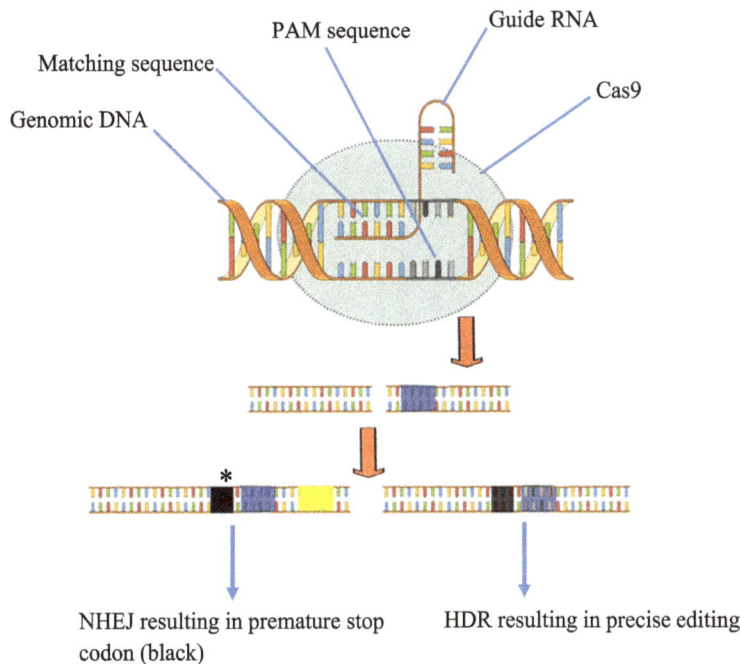

Fig. 3 CRISPR/Cas9 mechanism. The important components in the system include Cas9 and gRNA. The nuclease Cas9 acts as a molecular scissors to cut the DNA strands. The gRNA directs the Cas9 to cleave the DNA at a specific position. The joining of the DNA occurs either by NHEJ or HDR

forcommercially available kits/ plasmids and CRISPR/Cas9 construction, as few are mentioned in Table 2.

Numerous vectors are used for Cas9 according to the desired gene modification to be performed. The desired modifications include single strand break (SSB), double strand break (DSB), activation of gene expression, repression of gene expression and tagging of proteins knockout genes, these tools working so that any user can design construct with selectable marker, and different gene to be inserted according to their own demands. Many of them are freely accesible, but some are paid as well, depicted in Table 3.

In addition, miscellaneous online resources are available for the designing of sgRNAs which provide information about OTs without limiting the PAM or number of - mismatch bases, for finding potential off targets in any genome, identification and ranking all sgRNA targets sites according to off target quality, help in inquiry of guide sequences [32], and few of them are described in Table 4 with pros and corns.

CRISPR/Cas9 and disease resistance
Development of cancer models using CRISPR/Cas9

A correct cancer disease model is highly essential to study and understand cancer pathogenesis. The same complex genetic scenario, as in cancer has to be restructured in various models of animals and human cells. For this purpose,

Table 2 Commercial available kits/plasmids and services for CRISPR/Cas9 construction

Sr No.	Company Name	Web link
1	Addgene	www.addgene.org/crispr/guide/
2	Thermo Fisher Scientific	www.thermofisher.com/pk/en/home/life-science/genome-editing/geneart-crispr/crispr-libraries/lentiarray-crispr-libraries/lentiarray-cas9-lentivirus.html
3	ATUM	www.atum.bio/products/expression-vectors/mammalian?exp=5
4	Synthego	www.synthego.com/products/synthetic-sgrna/
5	GeneCopoeia	www.genecopoeia.com/product/transgenic-mouse/
6	Origene	http://www.origene.com/CRISPR-CAS9/
7	Clonetech	http://www.clontech.com/US/Products/Genome_Editing/CRISPR_Cas9/Resources/About_Guide-it_Kits
8	Sigma-Aldrich	https://www.sigmaaldrich.com/webapp/wcs/stores/servlet/LogonForm?storeId=11001
9	CHOPCHOP	https://chopchop.rc.fas.harvard.edu/
10	Active Motif	http://www.activemotif.com/catalog/1172/enchip

Table 3 Selective CRISPR/Cas9 plasmids

	Name	Gene/insert	Selectable marker	Purpose	Reference
1. CRISPR/Cas9 plasmids that create single stranded break (Mammalian)	pX335-U6-chimeric_BB-CBh-hSpCas9n (D10A)	Humanized S. pyogenes Cas9 (D10A) nickase	None	A human codon-optimized SpCas9 nickase and chimeric guide RNA expression plasmid	[28]
2. CRISPR/Cas9 plasmids that create double stranded break (Mammalian)	pX330-U6-chimeric_BB-CBh-hSpCas9	humanized S. pyogenes Cas9	None	A human codon-optimized SpCas9 and chimeric guide RNA expression plasmid	[28]
3. CRISPR/Cas9 plasmids which activate gene expression (Mammalian)	pSpCas9 (BB)-2A–Puro (PX459) V2.0	hSpCas9-2A-Puro V2.0 (Synthetic)	Puromycin	Cas9 from S. pyogenes with 2A-Puro, and cloning backbone for sgRNA (V2.0)	[31]
	SP-dCas9-VPR	SP-dCas9-VPR (Homo sapiens)	Neomycin (select with G418)	SP-dCas9 with VP64-p65-Rta (VPR) fused to its C-terminus; mammalian vector	[33]
	dCAS9-VP64_GFP	dCAS9(D10A, H840A)-VP64_2A_GFP (Synthetic)	GFP	Expresses dCas9-VP64 activator with 2A GFP	[34]
	lenti dCAS-VP64_Blast	dCAS9(D10A, N863A)-VP64_2A_Blast (Synthetic)	Blasticidin	3rd generation lenti vector encoding dCas9-VP64 with 2A Blast resistance marker (EF1a-NLS-dCas9 (N863)-VP64-2A-Blast-WPRE)	[34]
4. CRISPR/Cas9 plasmids which repress gene expression (Mammalian)	pSLQ1658-dCas9-EGFP	dCas9 fuse to EGFP (Homo sapiens)	Puromycin	Template for NLS-dCas9-NLS-EGFP fusion protein for CRISPR imaging (the recipient vector can be TetON 3G promoter system)	[35]
	pLV hUbC-dCas9-T2A-GFP	Humanized dead Cas9 T2A GFP (Other)	Zeocin	Co-expresses human optimized S. pyogenes dCas9 and GFP	[36]
	pJMP1	dCas9 (Other)	None	Bacillus subtilis dCas9 expression vector; integrates into lacA/ganA	[37]
5. CRISPR/Cas9 plasmid for tagging protein	Protein pFETCh_NCoA2	Human	Donor plasmid pFETCh_NCoA2	Donor vector for 3' FLAG tag of human NCoA2	[38]
	pFETCh_RAD21	Human	pFETCh_RAD21	Homology arms and 3X Flag with P2A Neo for 3' tagging of human RAD21	[38]

Table 4 Tools available for sgRNA designing

Tool	Website	Purpose	Input	Output	Available genomes	Pros	Cons	Reference
Atum	https://www.atum.bio/eCommerce/cas9/input	Candidate gRNA	DNA sequence, (max 10,000 bp) gene name, genomic region	Candidate guide sequences and off target loci	5	Uses ATUM scoring to minimize off-targets/all in one nickase ninja	Not free of cost	N/A
Benchling	https://benchling.com/crispr	Candidate gRNA	DNA sequence/gene name	Candidate guide sequences and off target loci	5	Free of cost		N/A
CRISPR design	http://crispr.mit.edu/	Used to find target sequences for a sequence or sequnces (batch mode), also provides in depth on/off target information	DNA sequence/FASTA files single or batch mode	Candidate guide sequences and off target loci	16	Helpful to generate many candidates with on/off information	Only handles short sequences up to 23–500 bp/slow to use/no efficacy merit/does not indicate identity of mismatches	[39]
CHOPCHOP	https://chopchop.rc.fas.harvard.edu/	To find target sequences for a single sequence/gene/transcript	DNA sequence/gene name/genome location	Candidate guide sequences and off target loci,	23	Good to generate multiple guides for a single target, free of cost	No on-target efficacy	[40]
Cas off finder	http://www.rgenome.net/cas-offinder/	Provides information about OTs without limiting the PAM or number of mismatch bases	sgRNA	Off target loci for guide sequences	20	Free of cost/easy to use	Does not give indication if OTs are in coding sequences	[41]
Fly CRISPR	http://tools.flycrispr.molbio.wisc.edu/targetFinder/	Candidate gRNA, software provides maximum stringency- (uses strict algorithm in cells lines) and minimum stringency; off target cleavage effects observed	DNA sequence	Candidate guide sequences and off target loci,	18	Free of cost	Slow to use	[42]
E-CRISP	http://www.e-crisp.org/E-CRISP/designcrispr.html	Finds target sequences for a single gene or sequence	DNA sequence/gene symbol	Candidate guide sequences and off target loci,	30	Free of cost	Numerous options may be confusing/no account for identity of mismatches	[43]
Cas OT	http://eendbzfgenetics.org/casot/	To find potential off targets in any genome	FASTA files	sgRNA and OT sites	User input	Free of cost/ First tool that identifies off-targetes in a user specified genome	No account for identity of mismatches	N/A
CRISPR ERA	http://crispr-era.stanford.edu/	Used for genome wide screening based on CRISPR, CRISPRi and CRISPRa	DNA sequence, gene name or TSS location	Candidate guide sequences and distances to TSS	9	Free of cost/can also be used for genome imaging and CRISPR synthetic circuit design		[44]
CCTop	http://crispr.cos.uni-heidelberg.de/	It helps in identifying and ranking all sgRNA targets sites according to off target quality	DNA sequence/FASTA file single/	Scores OTs and also ranks	45	Free of cost/easy to use	No on-target efficacy prediction	[45]

Table 4 Tools available for sgRNA designing (Continued)

Tool	Website	Purpose	Input	Output	Available genomes	Pros	Cons	Reference
			batch/ sequences 23 to 500 bp	sgRNA by OTs				
WU-CRISPR	http://crispr.wustl.edu/	Potential candidate gRNA	DNA sequence/ gene symbol	sgRNA list ranked by efficacy score	2 (Human and mouse)	Free of cost/easy to use	No account of identity of mismatches	[46]
GTscan	http://gt-scan.csiro.au/	Used to find target sequences and OTs for a single sequence	DNA sequence/ FASTA file	SgRNA, genomic sites with 0 to 3 mismatches	51	Free of cost/easy to use	Trouble in finding exact matches in genome	[47]
CRISPR direct	https://crispr.dbcls.jp/	To find target sequences for a single transcript/sequence	DNA sequence/ genome location/ transcript	Target sequence and position	20	Free of cost/rapid visual display of target sequence and OT information	No on-target efficacy	[48]
COD	http://cas9.wicp.net/	Used to find target sequences for an input sequence	DNA sequence up to 400 bp	Gene bank file/ CSC file/ OT scoring	27	Free of cost/easy to use/ OT scoring	Slow to use/no on-taget prediction	N/A
sgRNA scorer 2.0	https://crispr.med.harvard.edu/	Used to find target sequences/ OT using Casfinder	DNA sequence/ FASTA files upto 10 kb	Target sequence with activity score	14	Free of cost/ allows to identify target sites for any CRISPR system	Slow to use/OT prediction does not account identity	N/A
CRISPOR	http://crispor.tefor.net/	To find candidate guide sequences	DNA sequence 1000 bp	Guide sequence with specificity score/guides for OTs	146	Free of cost	N/A	[49]

CRISPR/Cas9 has proved to be an extremely valuable genetic tool for creating a same cancer-like conditions. The efficient CRISPR tool has expedited gene modification for the development of quick animal and human cellular models for oncogenic studies [50, 51]. Genome alterations are the driving force behind the processes that initiate human cancer. These cancer-initiating processes include chromosomal arrangements (deletions, duplications, inversions, translocations) and point mutations, which in turn inactivate tumor suppressor genes (TSGs) and convert proto-oncogenes into oncogenes [52]. The CRISPR/Cas9 system has been successfully used in established cell lines, organoids and patient-derived xenografts to engineer LOF(loss of function) mutations by NHEJ, GOF(gain of function) mutations by HDR and chromosomal re-arrangements by cutting at two distant loci [50, 52]. Several groups have used the CRISPR system to study hematological malignancies by CRISPR/Cas9 mediated editing of genes in hematopoietic cells and subsequent transplantation back into animals to assess tumorigenicity [53].

CRISPR/Cas9 has the potential to generate quick and efficient mouse models for cancer gene studies. Positive results were reported about the generation of pancreatic cancer in adult mice using a transfection-based multiplex delivery of CRISPR/Cas9 components. This allowed multiple genes in the individual cells to be edited. In addition, the authors also claimed to have modeled complex chromosomal arrangements, and a LOF mutation [54].

Mammalian hematopoietic stem cells (HSCs) have both multipotency and self-renewal abilities. The first term relates to the ability of these cells to give rise to a collection of blood cells, while the latter term indicates their ability to give rise to other HSCs without differentiation [55]. Mutations in these stem cells give rise to cancer. A research group modified five genes in a single mouse HSC. This was performed by the delivery of combinations of sgRNAs and Cas9 with a lentiviral vector. The modification of the genes resulted in clonal outgrowth and myeloid malignancy in the mice similar to the human disease [56].

KRAS is an important oncogene present in about 30% of human cancers [57]. It is the most common mutated oncogene in non-small cell lung cancer (NSCLC) in humans. A lung cancer model based on a mutation in the oncogene Kras was achieved by a research group. The genome of tumor suppressor genes was edited using CRISPR/Cas9 resulting in LOF of the TSGs. This editing resulted in the loss of function of the tumor suppressor genes similar to the human oncogenic condition [58]. The work on kras by scientists is the initiative step towards treatment of human disease by involving diverse genome engineering.

The Cre-loxP technology has been used by researchers to generate cancer models in mice. Using CRISPR/Cas9 a research group induced tumor formation in mice 3T3 cells similar to the Cre-loxP system. Mutations (Indels) were induced in two cancer suppressor genes: Pten and p53 [59]. Using CRISPR/Cas9 technology many human cellular models have been constructed for detailed cancer pathogenesis studies. A detailed description of recent research about the role of CRISPR/Cas9 in cancer disease modeling is given in Table 5.

Table 5 Role of CRISPR/Cas9 in cancer modeling

Type of cancer	Method of CRISPR/Cas9 delivery	Conclusion	Reference
Pancreatic cancer	Transfection based multiplexed delivery into mice	Editing of multiple gene sets in pancreatic cells of mice	[54]
Acute myeloid cancer (AML)	Lentiviral based delivery into Hematopoirtic stem cells	Loss of function in nine targeted genes analogous to AML	[56]
Liver cancer	Hydrodynamic injection into wild type mice	Mutation in the Pten and p53 genes leading to liver cancer in mice	[59]
Breast cancer	Plasmid transfection into JygMC (mouse cell line)	The stem cell marker Cripto-1 was shown to be as a breast target	[60]
Pancreatic cancer	Lentivirus/Adenovirus based delivery into somatic pancreatic cells of mice	Knockout of gene Lkb1	[61]
Lung cancer	Plasmid transfection into human cell line (HEK 293)	Chromosomal rearrangement among EML4 and ALK genes	[62]
Lung cancer	Lentivirus/Adenovirus mediated	Gain of function of KRS and loss of function of p53 and Lkb1	[63]
Colon cancer	Plasmid transfection into DLD1 and HCT116 cell lines (human)	Loss of function in protein kinase c subgroups	[64]
Colorectal cancer	Electropolation into organoids intestinal epithelium (human)	Loss of function and directed mutation in APC, SMAD4, TP 53 and KRAS genes	[65]
Gliobastoma Medulloblastoma	Postnatal PEI-mediated transfection and in utero electroporation into mice	Deletion of TSGs (Ptch1, Trp 53, Pten and Nf1)	[66]
Renal cancer	Renca (mouse cell line)	Knockout of TSG VHL to induce cancer	[67]

CRISPR/Cas9 in direct cancer gene therapy

Previous research has suggested the potential of CRISPR/Cas9 in the treatment of cancer. The ability of cancer cells to develop resistance to chemotherapy drugs is a primary cause of failure of chemotherapy. The application of the CRISPR/Cas9 system to inactivate drug resistance genes in a given cancer is a potential therapeutic strategy to increase the efficacy of chemotherapy.

For instance, Tang and Shrager suggested an approach using CRISPR-mediated genome editing in the treatment of epidermal growth factor receptor (EGFR)-mutant lung cancer. They proposed a sort of personalized molecular surgical therapy molecular. In the proposed technique, the CRISPR/Cas9 system comprising of Cas9 and sgRNA expression plasmid, and donor DNA plasmid will be packaged into viruses and delivered to patients. Intravascular delivery of CRISPR/Cas9 has been suggested by the authors for metastatic lung cancer and intratracheally for localized lung cancer [68].

For cancer, until now, the role of CRISPR/Cas9 has been predominantly about the generation of cancer models in animals and cell lines. These cancer models are and will be highly advantageous in understanding oncogenic pathways, new markers of cancer progression, identifying novel tumor suppressor genes, and will definitely provide an improved and efficient repertoire of strategies for cancer therapies. For instance, transcriptomic studies using CRISPR/Cas9 revealed a novel TSG "FOXA2" in pancreatic cancer, which was previously not known to function as a TSG [69].

Radiotherapy has also been used in the treatment of cancer for a while. However, poor radiation sensitivity has been reported in tumors having mutations in the p53 and p21 genes. Correction of these mutations in the cancer cells and interruption of the cellular radiation injury repair pathway may be a potential alternative way to augment radio-sensitivity. A combination of radiotherapy and CRISPR/Cas9-mediated gene therapy with synergistic anticancer effects may become a promising therapeutic strategy for cancer therapy [70]. Another aspect of CRISPR/Cas9 in cancer therapy is to enhance the host cells immune response to cancer. This could be possible through CRISPR/Cas9 mediated modification of T-cells. The reinfusion of genetically modified T-cells into cancer patients has shown promising results in clinical trials [71] and could be a way forward for anti-cancer therapies.

Another potential way to used CRISPR/Cas9 in cancer therapy could be the development of genetically engineered oncolytic viruses (OVs). These OVs have antitumor properties and can kill the cancer cells without causing any harm to the normal cells [72]. The killing of the cancer cells takes place via virus-mediated cytotoxicity or by an increased anticancer immune response. CRISPR/Cas9 can play an important role in oncolytic viral therapy by addition of cancer-specific promoter to genes that are indispensable for viral replication, and inducing mutations in viral genomes [73]. In both pre-clinical models and clinical trials promising results have been reported about the use of OVs in cancer therapy [72].

Recently, a research group in China headed by Lu You at Sichuan University has held clinical trials using CRISPR/Cas9 in a patient suffering from lung cancer. In this clinical trial, immune cells from the patient were removed and the Programmed death (PD-1) gene, which encodes for the protein PD-1 was disabled. This protein PD-1 is used by the cancerous cells to keep the host immune response in check. This is the first report of human trials using the CRISPR/Cas9 in clinical trials on human patients [126].

Genetic disorders and CRISPR/Cas9

The modification of germline is a conventional approach for the study of genome modification studies in animal models. Various researches in the past years have confirmed the efficiency of CRISPR/Cas9 as a probable method to overcome genetic diseases in humans via experimentation in animal and human cellular models. Targeted mutation using CRISPR/Cas9 can manipulate genetic material by deleting and replacing causal mutations, host mutations can also be induced that will provide protection to the host [74]. Regarding the various genetic diseases, CRISPR/Cas9 technology can be used with ease to treat monogenic diseases; where a correction in the culprit gene could reverse the genetic disease. On the other hand, polygenic diseases are not so straightforward, having multiple mutations in the genome; they possess a far strenuous challenge to treat in comparison to monogenic diseases.

Duchene muscular dystrophy (DMD) is an X-linked recessive disorder, and is caused by mutations in the dystrophin gene [75]. An mdx (point mutation in dystrophin gene) mouse model of Duchene muscular dystrophy was used in an experiment. The CRISPR editing in the germline resulted in the correction of the dystrophin gene mutation in the mosaic offsprings. The offsprings carried 2–100% of the corrected gene. Surprisingly; the extent of phenotype rescue surpassed the percentage of gene correction [76]. CRISPR/Cas9 has also been used to correct another genetic disease cataract in a mouse germline. The cataract phenotype is caused by a frame-shift mutation of one base pair deletion in exon 3 of Crygc (crystalline gamma c) [77].

Beta thalassemia is one of the most common genetic diseases in the world. Mutations in the human hemoglobin beta gene (HBB) give rise to this genetic defect [78]. Induced pluripotent stem cells (iPSCs) from human beta thalassemia patients were edited by a research group with a CRISPR/Cas9 system combined with the transposon *piggyback*. This resulted in the efficient correction of the HBB mutations; in the corrected IPSCs no off-target effects were detected and the cells exhibited normal karyotypes indicative of full pluripotency [79].

Another genetic disease sickle cell anemia affects around 300,000 neonates globally per year [80]. The disease occurs as a result of mutations in the sixth codon of the beta-globin gene [81]. To check the gene editing ability of CRISPR/Cas9 an experiment was performed by Li et al. [81]. They developed a novel hybrid reprogramming viral vector, rCLAE-R6 (HDAd/EBV) using Adenovirus/Epstein bar virus. Highly efficient footprint iPSCs were obtained after viral vector transduction of keratinocytes. After delivery of CRISPR/Cas9 with adenovirus, nucleoporation was done using a 70-nucleotide single-stranded oligodeoxynucleotide (ssODN) correction template. Furthermore, genome sequencing of the corrected iPSCs confirmed no off-target modifications, and no changes in tumor suppressor genes [81].

Tyrosinemia is a genetic disease caused by a mutation in the FAH gene in humans. The mutation leads to abnormalities in the enzyme fumarylacetoacetate hydrolase functioning and the enzyme cannot break down the amino acid tyrosine [82]. CRISPR/Cas9 was used in an experiment to correct the FAH mutation in liver cells in a mouse model of the human genetic disease tyrosinemia. Tail vein hydrodynamic injection was used for the delivery of CRISPR/Cas9 and homologous donor template into adult mice. The adopted therapeutic method may be applicable to human therapeutics, as it does not comprise of any embryo manipulations [83]. A description about the use of CRISPR/Cas9 in the correction of genetic diseases is given in Table 6.

Viral diseases and CRISPR/Cas9

The therapeutic challenge of viruses is captivating these obligate parasites rely on host metabolic machinery to replicate. It is a much arduous task to treat viruses as compare to bacteria due to their unique nature and machinery. Antiviral therapy targeting various viral proteins showed promising results, but anti-viral drug failure is becoming common, however, scientists have recently used the CRISPR/Cas9 phenomenon against a congregation of pathogenic viruses.

Herpesviruses

Herpesviruses include human simplex virus 1 (HSV-1), human cytomegalovirus and Epstein-barr virus. Human cytomegalovirus-1 causes cold sores and herpes simplex keratitis. Human cytomegalovirus causes conditions in immune-compromised people, while Epstein-barr virus causes Hodgkin's disease and Burkitt's lymphoma [86]. The CRISPR/Cas9 system has been used against the EBV. Cells derived from a patient with Burkitt's lymphoma with latent EBV infection (Raji cells) showed a marked reduction in proliferation and decline in viral load as well as restoration of the apoptosis pathway in the cells after treatment with CRISPR/Cas9 [87]. In another research, CRISPR/Cas9-mediated editing of EBV in human cells was done using two gRNAs to make a targeted deletion of 558 bp in the promoter region for the BART (Bam HI A rightward transcript), which codes for viral miRNA's. This resulted in the loss of BART miRNA expression and activity indicating the feasibility of CRISPR/Cas9-mediated editing of the EBV genome. No off-target cleavage was found by deep sequencing [88]. It was the first genetic evidence that the BART promoter drives the expression of the BART transcript, and also a new and efficient method for targeted editing of EBV genome in human cells.

Human papillomaviruses (HPV)

Human papillomaviruses (HPV) cause warts in humans; in addition, they are also oncogenic in nature. The majority of the cancers are caused by HPV16 and HPV18 including cervical cancer in females. The viral proteins E6 and E7 are the major contributors towards the oncogenic properties of the viruses; these proteins are encoded by the oncogenes E6 and E7 [89]. Kennedy et al. used HPV 16 and HPV 18 integrated HELA and SiHa cervical cancer cell lines for their CRISPR-associated editing of the E6 and E7 genes of HPV. They were able to induce mutations in the E6 and E7 genes rendering

Table 6 Overview of gene correction of genetic diseases using CRISPR/Cas9

Genetic disease	Method of CRISPR/Cas9 delivery	Conclusion/outcome	Reference
Tyrosinemia	Tail vein hydrodynamic injection into adult mice	Correction of Fah gene mutation (1 nt substitution)	[83]
Hemophillia A	Transfection based delivery into iPSCs	Inversion based correction of the blood coagulation factor VIII (F8) gene	[84]
Hemophillia B	Tail vein hydrodynamic injection into Fah mice	Correction of mutation in F9 gene	[85]
Cataract	Injection into Oocyte of mouse	Correction in mutation of CRYGC gene (1 nt insertion)	[77]
Sickle cell anemia	Adenovirus based transduction into human IPSCs	Correction in sixth codon of beta globin gene	[81]
Beta Thalassemia	Transfection and piggyback removal in IPSCs from patients	HBB mutations corrected (1 nt substitution 4 nt insertion)	[79]
Cystic fibrosis	Transfection into intestinal stem cells from patients	Correction of CFTR gene mutation (3 substitution)	[50]

them inactive and promoting the anti-tumor effect of p53 and Rbp. They employed a CRISPR/Cas9 system comprising of Cas9, E6 and E7 specific gRNAs [90]. Future research should pay emphasis on using CRISPR/Cas9 to not only inactivate potential cancer risk genes, but to also promote anti-tumor factors.

Hepatitis B virus

Hepatitis B virus is among the major viruses of health concern. It causes liver cirrhosis and hepatocellular carcinoma in humans [91]. Anti-viral therapy has a major disadvantage against the virus; due to the fact that the covalently closed circular DNA of the virus localizes in the nucleus of hepatocytes [92]. Promising results have been reported in using CRISPR/Cas9 against hepatitis B virus. [91].

Moreover, a research team designed eight gRNAs against HBV and showed that the CRISPR/Cas9 system significantly reduced the production of HBV core and HBsAg proteins in the Huh-7 hepatocyte-derived cellular carcinoma cells transfected with an HBV-expression vector. Further, this system could cleave intrahepatic HBV genome-containing plasmid and facilitate its clearance in vivo in a mouse model resulting in a reduction in serum HBsAg level [93].

For the simultaneous targeting of the three loci of the HBV genome, a multiplex all in one CRISPR/Cas9 nuclease and Cas9 nickase vector systems was used in an experiment. [94]. Transfection of the HBV expressing plasmid and vectors into HepG2 cell line was performed. Results indicated a reduction in the HBV replicative intermediates, and also a reduction in the surface and envelope antigens. DNA sequencing confirmed fragmentation of the viral genome and no off-target mutations were reported either. The all in one vector represent an adaptable methodology for simultaneous targeting of the three HBV domains and may be used for therapeutic purposes for HBV patients [94].

In another experiment, lentiviral transduction of Cas9 and HBV-specific gRNAs into human cell line HepAD was performed. Effective inhibition of the HBV DNA production was observed. Total HBV DNA levels were reduced by up to ~ 1000-fold while cccDNA levels were reduced by up to ~ 10-fold, and the majority of the residual viral DNA was mutationally inactivated [95].

In the most recent study of HBV and CRISPR, Zhen et al., targeted the HBsAg and HBx-encoding region of HBV. The experiment involved both cell culture and in vivo trials. The level of surface antigen was much reduced as indicated by ELISA. The HBV DNA levels and HBsAg expression in mouse liver were reduced as also shown by qPCR and immunohistochemistry respectively [96]. The encoding regions of the hepatitis virus must be the center of concentration for future research, in which

case inactivation of these encoding regions will certainly decrease the catastrophic effects of the hepatitis viruses.

Human immunodeficiency virus (HIV)

One of the most researched viruses in history is the HIV; the causative agent of acquired immunodeficiency syndrome (AIDS) in humans. For the past 30 years, AIDS has remained a major health concern [97]. Until much information has been gained about the pathogenesis replication and clinical manifestations of the virus, however, a complete therapeutic strategy has not been achieved so far. Presently, it is estimated that about 37 million people are infected with HIV globally, and each year there is a substantial increase in a number of the infected. In the past decade, AIDS related mortalities have been reduced due to the use of anti-retroviral therapy (ART) [98]. But, still, a proper cure of the virus has been unattainable.

There are two possible mechanisms of the inactivation of HIV gene expression using CRISPR/Cas9: 1. prior to virus integration into the host genome, Cas/9 can inactivate viral gene expression 2. Cas9 can cause disruption of the proviral element already integrated into the host genome. In general targeting of the long terminal repeats (LTR) of the virus has resulted in better results. The cause may be the presence of the conserved transactivation response (TAR) sequence among HIV-1 subtypes, hence LTR should be the preferred targeting of future anti-viral strategies using CRISPR/Cas9 [99].

CRISPR/Cas9 has been used in research for HIV treatment with mixed outcomes. Wang et al., used CRISPR/Cas9 against HIV proviral infection in cells to initiate sequence-specific cleavage. Replication of the HIV was inhibited by harnessing the T-cells with Cas9 and anti-viral guide RNA's, but the virus seemed to escape the inhibition. Sequencing results of the escaped HIV showed various nucleotide substitutions, deletions and insertions around the cleavage site indicative of NHEJ associated DNA repair, thus to some extent there is a limitation of the use of CRISPR/Cas9 against HIV [100].

Another interesting prospect in the battle against HIV is editing host cell factors that are deemed necessary for the HIV replication and infection in the T-cells. Examples of such host cell factors include CXCR4 (Chemokine receptor type 4) and CCR5 (Chemokine receptor type 5). For efficient entry of the virus into the cell, the envelope (Env) has to bind with these two receptors [101, 102]. Other factors are TNPO3 (transportin 3), required for viral replication, and LEDGF (lens epithelium derived growth factor), required for integration of the viral genome into host cells. In an experiment, electroporation of CRISPR/Cas9 ribonucleoproteins (RNPs) into primary CD4+ T cells resulted in CXCR4 or CCR5 knockout cells. These cells exhibited resistance to HIV infection in a tropism dependent manner. The knockout of LEDGF or TNPO3 resulted in reduced-infection, but impartial to any tropism. CRISPR/Cas9 ribonucleoproteins can furthermore, edit multiple genes simultaneously enabling studies of interactions among multiple hosts and viral factors [103].

In further research on the effectiveness of CRISPR/Cas9 on HIV, a research included the targeting of the LTR, Gag and Pol gene. An HIV-susceptible human T-cell line was used, and transduction of the gRNA and Cas9 was done. A clear inhibition was observed in the early HIV infection. However, the anti-viral potency was insufficient in multiple rounds of the wild type viral replication, indicating difficulties in treating HIV with CRISPR/Cas9 [104].

In a transgenic mouse model, Kaminski et al. used an adeno associated virus 9 vector (rAAV$_9$) expressing gRNAs and Cas9 for removing important segments of the HIV (5′ LTR and Gag gene). Tail vein injection in the mice exhibited cleavage of viral DNA and excision of a 978 bp DNA segment between LTR and Gag in various organs such as kidney liver, lung heart and also in blood lymphocytes. Retro-orbital inoculation excising of CRISPR/Cas9 resulted in of targeted DNA segment and also inhibited gene expression of the virus hence indicating for the first time, the in-vivo efficacy of CRISPR/Cas9 via rAAV$_9$ in a wide variety of cells and tissues that harbored copies of the HIV DNA [105].

Table 7 gives an insight into the use of CRISPR/Cas9 against viral diseases.

Future of CRISPR/Cas9 against viral diseases
The original antiviral role of CRISPR/Cas9 in prokaryotes makes it an interesting candidate to use against human - viruses. Many of the advancements regarding its role in antiviral therapy have already been discussed. For the development of antiviral therapies, CRISPR/Cas9 can be used to target the virus sequence for destruction or can be employed for the engineering of host sequences essential

for virus infection [74]. Furthermore, CRISPR/Cas9 can be used to knockout host factors that may be essential for virus survival, integration and replication [103]. In addition to much comprehensive research on antiviral therapy, another dimension is the use of CRISPR/Cas9 in the development of vaccines for viral diseases. CRISPR/Cas9 system into vaccine development has been reported by Liang et al., who combined both CRISPR/Cas9 and Cre/Lox system for the development of a pseudorabies vaccine for swines [109]. Over passage expance of time the perspective of vaccine manufacturing using CRISPR/Cas9 is certainly a point to ponder for further research.

Neurological disorders
These disorders are a menace to public health affecting millions of people worldwide. Potential treatment of neurological disorders may be futile, due to the chronic nature of the disorder and treatment ineffectiveness. Research is now being done on the potential role of CRISPR/Cas9 against neurological disorders. Huntington disease is a neurodegenerative disorder characterized by dementia, choreatic movements and behavior disturbances [110]. A novel CRISPR/Cas9-based gene editing approach was used against Huntington disease (HD) and resulted in the inactivation of HD-associated mutant HTT allele without affecting the normal allele [111].

Another neurological disorder Schizophrenia has also been tested upon using CRISPR/Cas9, using a mouse model a single intracranial injection of AAV2g9 vectors encoding guide RNAs targeting the schizophrenia risk gene MIR137 (encoding MIR137) was used. It resulted in brain-specific gene deletion with no detectable events in the liver. This engineered AAV vector is a promising platform for treating neurological disorders through gene therapy, gene silencing or editing modalities [112].

Table 7 Overview of CRISPR/Cas9 in virus genome modification

Virus	Method of delivery of CRISPR/Cas9	Conclusion/outcome	Reference
HSV-1	Transfection into HEK293 cells	Modification of ICP0 gene in different locations of genome	[106]
EBV	Nucleofaction into Burkhitt's lymphoma cell line	Complete virus clearance in 25% cells, partial in 50%	[87]
EBV	Transfection into HEK 293-BX1 and C666–1 cells	Loss of BART Micro RNA expression	[88]
HPV	Lentiviral transduction into HELA and SiHA cell lines	Indel mutations in the E6 and E7 genes	[90]
HBV	Transfection in to Huh cells	Cleavage of the HBV genome-expressing template	[93]
HBV	Hydrodynamic injection into C57BL/6 mice	Cleavage of the HBV genome-expressing template	[107]
HBV	Transfection into HepG2 cell line	Fragmentation of viral genome	[94]
HBV	Lentiviral transduction into HepAD cell line (Chronic HBV infection)	Inhibition of viral DNA production	[95]
HIV	Lentiviral transduction into SupT1 CD4+ T cell line	Inactivation of virus and acceleration of virus escape	[100]
HIV	Lentiviral transduction into T-cells	Inhibition of early phase viral infection, but anti-HIV potency was not consistent in multiple rounds	[104]
HIV	Retro-orbital injection into transgenic mice	Decrease of viral gene expression in T-cells	[105]
Polyomavirus (JCV)	Transfection into TC 620 cell line	Inactivation of T-antigen gene	[108]

The use of CRISPR/Cas9 against neurological disorders has immense potential to be explored by scientists. However, some limitations have to be addressed while using the system in neurological disorders. First of all, efficient delivery of the Cas9 nuclease and sgRNA to the brain is essential, and novel methods have to be introduced that can lead to efficient gene insertion and correction in the post-mitotic cells of the brain. In addition to devising therapeutic strategies, this genome editor can certainly be applied in attaining a comprehensive notion about the working and functionality of the brain, and to get a more lucid understanding of the mechanisms of neurological disorders [113].

Allergy and immunological diseases

CRISPR/Cas9 possesses potential against allergic and Mendelian disorders of the immune system. Janus Kinase 3 (JAK 3) deficiency in humans is characterized by normal but poor functioning B-lymphocytes, and the absence of natural killer cells (NKs) and T-lymphocytes. For correction of this immunological disorder, CRISPR/Cas9 was used in induced pluripotent stem cells. Correction of the JAK 3 mutation was made, resulting in restoration of normal T-lymphocyte development and number [114].

X-linked hyper immunoglobulin IgM syndrome is an immunological disorder of humans. It is caused by a mutation in the CD40 ligand and causes increased level of IgM. Kuo et al. have reported the correction of the mutation using CRISPR/Cas9 [115]. Another immunological disorder is X-linked chronic granulomatous disease (X-CGD) result due to mutation in the CYBB gene, this leads to improper functioning of the phagocytes. The NADPH oxidase system of the phagocytes of the patient is defective in this condition; as a result the phagocytes are unable to generate superoxide rendering them ineffective to kill pathogenic microbes [116]. Recently, CRISPR/Cas9 was used by a team of scientist who were successful in correcting the mutation in the CYBB gene of HPSCs from patients suffering from X-CGD [117].

Scientists are using methodologies, which provide a critical analysis of the use of CRISPR/Cas9 as a treatment for allergic and immunological diseases. Single nucleotide polymorphisms (SNPs) are known to contribute to allergic diseases such as asthma and allergic rhinitis [118, 119]. These SNPs can be modified using CRISPR/Cas9, however, much testing in experimental systems is necessary before advancing to human therapy. Additionally, hematopoietic cells remain the most common target for both allergic and immunological diseases, and can be corrected using CRISPR/Cas9 [115]. The main emphasis of CRISPR/Cas9 in relation to allergic diseases has been about the investigation of the potential role of particular genes. Using the technology, certain gene knockout models can be created, which will provide an evaluation of the role of certain genes in

allergic diseases and immunological disorders. Moreover, CRISPR/Cas9 is rapidly becoming the primary tool to create mutant mouse models of diseases, including allergic and immunologic diseases, due to the ease, precision, and flexibility of this technique.

Potential of CRISPR/Cas9 as antimicrobials

A diverse manner of using CRISPR/Cas9 could be putting it to use as an antimicrobial entity. Antibiotics have been used in the treatment of bacterial diseases for quite a while. They inhibit certain bacterial metabolic pathways and hence kill the microbe in different ways, but cannot target specific members of a microbial population. However, antibiotic resistance has been a major problem, and now the emergence of multidrug-resistant (MDR) bacteria is a ginormous menace.

Using CRISPR/Cas9 as an antimicrobial tool, Bikard et al. reported promising results that used a phagemid-based delivery of programmable, sequence-specific antimicrobials using the RNA-guided nuclease Cas9. The reprogrammed Cas9 only targeted the virulence genes of *Staphylococcus aureus* killing virulent strains, and did not kill avirulent strains. Much of the antibiotic resistance is caused by plasmids; the nuclease was also reprogrammed to target plasmid sequences in *S. aureus* with positive results. In a mouse skin model the CRISPR/Cas9 antimicrobials showed extreme potential in killing of *Staph aureus*. This technology creates opportunities to manipulate complex bacterial populations in a sequence-specific manner [120].

The true capability of CRISPR/Cas9 as an antimicrobial can be further exploited by developing delivery systems using phages that can help in the injection of cargo into diverse bacterial strains. However, broad host range phages are very rare and those that are known infect only single species within a genus. In molecular biology, phages have been serving as the first model system, but little is known in how to alter or expand the host range of the phages. This provides an excellent opportunity to develop enhanced phages that will have the ability to infect any host microbe. Alternatively, nanoparticles, or outer membrane vesicles may be used as delivery systems.

Gene drive and CRISPR the ultimate gene editing alliance?

A gene drive is a process by which an altered gene is introduced inside an animal population. The aim of gene drive is to get desired traits a population through natural reproduction alone. The use of novel gene drives resides in the use of CRISPR, the CRISPR technique has great potential in genome engineering. By using it scientists edit genes with precision, quickness, and economy, in addition it also has the potential of generating genetic alterations in wild animals that may persist in nature [127].

Gene drive research and its applications are progressing quickly. The CRISPR/Cas9 phenomenon became the holy grail of genome editing about 4–5 years ago, and the first reports of gene drive organisms (yeast, laboratory fruit flies and mosquitoes) were published in 2015 [128]. It will take some time for scientists to release genetically modified organisms (GMO's) with a gene drive system into the wild, till that happens the US National Academy of Sciences, Engineering and Medicine has recently approved comprehensive research for the betterment of gene drive and has encouraged carefully controlled field trials in the near future [129].

Gene drives have the potential to limit the spread of various diseases, to support the agriculture sector by reversing pesticides and herbicides resistance in insects and plants.. Till now there is no claim about the successful testing of any gene drive in the wild but in laboratory organisms like fruitfly and mosquitos, scientists have converted almost entire populations to carry a favored trait. In laboratory tests, different groups have already used CRISP for editing genes of mosquito species, these blood thirsty insects harbor the parasite that causes malaria, and so the gene drive can be used to prevent female mosquitoes from producing fertile eggs [129].

So far, gene drives have been tested and evaluated only in laboratories, and the main emphasis of research has been on mosquitoes that transmit infectious diseases, as well as lab animals such as mice. The objectives are numerous however, some of the pivotal ones include control of the size of the population, or to suppress it completely, the last but not least is its use to combat against infectious diseases. Gene drives therefore have the potential to reduce the occurrence of, and possibly eradicate various infectious diseases by upsetting their transmission chains [130].

Conclusions
Ever since CRISPR/Cas9 was introduced as the key aspect of genome engineering a plethora of advances have been made. Despite its easy adoption, the proper translation of this technology for clinical purposes has been cumbersome. The main emphasis on the utilization of this genome-editing tool has been to develop a control of the repair mechanisms in the targeted DNA. Despite recent advances in genome editing targeted in vivo gene integration has not been achieved specifically in non-dividing cells A recent development of much interest is homology-independent targeted integration (HITI) for CRISPR/Cas9, which allows robust knock-in in both dividing and non-dividing cells [28, 121–123].

Another limitation in the use of CRISPR/Cas9 has been off-target cleavage activity. However, experiments have proven that shortening the length of gRNA < 200 nucleotides can reduce off-target mutagenesis. [124]. A high fidelity variant Cas9 termed (Cas9-HFI) has been constructed with reduced off-targets. It was compared with wild type Cas9, it showed similar on target results and reduced off-targets [124]. Similar results were shown by Slaymaker et al. by the use of an "enhanced specificity" Cas9 [125]. In short, the use of altered Cas9 nucleases, which possess higher precision as compared to wild type Cas9 could be an appropriate tactic to curtail off-target cleavage.

In this review, many of the possibilities of CRISPR/Cas9 have been outlined in relation to not only understanding the various diseases but also devising ways of making efficient therapeutic cures using CRISPR/Cas9. What the future holds with CRSIPR/Cas9 is both fascinating and intriguing, however much further research is necessary to overcome the shortcomings at hand, to tackle any possible adverse effects on humans, and the ethical aspects of such experiments must not be overlooked.

Acknowledgments
We are grateful to USAID for provision of funds to conduct research work. Sehrish Khan was also supported by USAID under USPCAS-AFS.

Funding
Research related to CRISPR/Cas9 was funded by USAid under United States Pakistan Center for Advanced Studies in Agriculture and Food Security (USPCAS-AFS), University of Agriculture, Faisalabad, Pakistan.

Authors' contributions
The manuscript was originally drafted by SK, AA and HZ. Further improvements were done by MSM, SUR, SH and ZK. All authors read and approved the final manuscript.

Competing interests
The authors declare they have no competing interests.

Author details
[1]Institute of Microbiology University of Agriculture, Faisalabad, Pakistan. [2]Center of Agricultural Biochemistry and Biotechnology, University of Agriculture, Faisalabad, Pakistan. [3]Department of Biochemistry/U.S.-Pakistan Center for Advanced Studies in Agriculture and Food Security (USPCAS-AFS), University of Agriculture Faisalabad (UAF), Faisalabad 38040, Pakistan.

References
1. Harrow J, Nagy A, Reymond A, et al. Identifying protein-coding genes in genomic sequences. Genome Biol. 2009;324(6092):34–8.

2. Thomas KR, Capecchi MR. Introduction of homologous DNA sequences into mammalian cells induces mutations in the cognate gene. Nature. 1986; 324(6092):34–8.

3. Yu D, Ellis HM, Lee EC, Jenkins NA, Copeland NG, Court DL. An efficient recombination system for chromosome engineering in Escherichia Coli. Proc Natl Acad Sci U S A. 2000;97(11):5978–83.

4. Rouet P, Smih F, Jasin M. Introduction of double-strand breaks into the genome of mouse cells by expression of a rare-cutting endonuclease. Mol Cell Biol. 1994;14(12):8096–106.

5. Choulika A, Perrin A, Dujon B, Nicolas JF. Induction of homologous recombination in mammalian chromosomes by using the I-SceI system of Saccharomyces Cerevisiae. Mol Cell Biol. 1995;15(4):1968–73.

6. Sander JD, Joung JK. CRISPR-Cas systems for editing, regulating and targeting genomes. Nat Biotechnol. 2014;32(4):347–55.

7. Guha TK, Wai A, Hausner G. Programmable genome editing tools and their regulation for efficient genome engineering. 2017;15:146–60.

8. Sovova T, Kerins G, Demnerova K, Ovesna J. Genome editing with engineered nucleases in economically important animals and plants: state of the art in the research pipeline. Curr Issues Mol Biol. 2016;21:41–62.

9. Kim YG, Cha J, Chandrasegaran S. Hybrid restriction enzymes: zinc finger fusions to Fok I cleavage domain. Proc Natl Acad Sci U S A. 1996;93(3): 1156–60.

10. Beerli RR, Segal DJ, Dreier B, Barbas CF 3rd. Toward controlling gene expression at will: specific regulation of the erbB-2/HER-2 promoter by using polydactyl zinc finger proteins constructed from modular building blocks. Proc Natl Acad Sci U S A. 1998;95(25):14628–33.

11. Bonas U, Stall RE, Staskawicz B. Genetic and structural characterization of the avirulence gene avrBs3 from Xanthomonas campestris pv. Vesicatoria. Mol Gen Genet. 1989;218(1):127–36.

12. Puchta H, Fauser F. Synthetic nucleases for genome engineering in plants: prospects for a bright future. Plant J. 2014;78(5):727–41.

13. Petersen B, Niemann H. Molecular scissors and their application in genetically modified farm animals. Transgenic Res. 2015;24(3):381–96.

14. Zhang H, Li HC, Miao XX. Feasibility, limitation and possible solutions of RNAi-based technology for insect pest control. Insect Sci. 2013;20(1):15–30.

15. Lee J, Chung JH, Kim HM, Kim DW, Kim H. Designed nucleases for targeted genome editing. Plant Biotechnol J. 2016;14(2):448–62.

16. Makarova KS, Wolf YI, Alkhnbashi OS, Costa F, Shah SA, Saunders SJ, et al. An updated evolutionary classification of CRISPR-Cas systems. Nat Rev Microbiol. 2015;13(11):722–36.

17. Doudna JA, Charpentier E. Genome editing. The new frontier of genome engineering with CRISPR-Cas9. Science. 2014;346(6213):1258096.

18. van der Oost J, Westra ER, Jackson RN, Wiedenheft B. Unravelling the structural and mechanistic basis of CRISPR-Cas systems. Nat Rev Microbiol. 2014;12(7):479–92.

19. Wright AV, Nunez JK, Doudna JA. Biology and applications of CRISPR systems: harnessing Nature's toolbox for genome engineering. Cell. 2016;164(1–2):29–44.

20. Hsu PD, Lander ES, Zhang F. Development and applications of CRISPR-Cas9 for genome engineering. Cell. 2014;157(6):1262–78.

21. Bondy-Denomy J, Davidson AR. To acquire or resist: the complex biological effects of CRISPR–Cas systems. Trends Microbiol. 2014;22(4):218–25.

22. Gilbert LA, Larson MH, Morsut L, Liu Z, Brar GA, Torres SE, et al. CRISPR-mediated modular RNA-guided regulation of transcription in eukaryotes. Cell. 2013;154(2):442–51.

23. Du D, Qi LS. An Introduction to CRISPR Technology for Genome Activation and Repression in Mammalian Cells. Cold Spring Harb Protoc. 2016;2016(1): pdb top086835.

24. Qi LS, Larson MH, Gilbert LA, Doudna JA, Weissman JS, Arkin AP, et al. Repurposing CRISPR as an RNA-guided platform for sequence-specific control of gene expression. Cell. 2013;152(5):1173–83.

25. Kearns NA, Genga RM, Enuameh MS, Garber M, Wolfe SA, Maehr R. Cas9 effector-mediated regulation of transcription and differentiation in human pluripotent stem cells. Development. 2014;141(1):219–23.

26. Mali P, Aach J, Stranges PB, Esvelt KM, Moosburner M, Kosuri S, et al. CAS9 transcriptional activators for target specificity screening and paired nickases for cooperative genome engineering. Nat Biotechnol. 2013;31(9):833–8.

27. Maeder ML, Linder SJ, Cascio VM, Fu Y, Ho QH, Joung JK. CRISPR RNA-guided activation of endogenous human genes. Nat Methods. 2013;10(10):977–9.

28. Cong L, Ran FA, Cox D, Lin S, Barretto R, Habib N, et al. Multiplex genome engineering using CRISPR/Cas systems. Science. 2013;339(6121):819–23.

29. Zuris JA, Thompson DB, Shu Y, et al. Efficient delivery of genome-editing proteins In Vitro and In Vivo. Nat Biotechnol. 2015;33(1):73–80.

30. D'Astolfo DS, Pagliero RJ, Pras A, Karthaus WR, Clevers H, Prasad V, et al. Efficient intracellular delivery of native proteins. Cell. 2015;161(3):674–90.

31. Ran FA, Hsu PD, Wright J, Agarwala V, Scott DA, Zhang F. Genome engineering using the CRISPR-Cas9 system. Nat Protoc. 2013;8(11):2281–308.

32. Sanjana NE, Shalem O, Zhang F. Improved vectors and genome-wide libraries for CRISPR screening. Nat Methods. 2014;11(8):783–4.

33. Chavez A, Scheiman J, Vora S, Pruitt BW, Tuttle M, PRI E, et al. Highly efficient Cas9-mediated transcriptional programming. Nat Methods. 2015;12(4):326–8.

34. Konermann S, Brigham MD, Trevino AE, Joung J, Abudayyeh OO, Barcena C, et al. Genome-scale transcriptional activation by an engineered CRISPR-Cas9 complex. Nature. 2015;517(7536):583–8.

35. Chen B, Gilbert LA, Cimini BA, Schnitzbauer J, Zhang W, Li GW, et al. Dynamic imaging of genomic loci in living human cells by an optimized CRISPR/Cas system. Cell. 2013;155(7):1479–91.

36. Kabadi AM, Ousterout DG, Hilton IB, Gersbach CA. Multiplex CRISPR/Cas9-based genome engineering from a single lentiviral vector. Nucleic Acids Res. 2014;42(19):e147.

37. Peters JM, Colavin A, Shi H, Czarny TL, Larson MH, Wong S, et al. A comprehensive, CRISPR-based functional analysis of essential genes in bacteria. Cell. 2016;165(6):1493–506.

38. Savic D, Partridge EC, Newberry KM, Smith SB, Meadows SK, Roberts BS, et al. CETCh-seq: CRISPR epitope tagging ChIP-seq of DNA-binding proteins. Genome Res. 2015;25(10):1581–9.

39. Hsu PD, Scott DA, Weinstein JA, Ran FA, Konermann S, Agarwala V, et al. DNA targeting specificity of RNA-guided Cas9 nucleases. Nat Biotechnol. 2013;31(9):827–32.

40. Montague TG, Cruz JM, Gagnon JA, Church GM, Valen E. CHOPCHOP: a CRISPR/Cas9 and TALEN web tool for genome editing. Nucleic Acids Res. 2014;42(Web Server issue):W401–7.

41. Bae S, Park J, Kim J-S. Cas-OFFinder: a fast and versatile algorithm that searches for potential off-target sites of Cas9 RNA-guided endonucleases. Bioinformatics. 2014;30(10):1473–5.

42. Gratz SJ, Ukken FP, Rubinstein CD, Thiede G, Donohue LK. cummings AM, et al. highly specific and efficient CRISPR/Cas9-catalyzed homology-directed repair in drosophila. Genetics. 2014;196(4):961–71.

43. Heigwer F, Kerr G, Boutros M. E-CRISP: fast CRISPR target site identification. Nat methods. 2014;11(2):122–3.

44. Liu H, Wei Z, Dominguez A, Li Y, Wang X, Qi LS. CRISPR-ERA: a comprehensive design tool for CRISPR-mediated gene editing, repression and activation. Bioinformatics. 2015;31(22):3676–8.

45. Stemmer M, Thumberger T, Del Sol Keyer M, Wittbrodt J, Mateo JL. CCTop: An Intuitive, Flexible and Reliable CRISPR/Cas9 Target Prediction Tool. PLoS One. 2015;10(4):e0124633.

46. Wong N, Liu W, Wang X. WU-CRISPR: characteristics of functional guide RNAs for the CRISPR/Cas9 system. Genome Biol. 2015;16:218.

47. O'Brien A, Bailey TL. GT-Scan: identifying unique genomic targets. Bioinformatics. 2014;30(18):2673–5.

48. Naito Y, Hino K, Bono H, Ui-Tei K. CRISPRdirect: software for designing CRISPR/Cas guide RNA with reduced off-target sites. Bioinformatics. 2015;31(7):1120–3.

49. Haeussler M, Schonig K, Eckert H, Eschstruth A, Mianne J, Renaud JB, et al. Evaluation of off-target and on-target scoring algorithms and integration into the guide RNA selection tool CRISPOR. Genome Biol. 2016;17(1):148.

50. Schwank G, Koo BK, Sasselli V, Dekkers JF, Heo I, Demircan T, et al. Functional repair of CFTR by CRISPR/Cas9 in intestinal stem cell organoids of cystic fibrosis patients. Cell Stem Cell. 2013;13(6):653–8.

51. Yang H, Wang H, Shivalila CS, Cheng AW, Shi L, Jaenisch R. One-step generation of mice carrying reporter and conditional alleles by CRISPR/Cas-mediated genome engineering. Cell. 2013;154(6):1370–9.

52. Torres-Ruiz R, Rodriguez-Perales S. CRISPR-Cas9: A Revolutionary Tool for Cancer Modelling. Int J Mol Sci. 2015;16(9):22151–68.

53. Zhang H, McCarty N. CRISPR-Cas9 technology and its application in haematological disorders. Br J Haematol. 2016;175(2):208–25.

54. Maresch R, Mueller S, Veltkamp C, Ollinger R, Friedrich M, Heid I, et al. Multiplexed pancreatic genome engineering and cancer induction by transfection-based CRISPR/Cas9 delivery in mice. Nat Commun. 2016;7:10770.

55. Seita J, Weissman IL. Hematopoietic stem cell: self-renewal versus differentiation. Wiley Interdiscip Rev Syst Biol Med. 2010;2(6):640–53.

56. Heckl D, Kowalczyk MS, Yudovich D, Belizaire R, Puram RV, McConkey ME, et al. Generation of mouse models of myeloid malignancy with combinatorial genetic lesions using CRISPR-Cas9 genome editing. Nat Biotechnol. 2014;32(9):941–6.

57. O'Hagan RC, Heyer J. KRAS mouse models: modeling cancer harboring KRAS mutations. Genes Cancer. 2011;2(3):335–43.

58. Sanchez-Rivera FJ, Papagiannakopoulos T, Romero R, Tammela T, Bauer MR, Bhutkar A, et al. Rapid modelling of cooperating genetic events in cancer through somatic genome editing. Nature. 2014;516(7531):428–31.

59. Xue W, Chen S, Yin H, Tammela T, Papagiannakopoulos T, Joshi NS, et al. CRISPR-mediated direct mutation of cancer genes in the mouse liver. Nature. 2014;514(7522):380–4.

60. Castro NP, Fedorova-Abrams ND, Merchant AS, Rangel MC, Nagaoka T, Karasawa H, et al. Cripto-1 as a novel therapeutic target for triple negative breast cancer. Oncotarget. 2015;6(14):11910–29.

61. Chiou SH, Winters IP, Wang J, Naranjo S, Dudgeon C, Tamburini FB, et al. Pancreatic cancer modeling using retrograde viral vector delivery and in vivo CRISPR/Cas9-mediated somatic genome editing. Genes Dev. 2015; 29(14):1576–85.

62. Choi PS, Meyerson M. Targeted genomic rearrangements using CRISPR/Cas technology. Nat Commun. 2014;5:3728.

63. Platt RJ, Chen S, Zhou Y, Yim MJ, Swiech L, Kempton HR, et al. CRISPR-Cas9 knockin mice for genome editing and cancer modeling. Cell. 2014;159(2):440–55.

64. Antal CE, Hudson AM, Kang E, Zanca C, Wirth C, Stephenson NL, et al. Cancer-associated protein kinase C mutations reveal kinase's role as tumor suppressor. Cell. 2015;160(3):489–502.

65. Matano M, Date S, Shimokawa M, Takano A, Fujii M, Ohta Y, et al. Modeling colorectal cancer using CRISPR-Cas9-mediated engineering of human intestinal organoids. Nat Med. 2015;21(3):256–62.

66. Zuckermann M, Hovestadt V, Knobbe-Thomsen CB, Zapatka M, Northcott PA, Schramm K, et al. Somatic CRISPR/Cas9-mediated tumour suppressor disruption enables versatile brain tumour modelling. Nat Commun. 2015;6:7391.

67. Schokrpur S, Hu J, Moughon DL, Liu P, Lin LC, Hermann K, et al. CRISPR-mediated VHL knockout generates an improved model for metastatic renal cell carcinoma. Sci Rep. 2016;6:29032.

68. Tang H, Shrager JB. CRISPR/Cas-mediated genome editing to treat EGFR-mutant lung cancer: a personalized molecular surgical therapy. EMBO Mol Med. 2016;8(2):83–5.

69. Vorvis C, Hatziapostolou M, Mahurkar-Joshi S, Koutsioumpa M, Williams J, Donahue TR, et al. Transcriptomic and CRISPR/Cas9 technologies reveal FOXA2 as a tumor suppressor gene in pancreatic cancer. Am J Physiol Gastrointest Liver Physiol. 2016;310(11):G1124–37.

70. Yi L, Li J. CRISPR-Cas9 therapeutics in cancer: promising strategies and present challenges. Biochim Biophys Acta. 2016;1866(2):197–207.

71. Siggs OM. Dissecting mammalian immunity through mutation. Immunol Cell Biol. 2014;92(5):392–9.

72. Yuan M, Webb E, Lemoine NR, Wang Y. CRISPR-Cas9 as a powerful tool for efficient creation of oncolytic viruses. Viruses. 2016;8(3):72.

73. Xiao-Jie L, Hui-Ying X, Zun-Ping K, Jin-Lian C, Li-Juan J. CRISPR-Cas9: a new and promising player in gene therapy. J Med Genet. 2015;52(5):289–96.

74. Eid A, Mahfouz MM. Genome editing: the road of CRISPR/Cas9 from bench to clinic. Exp Mol Med. 2016;48(10):e265.

75. Nowak KJ, Davies KE. Duchenne muscular dystrophy and dystrophin: pathogenesis and opportunities for treatment. EMBO Rep. 2004;5(9):872–6. https://doi.org/10.1038/sj.embor.7400221.

76. Long C, McAnally JR, Shelton JM, Mireault AA, Bassel-Duby R, Olson EN. Prevention of muscular dystrophy in mice by CRISPR/Cas9-mediated editing of germline DNA. Science. 2014;345(6201):1184–8.

77. Wu Y, Liang D, Wang Y, Bai M, Tang W, Bao S, et al. Correction of a genetic disease in mouse via use of CRISPR-Cas9. Cell Stem Cell. 2013;13(6):659–62.

78. Galanello R, Origa R. Beta-thalassemia. Orphanet Journal of Rare Diseases. 2010;5:11. https://doi.org/10.1186/1750-1172-5-11.

79. Xie F, Ye L, Chang JC, Beyer AI, Wang J, Muench MO, et al. Seamless gene correction of beta-thalassemia mutations in patient-specific iPSCs using CRISPR/Cas9 and piggyBac. Genome Res. 2014;24(9):1526–33.

80. Tasan I, Jain S, Zhao H. Use of genome-editing tools to treat sickle cell disease. Hum Genet. 2016;135(9):1011–28.

81. Li C, Ding L, Sun CW, Wu LC, Zhou D, Pawlik KM, et al. Novel HDAd/EBV reprogramming vector and highly efficient ad/CRISPR-Cas sickle cell disease gene correction. Sci Rep. 2016;6:30422.

82. Russo PA, Mitchell GA, Tyrosinemia TRM. a review. Pediatr Dev Pathol. 2001; 4(3):212–21.

83. Yin H, Xue W, Chen S, Bogorad RL, Benedetti E, Grompe M, et al. Genome editing with Cas9 in adult mice corrects a disease mutation and phenotype. Nat Biotechnol. 2014;32(6):551–3.

84. Park CY, Lee DR, Sung JJ, Kim DW. Genome-editing technologies for gene correction of hemophilia. Hum Genet. 2016;135(9):977–81.

85. Guan Y, Ma Y, Li Q, Sun Z, Ma L, Wu L, et al. CRISPR/Cas9-mediated somatic correction of a novel coagulator factor IX gene mutation ameliorates hemophilia in mouse. EMBO Mol Med. 2016;8(5):477–88.

86. Van Diemen FR, Lebbink RJ. CRISPR/Cas9, a powerful tool to target human herpesviruses. Cell Microbiol. 2017;19(2)

87. Wang J, Quake SR. RNA-guided endonuclease provides a therapeutic strategy to cure latent herpesviridae infection. Proc Natl Acad Sci U S A. 2014;111(36):13157–62.

88. Yuen KS, Chan CP, Wong NH, Ho CH, Ho TH, Lei T, et al. CRISPR/Cas9-mediated genome editing of Epstein-Barr virus in human cells. J Gen Virol. 2015;96(Pt 3):626–36.

89. White MK. Hu W, Khalili K. The CRISPR/Cas9 genome editing methodology as a weapon against human viruses. Discov Med. 2015;19(105):255–62.

90. Kennedy EM, Kornepati AV, Goldstein M, Bogerd HP, Poling BC, Whisnant AW, et al. Inactivation of the human papillomavirus E6 or E7 gene in cervical carcinoma cells by using a bacterial CRISPR/Cas RNA-guided endonuclease. J Virol. 2014;88(20):11965–72.

91. Niederau C, Chronic h B. In 2014: great therapeutic progress, large diagnostic deficit. World Journal of Gastroenterology : WJG. 2014;20(33): 11595–617.

92. Ayoub WS, Keeffe EB. Review article: current antiviral therapy of chronic hepatitis B. Aliment Pharmacol Ther. 2011;34(10):1145–58.

93. Lin G, Zhang K, Li J. Application of CRISPR/Cas9 technology to HBV. Int J Mol Sci. 2015;16(11):26077–86.

94. Sakuma T, Masaki K, Abe-Chayama H, Mochida K, Yamamoto T, Chayama K. Highly multiplexed CRISPR-Cas9-nuclease and Cas9-nickase vectors for inactivation of hepatitis B virus. Genes Cells. 2016;21(11):1253–62.

95. Kennedy EM, Bassit LC, Mueller H, Kornepati AV, Bogerd HP, Nie T, et al. Suppression of hepatitis B virus DNA accumulation in chronically infected cells using a bacterial CRISPR/Cas RNA-guided DNA endonuclease. Virology. 2015;476:196–205.

96. Zhen S, Hua L, Liu YH, Gao LC, Fu J, Wan DY, et al. Harnessing the clustered regularly interspaced short palindromic repeat (CRISPR)/CRISPR-associated Cas9 system to disrupt the hepatitis B virus. Gene Ther. 2015;22(5):404–12.

97. Moss JA. HIV/AIDS Review. Radiol Technol. 2013;84(3):247–67. quiz p 68–70

98. Adejumo OA, Malee KM, Ryscavage P, Hunter SJ, Taiwo BO. Contemporary issues on the epidemiology and antiretroviral adherence of HIV-infected adolescents in sub-Saharan Africa: a narrative review. J Int AIDS Soc. 2015; 18(1):200–19.

99. Liao HK, Gu Y, Diaz A, Marlett J, Takahashi Y, Li M, et al. Use of the CRISPR/Cas9 system as an intracellular defense against HIV-1 infection in human cells. Nat Commun. 2015;6:6413.

100. Wang G, Zhao N, Berkhout B, Das AT. CRISPR-Cas9 can inhibit HIV-1 replication but NHEJ repair facilitates virus escape. Mol Ther. 2016;24(3):522–6.

101. Berson JF, Long D, Doranz BJ, Rucker J, Jirik FR, Doms RWA. Seven-transmembrane domain receptor involved in fusion and entry of T-cell-tropic human immunodeficiency virus type 1 strains. J Virol. 1996;70(9): 6288–95.

102. Feng Y, Broder CC, Kennedy PE, Berger EA. HIV-1 entry cofactor: functional cDNA cloning of a seven-transmembrane, G protein-coupled receptor. Science. 1996;272(5263):872–7.

103. Hultquist JF, Schumann K, Woo JM, Manganaro L, McGregor MJ, Doudna J, et al. A Cas9 ribonucleoprotein platform for functional genetic studies of HIV-host interactions in primary human T cells. Cell Rep. 2016;17(5):1438–52.

104. Ueda S, Ebina H, Kanemura Y, Misawa N, Koyanagi Y. Anti-HIV-1 potency of the CRISPR/Cas9 system insufficient to fully inhibit viral replication. Microbiol Immunol. 2016;60(7):483–96.

105. Kaminski R, Chen Y, Fischer T, Tedaldi E, Napoli A, Zhang Y, et al. Elimination of HIV-1 genomes from human T-lymphoid cells by CRISPR/Cas9 gene editing. Sci Rep. 2016;6:22555.

106. Lin C, Li H, Hao M, Xiong D, Luo Y, Huang C, et al. Increasing the efficiency of CRISPR/Cas9-mediated precise genome editing of HSV-1 virus in human cells. Sci Rep. 2016;6:34531.

107. Lin SR, Yang HC, Kuo YT, Liu CJ, Yang TY, Sung KC, et al. The CRISPR/Cas9 system facilitates clearance of the intrahepatic HBV templates in vivo. Mol Ther Nucleic Acids. 2014;e186:3.

108. Wollebo HS, Bellizzi A, Kaminski R, Hu W, White MK, Khalili K. CRISPR/Cas9 system as an agent for eliminating polyomavirus JC infection. PLoS One. 2015;10(9):e0136046.

109. Liang X, Sun L, Yu T, Pan Y, Wang D, Hu X, et al. A CRISPR/Cas9 and Cre/lox system based express vaccine development strategy against re-emerging pseudorabies virus. Sci Rep. 2016;18(6):19176.
110. Roos RA. Huntington's disease: a clinical review. Orphanet J Rare Dis. 2010;5:40.
111. Shin JW, Kim KH, Chao MJ, Atwal RS, Gillis T, MacDonald ME, et al. Permanent inactivation of Huntington's disease mutation by personalized allele-specific CRISPR/Cas9. Hum Mol Genet. 2016;
112. Murlidharan G, Sakamoto K, Rao L, Corriher T, Wang D, Gao G, et al. CNS-restricted transduction and CRISPR/Cas9-mediated gene deletion with an engineered AAV vector. Mol Ther Nucleic Acids. 2016;5(7):e338.
113. Heidenreich M, Zhang F. Applications of CRISPR-Cas systems in neuroscience. Nat Rev Neurosci. 2016;17(1):36–44.
114. Chang CW, Lai YS, Westin E, Khodadadi-Jamayran A, Pawlik KM, Lamb LS Jr, et al. Modeling human severe combined immunodeficiency and correction by CRISPR/Cas9-enhanced gene targeting. Cell Rep. 2015;12(10):1668–77.
115. Goodman MA, Moradi Manesh D, Malik P, Rothenberg ME. CRISPR/Cas9 in allergic and immunologic diseases. Expert Rev Clin Immunol. 2017;13(1):5–9.
116. Song E, Jaishankar GB, Saleh H, Jithpratuck W, Sahni R, Krishnaswamy G. Chronic granulomatous disease: a review of the infectious and inflammatory complications. Clinical and Molecular Allergy. 2011;9:10.
117. De ravin SS, Li L, Wu X, et al. CRISPR-Cas9 gene repair of hematopoietic stem cells from patients with X-linked chronic granulomatous disease. Sci Transl Med. 2017;9(372)
118. Wang M, Xing ZM, Lu C, Ma YX, Yu DL, Yan Z, et al. A common IL-13 Arg130Gln single nucleotide polymorphism among Chinese atopy patients with allergic rhinitis. Hum Genet. 2003;113(5):387–90.
119. Werner M, Herbon N, Gohlke H, Altmuller J, Knapp M, Heinrich J, et al. Asthma is associated with single-nucleotide polymorphisms in ADAM33. Clin Exp Allergy. 2004;34(1):26–31.
120. Bikard D, Euler CW, Jiang W, Nussenzweig PM, Goldberg GW, Duportet X, Fischetti VA, Marraffini LA. Exploiting CRISPR-Cas nucleases to produce sequence-specific antimicrobials. Nat Biotechnol. 2014;32(11): 1146–50.
121. Maruyama T, Dougan SK, Truttmann M, Bilate AM, Ingram JR, Ploegh HL. Inhibition of non-homologous end joining increases the efficiency of CRISPR/Cas9-mediated precise [TM: inserted] genome editing. Nat Biotechnol. 2015;33(5):538–42.
122. Basu S, Aryan A, Overcash JM, Samuel GH, Anderson MA, Dahlem TJ, et al. Silencing of end-joining repair for efficient site-specific gene insertion after TALEN/CRISPR mutagenesis in Aedes Aegypti. Proc Natl Acad Sci U S A. 2015;112(13):4038–43.
123. Suzuki K, Tsunekawa Y, Hernandez-Benitez R, Wu J, Zhu J, Kim EJ, et al. In vivo genome editing via CRISPR/Cas9 mediated homology-independent targeted integration. Nature. 2016;540(7631):144–9.
124. Klinestiver BP, Pattanayak V, Prw MS, Tsai SQ, Nguyen NT, Zheg Z, et al. High fidelity CRISPR/Cas9 nucleases with no detectable genome –wide off-target effects. Nature. 2016;529(7587):4905.
125. Slaymaker IM, Gao L, Zetsche B, Scott DA, Yan WX, Zhang F. Rationally engineered Cas9 nucleases with improved specificity. Science. 2016; 351(6268):84–8.
126. Cyranoski D. CRISPR gene-editing tested in a person for the first time. Nature. 2016;539(7630):479.
127. Gantz VM, Jasinskiene N, Tatarenkova O, Fazekas A, Macias VM, Bier E, James AA. Highly efficient Cas9-mediated gene drive for population modification of the malaria vector mosquito Anopheles stephensi. Proc Natl Acad Sci U S A. 2015;112:6736–43.
128. De carlo JE, Chavez A, Dietz SL, Esvelt KM, Church GM. Safeguarding CRISPR/Cas9 gene drives in yeast. Nat Biotechnol. 2015;33(1):1250–5.
129. Hammond A, Galizi R, Kyrou K, et al. A CRISPR-Cas9 gene drive system targeting female reproduction in the malaria mosquito vector Anopheles gambiae. Nat Biotechnol. 2016;34(1):78–83.
130. Gantz VM, Bier E. The mutagenic chain reaction: a method for converting heterozygous to homozygous mutations. Science. 2015;348:442–4.

2

Ubiquitination by HUWE1 in tumorigenesis and beyond

Shih-Han Kao[1,2]*, Han-Tsang Wu[6] and Kou-Juey Wu[1,2,3,4,5]* (iD)

Abstract

Ubiquitination modulates a large repertoire of cellular functions and thus, dysregulation of the ubiquitin system results in multiple human diseases, including cancer. Ubiquitination requires an E3 ligase, which is responsible for substrate recognition and conferring specificity to ubiquitination. HUWE1 is a multifaceted HECT domain-containing ubiquitin E3 ligase, which catalyzes both mono-ubiquitination and K6-, K48- and K63-linked poly-ubiquitination of its substrates. Many of the substrates of HUWE1 play a crucial role in maintaining the homeostasis of cellular development. Not surprisingly, dysregulation of HUWE1 is associated with tumorigenesis and metastasis. HUWE1 is frequently overexpressed in solid tumors, but can be downregulated in brain tumors, suggesting that HUWE1 may possess differing cell-specific functions depending on the downstream targets of HUWE1. This review introduces some important discoveries of the HUWE1 substrates, including those controlling proliferation and differentiation, apoptosis, DNA repair, and responses to stress. In addition, we review the signaling pathways HUWE1 participates in and obstacles to the identification of HUWE1 substrates. We also discuss up-to-date potential therapeutic designs using small molecules or ubiquitin variants (UbV) against the HUWE1 activity. These molecular advances provide a translational platform for future bench-to-bed studies. HUWE1 is a critical ubiquitination modulator during the tumor progression and may serve as a possible therapeutic target for cancer treatment.

Keywords: Ubiquitination, HUWE1, Tumorigenesis, Cancer therapeutics

Background

Amongst various post-translational modifications, ubiquitination is a common yet significant process in cells. Discovered in the 1980s by Goldstein [1], ubiquitination has since been modeled as a process that marks proteins for degradation [2, 3]. However, a growing body of evidence has shown that ubiquitination modulates disparate functions other than proteolysis, such as protein trafficking, signaling transduction, enzymatic activities, chromatin structure, nuclear localization, genome integrity [4–8]. Therefore, dysregulation of the ubiquitin system can lead to pathogenesis, including tumor development.

In this review, we briefly introduce the process of ubiquitination and the structure of HUWE1. Then, we address some of the substrates of HUWE1-mediated ubiquitination and their signaling and functional alterations in tumorigenesis and beyond. Finally, we summarize the clinical relevance, the underlying challenges of expanding the atlas of HUWE1 substrates and the possible application of HUWE1 in cancer therapeutics.

The process of ubiquitination

The attachment of ubiquitin (8.5 kDa) to a substrate protein requires the actions of three distinct enzymes and steps. The first step activates ubiquitin by forming a thioester linkage with ubiquitin-activating enzyme, E1. Subsequently, ubiquitin is transferred to an ubiquitin-conjugating enzyme, E2. Finally, an E3 ligase catalyzes the bonding between ubiquitin and a lysine residue of a target protein. The E3 ligases are responsible for substrate recognition and render substrate specificity. Therefore, E3 ligases are considered the most important components in this ubiquitin machinery. Ubiquitin ligases fall into three classes based on their structural domains: 1) the homologs to the E6-AP carboxyl terminus (HECT) domain, 2) the really interesting new gene (RING) domain, and 3) the U-box domain. While other E3 ligases act as adaptors to bring charged E2s close to substrates to facilitate ubiquitination, HECT-domain E3s

* Correspondence: shkao@mail.cmu.edu.tw; wukj@mail.cmu.edu.tw
[1]Research Center for Tumor Medical Science, China Medical University, No. 91, Hseuh-Shih Rd, Taichung 40402, Taiwan
Full list of author information is available at the end of the article

form a covalent thioester intermediate with ubiquitin during ubiquitination [9]. Many E3 ligases have been implicated in tumorigenesis because most of their known substrates are oncogenes or tumor suppressors. For instance, the Skp1/Cul1/F-box (SCF) complex represents a family of the multi-protein E3 ubiquitin ligase complex, which catalyzes ubiquitination of proteins and controls various cellular events, especially the cell cycle, by proteasomal degradation [10]. Dysregulation of the cell-cycle ubiquitin-proteasome system can result in perturbed cell growth and enhanced tumorigenesis. The F-box protein, Skp2, is the E3 ligase in the SCF complex responsible for substrate recognition and promotes the degradation of p27 Cdk inhibitor during S-phase [11]. Excessive amount of Skp2 results in a loss of p27 and this oncogenic role of Skp2, corresponding to up-regulation of Skp2 in tumor tissues, has been observed in a wide range of human cancers, including lung, breast, colorectal, head and neck squamous cell carcinoma (HNSCC) [12–14]. Inhibition of Skp2 has been demonstrated to potentially restrict cancer progression [12, 13]. On the contrary, the F-box protein, FBW7, is considered a tumor suppressor, as it degrades proto-oncogenes, such as Myc, cyclin E, Jun, Mcl-1, and Notch [14–19]. Therefore, understanding the modulation and the molecular mechanism of E3 ligases is of paramount importance in understanding tumor development and progression.

Interestingly, ubiquitin can be conjugated to a substrate in more than one form and different types of ubiquitination control diverse biological consequences [20]. The processes by which proteins are ubiquitinated on a single lysine residue by a single ubiquitin is called mono-ubiquitination. This modification has been found to regulate receptor internalization, degradation in lysosomes and protein recycling [21]. Aside from mono-ubiquitination, other well-established types of modification are K48-linked and K63-linked poly-ubiquitination. The conjugation of poly-ubiquitination is achieved via isopeptide bonds between the carboxylate at the C-terminal glycine of the distal ubiquitin and the ε–amine of an internal lysine of the proximal ubiquitin [22]. Whereas K48-linked polyubiquitin target proteins for proteasomal degradation, K63-linked polyubiquitin chains are involved in a wider variety of regulations, including signal transduction, protein localization, DNA repair, endocytosis, and protein-protein interaction [23–25]. Other types of ubiquitin linkage have been discovered as well, such as K6, K11, K27, K29, and K33 [26], increasing the versatility and the functional repertoire of ubiquitination.

Structure of HUWE1
The HECT domain-containing ubiquitin E3 ligase, HUWE1 (also known as HectH9, ARF-BP1, URE-B1, Mule, and LASU1), was first detected from a size-fractionated human brain cDNA library by Nagase et al. [27], and the full-length human HUWE1 was then identified by Liu et al., which they termed LASU1 [28]. Encoded by the *HUWE1* gene, the 482-kDa-sized HUWE1 contains two N-terminal domains, DUF908 and DUF913 (*domains of unknown functions*), similar to domains in an *S. cerevisiae* HECT ligase, Tom1, followed by a ubiquitin-associated (UBA) domain [28]. A WWE domain involved in the regulation of ubiquitin-dependent proteolysis [29] and a BH3 domain shared by all the Bcl-2 family members are also contained within HUWE1 [30]. At the C-terminus of HUWE1, there is a HECT domain which contains a catalytic cysteine residue for ubiquitin-thioester formation, and thus the HECT domain carries the enzymatic activity of this protein [31] (Fig. 1a). Structural studies have shown that the canonical HECT domain is composed of a bilobal architecture (the N-terminal (N) lobe and C-terminal (C) lobe) that separates the E2 binding region and the catalytic cysteine [32–34]. The N lobe of HECT is composed of 13 α–helices and 7 β–strands and the C lobe is comprised of 4 α–helices and 4 β–strands [31]. Crystal structural analysis of the HECT domain of HUWE1 reveals that helix α1 in the N lobe stabilizes the HECT domain and modulates the autoubiquitination ability of HUWE1 by reducing the rate of Ub addition to the HECT domain [31]. According to Pandya et al., removal of helix α1 may cause a more relaxed form of HUWE1 that exhibits greater intradomain flexibility, possibly leading to the increased enzymatic activity [31].

Highly conserved in mammals, the amino acid sequences of human and mouse HUWE1 are more than 90% identical [30], and expression of *HUWE1* is high in a considerable amount of mouse tissues, including cortex, hippocampus, eye, tongue, liver, kidney, adrenal gland, and fibroblasts [35]. Its ubiquitous expression suggests that HUWE1 may participate in quite a number of cellular functions. More importantly, while most HECT domain-containing E3s synthesize polyubiquitin chains with linkage preferences, HUWE1 is one of the few HECT E3s that can mediate both K48- and K63-linked ubiquitination [36–38]. Notably, HUWE1 can also assemble mono-ubiquitination on its substrates and the less-known K6-linked poly-ubiquitination [39–42], suggesting HUWE1 plays multiple regulatory roles via mono–/poly-ubiquitination and linkage diversities.

By functional enrichment, HUWE1 is highly associated with proliferation/differentiation, apoptosis, DNA repair, and stress response (Fig. 1b), but the impact of HUWE1 in other aspects of functions has been studied. In the next section, we introduce the substrates of HUWE1 and the signals that modulate HUWE1.

Substrates of HUWE1
MYC
Myc was one of the first proteins discovered to be a substrate of HUWE1. This proto-oncogene can act as a transcription activator or repressor, depending on the

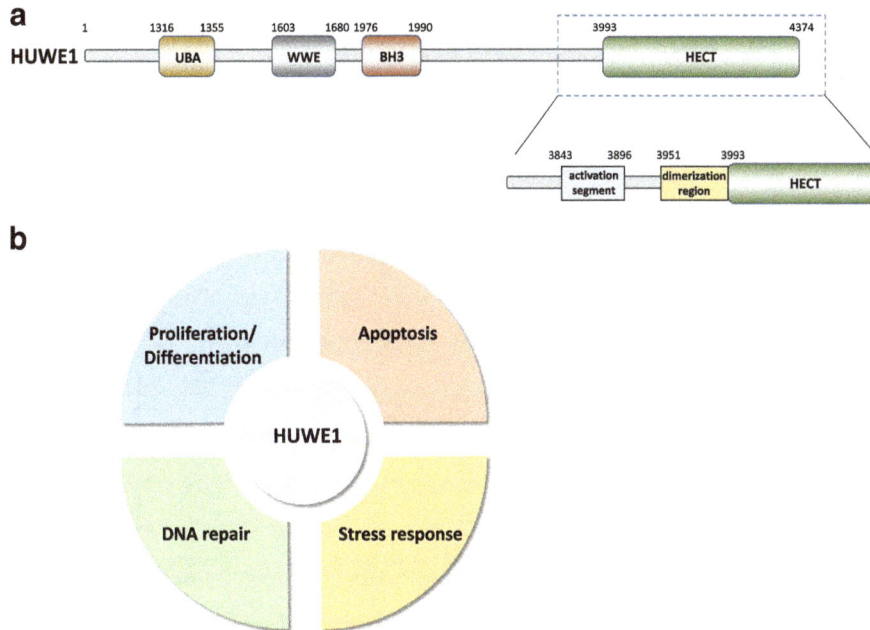

Fig. 1 The functional domains of HUWE1 and functional enrichment of HUWE1. **a** Schematic diagram of the structural features of HUWE1 protein. Huwe1 protein mainly contains four domains: 1) the UBA domain and 2) the WWE domain, 3) the BH3 domain, and 4) the HECT domain. The HECT domain contains a catalytic cysteine residue for the ubiquitin-thioester bond formation and therefore carries the enzymatic activity of HUWE1 protein. Crystal structural analysis shows that the activity of HUWE1 can be self-activated through an activation segment. HUWE1 proteins exhibit the dimerization ability using the region close to the N-terminus of the HECT domain. **b** Functional enrichment of HUWE1. Based on the substrates regulated by HUWE1, HUWE1 is involved in four major aspects of cellular regulation: Proliferation/differentiation, apoptosis, DNA repair, and stress response. Dysregulation of HUWE1, either through the impaired enzymatic activity or the aberrant expression of HUWE1, leads to disease development, such as tumor formation

components in the transcription complex. In the binary module of the complex, Myc, along with Max, binds to a specific DNA sequence, the E-box element (CACGTG), and activates transcription of a set of pro-growth genes [43]. However, when Myc forms a ternary complex with Max and Miz1, it represses transcription through interruption of the interaction between Miz1 and p300 histone acetyltransferase [44] and by recruiting a DNA methyltransferase, DNMT3a [45]. Increased levels of Myc in cells lead to cell growth, transformation, and tumorigenesis. One of the hallmarks of Myc-mediated cell transformation is the elevated activity of cyclin D-CDK4. On one hand, Myc transactivates CDK4, causing G1 progression in response to mitogenic signals [46]. On the other, genes of INK inhibitors (p15^{INK4b} and p18^{INK4c}) and CIP1/KIP1 (p21 and p27) are repressed by Myc, leading to enhanced cyclin D-CDK4 activity [47–49]. As a short-lived protein, Myc is known to be ubiquitinated by Skp2, FBW7, FBXO28, FBXL14 [50–53]. Ubiquitination of Myc by HUWE1, however, is far more complicated. In one model, c-Myc is K63-linked polyubiquitinated by HUWE1 at the C-terminus, which is required for recruitment of the coactivators, p300 [43] (Fig. 2). In this model, site-specific ubiquitination dictates the switch between transcription activation and

repression of Myc. Knockdown of HUWE1 reduces Myc functions in breast cancer cell lines and co-depletion of HUWE1 and Mnt, an antagonist of transactivation by Myc further abolished the colony formation in HeLa cells [54], suggesting an oncogenic role of HUWE1 in regulating Myc functions.

The related N-Myc, normally expressed in neural stem cells and neuroectodermal progenitors, needs timely withdrawal to initiate differentiation during neural development [55]. Premature disappearance of N-Myc results in precocious differentiation and disturbed cell cycle and N-Myc expression plays a key role during neuroblastoma differentiation [56, 57]. To ensure accurate expression of N-Myc, N-Myc protein degradation by the ubiquitin-proteasome system is essential to control the temporal expression of N-Myc [58, 59]. Liquid chromatography-tandem mass spectrometry (LC-MS/MS) results have identified that the HUWE1 is associated with N-Myc in neural cells and HUWE1-mediated N-Myc ubiquitination directs N-Myc degradation via K48-linkage assembly [60]. *Cyclin D2*, a downstream target gene of N-Myc, is decreased in N-Myc knockdown cells but increased in HUWE1-silenced cortices [60], demonstrating that this HUWE1-N-Myc pathway controls neural differentiation of mouse ES cells [60]. A follow-up study showed that the DLL3-Notch pathway is excessively activated by N-Myc

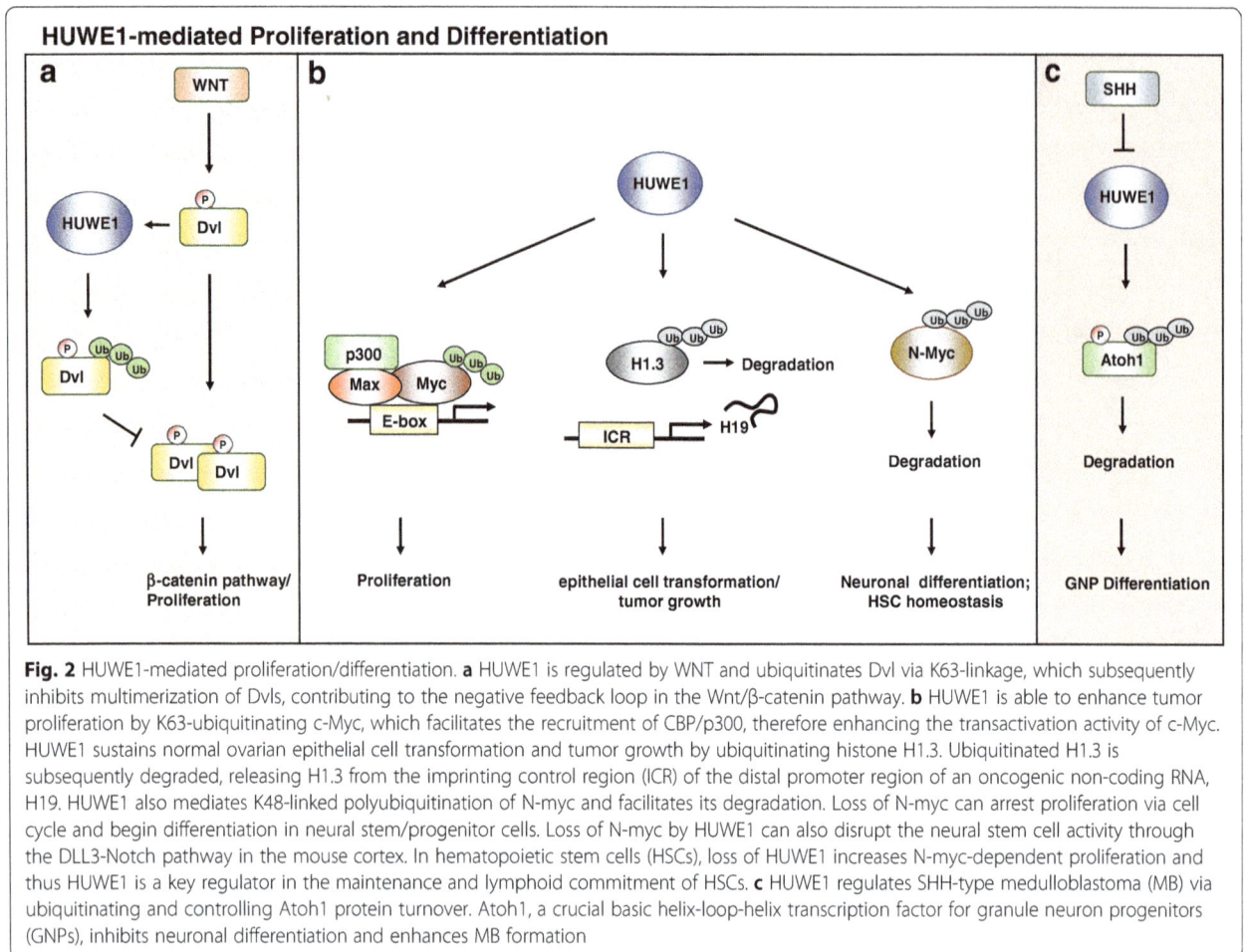

Fig. 2 HUWE1-mediated proliferation/differentiation. **a** HUWE1 is regulated by WNT and ubiquitinates Dvl via K63-linkage, which subsequently inhibits multimerization of Dvls, contributing to the negative feedback loop in the Wnt/β-catenin pathway. **b** HUWE1 is able to enhance tumor proliferation by K63-ubiquitinating c-Myc, which facilitates the recruitment of CBP/p300, therefore enhancing the transactivation activity of c-Myc. HUWE1 sustains normal ovarian epithelial cell transformation and tumor growth by ubiquitinating histone H1.3. Ubiquitinated H1.3 is subsequently degraded, releasing H1.3 from the imprinting control region (ICR) of the distal promoter region of an oncogenic non-coding RNA, H19. HUWE1 also mediates K48-linked polyubiquitination of N-myc and facilitates its degradation. Loss of N-myc by HUWE1 can arrest proliferation via cell cycle and begin differentiation in neural stem/progenitor cells. Loss of N-myc by HUWE1 can also disrupt the neural stem cell activity through the DLL3-Notch pathway in the mouse cortex. In hematopoietic stem cells (HSCs), loss of HUWE1 increases N-myc-dependent proliferation and thus HUWE1 is a key regulator in the maintenance and lymphoid commitment of HSCs. **c** HUWE1 regulates SHH-type medulloblastoma (MB) via ubiquitinating and controlling Atoh1 protein turnover. Atoh1, a crucial basic helix-loop-helix transcription factor for granule neuron progenitors (GNPs), inhibits neuronal differentiation and enhances MB formation

accumulation in the HUWE1-knockout mouse brain, leading to defected neurogenesis [61]. Zhao et al. have further demonstrated that human high-grade gliomas contain focal hemizygous deletions of the X-linked *HUWE1* gene and amplification of the *N-myc* locus [61]. HUWE1 also plays a role in hematopoietic stem cells (HSC) self-renewal, quiescence and lymphoid fate specification by regulating the expression of N-Myc [62]. Upregulation of N-Myc increased proliferation and stem cell exhaustion in HUWE1-knockout HSCs [62]. Together these data show that HUWE1 is important in both the development of neurogenesis and maintenance of HSC homeostasis by tightly controlling N-Myc expression (Fig. 2).

Contradictory to the observation that c-Myc forms polyubiquitin chains via K63 linkage [43], Zhao et al. have shown that both N-Myc and c-Myc can be ubiquitinated by HUWE1 through K48-mediated linkage and genetic knockout of *HUWE1* in embryonic stem (ES) cells can stabilize both N-Myc and c-Myc [60]. In their study, Zhao et al. used a truncated HUWE1, where c-Myc binds to HUWE1 less efficiently than N-Myc [60], which might be the reasons why contrasting observations are presented by different groups. It is thus possible that c-Myc can be

tagged with K48- and K63-linked ubiquitin moieties in vivo by HUWE1. This difference may emblem diverse biological influences in time- or context-dependent regulations of Myc by HUWE1.

Dvl

It has recently been verified that HUWE1 regulates Dishevelled (Dvl) multimerization in the Wnt signaling pathway [63]. HUWE1 promotes K63-linked poly-ubiquitination of Dvl at the DIX domain, inhibiting Dvl multimerization. Importantly, the interaction between HUWE1 and Dvl depends on Wnt3a stimulation or CK1 phosphorylation, and this leads to a negative feedback loop to inhibit Wnt signaling [63] (Fig. 2).

Atoh1

Medulloblastoma (MB) is the most common malignant pediatric brain tumor with a 20–30% incidence rate among all central nervous system (CNS) malignancies and an overall 5-year survival rate of 70–80% [64, 65]. Disruptions in cerebellar development have been shown to cause medulloblastoma [66]. Recent molecular analyses have divided medulloblastoma into four subgroups

(WNT, SHH, Group 3, and Group 4) whose genetic differences lead to distinct prognoses, temporal, and anatomical patterns of recurrence [67, 68]. Associated with the development of cerebellum, knockout of HUWE1 increases the proliferation of cerebellar granule cells in the external granule layer (EGL) of postnatal cerebella and results in disorganization of glial cells and granule neuron migration defects [69]. HUWE1 plays a significant role in Group 2 sonic hedgehog (SHH)-type of medulloblastoma by regulating the turnover of the basic helix-loop-helix (bHLH) transcription factor, Atoh1, which prevents differentiation of cerebellar granule neuron progenitors (GNPs) and enhances medulloblastoma (MB) formation [66, 70]. Upon SHH treatment, Atoh1 is stabilized, which can transform GNPs into MB-initiating cells by suppressing neuronal differentiation [70]. Conversely, when the ligand, SHH, is subtracted, HUWE1 is immediately recruited to facilitate Atoh1 ubiquitination and degradation in a phosphorylation-dependent manner [71] (Fig. 2). The high HUWE1 mRNA level correlates with a better survival in patients with SHH medulloblastoma and this prognostic role of HUWE1 may serve as a platform for a combination

therapy for SHH medulloblastoma where both SHH signaling and Atoh1 via the HUWE1 pathway are inhibited [71].

Miz1

Miz1 is a zinc-finger transcription factor which binds to the core promoter of several genes [72, 73] and regulates their expressions, including Bcl-2 [74], p15^{INK4b} [48], p21^{CIP1} [47]. Miz-1 is a negative regulator of tumor necrosis factor alpha (TNFα) signaling [75, 76]. Yang et al. have shown that upon TNFα stimulation, HUWE1 degrades Miz-1 protein and facilitates TNFα-induced JNK activation [77] (Fig. 3). Knockdown of HUWE1 restrained TNFα-induced JNK activation and cell death but the effect was abolished in Miz1$^{-/-}$ MEFs [77]. In another *HUWE1* knockout mouse model, HUWE1 deletion causes increased severity of skin tumors, which were induced by carcinogens, 7,12-dimethylbenz-(a)-anthracene (DMBA) and 12-O-tetradecanoylphorbol-13-acetate (PMA) [78]. HUWE1 deficiency results in an accumulation of the c-Myc/Miz1 complex and concomitant knockout of c-Myc could rescue HUWE1-deficient phenotype [78]. In vitro knockdown of MiZ1 could

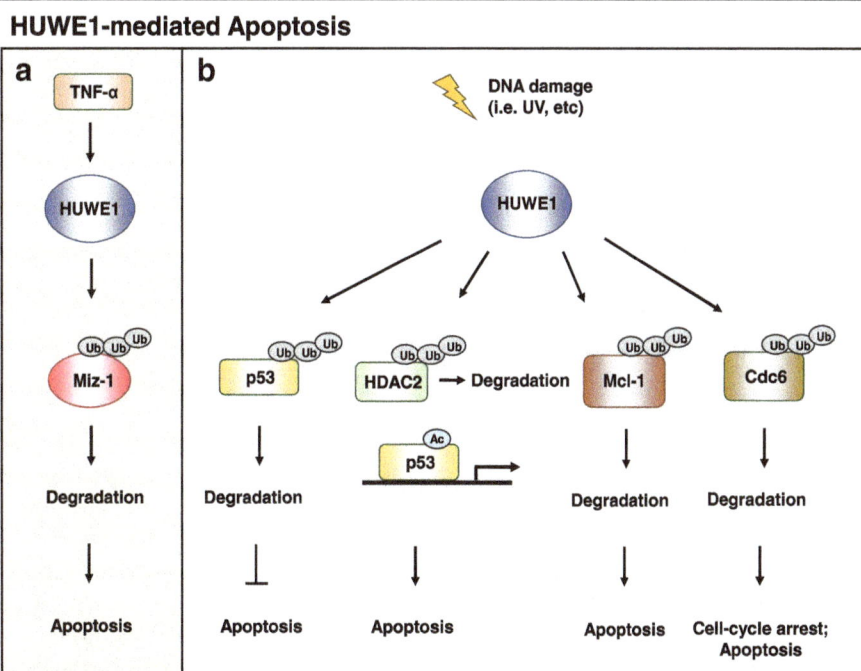

Fig. 3 HUWE1-mediated apoptosis. **a** Upon TNFα stimulation, HUWE1 can mediate K48-linked polyubiquitination of Miz-1, thereby facilitating the degradation of Miz-1 protein. Miz-1 suppresses TNFα-induced JNK activation and cell death. Reduced Miz-1 levels relieve this negative regulation on TNFα. **b** When DNA damage occurs, cells undergo cell-cycle arrest and apoptosis by enhancing the activities of p53, downregulating the expressions of anti-apoptotic molecules (i.e. Mcl-1) and the assembly of pre-replicative complex (Cdc6 in preRC). HUWE1 is an associating protein of the tumor suppressor, ARF, which plays a pivotal role in regulating p53 and inhibits the ubiquitin ligase activity of HUWE1. Expression of HUWE1 can directly ubiquitinate and degrade p53 in a Mdm2-independent way, thereby suppressing p53-dependent apoptosis. HUWE1 mediates polyubiquitination of HDAC2, which deacetylates p53 and affects p53 transcriptional activity. HUWE1 deficiency leads to accumulation of HDAC2 and compromised p53 acetylation and apoptotic response upon DNA damage. HUWE1 interacts with Mcl-1 through the BH3 domain, causing Mcl-1 degradation upon DNA damage. Cdc6 plays a key role in DNA replication and degradation of Cdc6 mediated by HUWE1 polyubiquitination occurs upon ultraviolet irradiation or DNA alkylation, resulting in cell-cycle arrest and apoptosis

reverse and reduce proliferation of HUWE1-deficient keratinocytes. Increased c-myc and Miz1 by HUWE1 depletion leads to a repression of *Cdkn2b* (p15^{INK4b}) and *Cdkn1a* (p21^{CIP1}), thereby enhancing tumorigenesis [78].

p53

Tumor suppressor p53 is a crucial coordinator in cellular responses to stress from oncogene activation, DNA damage, and hypoxia [79, 80]. The antiproliferative capability of p53 mediates cell cycle arrest, apoptosis, and even cellular senescence [81, 82]. While mutations of p53 are observed in more than half of human tumors [83], dysregulation of the ARF tumor-suppressor protein (p14^{ARF} in humans and p19^{ARF} in mouse), which increases and activates wild-type p53 by sequestering Mdm2 in the nucleolus [84] or by directly inhibiting the enzymatic activity of Mdm2 [85, 86], is a common characteristic in cancer as well. Chen et al. have identified HUWE1 (termed ARF-BP1 in their report) as a major associating protein of ARF in p53-null cells and ARF induces p53-independent growth suppression by inhibiting the ubiquitin ligase activity of HUWE1 [87]. In p53-wildtype cells, however, HUWE1 directly binds to and ubiquitinates p53, which facilitates p53 protein degradation and subsequently suppresses p53-dependent apoptosis [87] (Fig. 3). ARF induces p53 stabilization through negatively regulating HUWE1, which is independent of Mdm2 [87], suggesting that multiple E3 ligases are involved in regulating p53 turnover. Dysregulation of p53 ubiquitination is thus a pivotal mechanism in tumorigenesis. Recently, reports have shown that suppression of HUWE1 elevates the p53 protein levels in Myc-driven B cell lymphomas, leading to growth arrest and apoptosis [88]. Together these findings favor the notion that HUWE1 promotes tumorigenesis and may serve as a therapeutic target as a future research direction.

HDAC2

Histone deacetylases (HDACs) mediates a broad range of cellular functions by epigenetically modulating chromatin structure and gene transcription. While acetylation is mediated by histone acetyltransferase (HAT) and is thought to activate gene transcription, HDACs reverses this process and mediates transcriptional suppression [89]. There are four major classes of HDACs. Class I HDACs are HDAC1–3, and HDAC8, which are ubiquitously present in cells and possess the strongest HDAC activities. Thus, both histone and non-histone proteins can be the substrates of Class I HDACs. Class II HDACs are HDAC4–7 and HDAC9 and their expressions are tissue specific. Class III HDACs, often referred to as sirtuins, require NAD$^+$ as a cofactor and are homologous with yeast Sir2. The Class VI HDAC (HDAC11) is homologous with Class I and Class II HDACs, all of which are Zn^{2+}-dependent enzymes as opposed to Class III HDACs [90, 91].

Investigation of HUWE1 and its role in DNA damage using HDAC inhibitors (HDACis) has shown that HUWE1 specifically ubiquitinates HDAC2 and negatively regulates its stability [92]. In *HUWE1* knockout embryonic fibroblasts (MEFs), increased HDAC2 abrogates acetylation of p53, a critical modification for p53 transcriptional activity, and apoptosis is attenuated under cisplatin or the HDACi, NaBu, treatments [92]. Collectively, these data show that the HUWE1-HDAC2 pathway controls cell apoptosis via modulating the transcriptional activity of p53 (Fig. 3).

Mcl-1

In the transcription-independent pathway of apoptosis, the stress signal induces mitochondrial outer membrane permeabilization (MOMP) and prompts the release of proapoptotic factors of Bcl-2 homology (BH)3-only molecules, such as BAD, BID, BIM, PUMA, and NOXA while the anti-apoptotic members of the Bcl-2 family antagonizes this event [93–95]. Mcl-1 is an anti-apoptotic member of the Bcl-2 family proteins which is frequently upregulated in cancers to promote cell survival [96–99]. Under normal conditions, Mcl-1 associates with the proapoptotic BAK protein to maintain BAK in an inactive state whereas downregulation of Mcl-1 proteins is triggered by DNA damage, such as infection by viruses [100]. HUWE1 contains a BH3 domain for specific interaction with Mcl-1 and facilitates the degradation Mcl-1, thereby enhancing apoptosis in response to DNA damage [30] (Fig. 3). The well-conserved BH3 domain within HUWE1 mostly resembles that of Bak and therefore HUWE1 might compete with Bak to break up the Mcl-1/Bak complex, converting the fate of a cell toward death. Further validation is needed to confirm the relationship among Bak, HUWE1, and Mcl-1 in the mitochondria-mediated apoptotic pathway.

Regulation of HUWE1-induced Mcl-1 degradation, however, is not limited to DNA damage or viral infection. During obesity-associated hepatocellular carcinoma (HCC) development, expression of interleukin-6 (IL-6), which results from a chronic low-grade proinflammatory state in white adipose tissue and liver [101], helps to stabilize Mcl-1 via promotion of GSK3β inactivation and suppression of HUWE1 [102]. As a result, obesity suppresses hepatocyte apoptosis through Mcl-1 stabilization and promotes liver carcinogenesis [102]. Whether HUWE1 also mediates Mcl-1 degradation in other cell types, as an alternative major regulatory pathway to control tumorigenesis, remains to be determined.

Cdc6

DNA damage can influence cell cycle by not only promoting checkpoint functions but reducing re-replicating DNA as well to block mitosis of cells with erroneous DNA. The prereplication complex (preRC) is assembled during G1 to facilitate replication and Cdc6 is an essential regulator in this complex [103]. In later cell cycle stages, Cdc6 takes part in checkpoint activation if DNA replication is not properly completed [104–106]. Cdc6 proteins are rapidly degraded during each cell cycle by the E3 ligase, anaphase promoting complex (APC^{Cdh1}) [107]. Upon DNA damage, Cdc6 is also ubiquitinated and degraded by APC^{Cdh1} in a p53-dependent manner [108]. However, Cdc6 degradation can occur independently of both p53 and cell cycle when DNA damage is caused by ultraviolet (UV) irradiation or DNA alkylation by methyl methane sulfonate (MMS) and this poly-ubiquitination process is mediated by HUWE1 [103] (Fig. 3). As a result, Cdc6 is directed to the proteasomal degradation route and released from chromatin. It is tempting to postulate that in response to DNA damage, HUWE1 mediates Cdc6 degradation to inhibit new preRC assembly, but may keep functional acetylated p53 in abundance to push cells to undergo cycle arrest, and finally apoptosis.

BRCA1

Loss of BRCA1 is a common characteristic in breast and ovarian cancers and causes defects in DNA repair, especially double-strand breaks (DSBs) by homologous recombination (HR), resulting in genomic instability [109–111]. Although germline mutations of BRCA1 are a risk factor of hereditary breast and ovarian cancers among women, their occurrence is less frequent in sporadic cancers [112]. Instead, a decrease in BRCA1 protein levels is more commonly detected, implying that a deregulation of the machinery of proteasomal degradation may take part in BRCA1-mediated tumorigenesis. Enzymes that regulate the turnover of BRCA1 have recently been identified, including HERC2, SCF^{FBXO44} as the E3 ligases [113, 114], and E2T, as an ubiquitin-conjugating E2 enzyme [115]. It has been shown that HUWE1 associates with the BRCA1-Merit40/RAP80 complex [116] and together mediate the ubiquitination and degradation of BRCA1 (Fig. 4). Upon ionizing radiation or mitomycin treatment, knockdown of HUWE1 confers treatment resistance to breast cancer cells [117]. The antagonistic effect of HUWE1 on BRCA1 may suppress HR-dependent DSB repair, supporting the role of HUWE1 in DNA damage repair.

Polβ & Polλ

HUWE1 also participates in DNA-damage response as a tuning mechanism for base excision repair (BER), which requires a set of enzymes to recognize and remove DNA lesions induced by DNA damaging agents and restore the correct DNA information. BER DNA polymerases are enzymes filling in the one nucleotide gap to replace the excised one during BER. Pol β is the major human polymerase that catalyzes this gap-filling process; therefore, its under- or over-expression may lead to severe

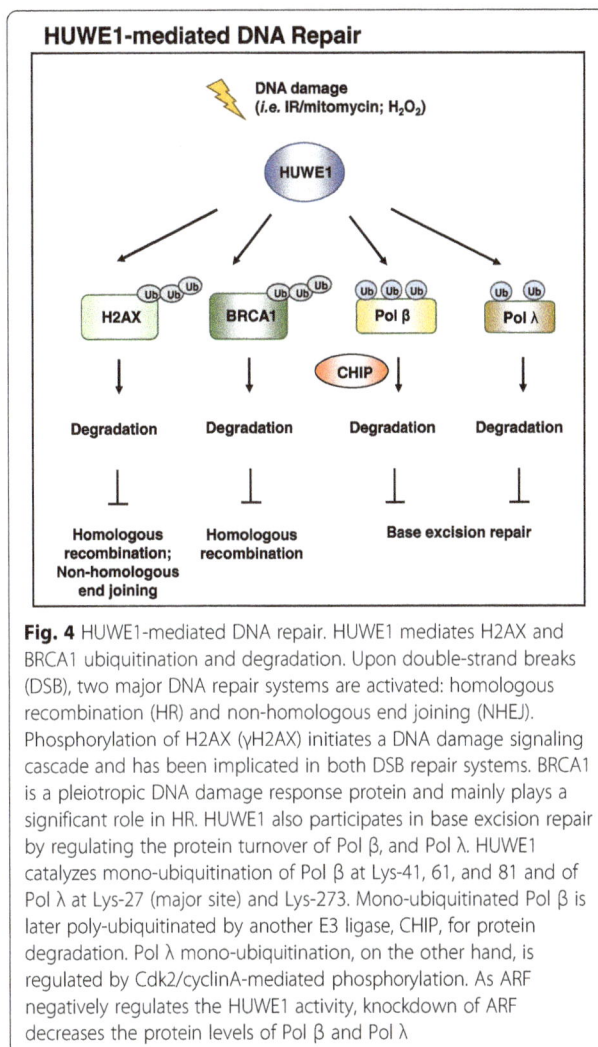

Fig. 4 HUWE1-mediated DNA repair. HUWE1 mediates H2AX and BRCA1 ubiquitination and degradation. Upon double-strand breaks (DSB), two major DNA repair systems are activated: homologous recombination (HR) and non-homologous end joining (NHEJ). Phosphorylation of H2AX (γH2AX) initiates a DNA damage signaling cascade and has been implicated in both DSB repair systems. BRCA1 is a pleiotropic DNA damage response protein and mainly plays a significant role in HR. HUWE1 also participates in base excision repair by regulating the protein turnover of Pol β, and Pol λ. HUWE1 catalyzes mono-ubiquitination of Pol β at Lys-41, 61, and 81 and of Pol λ at Lys-27 (major site) and Lys-273. Mono-ubiquitinated Pol β is later poly-ubiquitinated by another E3 ligase, CHIP, for protein degradation. Pol λ mono-ubiquitination, on the other hand, is regulated by Cdk2/cyclinA-mediated phosphorylation. As ARF negatively regulates the HUWE1 activity, knockdown of ARF decreases the protein levels of Pol β and Pol λ

mutagenesis and cancer susceptibility [118, 119]. In the absence of Pol β, however, Pol λ can compensate the functions of Pol β as both proteins share noteworthy enzymatic and structural similarities [120]. Interestingly, both Pol β and Pol λ can be ubiquitinated by HUWE1 and another E3 ligase, carboxyl terminus of Hsc70 interacting protein (CHIP) [39, 121].

In the case of Pol β, Parsons et al. observed that HUWE1 and ARF oppositely modulate the BER activity by controlling the stability of Pol β [39]. HUWE1 first catalyzes mono-ubiquitination at Lys-41, 61, and 81 of Pol β, which is subjected to CHIP-mediated poly-ubiquitination and subsequent degradation [39]. Double silencing of HUWE1 and CHIP only marginally elevates Pol β protein expression, suggesting that these two E3 ligases orchestrate Pol β degradation in the same pathway. Knockdown of ARF, which is known to inhibit the ubiquitination activity of HUWE1 [87], however, could increase the levels of mono-ubiquitinated Pol β [39]. While ARF knockdown slows down the rate of DNA repair, HUWE1 silencing conspicuously increases the repair efficacy of hydrogen peroxide-induced DNA lesions because of the enrichment of Pol β in the nucleus [39]. Hence, HUWE1, ARF and CHIP together modulate BER capacity by controlling the protein dynamics of Pol β [39] (Fig. 4). Similar to Pol β, ARF also modulates the steady state of Pol λ as knockdown of ARF decreases the protein levels of Pol λ [40]. HUWE1 ubiquitinates Pol λ at Lys-27 (major site) and Lys-273 (minor site), but unlike Pol β, a subsequent in vivo regulation by CHIP has not been further validated (Fig. 4). Nevertheless, ubiquitination of Pol λ is regulated by Cdk2/cyclinA-mediated phosphorylation [40]. Phosphorylation of Pol λ inhibits protein degradation by keeping Pol λ proteins on chromatin in the nucleus [40]. Increased ubiquitination and degradation by HUWE1 is observed when phosphorylation-deficient mutant of Pol λ is expressed, resulting in error-prone single-nucleotide incorporation upon 8-oxo-G DNA treatment [40]. It remains to be answered what stimulus is involved in activating each repair Pol and whether post-translational modifications (PTMs), such as phosphorylation, would contribute to Pol subcellular localization and degradation.

HAUSP (USP7)

HAUSP (USP7) is a USP type deubiquitinase that stabilizes many proteins via deubiquitination. Amongst its substrates, MDM2 and PTEN have been shown to be deubiquitinated by HAUSP to cause the stabilization or change of cellular localization, respectively, leading to tumorigenesis [122, 123]. Recent results have also shown that HUWE1 mediates K63-linked polyubiquitination of HAUSP to increase its deubiquitinase function [124]. In addition, K63-polyubiquitinated HAUSP serves as a scaffold to anchor HIF-1α, CBP, the mediator complex, and the super-elongation complex to enhance the gene transcription activity initiated by HIF-1α binding to the hypoxia response element in the promoters of HIF-1α target genes, including VEGF, Glut1, and Twist1 [124]. As HAUSP is shown to be a deubiquitinase of HIF-1α [124], the K63-linked polyubiquitination of HAUSP further enhances its ability to deubiquitinate HIF-1α. Therefore, K63-linked polyubiquitination of HAUSP improves both its deubiquitinase activity and its transcription complex scaffolding activity. These properties make HAUSP a unique HUWE1 substrate. Finally, as HIF-1α plays a major role in inducing tumor progression [125], K63-polyubiquination of HAUSP mediated by HUWE1 would contribute to the oncogenic function of HUWE1 (Fig. 5). As HUWE1 is induced by hypoxia [124], the inter-relationship between HUWE1 and HIF-1α will make HUWE1 a re-enforcing target in the complex hypoxia-induced tumorigenesis network.

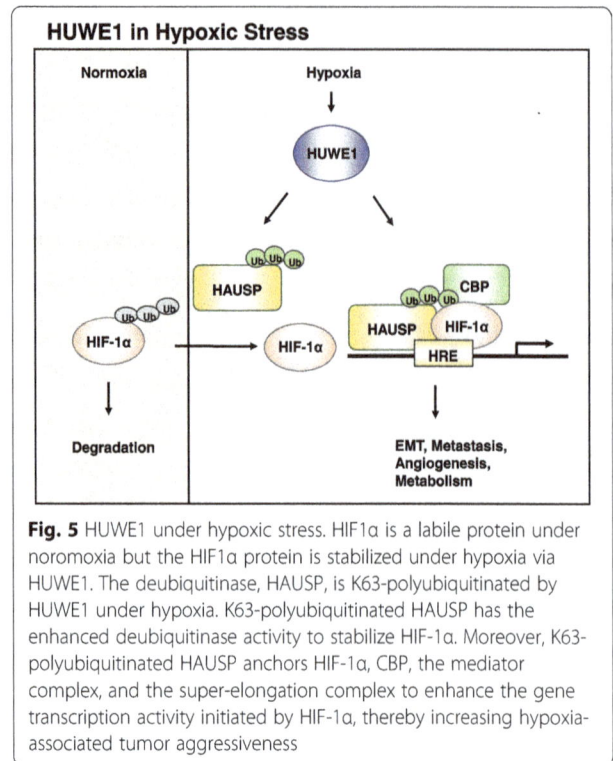

Fig. 5 HUWE1 under hypoxic stress. HIF1α is a labile protein under noromoxia but the HIF1α protein is stabilized under hypoxia via HUWE1. The deubiquitinase, HAUSP, is K63-polyubiquitinated by HUWE1 under hypoxia. K63-polyubiquitinated HAUSP has the enhanced deubiquitinase activity to stabilize HIF-1α. Moreover, K63-polyubiquitinated HAUSP anchors HIF-1α, CBP, the mediator complex, and the super-elongation complex to enhance the gene transcription activity initiated by HIF-1α, thereby increasing hypoxia-associated tumor aggressiveness

Tiam1

It has recently been shown that HUWE1 may participate in cell movement through HGF-induced RAC signaling [126]. T lymphoma invasion and metastasis inducing protein 1 (Tiam1) serves as a guanine nucleotide exchange factor (GEF) for the activation of the small GTPase, Rac [127]. *Tiam1* deficiency leads to increased apoptosis during the initiation of Ras-induced skin tumors and reduced proliferation during promotion [128]. The impaired Tiam1-mediated Rac activity leads to decreased levels of intracellular reactive oxygen speicies (ROS), which, in turn, blocks ERK phosphorylation and activation [129]. Nevertheless, the few tumors arising from $Tiam1^{-/-}$ mice are more malignant and invasive compared to those from Tiam$^{+/+}$ mice [128], raising the possibility that Tiam-Rac regulates different aspects of Ras-induced tumorigenesis. It turns out that Rac activation has dual roles in cell movement. Tiam1-Rac can enhance lamellipodia and invadopodia formation in breast cancer at a low cell density [130] but it can also promote E-cadherin-mediated adhesion in MDCKII cells [131, 132]. In accordance with the role of Tiam1 in maintaining the cell junction structure, Vaughan et al. have shown that in response to HGF, Tiam1 can be ubiquitinated at Lys-595 by HUWE1, resulting in Tiam1 degradation and disassembly of cell junctions, increasing cell migration and invasion in lung carcinoma cells [126]. HGF-induced Rac1-mediated cell migration is regulated by another HECT E3 ligase, HECT domain and Ankyrin repeat containing E3 ubiquitin-protein ligase 1 (HACE1), which degrades Rac itself [133]. Thus, ubiquitination can act as a rapid response mechanism to mitogens to ready the cells for possible movement.

MyoD

HUWE1 is involved in myogenesis by regulating the stability of MyoD, which is one of the master transcription factors determining myoblast proliferation and myotube differentiation [134]. The transcriptional activity of MyoD is regulated at both the epigenetic level and post-translational level [135, 136]. MyoD degradation is mainly mediated by a muscle-specific E3 ligase, MAFbx/AT-1 [137], but a growing line of evidence has shown that other E3 ligases may be involved. Tom1, a homolog of HUWE1 in *S. cerevisiae*, serves as the MyoD E3 ligase and human HUWE1 in mammalian cells mediates the ubiquitination of the N-terminal residue lysines of MyoD [138]. As myogenesis is mainly regulated by fibroblast growth factor (FGF), it remains to be determined whether HUWE1 is affected by FGF, thereby influencing MyoD expression and the cell fate of myoblasts.

Histones

HUWE1 ubiquitinates multiple histones (H1, H2A, H2B, H3, and H4) during spermatogenesis. To evolve into elongated mature forms, spermatids require degradation of a fraction of proteins, including histones. Loss of histones by HUWE1-mediated ubiquitination subsequently causes chromatin condensation into the narrow head of the mature spermatids [28]. HUWE1-mediated ubiquitination of specific histones can be detected in other physiological scenarios. HUWE1 mediates ubiquitination and degradation of histone H1.3 has been reported to regulate normal ovarian epithelial cell transformation and tumor growth [139]. H1.3 is a specific repressor for the noncoding oncogene H19 in ovarian cancer, where H1.3 overexpression occupies the H19 regulator region encompassing the imprinting control region (ICR), along with increased DNA methylation and reduced binding of the insulator protein CTCF at the ICR [140]. HUWE1 thus controls the H1.3-H19 cascade to promote ovarian tumorigenesis [139] (Fig. 2). Another histone that can be ubiquitin-modified by HUWE1 is H2AX, which is maintained at a low level in resting cells [141] but stabilized and phosphorylated to produce γH2AX at DNA double-strand breaks (DSBs) [142]. Atsumi et al. have shown that H2AX is poly-ubiquitinated by HUWE1 and subject to degradation. Upon DSBs, H2AX is dissociated from HUWE1 and enhances incorporation with chromatin regulated by SIRT6 and SNF2H [142] (Fig. 4). It would not be surprising if HUWE1 may contribute to modulation of other specific histones, although physiologic cues have not yet been found.

Clinical relevance and therapeutic strategies

HUWE1 controls the expressions or activities of many pivotal downstream proteins. Numerous studies have shown that HUWE1 can be either oncogenic or tumor suppressing, depending on the leading substrates that it regulates in the context [see "Substrates of HUWE1"]. HUWE1 is often found over-expressed in cancers of breast, lung, prostate, colon, larynx, stomach, and uterus but under-expressed in brain tumors [43, 143]. In SHH-type medulloblastoma, high expression of HUWE1 correlates with a better survival outcome [71], indicating that HUWE1 potentially serves as a tumor suppressor and a prognostic marker in brain tumors. The small-molecule therapeutic by GDC-0449, a drug that targets the serpentine receptor Smoothened (SMO), has been used to treat a patient with advanced medulloblastoma, in which a rapid yet transient regression and an incomplete response to inhibition of the hedgehog (Hh) pathway were observed [144]. Drug resistance against GDC-0449 likely results from SMO mutation in the Hh signaling pathway [145]. Therefore, a combination therapy downregulating both SHH signaling and Atoh1 by HUWE1 should be taken into consideration for brain tumors therapy, which may be a more promising therapeutic avenue.

In tumors where HUWE1 acts as an oncogene, blockage of the enzymatic activity of HUWE1 or a direct inhibition of HUWE1 expression is useful in counteracting pathways governing cell proliferation. Being one of the well-known substrates of HUWE1, Myc provides the major pro-proliferative signaling for cancer cells and indeed, several avenues to block Myc and its signaling transduction have been designed [146–148]. Recently, a high-throughput screening of small molecules was conducted to identify two HUWE1 inhibitors, BI8622 and BI8626 [149]. Peter et al. exploited the fact that the HECT-domain of HUWE1 can autoubiquitinate and small molecules that block autoubiquitination fluorescence signals can be selected as potential inhibitors of HUWE1 in vitro [149]. Their findings show that inhibition of HUWE1 accumulates Miz1, thereby repressing Myc-activated target genes in colorectal cancer cells [149]. In accordance, in Myc-driven B cell lymphomas, HUWE1 inhibition by its specific siRNA increases p53 levels and reduces the transcriptional activity of Myc, thereby inducing apoptosis in tumors cells [88]. Thus, a direct downregulation of HUWE1 by antisense oligonucleotide (ASO) therapy delivered with nanoparticles to enhance transfection efficiency may be further applied in therapeutic intervention of cancer.

Zhang et al. have lately developed another high-throughput system-wide platform using the phage-displayed ubiquitin variants (UbV) that inhibit or activate HECT E3s [150]. They further demonstrated by structural analysis that UbV inhibitors occupy the E2-binding site whereas the UbV

Table 1 Substrates of HUWE1-mediated ubiquitination

Targets	Ubiquitination Type and Linkage	Ubiquitination Effects	Functional Alteration by ubiquitination	References
c-Myc	K63-linked poly-ubiquitination	c-Myc transactivation	Increased cell proliferation	[43]
N-Myc	K48-linked poly-ubiquitination	Degradation	Dysregulated neural differentiation; Perturbed HSC self-renewal	[60–62]
Dvl	K63-linked poly-ubiquitination	Inhibit Dvl multimerization	Negative feedback loop to Wnt signaling	[63]
Atoh1	Poly-ubiquitination	Phosphorylation-dependent degradation	Increased neuronal differentiation	[71]
Mcl-1	Poly-ubiquitination	Degradation	Increased DNA-damage induced apoptosis; Increased hepatocyte apoptosis	[77]
p53	Poly-ubiquitination	Degradation	Reduced cell growth arrest; Increased anti-apoptosis	[87]
HDAC2	Poly-ubiquitination	Degradation	Apoptosis	[92]
Miz1; c-Myc/Miz1	K48-linked poly-ubiquitination	Degradation	JNK activation and apoptosis; Ras signaling suppression;	[30, 102]
Cdc6	Poly-ubiquitination	Degradation	Released from chromatin; Inhibition of preRC assembly	[103]
BRCA1	Poly-ubiquitination	Degradation	Reduced DNA repair	[116, 117]
Pol β	Mono-ubiquitination	Degradation	Decreased DNA repair	[39]
Pol λ	Mono-ubiquitination	Degradation	Decreased DNA repair; Reduced chromatin binding	[40]
HAUSP	K63-linked poly-ubiquitination	Enhanced HAUSP deubiquitase activity; enhanced transactivation	EMT, chromatin modification	[124]
TIAM1	Poly-ubiquitination	Degradation	Enhanced migration, invasion	[126]
MyoD	Poly-ubiquitination	Degradation	Myogenesis	[138]
H1.3	Poly-ubiquitination	Degradation	Ovarian epithelial cell transformation; Tumor growth	[139]
H2AX	Poly-ubiquitination	Degradation	Decreased DNA repair	[142]

activators bind to a ubiquitin-binding exosite [150]. The HUWE1 inhibitors (HU.1 and HU.2) they identified reduced in vitro autoubiquitination and stabilized the protein levels of HUWE1 and c-Myc. Further application of HU.1 and HU.2 in cancer therapy needs to be tested. Interestingly, the crystal structure of the C-terminal part of HUWE1, which encompasses the catalytic domain, shows an asymmetric auto-inhibited dimer and an activation segment (residues 3843–3895) [151] (Fig. 1a). Interaction between the tumor suppressor p14ARF and the activation segment promotes oligomerization of HUWE1, therefore shifting the conformational equilibrium of HUWE1 toward the inactive state [151]. Together with Zhang's finding [150], these data reveal that the activity of HUWE1 is largely determined by its conformation. Disruption of the proper enzymatic conformation of HUWE1 should be taken into consideration when small molecule inhibitors or peptides are developed as a novel therapeutic intervention in the future, which will fulfill the principal rule of precision medicine based on tumor types, genetic contents, and molecular/cellular presentations.

Challenges, perspectives, and conclusion

As more findings have demonstrated the significance of post-translational modification in cancer regulation, molecular pathways which play a role in this process may serve as not only a biomarker of cancer progression but also a possible target for cancer therapy. Undoubtedly, HUWE1 is such a candidate E3 ligase that mediates ubiquitination and has shown significant implication in clinical applications. However, a precise understanding of the HUWE1 mechanism lies heavily on the identification of its substrates, which also poses technical challenges in certain aspects. First, ubiquitination is a tightly controlled, highly coordinated, and dynamic process which involves E3 ligases and deubiquitinating enzymes (DUBs) in response to environmental changes. The dynamic nature of ubiquitination is manifested by the weak physical interaction between an E3 ligase and its substrate and rapid dissociation rate. Traditional immunoprecipitation followed by mass spectrometry may only fill in a piece of the map without comprehensively identifying the substrates. Second, the fact that a single E3 ligase targets multiple substrates and a particular substrate is regulated by several E3 ligases provide significant degrees of redundancy and this web-like regulations between E3 ligases and substrates under different temporal and spatial conditions make the cellular analysis difficult [152]. Third, although the WW domains of NEDD4 family E3 ligases associate with proline rich PPxY (PY) motifs or phosphoserine/threonine residues in their substrates [153], other HECT E3 ligases, including HUWE1, have not been shown to bind specifically to a certain consensus motif. Recently, systemic and quantitative approaches using monoclonal antibodies that recognize diglycine (diGly)-isopeptide have been utilized to characterize ubiquitin-modified proteome [154, 155]. Most of the identified substrates of HUWE1 discovered so far have K48-linkage or K63-linkage polyubiquitins (Table 1). Michel et al. have used K6-linkage-specific "affimer" to identify HUWE1 as a main E3 ligase for this chain type [42]. These bettered "ubiquitome" techniques can enhance the breadth and depth of HUWE1 studies. Further characterization on the signaling pathways that modulate the activity or the expression of HUWE1 as well as the chain types of its downstream targets may assist us to understand the underlying mechanism of tumorigenesis and metastasis. In sum, these molecular and cellular researches can later be applied to translational studies as new therapeutic approaches for tumor treatment.

Abbreviations
BER: Base excision repair; CHIP: Carboxyl terminus of Hsc70 interacting protein; DSBs: Double-strand breaks; Dvl: Dishevelled; GNPs: Granule neuron progenitors; HDACis: HDAC inhibitors; HDACs: Histone deacetylases; HECT: Homologs to the E6-AP carboxyl terminus; HR: Homologous recombination; HSC: Hematopoietic stem cells; HUWE1: HECT, UBA and WWE domain containing 1, E3 ubiquitin protein ligase; MB: Medulloblastoma; NHEJ: Non-homologous end joining; preRC: Prereplication complex; SCF: Skp1/Cul1/F-box; SHH: Sonic hedgehog; UBA: Ubiquitin-associated

Funding
This work was supported by the "Drug Development Center, China Medical University" from The Featured Areas Research Center Program within the framework of the Higher Education Sprout Project by the Ministry of Education (MOE) in Taiwan. This work was also supported in part to K.J.W. by Ministry of Science and Technology Summit grant (MOST 107–2745-B-039-001, MOST 106–2745-B-039-001); and to S.H.K by Ministry of Science and Technology (MOST 105–2320-B-039-063) and China Medical University (CMU 103-RAP-03).

Authors' contributions
The manuscript was prepared by SHK and KJW. The figures were drawn by SHK and HTW. All authors have read and approved the manuscript.

Competing interests
The authors declare that they have no competing interests.

Author details
[1]Research Center for Tumor Medical Science, China Medical University, No. 91, Hseuh-Shih Rd, Taichung 40402, Taiwan. [2]Drug Development Center, China Medical University, Taichung 40402, Taiwan. [3]Institute of New Drug Development, Taichung 40402, Taiwan. [4]Graduate Institutes of Biomedical Sciences, China Medical University, Taichung 40402, Taiwan. [5]Departmet of Medical Research, China Medical University Hospital, Taichung 40402, Taiwan. [6]Department of Cell and Tissue Engineering, Changhua Christian Hospital, Changhua City 500, Taiwan.

References

1. Goldstein G, Scheid M, Hammerling U, Schlesinger DH, Niall HD, Boyse EA. Isolation of a polypeptide that has lymphocyte-differentiating properties and is probably represented universally in living cells. Proc Natl Acad Sci U S A. 1975;72:11–5.

2. Hershko D, Bornstein G, Ben-Izhak O, Carrano A, Pagano M, Krausz MM, et al. Inverse relation between levels of p27(Kip1) and of its ubiquitin ligase subunit Skp2 in colorectal carcinomas. Cancer. 2001;91:1745–51.

3. Schwartz DC, Hochstrasser M. A superfamily of protein tags: ubiquitin, SUMO and related modifiers. Trends Biochem Sci. 2003;28:321–8.

4. Bennett EJ, Harper JW. DNA damage: ubiquitin marks the spot. Nat Struct Mol Biol. 2008;15:20–2.

5. Katzmann DJ, Odorizzi G, Emr SD. Receptor downregulation and multivesicular-body sorting. Nat Rev Mol Cell Biol. 2002;3:893–905.

6. Haglund K, Dikic I. Ubiquitylation and cell signaling. EMBO J. 2005;24:3353–9.

7. Mukhopadhyay D, Riezman H. Proteasome-independent functions of ubiquitin in endocytosis and signaling. Science. 2007;315:201–5.

8. Swatek KN, Komander D. Ubiquitin modifications. Cell Res. 2016;26:399–422.

9. Bedford L, Lowe J, Dick LR, Mayer RJ, Brownell JE. Ubiquitin-like protein conjugation and the ubiquitin-proteasome system as drug targets. Nat Rev Drug Discov. 2011;10:29–46.

10. Koepp DM, Harper JW, Elledge SJ. How the cyclin became a cyclin: regulated proteolysis in the cell cycle. Cell. 1999;97:431–4.

11. Carrano AC, Eytan E, Hershko A, Pagano M. SKP2 is required for ubiquitin-mediated degradation of the CDK inhibitor p27. Nat Cell Biol. 1999;1:193–9.

12. Chan C-H, Morrow JK, Li C-F, Gao Y, Jin G, Moten A, et al. Pharmacological inactivation of Skp2 SCF ubiquitin ligase restricts cancer stem cell traits and cancer progression. Cell. 2013;154:556–68.

13. Wu L, Grigoryan AV, Li Y, Hao B, Pagano M, Cardozo TJ. Specific small molecule inhibitors of Skp2-mediated p27 degradation. Chem Biol. 2012;19:1515–24.

14. Yada M, Hatakeyama S, Kamura T, Nishiyama M, Tsunematsu R, Imaki H, et al. Phosphorylation-dependent degradation of c-Myc is mediated by the F-box protein Fbw7. EMBO J. 2004;23:2116–25.

15. Nateri AS, Riera-Sans L, Da Costa C, Behrens A. The ubiquitin ligase SCFFbw7 antagonizes apoptotic JNK signaling. Science. 2004;303:1374–8.

16. Fuchs SY, Xie B, Adler V, Fried VA, Davis RJ, Ronai Z. C-Jun NH2-terminal kinases target the ubiquitination of their associated transcription factors. J Biol Chem. 1997;272:32163–8.

17. Oberg C, Li J, Pauley A, Wolf E, Gurney M, Lendahl U. The notch intracellular domain is ubiquitinated and negatively regulated by the mammalian Sel-10 homolog. J Biol Chem. 2001;276:35847–53.

18. Koepp DM, Schaefer LK, Ye X, Keyomarsi K, Chu C, Harper JW, et al. Phosphorylation-dependent ubiquitination of cyclin E by the SCFFbw7 ubiquitin ligase. Science. 2001;294:173–7.

19. Inuzuka H, Shaik S, Onoyama I, Gao D, Tseng A, Maser RS, et al. SCF(FBW7) regulates cellular apoptosis by targeting MCL1 for ubiquitylation and destruction. Nature. 2011;471:104–9.

20. Dwane L, Gallagher WM, Ní Chonghaile T, O'Connor DP. The emerging role of non-traditional ubiquitination in oncogenic pathways. J Biol Chem. 2017; 292:3543–51.

21. Haglund K, Sigismund S, Polo S, Szymkiewicz I, Di Fiore PP, Dikic I. Multiple monoubiquitination of RTKs is sufficient for their endocytosis and degradation. Nat Cell Biol. 2003;5:461–6.

22. Komander D, Rape M. The ubiquitin code. Annu Rev Biochem. 2012;81:203–29.

23. Silva GM, Finley D, Vogel C. K63 polyubiquitination is a new modulator of the oxidative stress response. Nat Struct Mol Biol. 2015;22:116–23.

24. Deng L, Wang C, Spencer E, Yang L, Braun A, You J, et al. Activation of the IkappaB kinase complex by TRAF6 requires a dimeric ubiquitin-conjugating enzyme complex and a unique polyubiquitin chain. Cell. 2000;103:351–61.

25. Mallette FA, Richard S. K48-linked ubiquitination and protein degradation regulate 53BP1 recruitment at DNA damage sites. Cell Res. 2012;22:1221–3.

26. Michel MA, Elliott PR, Swatek KN, Simicek M, Pruneda JN, Wagstaff JL, et al. Assembly and specific recognition of k29- and k33-linked polyubiquitin. Mol Cell. 2015;58:95–109.

27. Nagase T, Ishikawa K, Nakajima D, Ohira M, Seki N, Miyajima N, et al. Prediction of the coding sequences of unidentified human genes. VII. The complete sequences of 100 new cDNA clones from brain which can code for large proteins in vitro. DNA Res. 1997;4:141–50.

28. Liu Z, Oughtred R, Wing SS. Characterization of E3Histone, a novel testis ubiquitin protein ligase which ubiquitinates histones. Mol Cell Biol. 2005;25:2819–31.

29. Aravind L. The WWE domain: a common interaction module in protein ubiquitination and ADP ribosylation. Trends Biochem Sci. 2001;26:273–5.

30. Zhong Q, Gao W, Du F, Wang X. Mule/ARF-BP1, a BH3-only E3 ubiquitin ligase, catalyzes the polyubiquitination of mcl-1 and regulates apoptosis. Cell. 2005;121:1085–95.

31. Pandya RK, Partridge JR, Love KR, Schwartz TU, Ploegh HL. A structural element within the HUWE1 HECT domain modulates self-ubiquitination and substrate ubiquitination activities. J Biol Chem. 2010;285:5664–73.

32. Huang L, Kinnucan E, Wang G, Beaudenon S, Howley PM, Huibregtse JM, et al. Structure of an E6AP-UbcH7 complex: insights into ubiquitination by the E2-E3 enzyme cascade. Science. 1999;286:1321–6.

33. Ogunjimi AA, Briant DJ, Pece-Barbara N, Le Roy C, Di Guglielmo GM, Kavsak P, et al. Regulation of Smurf2 ubiquitin ligase activity by anchoring the E2 to the HECT domain. Mol Cell. 2005;19:297–308.

34. Verdecia MA, Joazeiro CAP, Wells NJ, Ferrer J-L, Bowman ME, Hunter T, et al. Conformational flexibility underlies ubiquitin ligation mediated by the WWP1 HECT domain E3 ligase. Mol Cell. 2003;11:249–59.

35. Froyen G, Belet S, Martinez F, Santos-Rebouças CB, Declercq M, Verbeeck J, et al. Copy-number gains of HUWE1 due to replication- and recombination-based rearrangements. Am J Hum Genet. 2012;91:252–64.

36. Wang G, Gao Y, Li L, Jin G, Cai Z, Chao J-I, et al. K63-linked ubiquitination in kinase activation and cancer. Front Oncol. 2012;2:5.

37. French ME, Klosowiak JL, Aslanian A, Reed SI, Yates JR, Hunter T. Mechanism of ubiquitin chain synthesis employed by a HECT domain ubiquitin ligase. J Biol Chem. 2017;292:10398–413.

38. Fang NN, Chan GT, Zhu M, Comyn SA, Persaud A, Deshaies RJ, et al. Rsp5/Nedd4 is the main ubiquitin ligase that targets cytosolic misfolded proteins following heat stress. Nat Cell Biol. 2014;16:1227–37.

39. Parsons JL, Tait PS, Finch D, Dianova II, Edelmann MJ, Khoronenkova SV, et al. Ubiquitin ligase ARF-BP1/mule modulates base excision repair. EMBO J. 2009;28:3207–15.

40. Markkanen E, van Loon B, Ferrari E, Parsons JL, Dianov GL, Hübscher U. Regulation of oxidative DNA damage repair by DNA polymerase λ and MutYH by cross-talk of phosphorylation and ubiquitination. Proc Natl Acad Sci U S A. 2012;109:437–42.

41. Choe KN, Nicolae CM, Constantin D, Imamura Kawasawa Y, Delgado-Diaz MR, De S, et al. HUWE1 interacts with PCNA to alleviate replication stress. EMBO Rep. 2016;17:874–86.

42. Michel MA, Swatek KN, Hospenthal MK, Komander D. Ubiquitin linkage-specific Affimers reveal insights into K6-linked ubiquitin signaling. Mol Cell. 2017;68:233–246.e5.

43. Adhikary S, Marinoni F, Hock A, Hulleman E, Popov N, Beier R, et al. The ubiquitin ligase HectH9 regulates transcriptional activation by Myc and is essential for tumor cell proliferation. Cell. 2005;123:409–21.

44. Vervoorts J, Lüscher-Firzlaff JM, Rottmann S, Lilischkis R, Walsemann G, Dohmann K, et al. Stimulation of c-MYC transcriptional activity and acetylation by recruitment of the cofactor CBP. EMBO Rep. 2003;4:484–90.

45. Brenner C, Deplus R, Didelot C, Loriot A, Viré E, De Smet C, et al. Myc represses transcription through recruitment of DNA methyltransferase corepressor. EMBO J. 2005;24:336–46.

46. Hermeking H, Rago C, Schuhmacher M, Li Q, Barrett JF, Obaya AJ, et al. Identification of CDK4 as a target of c-MYC. Proc Natl Acad Sci U S A. 2000; 97:2229–34.

47. Seoane J, Le H-V, Massagué J. Myc suppression of the p21(Cip1) Cdk inhibitor influences the outcome of the p53 response to DNA damage. Nature. 2002;419:729–34.

48. Staller P, Peukert K, Kiermaier A, Seoane J, Lukas J, Karsunky H, et al. Repression of p15INK4b expression by Myc through association with Miz-1. Nat Cell Biol. 2001;3:392–9.

49. Yang W, Shen J, Wu M, Arsura M, FitzGerald M, Suldan Z, et al. Repression of transcription of the p27(Kip1) cyclin-dependent kinase inhibitor gene by c-Myc. Oncogene. 2001;20:1688–702.

50. von der Lehr N, Johansson S, Wu S, Bahram F, Castell A, Cetinkaya C, et al. The F-box protein Skp2 participates in c-Myc proteosomal degradation and acts as a cofactor for c-Myc-regulated transcription. Mol Cell. 2003;11:1189–200.

51. Cepeda D, Ng H-F, Sharifi HR, Mahmoudi S, Cerrato VS, Fredlund E, et al. CDK-mediated activation of the SCF(FBXO) (28) ubiquitin ligase promotes

MYC-driven transcription and tumourigenesis and predicts poor survival in breast cancer. EMBO Mol Med. 2013;5:1067–86.

52. Fang X, Zhou W, Wu Q, Huang Z, Shi Y, Yang K, et al. Deubiquitinase USP13 maintains glioblastoma stem cells by antagonizing FBXL14-mediated Myc ubiquitination. J Exp Med. 2017;214:245–67.

53. Welcker M, Orian A, Jin J, Grim JE, Grim JA, Harper JW, et al. The Fbw7 tumor suppressor regulates glycogen synthase kinase 3 phosphorylation-dependent c-Myc protein degradation. Proc Natl Acad Sci U S A. 2004;101:9085–90.

54. Walker W, Zhou Z-Q, Ota S, Wynshaw-Boris A, Hurlin PJ. Mnt-max to Myc-max complex switching regulates cell cycle entry. J Cell Biol. 2005; 169:405–13.

55. Stanton BR, Perkins AS, Tessarollo L, Sassoon DA, Parada LF. Loss of N-myc function results in embryonic lethality and failure of the epithelial component of the embryo to develop. Genes Dev. 1992;6:2235–47.

56. Knoepfler PS, Cheng PF, Eisenman RN. N-myc is essential during neurogenesis for the rapid expansion of progenitor cell populations and the inhibition of neuronal differentiation. Genes Dev. 2002;16:2699–712.

57. Guglielmi L, Cinnella C, Nardella M, Maresca G, Valentini A, Mercanti D, et al. MYCN gene expression is required for the onset of the differentiation programme in neuroblastoma cells. Cell Death Dis. 2014;5:e1081.

58. Otto T, Horn S, Brockmann M, Eilers U, Schüttrumpf L, Popov N, et al. Stabilization of N-Myc is a critical function of aurora a in human neuroblastoma. Cancer Cell. 2009;15:67–78.

59. Xiao D, Yue M, Su H, Ren P, Jiang J, Li F, et al. Polo-like Kinase-1 regulates Myc stabilization and activates a feedforward circuit promoting tumor cell survival. Mol Cell. 2016;64:493–506.

60. Zhao X, Heng JI-T, Guardavaccaro D, Jiang R, Pagano M, Guillemot F, et al. The HECT-domain ubiquitin ligase Huwe1 controls neural differentiation and proliferation by destabilizing the N-Myc oncoprotein. Nat Cell Biol. 2008;10:643–53.

61. Zhao X, D' Arca D, Lim WK, Brahmachary M, Carro MS, Ludwig T, et al. The N-Myc-DLL3 cascade is suppressed by the ubiquitin ligase Huwe1 to inhibit proliferation and promote neurogenesis in the developing brain. Dev Cell. 2009;17:210–21.

62. King B, Boccalatte F, Moran-Crusio K, Wolf E, Wang J, Kayembe C, et al. The ubiquitin ligase Huwe1 regulates the maintenance and lymphoid commitment of hematopoietic stem cells. Nat Immunol. 2016;17:1312–21.

63. de Groot REA, Ganji RS, Bernatik O, Lloyd-Lewis B, Seipel K, Šedová K, et al. Huwe1-mediated ubiquitylation of dishevelled defines a negative feedback loop in the Wnt signaling pathway. Sci Signal. 2014;7:ra26.

64. Packer RJ, Zhou T, Holmes E, Vezina G, Gajjar A. Survival and secondary tumors in children with medulloblastoma receiving radiotherapy and adjuvant chemotherapy: results of Children's oncology group trial A9961. Neuro-Oncology. 2013;15:97–103.

65. Ning MS, Perkins SM, Dewees T, Shinohara ET. Evidence of high mortality in long term survivors of childhood medulloblastoma. J Neuro-Oncol. 2015;122:321–7.

66. Roussel MF, Hatten ME. Cerebellum development and medulloblastoma. Curr Top Dev Biol. 2011;94:235–82.

67. Ramaswamy V, Remke M, Bouffet E, Faria CC, Perreault S, Cho Y-J, et al. Recurrence patterns across medulloblastoma subgroups: an integrated clinical and molecular analysis. Lancet Oncol. 2013;14:1200–7.

68. Shih DJH, Northcott PA, Remke M, Korshunov A, Ramaswamy V, Kool M, et al. Cytogenetic prognostication within medulloblastoma subgroups. J Clin Oncol. 2014;32:886–96.

69. D'Arca D, Zhao X, Xu W, Ramirez-Martinez NC, Iavarone A, Lasorella A. Huwe1 ubiquitin ligase is essential to synchronize neuronal and glial differentiation in the developing cerebellum. Proc Natl Acad Sci U S A. 2010;107:5875–80.

70. Ayrault O, Zhao H, Zindy F, Qu C, Sherr CJ, Roussel MF. Atoh1 inhibits neuronal differentiation and collaborates with Gli1 to generate medulloblastoma-initiating cells. Cancer Res. 2010;70:5618–27.

71. Forget A, Bihannic L, Cigna SM, Lefevre C, Remke M, Barnat M, et al. Shh signaling protects Atoh1 from degradation mediated by the E3 ubiquitin ligase Huwe1 in neural precursors. Dev Cell. 2014;29:649–61.

72. Bédard M, Roy V, Montagne M, Lavigne P. Structural insights into c-Myc-interacting zinc finger Protein-1 (Miz-1) delineate domains required for DNA scanning and sequence-specific binding. J Biol Chem. 2017;292:3323–40.

73. Barrilleaux BL, Burow D, Lockwood SH, Yu A, Segal DJ, Knoepfler PS. Miz-1 activates gene expression via a novel consensus DNA binding motif. PLoS One. 2014;9:e101151.

74. Saito M, Novak U, Piovan E, Basso K, Sumazin P, Schneider C, et al. BCL6 suppression of BCL2 via Miz1 and its disruption in diffuse large B cell lymphoma. Proc Natl Acad Sci U S A. 2009;106:11294–9.

75. Liu J, Zhao Y, Eilers M, Lin A. Miz1 is a signal- and pathway-specific modulator or regulator (SMOR) that suppresses TNF-alpha-induced JNK1 activation. Proc Natl Acad Sci U S A. 2009;106:18279–84.

76. Liu J, Yan J, Jiang S, Wen J, Chen L, Zhao Y, et al. Site-specific ubiquitination is required for relieving the transcription factor Miz1-mediated suppression on TNF-α-induced JNK activation and inflammation. Proc Natl Acad Sci U S A. 2012;109:191–6.

77. Yang Y, Do H, Tian X, Zhang C, Liu X, Dada LA, et al. E3 ubiquitin ligase mule ubiquitinates Miz1 and is required for TNFalpha-induced JNK activation. Proc Natl Acad Sci U S A. 2010;107:13444–9.

78. Inoue S, Hao Z, Elia AJ, Cescon D, Zhou L, Silvester J, et al. Mule/Huwe1/Arf-BP1 suppresses Ras-driven tumorigenesis by preventing c-Myc/Miz1-mediated down-regulation of p21 and p15. Genes Dev. 2013; 27:1101–14.

79. Bykov VJN, Eriksson SE, Bianchi J, Wiman KG. Targeting mutant p53 for efficient cancer therapy. Nat Rev Cancer. 2018;18:89–102.

80. Leszczynska KB, Foskolou IP, Abraham AG, Anbalagan S, Tellier C, Haider S, et al. Hypoxia-induced p53 modulates both apoptosis and radiosensitivity via AKT. J Clin Invest. 2015;125:2385–98.

81. Lowe SW, Sherr CJ. Tumor suppression by Ink4a-Arf: progress and puzzles. Curr Opin Genet Dev. 2003;13:77–83.

82. Vogelstein B, Lane D, Levine AJ. Surfing the p53 network. Nature. 2000; 408:307–10.

83. Muller PAJ, Vousden KH. Mutant p53 in cancer: new functions and therapeutic opportunities. Cancer Cell. 2014;25:304–17.

84. Weber JD, Taylor LJ, Roussel MF, Sherr CJ, Bar-Sagi D. Nucleolar Arf sequesters Mdm2 and activates p53. Nat Cell Biol. 1999;1:20–6.

85. Honda R, Yasuda H. Association of p19(ARF) with Mdm2 inhibits ubiquitin ligase activity of Mdm2 for tumor suppressor p53. EMBO J. 1999;18:22–7.

86. Sherr CJ. The INK4a/ARF network in tumour suppression. Nat Rev Mol Cell Biol. 2001;2:731–7.

87. Chen D, Kon N, Li M, Zhang W, Qin J, Gu W. ARF-BP1/mule is a critical mediator of the ARF tumor suppressor. Cell. 2005;121:1071–83.

88. Qi C-F, Kim Y-S, Xiang S, Abdullaev Z, Torrey TA, Janz S, et al. Characterization of ARF-BP1/HUWE1 interactions with CTCF, MYC, ARF and p53 in MYC-driven B cell neoplasms. Int J Mol Sci. 2012;13:6204–19.

89. Strahl BD, Allis CD. The language of covalent histone modifications. Nature. 2000;403:41–5.

90. Haberland M, Montgomery RL, Olson EN. The many roles of histone deacetylases in development and physiology: implications for disease and therapy. Nat Rev Genet. 2009;10:32–42.

91. Ceccacci E, Minucci S. Inhibition of histone deacetylases in cancer therapy: lessons from leukaemia. Br J Cancer. 2016;114:605–11.

92. Zhang J, Kan S, Huang B, Hao Z, Mak TW, Zhong Q. Mule determines the apoptotic response to HDAC inhibitors by targeted ubiquitination and destruction of HDAC2. Genes Dev. 2011;25:2610–8.

93. Green DR, Kroemer G. Cytoplasmic functions of the tumour suppressor p53. Nature. 2009;458:1127–30.

94. Leu JI-J, Dumont P, Hafey M, Murphy ME, George DL. Mitochondrial p53 activates Bak and causes disruption of a Bak-Mcl1 complex. Nat Cell Biol. 2004;6:443–50.

95. Perciavalle RM, Stewart DP, Koss B, Lynch J, Milasta S, Bathina M, et al. Anti-apoptotic MCL-1 localizes to the mitochondrial matrix and couples mitochondrial fusion to respiration. Nat Cell Biol. 2012;14:575–83.

96. Luedtke DA, Niu X, Pan Y, Zhao J, Liu S, Edwards H, et al. Inhibition of mcl-1 enhances cell death induced by the Bcl-2-selective inhibitor ABT-199 in acute myeloid leukemia cells. Signal Transduct Target Ther. 2017;2:17012.

97. Merino D, Whittle JR, Vaillant F, Serrano A, Gong J-N, Giner G, et al. Synergistic action of the MCL-1 inhibitor S63845 with current therapies in preclinical models of triple-negative and HER2-amplified breast cancer. Sci Transl Med. 2017;9 https://doi.org/10.1126/scitranslmed.aam7049.

98. Tong J, Wang P, Tan S, Chen D, Nikolovska-Coleska Z, Zou F, et al. Mcl-1 degradation is required for targeted therapeutics to eradicate Colon Cancer cells. Cancer Res. 2017;77:2512–21.

99. Campbell KJ, Dhayade S, Ferrari N, Sims AH, Johnson E, Mason SM, et al. MCL-1 is a prognostic indicator and drug target in breast cancer. Cell Death Dis. 2018;9:19.

100. Cuconati A, Mukherjee C, Perez D, White E. DNA damage response and MCL-1 destruction initiate apoptosis in adenovirus-infected cells. Genes Dev. 2003;17:2922–32.

101. Sun S, Ji Y, Kersten S, Qi L. Mechanisms of inflammatory responses in obese adipose tissue. Annu Rev Nutr. 2012;32:261–86.

102. Gruber S, Straub BK, Ackermann PJ, Wunderlich CM, Mauer J, Seeger JM, et al. Obesity promotes liver carcinogenesis via mcl-1 stabilization independent of IL-6Rα signaling. Cell Rep. 2013;4:669–80.

103. Hall JR, Kow E, Nevis KR, Lu CK, Luce KS, Zhong Q, et al. Cdc6 stability is regulated by the Huwe1 ubiquitin ligase after DNA damage. Mol Biol Cell. 2007;18:3340–50.

104. Clay-Farrace L, Pelizon C, Santamaria D, Pines J, Laskey RA. Human replication protein Cdc6 prevents mitosis through a checkpoint mechanism that implicates Chk1. EMBO J. 2003;22:704–12.

105. Lau E, Zhu C, Abraham RT, Jiang W. The functional role of Cdc6 in S-G2/M in mammalian cells. EMBO Rep. 2006;7:425–30.

106. Oehlmann M, Score AJ, Blow JJ. The role of Cdc6 in ensuring complete genome licensing and S phase checkpoint activation. J Cell Biol. 2004;165:181–90.

107. Petersen BO, Wagener C, Marinoni F, Kramer ER, Melixetian M, Lazzerini Denchi E, et al. Cell cycle- and cell growth-regulated proteolysis of mammalian CDC6 is dependent on APC-CDH1. Genes Dev. 2000;14:2330–43.

108. Duursma A, Agami R. p53-dependent regulation of Cdc6 protein stability controls cellular proliferation. Mol Cell Biol. 2005;25:6937–47.

109. Jasin M. Homologous repair of DNA damage and tumorigenesis: the BRCA connection. Oncogene. 2002;21:8981–93.

110. Xu X, Weaver Z, Linke SP, Li C, Gotay J, Wang XW, et al. Centrosome amplification and a defective G2-M cell cycle checkpoint induce genetic instability in BRCA1 exon 11 isoform-deficient cells. Mol Cell. 1999;3:389–95.

111. Venkitaraman AR. Cancer susceptibility and the functions of BRCA1 and BRCA2. Cell. 2002;108:171–82.

112. King M-C, Marks JH, Mandell JB, New York Breast Cancer Study Group. Breast and ovarian cancer risks due to inherited mutations in BRCA1 and BRCA2. Science. 2003;302:643–6.

113. Wu W, Sato K, Koike A, Nishikawa H, Koizumi H, Venkitaraman AR, et al. HERC2 is an E3 ligase that targets BRCA1 for degradation. Cancer Res. 2010; 70:6384–92.

114. Lu Y, Li J, Cheng D, Parameswaran B, Zhang S, Jiang Z, et al. The F-box protein FBXO44 mediates BRCA1 ubiquitination and degradation. J Biol Chem. 2012;287:41014–22.

115. Ueki T, Park J-H, Nishidate T, Kijima K, Hirata K, Nakamura Y, et al. Ubiquitination and downregulation of BRCA1 by ubiquitin-conjugating enzyme E2T overexpression in human breast cancer cells. Cancer Res. 2009;69:8752–60.

116. Shao G, Patterson-Fortin J, Messick TE, Feng D, Shanbhag N, Wang Y, et al. MERIT40 controls BRCA1-Rap80 complex integrity and recruitment to DNA double-strand breaks. Genes Dev. 2009;23:740–54.

117. Wang X, Lu G, Li L, Yi J, Yan K, Wang Y, et al. HUWE1 interacts with BRCA1 and promotes its degradation in the ubiquitin-proteasome pathway. Biochem Biophys Res Commun. 2014;444:290–5.

118. Cabelof DC, Guo Z, Raffoul JJ, Sobol RW, Wilson SH, Richardson A, et al. Base excision repair deficiency caused by polymerase beta haploinsufficiency: accelerated DNA damage and increased mutational response to carcinogens. Cancer Res. 2003;63:5799–807.

119. Chan K, Houlbrook S, Zhang Q-M, Harrison M, Hickson ID, Dianov GL. Overexpression of DNA polymerase beta results in an increased rate of frameshift mutations during base excision repair. Mutagenesis. 2007;22:183–8.

120. Braithwaite EK, Prasad R, Shock DD, Hou EW, Beard WA, Wilson SH. DNA polymerase lambda mediates a back-up base excision repair activity in extracts of mouse embryonic fibroblasts. J Biol Chem. 2005;280:18469–75.

121. Markkanen E, van Loon B, Ferrari E, Hübscher U. Ubiquitylation of DNA polymerase λ. FEBS Lett. 2011;585:2826–30.

122. Cummins JM, Vogelstein B. HAUSP is required for p53 destabilization. Cell Cycle. 2004;3:689–92.

123. Song MS, Salmena L, Carracedo A, Egia A, Lo-Coco F, Teruya-Feldstein J, et al. The deubiquitinylation and localization of PTEN are regulated by a HAUSP-PML network. Nature. 2008;455:813–7.

124. Wu H-T, Kuo Y-C, Hung J-J, Huang C-H, Chen W-Y, Chou T-Y, et al. K63-polyubiquitinated HAUSP deubiquitinates HIF-1α and dictates H3K56 acetylation promoting hypoxia-induced tumour progression. Nat Commun. 2016;7 Cited 22 May 2017 . Available from: http://www.ncbi.nlm.nih.gov/pmc/articles/PMC5155157/

125. Yang M-H, Wu M-Z, Chiou S-H, Chen P-M, Chang S-Y, Liu C-J, et al. Direct regulation of TWIST by HIF-1alpha promotes metastasis. Nat Cell Biol. 2008; 10:295–305.

126. Vaughan L, Tan C-T, Chapman A, Nonaka D, Mack NA, Smith D, et al. HUWE1 ubiquitylates and degrades the RAC activator TIAM1 promoting cell-cell adhesion disassembly, migration, and invasion. Cell Rep. 2015;10:88–102.

127. Michiels F, Habets GG, Stam JC, van der Kammen RA, Collard JG. A role for Rac in Tiam1-induced membrane ruffling and invasion. Nature. 1995;375:338–40.

128. Malliri A, van der Kammen RA, Clark K, van der Valk M, Michiels F, Collard JG. Mice deficient in the Rac activator Tiam1 are resistant to Ras-induced skin tumours. Nature. 2002;417:867–71.

129. Rygiel TP, Mertens AE, Strumane K, van der Kammen R, Collard JG. The Rac activator Tiam1 prevents keratinocyte apoptosis by controlling ROS-mediated ERK phosphorylation. J Cell Sci. 2008;121:1183–92.

130. Bourguignon LY, Zhu H, Shao L, Chen YW. Ankyrin-Tiam1 interaction promotes Rac1 signaling and metastatic breast tumor cell invasion and migration. J Cell Biol. 2000;150:177–91.

131. Malliri A, van Es S, Huveneers S, Collard JG. The Rac exchange factor Tiam1 is required for the establishment and maintenance of cadherin-based adhesions. J Biol Chem. 2004;279:30092–8.

132. Hordijk PL, ten Klooster JP, van der Kammen RA, Michiels F, Oomen LC, Collard JG. Inhibition of invasion of epithelial cells by Tiam1-Rac signaling. Science. 1997;278:1464–6.

133. Castillo-Lluva S, Tan C-T, Daugaard M, Sorensen PHB, Malliri A. The tumour suppressor HACE1 controls cell migration by regulating Rac1 degradation. Oncogene. 2013;32:1735–42.

134. Berkes CA, Tapscott SJ. MyoD and the transcriptional control of myogenesis. Semin Cell Dev Biol. 2005;16:585–95.

135. Kay PH, Pereira E, Marlow SA, Turbett G, Mitchell CA, Jacobsen PF, et al. Evidence for adenine methylation within the mouse myogenic gene Myo-D1. Gene. 1994;151:89–95.

136. Sartorelli V, Puri PL, Hamamori Y, Ogryzko V, Chung G, Nakatani Y, et al. Acetylation of MyoD directed by PCAF is necessary for the execution of the muscle program. Mol Cell. 1999;4:725–34.

137. Tintignac LA, Lagirand J, Batonnet S, Sirri V, Leibovitch MP, Leibovitch SA. Degradation of MyoD mediated by the SCF (MAFbx) ubiquitin ligase. J Biol Chem. 2005;280:2847–56.

138. Noy T, Suad O, Taglicht D, Ciechanover A. HUWE1 ubiquitinates MyoD and targets it for proteasomal degradation. Biochem Biophys Res Commun. 2012;418:408–13.

139. Yang D, Sun B, Zhang X, Cheng D, Yu X, Yan L, et al. Huwe1 sustains normal ovarian epithelial cell transformation and tumor growth through the histone H1.3-H19 Cascade. Cancer Res. 2017;77:4773–84.

140. Medrzycki M, Zhang Y, Zhang W, Cao K, Pan C, Lailler N, et al. Histone h1.3 suppresses h19 noncoding RNA expression and cell growth of ovarian cancer cells. Cancer Res. 2014;74:6463–73.

141. Atsumi Y, Fujimori H, Fukuda H, Inase A, Shinohe K, Yoshioka Y, et al. Onset of quiescence following p53 mediated down-regulation of H2AX in normal cells. PLoS One. 2011;6:e23432.

142. Atsumi Y, Minakawa Y, Ono M, Dobashi S, Shinohe K, Shinohara A, et al. ATM and SIRT6/SNF2H mediate transient H2AX stabilization when DSBs form by blocking HUWE1 to allow efficient γH2AX foci formation. Cell Rep. 2015;13:2728–40.

143. Confalonieri S, Quarto M, Goisis G, Nuciforo P, Donzelli M, Jodice G, et al. Alterations of ubiquitin ligases in human cancer and their association with the natural history of the tumor. Oncogene. 2009;28:2959–68.

144. Rudin CM, Hann CL, Laterra J, Yauch RL, Callahan CA, Fu L, et al. Treatment of medulloblastoma with hedgehog pathway inhibitor GDC-0449. N Engl J Med. 2009;361:1173–8.

145. Yauch RL, Dijkgraaf GJP, Alicke B, Januario T, Ahn CP, Holcomb T, et al. Smoothened mutation confers resistance to a hedgehog pathway inhibitor in medulloblastoma. Science. 2009;326:572–4.

146. Hart JR, Garner AL, Yu J, Ito Y, Sun M, Ueno L, et al. Inhibitor of MYC identified in a Kröhnke pyridine library. Proc Natl Acad Sci U S A. 2014;111: 12556–61.

147. Delmore JE, Issa GC, Lemieux ME, Rahl PB, Shi J, Jacobs HM, et al. BET bromodomain inhibition as a therapeutic strategy to target c-Myc. Cell. 2011;146:904–17.

148. Brockmann M, Poon E, Berry T, Carstensen A, Deubzer HE, Rycak L, et al. Small molecule inhibitors of aurora-a induce proteasomal degradation of N-myc in childhood neuroblastoma. Cancer Cell. 2013;24:75–89.

149. Peter S, Bultinck J, Myant K, Jaenicke LA, Walz S, Müller J, et al. Tumor cell-specific inhibition of MYC function using small molecule inhibitors of the HUWE1 ubiquitin ligase. EMBO Mol Med. 2014;6:1525–41.

150. Zhang W, Wu K-P, Sartori MA, Kamadurai HB, Ordureau A, Jiang C, et al. System-wide modulation of HECT E3 ligases with selective ubiquitin variant probes. Mol Cell. 2016;62:121–36.

151. Sander B, Xu W, Eilers M, Popov N, Lorenz S. A conformational switch regulates the ubiquitin ligase HUWE1. elife. 2017;6 https://doi.org/10.7554/eLife.21036.

152. Iconomou M, Saunders DN. Systematic approaches to identify E3 ligase substrates. Biochem J. 2016;473:4083–101.

153. Shearwin-Whyatt L, Dalton HE, Foot N, Kumar S. Regulation of functional diversity within the Nedd4 family by accessory and adaptor proteins. BioEssays. 2006;28:617–28.

154. Kim W, Bennett EJ, Huttlin EL, Guo A, Li J, Possemato A, et al. Systematic and quantitative assessment of the ubiquitin-modified proteome. Mol Cell. 2011;44:325–40.

155. Wagner SA, Beli P, Weinert BT, Nielsen ML, Cox J, Mann M, et al. A proteome-wide, quantitative survey of in vivo ubiquitylation sites reveals widespread regulatory roles. Mol Cell Proteomics. 2011;10:M111.013284.

3

Identification of target genes in cardiomyopathy with fibrosis and cardiac remodeling

Jianquan Zhao[1*], Tiewei Lv[2], Junjun Quan[2], Weian Zhao[2], Jing Song[3], Zhuolin Li[4], Han Lei[4], Wei Huang[4] and Longke Ran[3*]

Abstract

Background: Identify genes probably associated with chronic heart failure and predict potential target genes for dilated cardiomyopathy using bioinformatics analyses.

Methods: Gene expression profiles (series number GSE3585 and GSE42955) of cardiomyopathy patients and healthy controls were downloaded from the Expression Omnibus Gene (GEO) database. Differential expression of genes (DEGS) between the two groups of total 14 cardiomyopathy patients and 10 healthy controls were subsequently identified by limma package of R. Database for Annotation, Visualization, and Integrated Discovery (DAVID Tool), which is an analysis of enriched biological processes. Search Tool for the Retrieval Interacting Genes (STRING) was used as well for the analysis of protein-protein interaction network (PPI). Prediction of the potential drugs was suggested based on the preliminarily identified genes using Connectivity Map (CMap).

Results: Eighty-nine DEGs were identified (57 up-regulated and 32 down-regulated). The most enrichment Gene Ontology (GO) terms ($P < 0.05$) contain genes involved in extracellular matrix (ECM) and biological adhesion signal pathways ($P < 0.05$, ES > 1.5) such as ECM-receptors, focal adhesion and transforming growth factor beta (TGF-β), etc. Fifty-one differentially expressed genes were found to encode interacting proteins. Eleven key genes along with related transcription factors were identified including CTGF, POSTN, CORIN, FIGF, etc.

Conclusion: Bioinformatics-based analyses reveal the targeted genes probably associated with cardiomyopathy, which provide clues for pharmacological therapies aiming at the targets.

Keywords: Dilated cardiomyopathy, Bioinformatics, Microarray, Heart failure

Background

Patients with dilated cardiomyopathy (DCM) often presents with progressive congested heart failure, arrhythmia and thromboembolic disease in forms of left ventricular mural thrombus and/or strike [1]. DCM is seen as a major cause of heart failure apart from coronary heart disease and hypertension [2]. Heart failure is a progressive chronic disease with a 5-year-suvival rate less than 50% [3]. The histologically confirmed diagnosis indicated that prevalence of

DCM is 14 to 52% among population proven previous history of myocarditis [4]. High morbidity and mortality underscore the necessity of deeper investigation of the underlying mechanism responsible for development of heart failure in DCM [5]. B-type natriuretic peptides (BNP) is a commonly used biomarker so far for diagnosis of DCM. However, the biomarkers are not so specific since the increased levels of the biomarkers sometimes indicate variety of cardiovascular diseases caused by heterogenetic etiologies, and cannot be explained by impaired left ventricular function alone [6]. The major goal for the treatment of DCM is to reduce the mortality and morbidity rate, to relief symptoms, and to prevent or, in some extent, reverse ventricular remodeling [7]. Fett et al. reported the necessity of application of polymerase chain

* Correspondence: jqzhaocqmu@163.com; qzhaocqmu@163.com; longkeran@aliyun.com
[1]Department of Cardiology, Bayannaoer City Hospital, 35 Xinhua District, Bayannaoer 015000, Inner Mongolia, China
[3]Department of Bioinformatics, Chongqing Medical University, 1 Yixueyuan Road, Yuzhong District, Chongqing 400016, China
Full list of author information is available at the end of the article

reaction (PCR) prior to the immunosuppressive therapy [8]. Hamshere *at el* provided a therapy by administration of granulocyte colony-stimulating factor (G-CSF) with intracoronary autologous bone marrow-derived cells (BMCs) to improve left ventricular systolic function in patients with DCM [9]. Beta-blocker and pace maker inhibitor ivabradine has been proved to have positive effects in reversing cardiac remodeling. However, reactions to beta-blocker or ivabradine vary based on the cases. In some individuals the left ventricular ejection fraction is improved significantly as a result of reversed of attenuated remodeling while in the others it remains [10]. More studies are needed to focus on treatment that improves the outcome of patients with DCM, to precisely make the diagnosis of the disease based on screening of biomarkers. These studies can improve prognosis of patients by lowering the risk of development of heart failure and relevant complications. So it is crucial to understand the mechanism and find biomarkers with a good specificity and sensitivity.

Gene chip microarray database has an open access. Gene chip technique is a widely used approach in analyzing gene function in post-genome era [11]. It is a High-throughput sequencing technique with optimal specificity and sensitivity. Previous studies have partially demonstrated the mechanism underlying DCM by this approach [12, 13]. In this study, two platforms (GPL96 and GPL6244) are incorporated to analyze differential expression genes, enrichment of GO terms or pathways and protein-protein interactions in DCM and predict potential targets and drugs for a better treatment of the disease.

Methods
Microarray gene expression
Gene expression profiles with series number GSE3585 based on platform GPL96 and series number GSE42955 on platform GPL6244 were downloaded from the Expression Omnibus Gene (GEO) database (http://www.ncbi.nlm.nih.gov/geo/). Data of seven cardiomyopathy patients and seven healthy controls were randomly selected from each platform, respectively. The total sample of the two patient groups is 14 and the healthy controls are 10 subjects. The samples from all selected subjects had been hybridized on the Affymetrix Human Genome U133A array on a GPL96/GPL6244 platform (Affymetrix, Santa Clara, CA, USA).

Identification of Differential Expressed Genes (DEG)
Limma of R/bio-conductor was used for screening of the DEGs (settings: $P < 0.05$, log2 (Fold Change)>/=1). Fifty-seven up-regulated (gene set A) and 32 down-regulated (gene set B) genes were identified. Hierarchical clustering and visualization were made by Heat-map package of R.

Enrichment analysis of significant modules
The Database for Annotation, Visualization and Integrated Discovery (DAVID) [14] provides a non-line comprehensive set of functional annotation tools for biological interpretation of large gene lists. DAVID was used here to group the functions of DEGs in modules, identify enriched biological processes and cellular components, and identify the pathways associated with the DEGs in the most significant modules. Function and pathway terms were retrieved from the Gene Ontology ($p < 0.05$, Benjamin< 0.01) and the Kyoto Encyclopedia of Genes and Genomes (KEGG) ($p < 0.05$, Benjamin< 0.01) databases, respectively.

Analysis of protein-protein interaction network
The topological properties of the PPI networks were analyzed using Network Analyzer available in Cytoscape. Search Tool for the Retrieval Interacting Genes 10.0 (http://string-db.org/) [15] provide online analysis of interactions among DEG-encoding proteins. The network of interactions was then imported into Cytoscape [16], degree ≥5 was set to filter crucial proteins in the middle of the network.

Analysis of transcription factors
PASTAA [17] was used for predictive analysis of transcription factors of DCMs, P value calculated from hyper geometric distribution was used to evaluate the correlation between the DCMs and transcription factor. TRAP [18] was used to predict the correlation. Geneset C,D was uploaded to the database and JASPAR, (version 2016) [19] was used to predict the DNA binding site.

Acquisition of target genes of drugs
Connectivity map [20] is an online implement that provides gene transcription-expression profile of thousands of genomes reflecting how cultured mammalian cell react to administration of 1309 kinds of bioactive modules in terms of gene-expression. CMap was used to identify potential unknown effect of existing drugs. Up-regulated gene set (gene set A) and down-regulated gene set (gene set B) were uploaded to CMap, EBAYES was used to calculate P-value, PEBAYES-value< 0.05 was considered significant, and could be a potential molecule in treatment of DCM. The half maximal inhibitory concentration (IC50) is a measure of the effectiveness of a substance in inhibiting a specific biological or biochemical function. In previous studies effectiveness of different drugs were demonstrated and published. Thus, results obtained by CMap were uploaded to NCBI PubChem database for verification.

Results

Identification of DCGs

Compared to the control group, 89 differential expression genes (DEG) are identified in the DCM group (57 up-regulated and 32 down-regulated), Fig. 1 is the hierarchical clustering heat-map.

Functional enrichment analysis

In GO functional and enrichment analysis, the most enriched GO terms associated with up-regulated genes are extracellular matrix concerning CC ($P = 3.810^{-11}$), extracellular region ($P = 5 \times 10^{-14}$) and biological adhesion ($P = 1.5 \times 10^{-6}$), the most enriched GO terms associated with down-regulated genes are response to injury

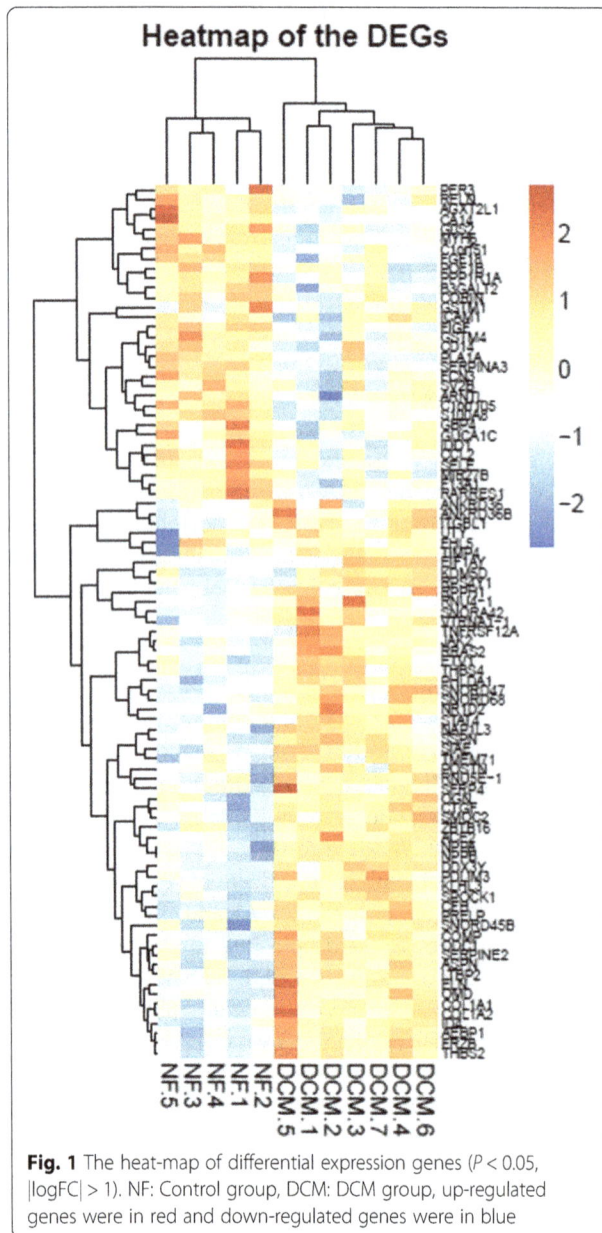

Fig. 1 The heat-map of differential expression genes ($P < 0.05$, |logFC| > 1). NF: Control group, DCM: DCM group, up-regulated genes were in red and down-regulated genes were in blue

concerning MF ($P = 1.5 \times 10^{-6}$) and extracellular region ($P = 5 \times 10^{-14}$) concerning CC.

The results of functional annotation about KEGG pathways are shown in Fig. 2. COL1A1, COL1A2, COMP, THBS2, and THBS4, RELN participate in the pathways associated with ECM-receptor interaction and focal adhesion. COMP, THBS2 and THBS4 are significantly enriched in all three pathways.

Topological analysis of PPI networks

Fifty-one significantly enriched gene were updated to STRING to construct the PPI network, and the PPI network was subsequently imported in Cytoscape to construct sub-networks. In sub-network 1, CTGF, COL1A1 (proteins with the highest degree of 8) and protein adjacent to them (COL1A2, THBS2, THBS4, POSTN, COMP, FIGF, PRELP) are highlighted. In sub-network 2 RPS4Y1 is in the central position. Sub-network three exhibit the three proteins with highest LogFC among all the sub-networks, as is all shown in Fig. 3. Table 1 shows fold changes of 11 DCMs and relevant P value, respectively. Figure 4 shows expression level of selected 11 genes between control and DCM samples. Among the 11 genes, nine of them are up-regulated while two are down-regulated.

Analysis of transcription factor

Transcription factor that modulate gene expression in DCM predicted by PASTAA is shown in Table 2. As shown in the Fig. 5a, Tef-1 and TFIIA transcription factor families play an important role in up-regulation of gene expression. TBP and TFIIA show features of constitutive expression as widely existing in transcription. By contrast, as shown in Fig. 5b, CORIN, FIGF of Myb families and Hnf-4 family are predicted to play an important role in down-regulation of gene expression. Figure 6 shows the transcription factor-binding site predicted by JASPAR.

Acquisition of target genes of drugs

Gene set A and B was uploaded to Connectivity Map to search for potential drugs, Table 3 shows predicted drug molecules that may induce/inhibit DCM-associated gene expression. Predicted molecule in Table 2 was uploaded to NCBI PubChem database to search for target genes of receptors. 19 target genes are significantly correlated with DCM, as shown in Table 4. Numbers in the brackets stand for the count of drugs. CTGF, POSTN, CORIN, FIGH have higher amount of drugs. Collagen family and THBS2, THBS4 are also ranked highly.

Discussion

Microarray analysis, an optimal approach to identify differentially expressed gene, helps to define an early diagnosis and lower misdiagnosis rate [21]. So far, the application

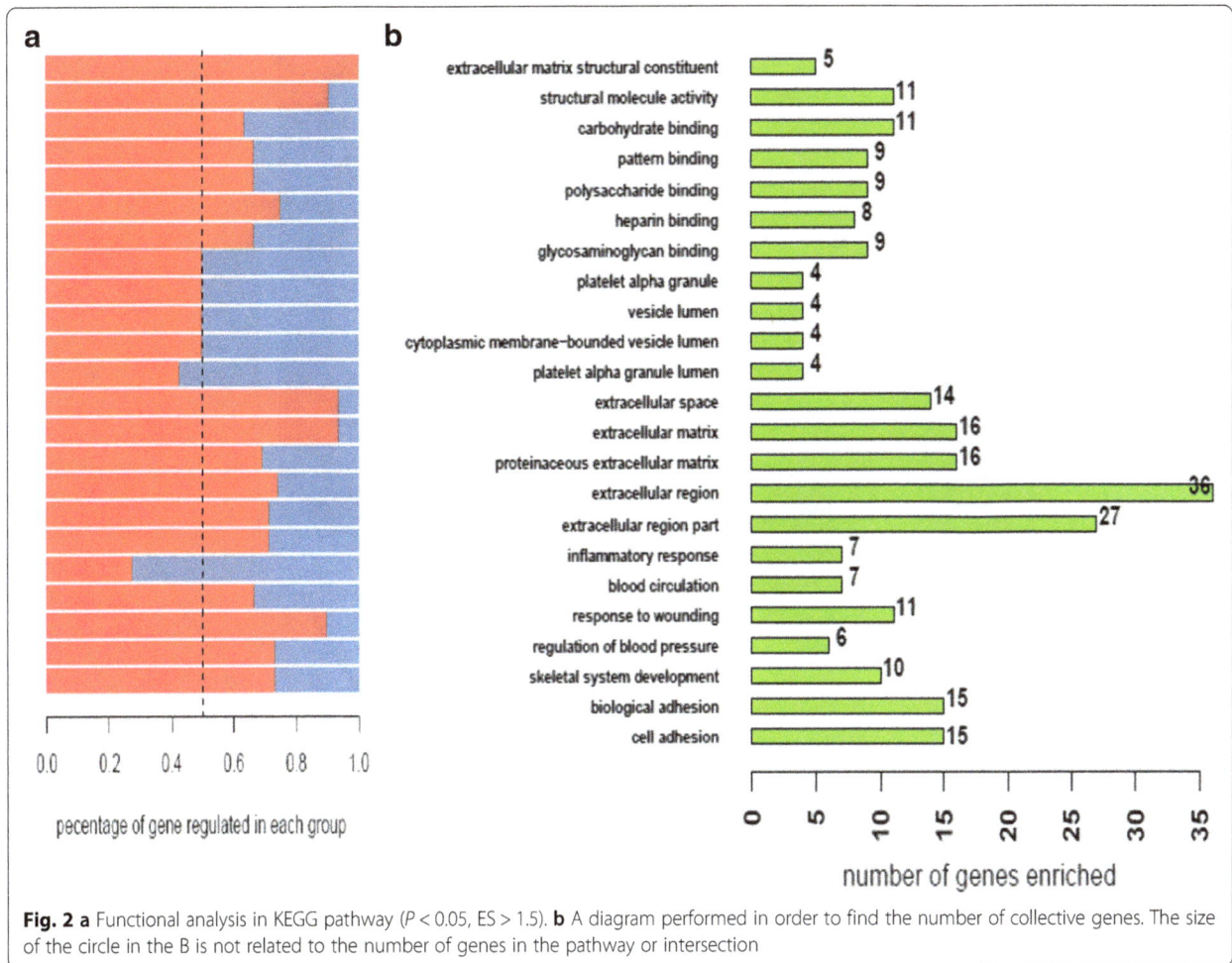

Fig. 2 a Functional analysis in KEGG pathway (*P* < 0.05, ES > 1.5). **b** A diagram performed in order to find the number of collective genes. The size of the circle in the B is not related to the number of genes in the pathway or intersection

of microarray analysis has revealed considerable bioprocesses associated with DCM. Barth et al [5] predicted and constructed a gene set including 27 genes differentially expressed, among which 25 were later confirmed. Micaela et al [22] analyzed ion channel-associated gene differential expression. They reported that ion channel-associated gene such as SCN2B. KCNJ5, CLIC2 play an important role in related bioprocesses. The present study aims at underlining the effects of regulation by transcription factors on differential gene expression. Effectiveness of target gene set is confirmed by referring to existing database.

By comparing differentially expressed genes in DCM samples with that from healthy controls, we predict that CORIN, FIGF, CTGF, COL1A1, COL1A2, THBS4, THBS4, POSTN, COMP, PRELP and RPS4Y1 may play a role in development of DCM. By the way, CORIN (encoding production could convert pro-ANP to bioactive ANP) is one of the known marker genes, the purpose of this study is to explore the mechanism underlying the differential expression level.

Cardiac remodeling characterized by collagen deposition in extracellular matrix [23] and myocardial fibrosis leading to heart failure [24, 25]. Expression level changes of genes encoding proteins associated with: 1) ECM-receptor interaction, 2) focal adhesion, 3) TGF-beta signaling pathway may play an integral role in development of systolic dysfunction. Up-regulation of CTGF in TGF-beta signaling pathway can lead to an increased deposition of type 3 collagen (COL3A1) and type 1 collagen (COL1A1, COL1A2 and COL1A3) [26, 27]. Furthermore, excessive collagen may cause myocardial fibrosis and heart failure. THBS2 and THBS4, existing in all three pathways that encode fibronectin are also modulated by CTGF. Previous study shows that up-regulation of THBS1 and THBS4 may lead to matri-cellular protein deposition, and subsequently resulting in DCM, heart failure or death. FIGF (also known as vascular endothelial growth factor-D; VEGF-D) in ECM-receptor interaction may also participate in the pathology of DCM. Gong X et al. [28] reported that VEGF preserve cardiac function after intra-myocardial transplantation in a DCM mouse by reducing cellular apoptosis and myocardial fibrosis in addition to enhanced angiogenesis, indicating that down-regulation of FIGF may improve cardiac function and preserve myocardial cells.

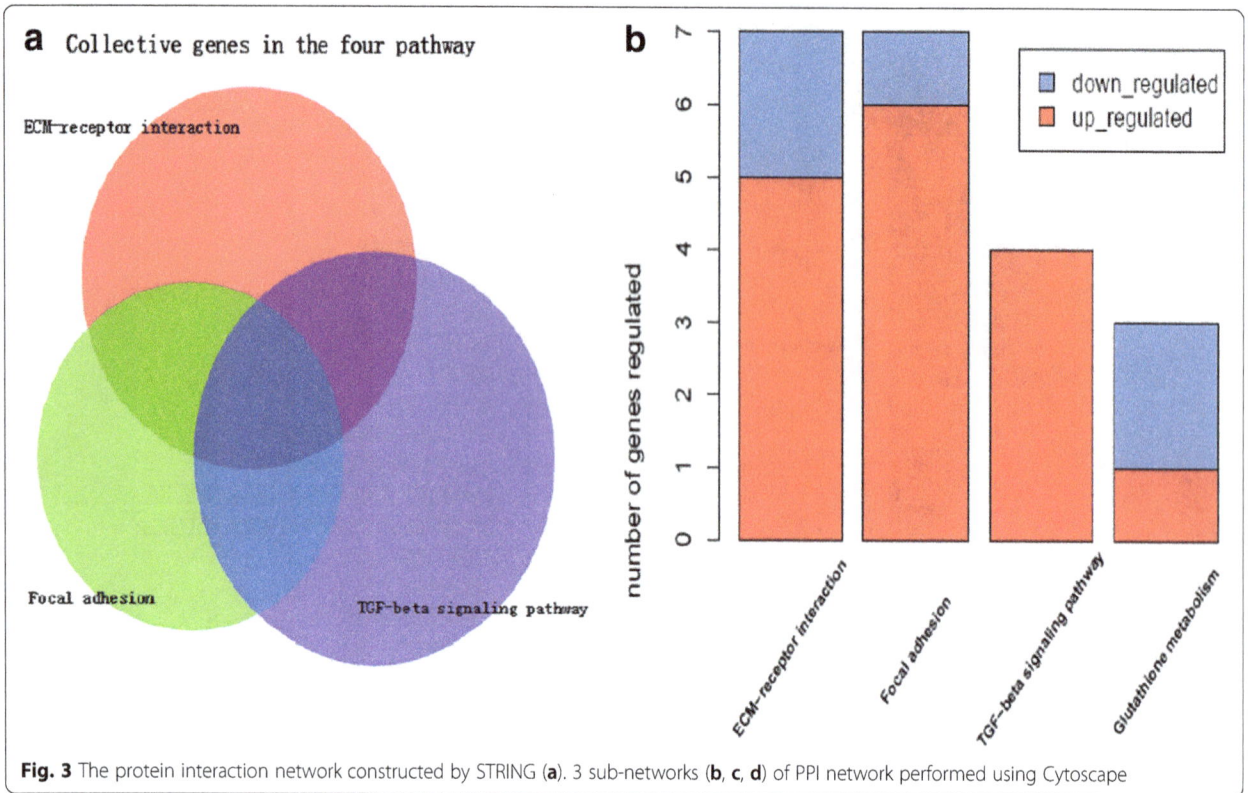

Fig. 3 The protein interaction network constructed by STRING (**a**). 3 sub-networks (**b**, **c**, **d**) of PPI network performed using Cytoscape

Differential expression gene exhibit up-regulation in GO terms of extracellular matrix and focal adhesion [29]. Mal-regulation of extracellular matrix is associated with progression of cardiac remodeling and heart failure. COMP encodes a non-collagen protein in ECM and previous studies have demonstrated that abnormal expression of COMP result in myocardial cell apoptosis and loss of myofilament [30]. COMP, COL1A1, COL1A2 and PRELP are up-regulated in ECM-receptor interaction and focal adhesion, inducing a component change in extracellular matrix [31].

POSTN bond with heparin, and is showed in the PPI network co-expressed with COL1A1, COL1A2, THBS4 and CTGF. High impression level of POSTN in myocardial fibroblast contributes to cardiac remodeling [32]. Therefore, highly co-expression of both POSTN and CTGF (regulate heparin in fibroblasts) may be associated with antagonism. However, it is unknown whether

Table 1 The expression level of 11 DEGs

Gene	Control Mean ± SD(log)	DCM Mean ± SD(log)	Log2 (Fold change)	P-value
collagen, type I, alpha 1(COL1A1)	9.46 ± 0.56	11.04 ± 0.72	1.50	0.001
collagen, type I, alpha 2(COL1A2)	8.73 ± 0.38	10.29 ± 1.00	1.50	0.004
cartilage oligomeric matrix protein(COMP)	6.50 ± 0.24	7.86 ± 0.68	1.32	5.18×10^{-4}
connective tissue growth factor(CTGF)	8.51 ± 0.76	10.49 ± 0.52	1.93	1.50×10^{-4}
periostin, osteoblast specific factor(POSTN)	10.09 ± 0.68	11.38 ± 0.89	1.48	0.007
thrombospondin 2(THBS2)	9.27 ± 0.25	10.39 ± 0.60	1.08	0.001
thrombospondin 4(THBS4)	10.53 ± 0.78	10.76 ± 0.73	1.47	3.13×10^{-4}
corin, serine peptidase(CORIN)	8.57 ± 0.94	6.72 ± 1.15	−1.86	0.008
c-fos induced growth factor (vascular endothelial growth factor D)(FIGF)	8.78 ± 0.47	8.15 ± 0.53	−1.23	0.035
ribosomal protein S4, Y-linked 1(RPS4Y1)	8.10 ± 1.16	9.46 ± 1.90	1.38	0.039
proline/arginine-rich end leucine-rich repeat protein(PRELP)	9.71 ± 0.44	10.81 ± 0.55	1.10	0.002

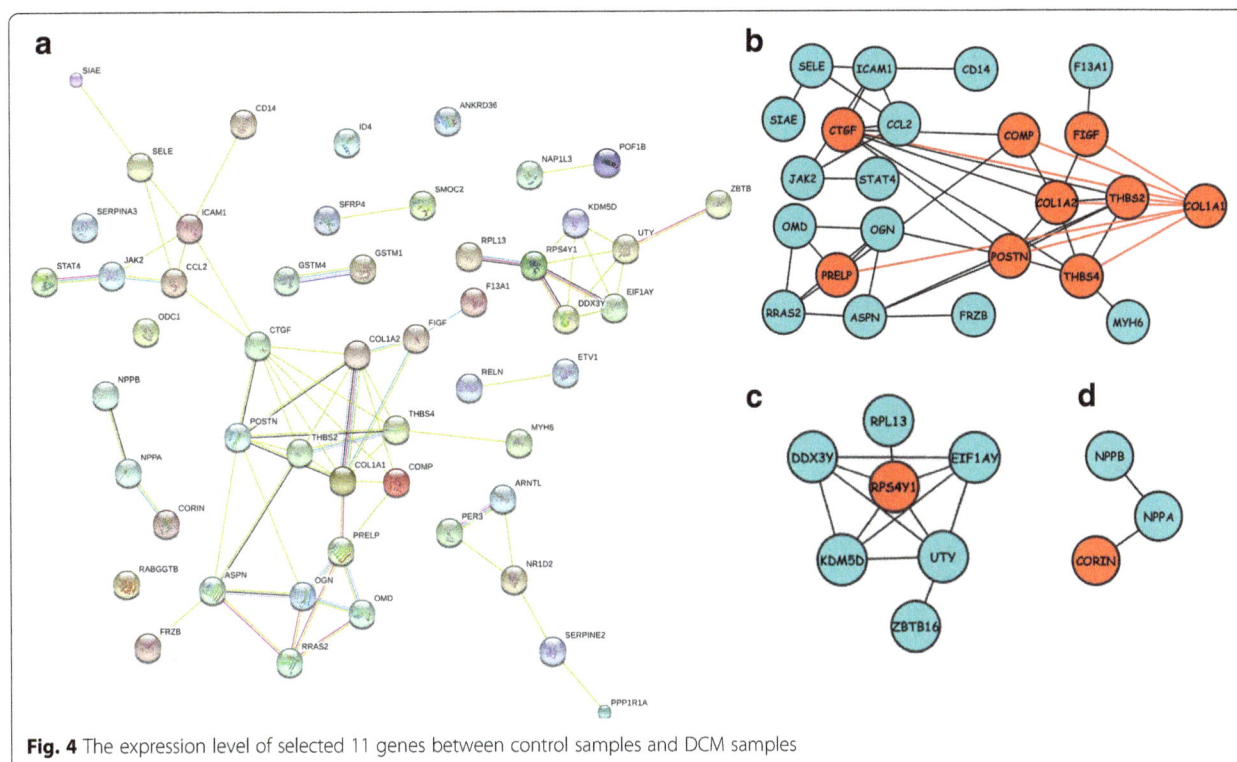

Fig. 4 The expression level of selected 11 genes between control samples and DCM samples

Table 2 Results of PASTAA analysis

Rank	Matrix	Transcription Factor	Association Score	P-Value
a. TFs predicted to regulate up-regulated genes				
1	TATA_01	Tbp	4.51	2.22E-04
2	TEF1_Q6	Tef-1	4.1	5.01E-04
3	TFIIA_Q6	Tflla-alpha/beta, Tflla-gamma	3.252	2.81E-03
4	NFKAPPAB_01	Rela	2.876	6.51E-03
5	NRL_HAND	N/A	2.865	6.75E-03
6	GFI1_01	Gfi1	2.85	7.00E-03
7	ALPHACP1_01	N/A	2.718	9.92E-03
8	CREL_01	C-rel	2.587	1.15E-02
9	TAL1BETAITF2_01	Itf-2, Tal-1beta	2.553	1.22E-02
10	NFY_01	N/A	2.509	1.44E-02
b. TFs predicted to regulate down-regulated genes				
1	VMYB_01	V-myb	3.123	6.94E-04
2	HNF4ALPHA_Q6	Hnf-4, Hnf-4alpha	3.043	9.08E-04
3	MYB_Q3	C-myb	2.646	4.16E-03
4	MYB_Q5_01	B-myb, C-myb	2.646	4.16E-03
5	CDC5_01	Cdc5	2.425	6.93E-03
6	CEBP_Q2	C/ebp, C/ebpalpha	2.425	6.93E-03
7	AP1_Q4_01	Fosb, Fra-1	2.123	1.23E-02
8	ZTA_Q2	N/A	2.123	1.23E-02
9	AP1_Q2_01	Fosb, Fra-1	2.044	1.23E-02
10	COUP_01	Coup-tf1, Hnf-4alpha1	2.044	1.23E-02

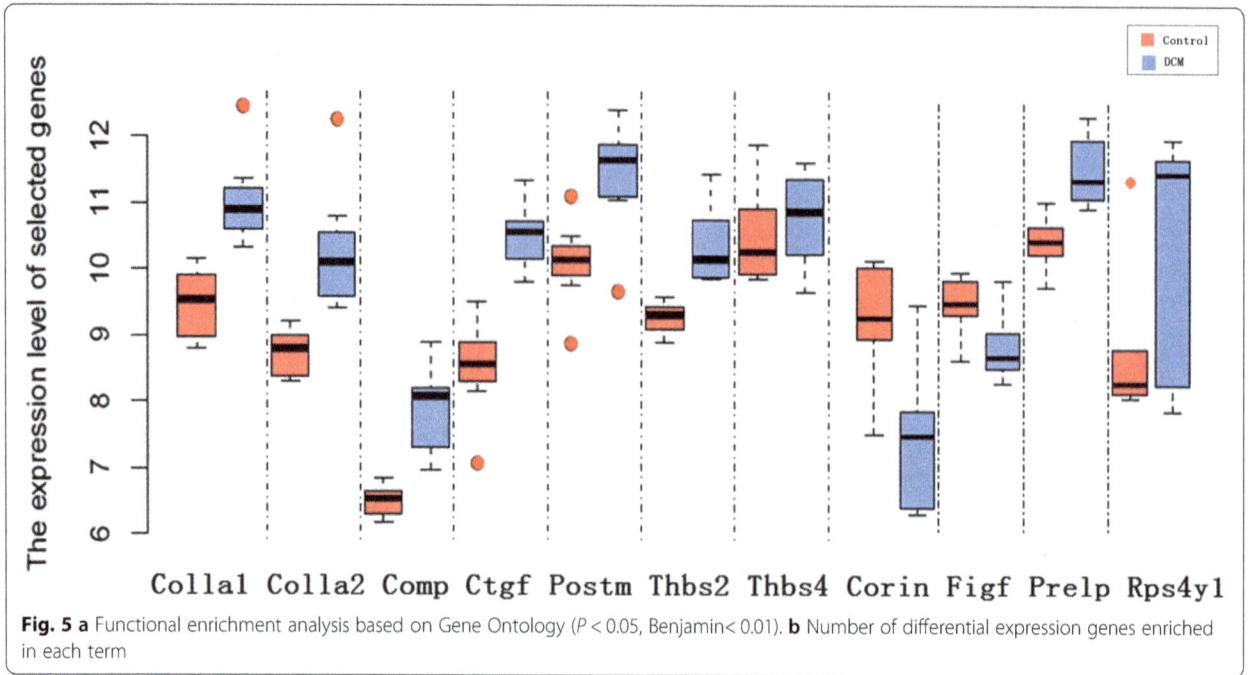

Fig. 5 a Functional enrichment analysis based on Gene Ontology (*P* < 0.05, Benjamin< 0.01). **b** Number of differential expression genes enriched in each term

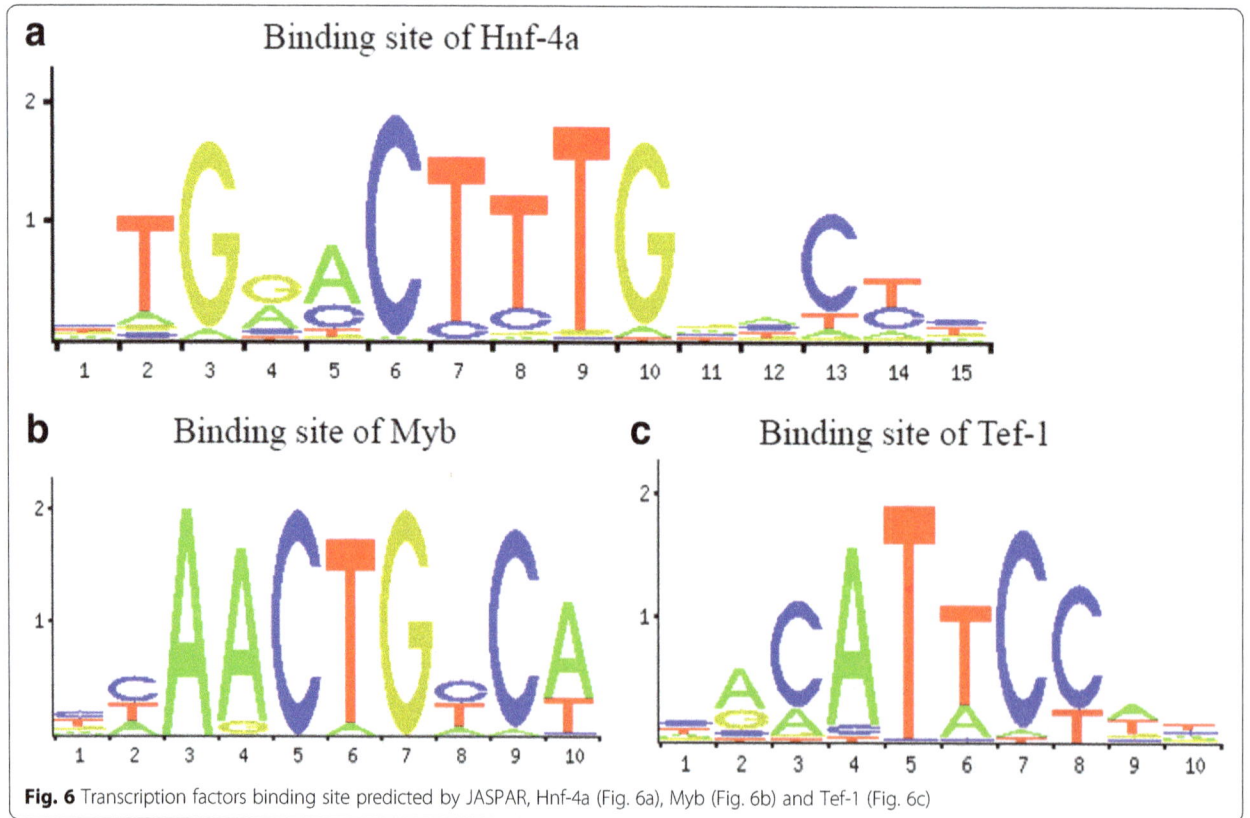

Fig. 6 Transcription factors binding site predicted by JASPAR, Hnf-4a (Fig. 6a), Myb (Fig. 6b) and Tef-1 (Fig. 6c)

Table 3 Chemical compounds identified by Connectivity map and list the top 20 ranked by P-value

rank	cmap name	Mean	n	enrichment	P-value
1	tridihexethyl	−0.64	4	−0.883	0.00044
2	Prestwick-682	−0.509	4	−0.848	0.00097
3	fluoxetine	−0.494	4	−0.806	0.00271
4	pirlindole	−0.668	3	−0.884	0.00312
5	methyldopa	0.382	5	0.732	0.00318
6	ciclacillin	0.494	4	0.789	0.00391
7	sulfadiazine	0.565	5	0.717	0.00409
8	khellin	−0.418	5	−0.708	0.00467
9	PNU-0251126	−0.358	6	−0.656	0.00467
10	metampicillin	0.389	5	0.704	0.00537
11	CP-645525-01	−0.558	3	−0.861	0.00553
12	minoxidil	−0.446	5	−0.694	0.00597
13	spiradoline	−0.478	4	−0.756	0.00718
14	PHA-00816795	−0.719	2	−0.942	0.00722
15	acenocoumarol	0.509	5	0.687	0.00741
16	cefotaxime	0.561	5	0.682	0.00845
17	metrizamide	0.487	4	0.731	0.01044
18	Y-27632	−0.674	2	−0.922	0.01223
19	bacampicillin	−0.354	4	−0.718	0.01271
20	levocabastine	0.274	4	0.718	0.01297

Mean:the arithmetic mean of the connectivity scores for corresponding instances, N:The number of instances, Enrichment: The degree of enrichment of the given instance in all instances, P-value:an estimate of the likelihood that the enrichment of a set of predicted potential drugs of all CMap drugs would be observed by chance

POSTN is regulated by CTGF. The co-expression of RPS4Y1, DDX3Y, EIF1AY and RPL13 were discovered. Heidecker et al. [33] demonstrated that they are associated with idiopathic DCM, but the expression level differentiates significantly and the mechanism remains unclear.

Transcription factors may affect the differential expression genes in DCM. Tef-1 (also known as TEAD1, TCF-13), a transcription enhancer, promotes the expression of troponin, myosin and actin [34, 35]. TFIIA, a member of TF family, exists ubiquitously in global tissues, participating in the formation of transcription initiation complex as an intra-nuclear protein [36]. It may trigger the up-regulation of differentially expressed genes. MYB [37], known as a transcription activator, encodes transcription factors of myb family. MYB has 1) a N-terminal DNA binding domain, 2) a transcription activating domain in the center [38] 3) a C-terminal domain associated with inhibition of transcription. The C-domain may be responsible for down-regulation of FIGF and CORIN. Hnf-4 transcription factor family is mainly expressed in kidney and liver [39]. Given that it is a transcription activator, the inhibition may down-regulate the expression of CORIN, FIGF and subsequentially the down-regulation of ANP level.

Re-localization of drugs is a cost-effective approach so that the development of CMap is engaged in efficiently predicting potential targets that drugs can aim at. Tridihexethyl, fluoxetine and pirlindole can inactivate G-protein-coupled receptor. Fluoxetine, methyldopa and sulfadiazine can inactivate cystic fibrosis trans-membrane conductance regulator and sequentially down-regulate the expression of Collagen, THBS, COMP and PRELP. Methyldopa, sulfadiazine and khellin may further regulate the gene expression by regulating the translation. Besides, up-regulated CTGF, POSTN and down-regulated CORN, FIGF are seen as the major targets in CMap prediction, indicating that combination of multiple drugs may achieve a better treatment.

However, up or down regulation of specific genes may not be responsible for pathogenesis of the relevant diseases [40, 41]. They may be only a downstream reaction or byproducts, such as s NPPB(logFC> 4.2)or NPPA(logFC> 2.5)in DCM. Age, gender, multi-drug therapy, etiology and individual variation may also cause differential gene expression. That is the limitation of the present study. In addition, we all know now that myofibril gene (protein) mutations are associated with the development of various cardiomyopathies including DCM. It is necessary in the future to carry out more analyses including the above-mentioned factors and myofibril protein mutations. Besides, differentially expressed genes in the same expression profile vary among different filters. These factors have also been taken into consideration in drawing any conclusions.

Conclusions

Bioinformatics-based analyses reveal the targeted genes probably associated with cardiomyopathy, which provide clues for pharmacological therapies aiming at the targets. Further studies considering other factors such as age, gender, multi-drug therapy, etiology and individual variation should be carried out in the future and bench work experiments should be performed to verify the relationship between the DEGs and the development of DCM.

Table 4 The genes targeted by the 20 potential drugs from CMap

CTGF (14) UP	POSTN (11) UP	COMP (8) UP	COL1A1 (8) UP	COL1A2 (8) UP
THBS2 (8) UP	THBS4 (8) UP	PRELP (7) UP	STAT4 (3) UP	FRZB (3) UP
RPS4Y1 (3) UP	ID4 (2) UP	ASPN (2) UP	SSPN (2) UP	
CORIN (7) DOWN	FIGF (5) DOWN	FCN3 (3) DOWN	CCL2 (2) DOWN	CD14 (1) DOWN

The number in the parentheses represent the number of associated CMap drugs, UP and DOWN represent up or down-regulated of corresponding gene

Abbreviations

BMCs: Bone marrow-derived cells; BNP: B-type natriuretic peptides; CMap: Connectivity map; DAVID: Visualization and integrated discovery; DCM: Dilated cardiomyopathy; DEGS: Differential expression of genes; ECM: Extracellular matrix; G-CSF: Granulocyte colony-stimulating factor; GEO: Expression Omnibus Gene; GO: Gene ontology; KEGG: The Kyoto Encyclopedia of Genes and Genomes; PCR: Polymerase chain reaction; PPI: Protein-protein interaction network; STRING: Search tool for the retrieval interacting genes; TGF-β: Transforming growth factor beta

Acknowledgements

We would like to give our sincere appreciation to the editor and reviewers of the journal for their helpful comments on this article.

Authors' contributions

TL and JQ carried out microarray gene expression and identified differential expressed genes. JS and ZL analyzed significant modules. HL and WZ analyzed transcription factors. WH acquired the target genes of drugs and analyzed protein-protein interaction network. The manuscript was prepared by JZ and LR. All authors read and approved the manuscript.

Competing interests

The authors declare that they have no competing interests.

Author details

[1]Department of Cardiology, Bayannaoer City Hospital, 35 Xinhua District, Bayannaoer 015000, Inner Mongolia, China. [2]Department of Cardiology, Children's hospital, Chongqing Medical University, Chongqing, China. [3]Department of Bioinformatics, Chongqing Medical University, 1 Yixueyuan Road, Yuzhong District, Chongqing 400016, China. [4]Department of Vascular Cardiology, the First Affiliated Hospital of Chongqing, Medical University, Chongqing, China.

References

1. Xiao HB, Brecker SJ, Gibson DG. Effects of abnormal activation on the time course of the left ventricular pressure pulse in dilated cardiomyopathy. Br Heart J. 1992;68:403–7.
2. Meder B, Rühle F, Weis T, Homuth G, Keller A, Franke J, Peil B, Bermejo JL, Frese K, Huge A. A genome-wide association study identifies 6p21 as novel risk locus for dilated cardiomyopathy. Eur Heart J. 2014;35:1069–77.
3. Pinto YM, Elliott PM, Arbustini E, Adler Y, Anastasakis A, Böhm M, Duboc D, Gimeno J, de Groote P, Imazio M. Proposal for a revised definition of dilated cardiomyopathy, hypokinetic non-dilated cardiomyopathy, and its implications for clinical practice: a position statement of the ESC working group on myocardial and pericardial diseases. Eur Heart J. 2016;37(23):1850–8.
4. d'Ambrosio A, Patti G, Manzoli A, Sinagra G, Di Lenarda A, Silvestri F, Di Sciascio G. The fate of acute myocarditis between spontaneous improvement and evolution to dilated cardiomyopathy: a review. Heart. 2001;85:499–504.
5. Barth AS, Kuner R, Buness A, Ruschhaupt M, Merk S, Zwermann L, Kääb S, Kreuzer E, Steinbeck G, Mansmann U. Identification of a common gene expression signature in dilated cardiomyopathy across independent microarray studies. J Am Coll Cardiol. 2006;48:1610–7.
6. Yung CK, Halperin VL, Tomaselli GF, Winslow RL. Gene expression profiles in end-stage human idiopathic dilated cardiomyopathy: altered expression of apoptotic and cytoskeletal genes. Genomics. 2004;83:281–97.
7. de Groote P, Pinet F, Bauters C. New technologies, new therapies: toward personalized medicine in heart failure patients? Eur Heart J. 2012;
8. Fett JD. Inflammation and virus in dilated cardiomyopathy as indicated by endomyocardial biopsy. Int J Cardiol. 2006;112:125–6.
9. Hamshere S, Arnous S, Choudhury T, Choudry F, Mozid A, Yeo C, Barrett C, Saunders N, Gulati A, Knight C. Randomized trial of combination cytokine

10. and adult autologous bone marrow progenitor cell administration in patients with non-ischaemic dilated cardiomyopathy: the REGENERATE-DCM clinical trial. Eur Heart J. 2015;36(44):3061–9.
10. Xie X, Wu B, Chen Y, Li W, Hu X, Chen J. Peripheral endothelial function may predict the effectiveness of beta-blocker therapy in patients with idiopathic dilated cardiomyopathy. Int J Cardiol. 2016;221:128–33.
11. Jo B-S, Koh I-U, Bae J-B, Yu H-Y, Jeon E-S, Lee H-Y, Kim J-J, Choi M, Choi SS. Methylome analysis reveals alterations in DNA methylation in the regulatory regions of left ventricle development genes in human dilated cardiomyopathy. Genomics. 2016;108:84–92.
12. Liu Y, Morley M, Brandimarto J, Hannenhalli S, Hu Y, Ashley EA, Tang WH, Moravec CS, Margulies KB, Cappola TP, Li M. MAGNet consortium. RNA-Seq identifies novel myocardial gene expression signatures of heart failure. Genomics. 2015;105(2):83–9. https://doi.org/10.1016/j.ygeno.2014.12.002.
13. Barth AS, Kuner R, Buness A, Ruschhaupt M, Merk S, Zwermann L, Kääb S, Kreuzer E, Steinbeck G, Mansmann U, Poustka A, Nabauer M, Sültmann H. Identification of a common gene expression signature in dilated cardiomyopathy across independent microarray studies. J Am Coll Cardiol. 2006;48(8):1610–7.
14. Dennis G, Sherman BT, Hosack DA, Yang J, Gao W, Lane HC, Lempicki RA. DAVID: Database for annotation, visualization, and integrated discovery. Genome Biol. 2003;4:1.
15. Franceschini A, Szklarczyk D, Frankild S, Kuhn M, Simonovic M, Roth A, Lin J, Minguez P, Bork P, Von Mering C. STRING v9. 1: protein-protein interaction networks, with increased coverage and integration. Nucleic Acids Res. 2013; 41:D808–15.
16. Shannon P, Markiel A, Ozier O, Baliga NS, Wang JT, Ramage D, Amin N, Schwikowski B, Ideker T. Cytoscape: a software environment for integrated models of biomolecular interaction networks. Genome Res. 2003;13:2498–504.
17. Roider HG, Manke T, O'Keeffe S, Vingron M, Haas SA. PASTAA: identifying transcription factors associated with sets of co-regulated genes. Bioinformatics. 2009;25:435–42.
18. Wang L, Zhu L, Luan R, Wang L, Fu J, Wang X, Sui L. Analyzing gene expression profiles in dilated cardiomyopathy via bioinformatics methods. Braz J Med Biol Res. 2016;49
19. Sandelin A, Wasserman WW. Constrained binding site diversity within families of transcription factors enhances pattern discovery bioinformatics. J Mol Biol. 2004;338:207–15.
20. Lamb J, Crawford ED, Peck D, Modell JW, Blat IC, Wrobel MJ, Lerner J, Brunet J-P, Subramanian A, Ross KN. The connectivity map: using gene-expression signatures to connect small molecules, genes, and disease. Science. 2006;313:1929–35.
21. Ivandic BT, Mastitsky SE, Schönsiegel F, Bekeredjian R, Eils R, Frey N, Katus HA, Brors B. Whole-genome analysis of gene expression associates the ubiquitin-proteasome system with the cardiomyopathy phenotype in disease-sensitized congenic mouse strains. Cardiovasc Res. 2012;94:87–95.
22. Rosello-Lleti E, Navarro MM, Ortega A, Tarazon E, Sanchez D, Lazaro IS, Almenar L, Salvador A, Portoles M, Otero MR. Differential gene expression of cardiac chloride and potassium ion channels in human dilated non-ischemic cardiomyopathy. Eur Heart J. 2013;34:P4194.
23. Tsoutsman T, Wang X, Garchow K, Riser B, Twigg S, Semsarian C. CCN2 plays a key role in extracellular matrix gene expression in severe hypertrophic cardiomyopathy and heart failure. J Mol Cell Cardiol. 2013;62: 164–78.
24. Touvron M, Escoubet B, Mericskay M, Angelini A, Lamotte L, Santini MP, Rosenthal N, Daegelen D, Tuil D, Decaux J-F. Locally expressed IGF1 propeptide improves mouse heart function in induced dilated cardiomyopathy by blocking myocardial fibrosis and SRF-dependent CTGF induction. Disease Models and Mechanisms. 2012;5:481–91.
25. Koshman YE, Sternlicht MD, Kim T, O'Hara CP, Koczor CA, Lewis W, Seeley TW, Lipson KE, Samarel AM. Connective tissue growth factor regulates cardiac function and tissue remodeling in a mouse model of dilated cardiomyopathy. J Mol Cell Cardiol. 2015;89:214–22.
26. Thiele B-J, Doller A, Kähne T, Pregla R, Hetzer R, Regitz-Zagrosek V. RNA-binding proteins heterogeneous nuclear ribonucleoprotein A1, E1, and K are involved in post-transcriptional control of collagen I and III synthesis. Circ Res. 2004;95:1058–66.
27. Zhao H-p LD, Zhang W, Zhang L, S-m W, Ma C-m, Qin C, L-f Z. Protective action of tetramethylpyrazine phosphate against dilated cardiomyopathy in cTnTR141W transgenic mice. Acta Pharmacol Sin. 2010;31:281–8.

28. Gong X, Wang P, Wu Q, Wang S, Yu L, Wang G. Human umbilical cord blood derived mesenchymal stem cells improve cardiac function in cTnT R141W transgenic mouse of dilated cardiomyopathy. Eur J Cell Biol. 2016;95:57–67.
29. Louzao-Martinez L, Vink A, Harakalova M, Asselbergs FW, Verhaar MC, Cheng C. Characteristic adaptations of the extracellular matrix in dilated cardiomyopathy. Int J Cardiol. 2016;220:634–46.
30. Huang Y, Xia J, Zheng J, Geng B, Liu P, Yu F, Liu B, Zhang H, Xu M, Ye P. Deficiency of cartilage oligomeric matrix protein causes dilated cardiomyopathy. Basic Res Cardiol. 2013;108:1–21.
31. Li H, Cui Y, Luan J, Zhang X, Li C, Zhou X, Shi L, Wang H, Han J. PRELP (proline/arginine-rich end leucine-rich repeat protein) promotes osteoblastic differentiation of preosteoblastic MC3T3-E1 cells by regulating the β-catenin pathway. Biochem Biophys Res Commun. 2016;470:558–62.
32. Guan J, Liu W-Q, Xing M-Q, Shi Y, Tan X-Y, Jiang C-Q, Dai H-Y. Elevated expression of periostin in diabetic cardiomyopathy and the effect of valsartan. BMC Cardiovasc Disord. 2015;15:90.
33. Heidecker B, Lamirault G, Kasper EK, Wittstein IS, Champion HC, Breton E, Russell SD, Hall J, Kittleson MM, Baughman KL. The gene expression profile of patients with new-onset heart failure reveals important gender-specific differences. Eur Heart J. 2009;
34. Benhaddou A, Keime C, Ye T, Morlon A, Michel I, Jost B, Mengus G, Davidson I. Transcription factor TEAD4 regulates expression of myogenin and the unfolded protein response genes during C2C12 cell differentiation. Cell Death Differ. 2012;19:220–31.
35. Jiang S-W, Trujillo MA, Sakagashira M, Wilke RA, Eberhardt NL. Novel human TEF-1 isoforms exhibit altered DNA binding and functional properties. Biochemistry. 2000;39:3505–13.
36. Høiby T, Zhou H, Mitsiou DJ, Stunnenberg HG. A facelift for the general transcription factor TFIIA. Biochimica et Biophysica Acta (BBA)-Gene Structure and Expression. 2007;1769:429–36.
37. Chen Y, Xu H, Liu J, Zhang C, Leutz A, Mo X. The c-Myb functions as a downstream target of PDGF-mediated survival signal in vascular smooth muscle cells. Biochem Biophys Res Commun. 2007;360:433–6.
38. Vargova K, Curik N, Burda P, Basova P, Kulvait V, Pospisil V, Savvulidi F, Kokavec J, Necas E, Berkova A. MYB transcriptionally regulates the miR-155 host gene in chronic lymphocytic leukemia. Blood. 2011;117:3816–25.
39. Chartier FL, Bossu J-P, Laudet V, Fruchart J-C, Laine B. Cloning and sequencing of cDNAs encoding the human hepatocyte nuclear factor 4 indicate the presence of two isoforms in human liver. Gene. 1994;147:269–72.
40. Fan S, Li X, Tie L, Pan Y, Li X. KIAA0101 is associated with human renal cell carcinoma proliferation and migration induced by erythropoietin. Oncotarget. 2016;7(12):13520–37. https://doi.org/10.18632/oncotarget.5876.
41. Qiu LL, Xu L, Guo XM, Li ZT, Wan F, Liu XP, Chen GH, Chang GB. Gene expression changes in chicken NLRC5 signal pathway associated with in vitro avian leukosis virus subgroup J infection. Genet Mol Res. 2016;15(1) https://doi.org/10.4238/gmr.15017640.

4

Genetic influence alters the brain synchronism in perception and timing

Victor Marinho[1,2,3*], Thomaz Oliveira[1,2], Juliete Bandeira[1], Giovanny R. Pinto[2,3], Anderson Gomes[2], Valéria Lima[2], Francisco Magalhães[1,3], Kaline Rocha[1,3], Carla Ayres[1], Valécia Carvalho[1,3], Bruna Velasques[4], Pedro Ribeiro[4], Marco Orsini[5], Victor Hugo Bastos[6], Daya Gupta[7] and Silmar Teixeira[1,3]

Abstract

Background: Studies at the molecular level aim to integrate genetic and neurobiological data to provide an increasingly detailed understanding of phenotypes related to the ability in time perception.

Main Text: This study suggests that the polymorphisms genetic *SLC6A4* 5-HTTLPR, *5HTR2A* T102C, *DRD2/ANKK1*-Taq1A, *SLC6A3* 3'-UTR VNTR, *COMT* Val158Met, *CLOCK* genes and *GABRB2* A/C as modification factor at neurochemical levels associated with several neurofunctional aspects, modifying the circadian rhythm and built-in cognitive functions in the timing. We conducted a literature review with 102 studies that met inclusion criteria to synthesize findings on genetic polymorphisms and their influence on the timing.

Conclusion: The findings suggest an association of genetic polymorphisms on behavioral aspects related in timing. However, order to confirm the paradigm of association in the timing as a function of the molecular level, still need to be addressed future research.

Keywords: Time perception, Genetic polymorphisms, Serotonin, Dopamine, Circadian rhythm, GABA

Background

The interindividual differences in the time perception are evident in daily actions and their neurobiological aspects (i.e. walking, talking, reward tasks, executive functions, and cognition), with neurotransmitters acting in synchronization of the Central Nervous System (CNS). Neurotransmitters actions help to synchronize stimuli [1, 2], and trigger responses on time scales that range from the milliseconds (motor coordination), seconds to minutes (conscious time perception) and hours of the day (circadian rhythms) [3, 4]. It has been known that the genetic makeup enables the coding of different environmental stimuli, modulated through the action of the serotonergic, dopaminergic, GABAergic neurotransmission as well as circadian oscillations [5].

The hypothesis that the genetic polymorphisms in the expression of neurotransmitter systems and in circadian rhythm influences the perceptual capacity [6], promoted an increase in the number of genetic research to understand the molecular underpinnings of the temporal processing. To evaluate the genetic factors in temporal processing, Balci et al. [7] and Meck et al. [8] analyzed the effects of *5HTR2A*, *SLC6A4*, *SLC6A3* and *DRD2* expression on peak interval (PI) or non-reward procedures in rats. Results showed that rats genetically knockout for *5HTR2A*, *SLC6A4*, *SLC6A3*, and *DRD2* have less precision in the performance of PI activities when compared to control rats. This supports the importance of the role of several gene products in the phenotypic behavior associated with processing time intervals.

Genotypic investigations regarding brain function associated with timing are passive to determination of endophenotypes [9]. The literature seeks to trace a genetic profile of association with psychometric functions and behavioral performances, for example, fear conditioning, timing tasks by means of visual, tactile or auditory stimuli in humans or other species (Table 1) [10–

---

* Correspondence: victormarinhophb@hotmail.com
[1]Neuro-innovation Technology & Brain Mapping Laboratory, Federal University of Piauí, Av. São Sebastião n° 2819 – Nossa Sra. de Fátima –, Parnaíba, PI CEP 64202-020, Brazil
[2]Genetics and Molecular Biology Laboratory, Federal University of Piauí, Parnaíba, Brazil
Full list of author information is available at the end of the article

Table 1 Summary of genetic studies investigating the impact of time perception

Genotyping	Protocol	Stimulus	Duration	Results
SLC6A3 5-HTTLPR	Group: 273 young healthy. Cognitive tasks: (memory and Face Identity Perception tasks).	Visual Face images	Seconds range, varied for each participant.	There was neither an association between the 5HTTLPR genotype and cognitive tasks, but there might be a tendency for better performance of SL as compared with SS carriers for fEP [24].
SLC6A4 5-HTTLPR, 5HT2A T102C, DRD2/ANKK1-Taq1A, SLC6A3 3'-UTR VNTR, COMT Val158Met, MAOA VNTR, and CLOCK genes.	Group: 647 healthy individuals, Questionnaire. Cognitive test. Production and Discrimination tasks.	Visual Auditory	1 s, 3 s, 6 s, 12 s, 15 s	Stability of an individual's temporal accuracy and precision across in supra-second intervals (ranging from 3 s to 15 s) in the cognitive tasks and time perception tasks. Female participants are more likely to underestimate time production task when an explicit counting strategy is not employed [6].
COMT Val158Met, 5HTR2A T102C.	Group: 90 healthy Japanese. Cognitive tasks and fMRI study.	Visual	2 s, 3 s	Results demonstrate that the COMT genotypes are related to recognition accuracy, whereas the 5HTR2A genotypes are associated with RTs for recognition. In addition, strong connectivity in the cingulo-frontal networks is closely linked to a better working memory performance, regardless of the genotypes [98].
COMT Val158Met, SLC6A3 3'UTR VNTR and DRD4 exon 3 VNTR.	Group: 52 healthy Estonians. Cognitive tasks and Discrimination task.	Visual	23 ms, 70 ms, 105 ms, 735 ms,	SLC6A3 variability no showed difference in study. COMT Val158Met and DRD4 exon 3 VNTR differ in their effects on attentional functions as explicated in long-SOA metacontrast [20].
DRD2/ANKK1-Taq1A.	Group: 25 healthy individuals. Temporal or color Discrimination task and fMRI acquisition	Visual	350 ms, 400 ms, 450 ms, 550 ms, 600 ms, 650 ms; 1,4 s, 1,8 s, 2 s, 2,2 s, 2,4 s, 2,6 s.	A1 carriers of the Taq1A polymorphism exhibited worse performance on temporal task. However, greater activation in the striatum and right dorsolateral prefrontal cortex, as well as reduced volume in the cerebellar [22].
DRD2/ANKK1-Taq1A and COMT Val158Met.	Group: 41 healthy individuals. Time perception tasks. Fixed-intervals tasks.	Visual	10s, 17 s.	DRD2/ANKK1-Taq1A in the striatum and COMT Val158Met, affecting the breakdown of dopamine in the prefrontal cortex— to interval timing and reward magnitude modulation of decision thresholds [7].
COMT Val158Met, SLC6A3 3'-UTR VNTR.	Group: 95 healthy individuals. 64-channel EEG study. Continuous performance test.	Visual	450 ms, 600 ms, 750 ms, 900 ms.	Effects of SLC6A3 and COMT on the occipito-temporal activity in CNV. In addition, there was a trend towards an interaction between the two polymorphisms [19].
SLC6A3 +/+ rats SLC6A3 −/− rats SLC6A3 +/− rats	Group: DAT-mutant rat. Peak interval task. Administration: Methamphetamine hydrochloride.	Visual	15 s, 20s, 45 s, 140 s, 200 s.	Complete loss of temporal control and altered sensitivity to drugs. Lower threshold for initiating responding in the timing task [8].
DRD2/ANKK1-Taq1A and COMT Val158Met.	Group: 65 healthy individuals. Temporal discrimination task and motor tempo task.	Visual	500 ms, 2 s	DRD2/ANKK1-Taq1A (A1+ allele) was associated with variability for the 500 ms duration only, whereas the COMT Val158Met (Val/Val) was associated with variability for the 2000 ms duration only. Additionally, the DRD2/ANKK1-Taq1A was associated with slower preferred motor time [21].
SLC6A3 +/+ rats SLC6A3 −/− rats SLC6A3 +/− rats	Group: KD rat and WT rat. Peak interval task and administration of the Raclopride.	Visual	20s, 40s, 60s, 80s, 100 s, 120 s.	DAT KD rats responded at higher levels in peak trials than WT rats in all conditions, but particularly during the fixed-interval 30 peak trials [1].
SLC6A4 5-HTTLPR, 5HT2A T102C, DRD2/ANKK1-Taq1A, SLC6A3 3'-UTR VNTR and COMT Val158Met.	Group: 44 healthy individuals. Discrimination task.	Visual Auditory	Combinations of supra seconds.	No differences between time representation and dopamine-genes. However, show association between serotinine-related genes and parameters derived from psychometric functions PSE [13].
DRD2/ANKK1-Taq1A	Group: Transgenic rat C57BL/6-CB. Peak interval tasks.	No	Fixed-interval: 24 s.	Overexpression of D2 receptors in the striatum caused a reduction in operant response rate, a broadening of the distribution of operant responses in time and an increase in the latency of the peak in response rate, consistent with an impairment in timing accuracy. The progressive ratio operant task confirmed that D2 overexpressing rats exhibited reduced operant motivation [23].

fEP face identity perception, *RT* response time, *SOA* Stimulus onset asynchrony, *CNV* Contingent negative variation, *KD* Knockdown, *WT* Wild type, *PSE* Point of subjective equality

12]. In principle, human cognitive performance is highly variable and under strong genetic control. Moreover, qualitative or quantitative genetic changes promote underestimation or overestimation of time according to the Scalar Expectancy Theory (SET) [5, 13, 14]. This is accounted by the interference in the number of oscillations captured per time unit from the internal clock [15, 16], and judgments of time intervals may result from changes in the pulse flow from an internal pacemaker in the presence of an event [17]. Consequently, genetic polymorphisms increase or decrease the speed of the internal clock, modulating the neurotransmission of the pulses and reactions to stimuli that determine the synchronism in motor and cognitive activities [11, 13, 18].

Therefore, the individual variability in the coding of the time intervals resulting from single nucleotide polymorphisms (SNPs) and numbers of tandem repeat variations (VNTRs) modifies timing process [19, 20]. In summary, studies suggest that the *SLC6A4* 5-HTTLPR, *5HTR2A* T102C, *DRD2/ANKK1*-Taq1A, *SLC6A3* 3'-UTR VNTR, *COMT* Val158Met, *CLOCK* genes and *GABRB2* A/C (rs6556547) expression in the cortical and subcortical areas influence the time judgment. Thus, it becomes relevant for neurogenetics to elucidate endophenotypes associated with the perception of the sub-second and supra-second intervals [6, 11, 13, 18, 21].

Finally, we presented a state-of-the-art for genetic polymorphisms and time perception, highlighting the main discoveries, and addressing further directions for clinically relevant neuroscience research. Although we have some papers not directly related to genetic influence on the time perception; these additional studies demonstrate behavioral phenotypes related to cognition and executive function, both have a key role in time intervals synchronization. These studies support neurochemical changes caused by differential gene expression, as well as a relationship with cognitive modulations embedded in ability to synchronize the time intervals.

Genetic of the serotoninergic system on the neurobiological aspects inbuilt in timing

Analyses of neural and genetic mechanisms have contributed to the understanding of how the time-trial process occurs [19]. Sysoeval, Tonevitsky and Wackermann [13] investigated differences in the neurobiological basis in perceiving stimuli through polymorphisms analysis (*SLC6A4* 5-HTTLPR, *5HTR2A* T102C, *DRD2/ANKK1*-Taq1A, *SLC6A3* 3'-UTR VNTR and *COMT* Val158Met) concomitantly with time discrimination tasks. Since the results do not reveal consistencies in data from the studies of genetic polymorphisms related to the dopaminergic system, it may be inferred that increased or decreased serotonin expression also influences the processing of time intervals. The results demonstrated that chemical modulations in the CNS in perceptive activities relates to serotonin concentration in the coding second to minutes duration intervals. Genetic polymorphisms in neurotransmission predispose participants to different behavioral phenotypes, and consequently we infer inappropriate recruitment, decrease or increase of neurotransmitters levels, which causes modulations of neural inputs in the timing circuits.

In particular, a biomarker of serotoninergic expression related to individual variability in cognition, the *SLC6A4* gene located in 17q11.2, encode a transmembrane protein that transports serotonin from synaptic spaces. An In/Del polymorphism exists within the 5´ region flanking the regulatory region of the *SLC6A4* gene, a highly polymorphic region (5-HTTLPR) associated with levels of transport and serotonin uptake. The genotypes related to *SLC6A4* 5-HTTLPR, the short allele (S) show decreased serotonin reabsorption compared to the long allele (L) [25, 26]. The allelic differences are associated with a decrease in the availability of serotonin. Individuals carrying the short allele have increased extracellular serotonergic levels compared to those with two copies of the long allele [27]. Fallgatter et al. [10] confirmed that individuals with one or two copies of the *SLC6A4* 5-HTTLPR short allele have greater brain activity and less error in memory and timing stimulus activities. Therefore, Heinz et al. [28] reported that the healthy carriers of short alleles of the *SLC6A4* 5-HTTLPR have increased amygdaloid neuron activation and the connection of neural inputs between the amygdala and the ventromedial prefrontal cortex than homozygous individuals for the long allele. It has been shown that genetic variations that encode serotonin play a central role in social learning neurobiology, the system of emotions and decision making.

Additionally, neurochemistry influences working memory, which is a system of limited capacity that permeates almost all levels of cognition, ranging from perceptive awareness to intelligence [29]. Thus, cortical and subcortical signaling is influenced by the receptors differential expression of receptors in regions of the brain that are involved in perceptual processing and executive functions. Accordingly, Crisan et al. [30] investigated the effects of *SLC6A4* 5-HTTLPR polymorphism concomitant with neuroimaging tools, through tasks that measure decision-making on economic risks in healthy financial market volunteers. The results of genotyping in the 5-HTTLPR region in this retrospective study indicate that carriers of the short alleles, same in heterozygosity, exhibit better performance in financial activities and a lower percentage of economic losses compared to homozygotes for the long allele. The relationship of *SLC6A4* 5-HTTLPR polymorphism with variable serotonin expression has been associated with neuropsychiatric conditions [11], social anxiety disorder [31], aggressiveness [32], depression [33] and impulsivity [34], diseases that contribute to the deficit in the time perception. However, genetic studies associated with cognitive parameters are not only linked to *SLC6A4* 5-HTTLPR [35], but the studies by Burt and Mikolajewski [36] show that that subjects make less harmful decisions, besides an adjuvant action of variations in the *5HTR2A* gene on cognitive aspects.

The *5HTR2A* gene located at 13q14–21 encodes the expression of postsynaptic type 2A (5-HT2A) serotonin receptors, which signal via diacylglycerol and triphosphate inositol during serotonergic stimulation. The *5HTR2A* gene influences the perceptual capacity of stimuli and executive functions [36], and are associated with impulsivity disorders in motor and cognitive planning tasks, likely from deficient connections as well as a decrease of serotonergic receptors in brain regions that perform these activities (i.e. prefrontal cortex and limbic system) [36, 37]. The *5HTR2A* T102C polymorphism corresponds to a thymine (T) shift by a cytosine (C) at position 102 of the codon in the promoter region of the gene and determines changes in the amino acid coding that make up the 2A receptors. Genotypes with TT alleles have higher expression of 5-HT2A than homozygous CC and heterozygous TC [38]. The genotypes studies at a molecular level in conjunction with pharmacological models suggests that the *5HTR2A* T102C polymorphism modulates the timing activity of visual stimuli in work memory tasks [39]. The ability to influence the perception of visual stimuli is because 5-HT2A receptors are highly expressed in the visual cortex [40]. Thus, the alterations in the density of the occipital cortex due to genetic variations decrease the expression of 5-HT2A, which facilitate the appearance of deficiencies in time interpretation and in risk of neurological diseases [41, 42].

Genetic aspects of the dopaminergic system in timing

The control in the human ability to judge the time intervals originated of the external stimuli has as one of the bases, the dopaminergic system [11, 43]. Among the genes that influence dopaminergic neurotransmission, the *DRD2* gene located in 11q23.2, encodes a G protein-coupled receptor in postsynaptic neurons, playing a key role in neurotransmission, besides influencing several behavioral phenotypes [44, 45]. In particular, SNP *DRD2/ANKK1*-Taq1A triggers glutamate changes by lysine (Glu713Lys) in *ANKK1*, altering the function of the *DRD2* promoter region and expression of the D2-type receptors. In view of the foregoing, two alleles (A1 and A2) can be identified, the presence of one or two alleles A1 is associated with the reduction of 20 to 40% of the D2 receptor in areas of the striatum, region essential in the encoding of neural inputs in the timing [13, 46]. The transient expression of D2 receptors have been demonstrated to cause a deficit in neural mechanisms in the indirect pathway activation of the prefrontal cortex, motor cortex, and premotor, consequently, thus impairs the acquisition of temporal control, and results in underestimation during timed-motor tasks [7].

Furthermore, molecular influence on dopaminergic neurotransmission in presynaptic terminals is mediated by *SLC6A3* gene located in 5p15.3, important to the chemical regulation between dopaminergic circuits and pathways related to cognition and time perception [47].

In this context, the polymorphism of the repeats in tandem *SLC6A3* 3'-UTR VNTR located in the 15 exon of the 3′ untranslated region, contains serial repetitions of 40 bp ranging from 3-repeats (3R) to 13-repeats. (13R), and the 9-repeats (9R) and 10-repeats (10R) series are the most common alleles in the general population. Consistent with the dopamine transporter (DAT) functionality, carriers of a 9R allele exhibit lower DAT protein encoding in the prefrontal cortex when compared to their 10R homozygous homologues. Although the protein structure is not altered, it is thought that function is affected by regulating mRNA stability, transport and protein synthesis [47]. The functional alleles 10R and 9R alter the related phenotypes with planning and execution processes of working memory tasks, stimuli perception and increase the risk of neurological diseases [48–50] because of patients with a 9R allele exhibit less DAT activity than their homozygotes 10R. In the prefrontal cortex and caudate nucleus, and thus modulate dopamine levels in the CNS during the processing of temporal and cognitive information [51, 52].

The studies are also based on the influence of dopamine-degrading enzymes, especially the *COMT* gene located in 22q11, which encodes dopaminergic degradation in the synaptic cleft. The *COMT* gene encodes the enzyme catechol-o-methyltransferase (COMT enzyme) that catalyzes the transfer of a methyl group from S-adenosylmethionine to catecholamines [11]. The level of degradation is modified by means of the *COMT* Val158Met polymorphism, known to influence enzymatic activity in the prefrontal cortex, increasing the dopaminergic levels and thus deregulating the nigrostriatal circuit in the time delay of supra seconds. Carriers of the Met allele (L) are more visualized in time-stamping studies by means of motor and cognitive tasks in patients with Parkinson's disease [18]. Carriers of the Met allele (L) have relatively low COMT enzyme activity and, presumably, have greater availability of dopamine. While the carriers of the Val allele (H) have a relatively high activity of COMT enzyme, and less availability of dopamine [11, 53]. The *COMT* Val158Met polymorphism has been associated with impairments in working memory [11], emotional problems [54], reduced attention levels [20], and associated with a risk of neurological diseases [55, 56]. Thus, the influence on the perception of time due to these neurological disorders is presumed to act in brain areas responsible for coding processes of time intervals, and in cognitive functions embedded in the timing.

Bartholomew et al. [6] have shown the hypothesis of genetic polymorphisms influencing the time interpretation and express complex human phenotypes. The authors reported that genetic polymorphisms contribute to individual variability in neurobiological aspects at internal clock speed. In the study methodology, 647 healthy individuals were analyzed in production and discrimination of time intervals, however, only 148 individuals were examined based on Genome-wide association study (GWAS) to see if any genetic polymorphism is associated with a trait. GWAS typically focus on associations between SNPs and human traits for different phenotypes in timing. The authors used the *DRD2/ANKK1*-Taq1A, *SLC6A3* 3'-UTR VNTR, and *COMT* Val158Met, which are correlated with precision in judging of time intervals. The genotypes were chosen based on the minor allele frequency (MAF) greater than 5%, and thus, the neurobiological data related to MAF identified common variations that may contribute to the understanding of the human behavioral phenotype in time coding.

Meck et al. [8], based on molecular influence on dopaminergic neurotransmission, the authors assessed behavioral phenotype in knockout rats for the *SLC6A3* and *COMT* gene and under the influence of drug. The authors concluded that the circuits of the prefrontal cortex and striatum have less activation during the encoding of stimuli, which is due to changes in the neurotransmitter levels due alterations in COMT enzyme and DAT. On the basis of this, we propose that the genetic polymorphisms *SLC6A3* 3'-UTR VNTR and *COMT* Val158Met alter the internal clock speed by decreasing accuracy in judging time intervals. Thus, the neural substrates underlying the three clock stages (clock phase, memory phase, and decision) can be modulated according to the genetic polymorphisms, which is likely due to changes in dopaminergic pathways. According to this model, dopamine participates mainly in the clock phase. An increase in dopaminergic signaling accelerates the accumulation of impulses over time and modifies the coding process of accumulated information, and consequently distorts judgment time [5].

Transport, receptors and dopaminergic degradation have been shown to be critical for the time interval in humans and animals [57]. Experiments with genetically knockout mice for *SLC6A3* and *DRD2* have increased levels of dopamine in the prefrontal cortex and neural inputs deficient in neurotransmitter via the nigrostriatal pathway. Elevated levels of the neurotransmitter imply impairment both in the time interval and in the motivation to work for food rewards [23]. In association with these characteristics, it was shown that deficits in time accuracy appear to be mediated by deficiencies in the systems of motivation, working memory or sustained attention. In general, the overall alteration of DAT and D2 receptor expression through *SLC6A3* 3'-UTR VNTR and *DRD2/ANKK1*-TAq1A results in underestimation in timing of behavior. It is inferred that the resulting effect does not resemble the effect of clock speed induced by injections of drug dopaminergic agonists when rats are trained by peak interval (PI) [58].

Influence of clock genes in the timing

The innate preference in the morning or evening is one of the characteristics determined by the circadian rhythm phase. From this circadian synchronization, our brain as an efficient machine in the orchestration of time scales encodes physiological information and cognitive behaviors [58, 59]. In mammals, this system is organized by a central clock located in the suprachiasmatic nucleus (SCN) of the hypothalamus, in addition to a series of peripheral oscillators present in the liver, lungs, adrenal glands, and other tissues [59–61].

The SCN regulates the biological rhythms of the organism through self-regulated transcription-translation loops of the so-called *CLOCK* genes in a 24-h period, with the *CLOCK*, *ARNTL*, *PER* (1, 2 and 3) and *CRY* (1 and 2) [62, 63]. Briefly, the CLOCK/ARNTL protein complex expresses negative regulators PER1–3 and CRY1–2 proteins, since they inhibit the expression of the CLOCK/ARNTL heterodimer. The CLOCK/ARNTL heterodimer controls the genetic expression acting in the physiology of the organism and, thus, the modulation of heterodimer levels leads to the rhythmicity of various metabolic and cognitive functions [59, 64, 65].

The control of CLOCK-ARNTL heterodimer levels exhibits time-dependent fluctuations, and thus modulate the synchronization capability of shorter intervals, such as second-to-minutes [65, 66]. Agostino and Cheng [58] provided experimental evidence showing changes in dopaminergic levels in rat striatum as a function of the circadian cycle, with lower levels of dopamine during the day and a peak at night. This occurs due to regulators in the promoter region of the *SLC6A3*, *DRD1* and *MAOA* genes, demonstrating that the expression of these components is linked to cycles of luminosity and metabolic variations [58]. Rats with modulations in the dopaminergic, levels in the dorsal striatum for lack of melatonin have an impact on the stimuli perception in fixed interval tasks. In addition, the lack of melatonin has been associated with circadian clock components, focusing on the *PER2* gene. The genetic expression of *PER2* is involved in the circadian regulation of dopaminergic metabolism through dorsal striatum and substantia nigra pars compacta (SNpc) oscillations [58].

Therefore, it is increasingly accepted that the variations in genetic components of circadian rhythm affect the rhythmicity of the organism in timing as well as environmental changes [59, 67]. In exemplification, workers who abruptly change their work shift may present mood problems, social and work activities, as well as favor the development of deficient cognitive functions [68, 69]. It has been shown that the *PER2* gene effect on insomnia was relatively stronger than environmental factors such as high stress at work. Thus, it is suggested that the genetic susceptibility of the individual should be considered for the sleep problems control [70]. In the context, Song et al. [71], in a Korean population, demonstrated that in addition to the involvement of the *PER2* gene, a synergistic action with other circadian genes may increase the risk of the diurnal preference toward evening [71]. Given the influence of genetic variations related to the circadian rhythm on sleep homeostasis, it is easier to understand how endogenous rhythmicity influences the interval timing, as changes in the sleep-wake cycle influence the processing of shorter time intervals. Späti et al. [66], analyzed the time perception of individuals who experienced sleep deprivation, and their findings showed that sustained wakefulness distorts the timing interval through pacemaker pulse oscillations over a 24-h period, with an exponential increase and saturation in the rate of the pacemaker with time constant of 18.2 h.

Neural synchronism deficient in the coding of the time intervals led by circadian dysregulation was studied by means of time estimation tasks with rats under conditions of 24 h in the dark (D/D) or 24 h in the daylight (L/L), different of the normal homeostatic condition of 12 h light / 12 h dark (L/D) [72]. Agostino et al. [72] observed that the group trained in the DD condition showed higher precision, whereas in the L/L condition the rats lost temporal control. This evidence is important in view of the fact that the light is the main cue for circadian rhythm. The time perception, in addition to varying with the time of day, is strongly correlated with circadian variations in body temperature and serum melatonin levels [73]. The circadian rhythm is indicated as a regulator of the interval timing by means of modulations in the dopamine levels, which is implicated as a key neurotransmitter responsible for the pacemaker-accumulator operation [67]. In fact, the processing of timing interval involves the interaction of cortico-striatal circuits through the dopaminergic-glutamatergic pathways. With this, alteration in dopaminergic neurotransmission during the day caused by circadian dysfunctions strongly influences the timing interval. However, the changes in neurotransmitter levels were shown to be reversed by levodopa injections in rats with circadian timing disruptions. So, it is suggested that a daily increase in dopamine is required for the accurate performance of timekeeping tasks [74].

Polymorphisms in different genomic regions are not only responsible for the stable changes throughout the organism, but also have the potential to modulate neural coding for interval timing [75]. In summary, the circadian genes expression in the striatum and substantia nigra, important structures involved in temporal processing and dopaminergic neurotransmission, influence neural oscillations when L/L conditions are induced [74]. If on the one hand, circadian changes alter the expression of dopamine and consequently the timing interval, dopamine-associated polymorphisms have also been implicated in circadian changes, showing a clear synergism between two systems [76].

Genetic of the GABAergic system have an impact on neurobiological aspects inbuilt in the time perception

The β2 GABA$_A$ subunit receptor is a multiple subunit chloride channel receptor that mediates the action of gamma-aminobutyric acid (GABA), a fast inhibitor of synaptic transmission in the CNS. The receptor is expressed by the *GABRB2* gene, located at 9q22.1-q22.3, which plays a role in modulating synapses and maintains the excitation-inhibition balance in the brain [77]. Different genetic polymorphisms alter the expression or function of elements of GABAergic neurotransmissions, such as the SNP *GABRB2* A/C type intronic polymorphism that decrease the expression of messenger RNA (mRNA) required for the synthesis of β2 subunit. This polymorphism decreases GABA concentration at the postsynaptic level and has thus been associated with changes in memory and attention, both influencing time-interval processing [5, 78]. It has been argued that *GABRB2* A/C modulates β2 subunit activity of the GABA$_A$ receptor in various time interval regions, specifically the visual cortex, frontal cortex, dopaminergic circuit associations and striatal-thalamic-cortical [79]. In this sense, it modifies the temporal processing of information obtained from the activity of sensory receptors, which is responsible for capturing and redirecting information to be interpreted in executive actions proposed in the classical pacemaker-accumulator model, this is consistent with the role of neural oscillations in synchronizing parts of distributed modular clocks in the brain (Fig. 1) [80–84].

Experimental evidence suggests that GABAergic fast inhibitory neurotransmission – mediated by GABA$_A$ receptor subtype – plays a key role in beta oscillations as shown by a study of the primary motor cortex of rats [85]. Furthermore, linkage and association mapping between genetic polymorphisms (microsatellite and single-nucleotide polymorphisms) shows significant dependence of beta-range oscillation phenotypes with GABAA gene location in chromosome 4 [85, 86]. More experimental evidence directly implicates GABAergic transmission in timing functions of the brain. In a psychophysics study, measuring visual interval estimation and reproduction, it was shown that the elevated levels of GABA in the visual cortex lead to the underestimation of visual intervals [77].

Kononowicz and Van Rijn [87] showed that subjective timing of millisecond intervals does not depend on changes indexed by the evoked potential known as contingent negative variation, and that the subjective experience of time is better reflected by distinct features of

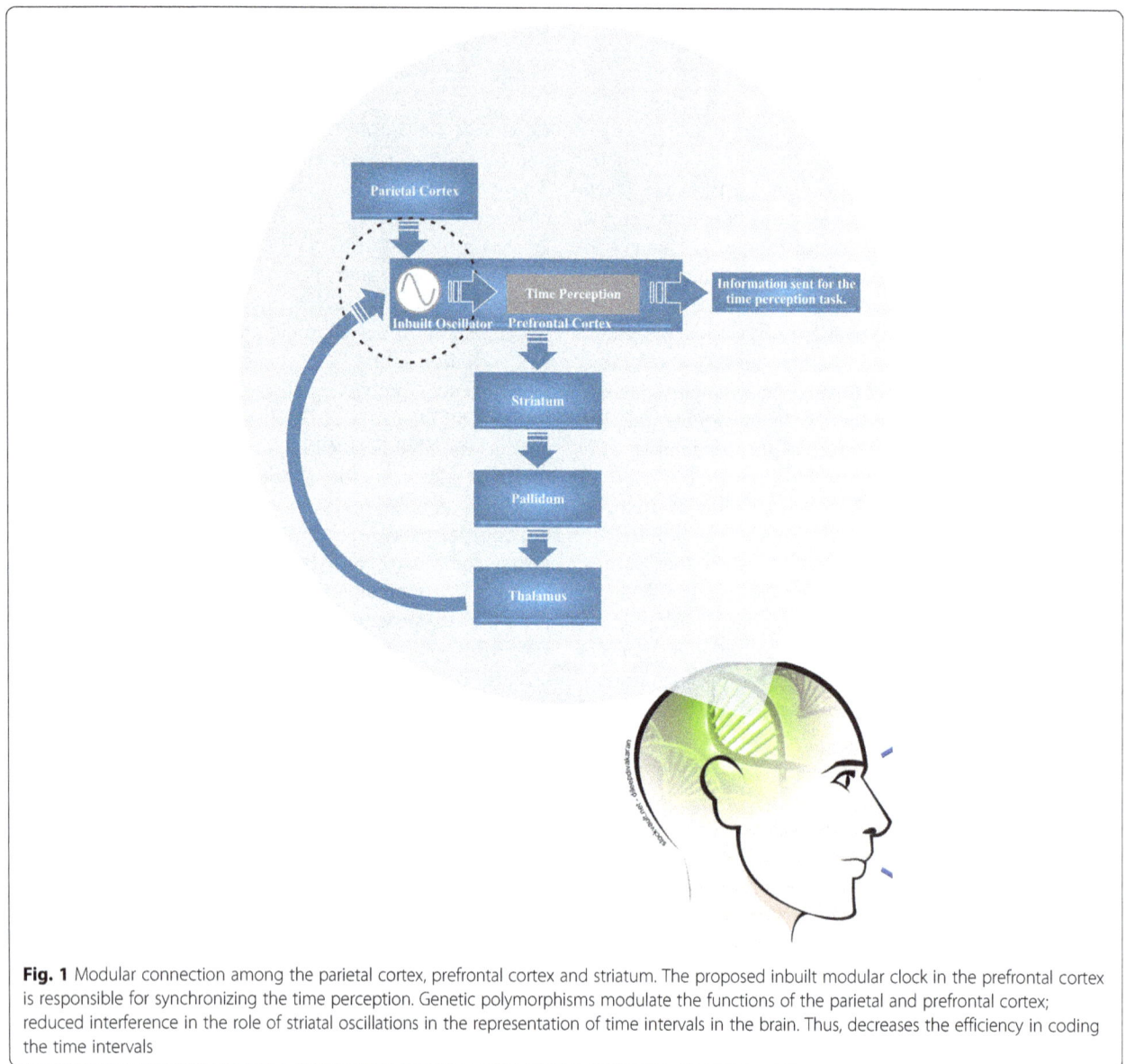

Fig. 1 Modular connection among the parietal cortex, prefrontal cortex and striatum. The proposed inbuilt modular clock in the prefrontal cortex is responsible for synchronizing the time perception. Genetic polymorphisms modulate the functions of the parietal and prefrontal cortex; reduced interference in the role of striatal oscillations in the representation of time intervals in the brain. Thus, decreases the efficiency in coding the time intervals

evoked potentials occurring after offset of comparison interval in a time estimation task [87]. In addition, the authors demonstrated that the neural responses evoked from GABAergic connections predicted the subjective perception of the comparison interval, with evoked responses more similar to the normal interval, independently of the duration presented [87, 88]. Furthermore, experimental evidences by means of computational modeling demonstrate GABAergic neurons inhibitory to the production of gamma oscillations in electroencephalography [89], as well as the GABA performance in the visual cortex for the differences in the individual phenotypes, as consequence of the decrease of the threshold of synchronization of visual stimuli [77, 87, 88].

Van Loon et al. [89] analyzed differences in the processing of visual stimuli due to the synchronism of

GABAergic neurons, implying, therefore, that GABA acts as a mediator in the perception of visual intervals. Thus, experiments with pharmacological modeling of GABAergic agonists and antagonists in accordance with genomic analyses are suggested to elucidate the role of GABAergic system in time discrimination tasks [77, 90]. Furthermore, GABAergic activity is susceptible to the modulation of time perception and the polymorphic form *GABRB2* A/C and its haplotypes have the capacity to influence the risk of neurological diseases (i.e., Parkinson's Disease, Schizophrenia, Bipolar Disorder), which affect the processing of time intervals by the brain in laboratory-controlled tasks or in the performance of everyday activities [78, 91]. In addition, the study by Oblack, Gibbs, and Blat [92] has shown that the neurobiological aspects related to the perceptual capacity of time in autistic subjects is deficient, which is associated with elevations of GABAergic activity in the visual cortex and auditory cortex. Moreover, these results may reveal underestimation of the time in relation to the timing of the stimuli [89, 90].

Another aspect of the GABA as an inhibitor of synaptic transmission in the CNS, is demonstrated through postsynaptic polarization, and decrease of intracellular Ca_{2+} levels in the medium spiny neurons. This occurs by means of GABAergic loops that are also important for interval timing mechanisms, among which are the glutamic acid decarboxylase (GAD), an enzyme that converts glutamate to GABA. The GAD1 gene encodes the GAD67 in both the cell body and nerve terminals. GAD65, on the other hand, is encoded by the GAD2 gene and is restricted to the nerve terminals [78, 93]. It can be hypothesized that reduced inhibitory transmission in the brain may play a role in timing based on the level these two isoforms, GAD65 and GAD67. Reduced synthesis of GABA due to inhibition or decreased levels of GAD may result in neural inputs deficits inbuilt in neurobiological aspects in timing, such as stimulus perception, decision-making and memory. Clearly, a dysregulation of glutamate and GABA metabolism in the brain may contribute to neurological diseases that affect the time judgment (for example, Anxiety disorders and Depression) [77, 93].

Few studies have evaluated the hypothesis of the genetic interaction of GABRB2 A/C on the interindividual variability of behavioral phenotypes related to a timing error in healthy individuals or in patients with some neurological disease. However, few state-of-the-art demonstrates studies studied electrophysiological measures of neural firing in monkeys the GABAergic performance in the coding and timing of stimuli [94–96]. Interestingly, they showed that the perceived duration is a consequence of the magnitude of the neuronal response at visual time-intervals in GABAergic circuits. The findings suggest a link between electrophysiological results due to inhibition of the specific sensory excitatory activity of the optical pathways of visual stimulation [89, 97, 98]. It may be that the prediction of the error as a function of the perceptual capacity is determined by local calcium limitations in the activation of the GABA receptors in the visual cortex, which affects the excitation-inhibition equilibrium [99].

Limitations of existing research

Some factors, such as sensory modality, intensity, size, complexity, familiarity are not standardized in the various studies of the time perception, making it impossible to completely determine the association with genetic polymorphisms in the neural inputs during time coding. Limitations involved on population size and further studies with larger samples are needed to determine

whether such genetic polymorphisms alone may or may not help explain the interindividual differences in timing. A limitation of this study, are few works that relate genetics on time perception, in particular, the variation referring to the neurotransmitter GABA. The presented studies suggest an applicability of the GABRB2 variants in the timing since it modifies in the inbuilt oscillator in executive functions essential in the judgment of the time.

Conclusion

The study of genetic polymorphisms is not only relevant to health, but also to various behavioral phenotypes that alter the temporal judgment. Thus, more studies are needed to substantiate the genotypic contributions on performance in temporal activities, by understanding the neurobiological mechanisms at the molecular and biochemical level behind timing synchronism. In summary, levels of neurotransmitters such as serotonin and dopamine are regulated by SLC6A4, 5HTR2A, DRD2/ANKK1, SLC6A3, and COMT gene that modulate the chemistry of the neural bases in the prefrontal circuits [100], associated with studies of cognition and working memory [101], learning and repetitive motor tasks in relation to a visual stimulus [102]. Regarding the CLOCK genes, corticosteroid changes due to alterations in PER2 expression promoted impacts in the time interval, as it acts on the dopaminergic metabolism due to the influence of circadian variations induced by changes in the light / dark cycle.

Furthermore, few studies have analyzed the GABRB2 A/C polymorphism in time perception tasks, and our hypothesis of acting on time intervals is supported by changes in the processing of perceptual process information in the visual cortex, suggested by changes in neural oscillations. In circadian pacemakers, for example, the SCN, due to limitations in the activation of GABA receptors in the visual cortex, affects the excitation-inhibition balance in the visual stimuli perception. Thus, genetic and cognitive information provide the means that direct the mechanisms underlying the perceptual behavior of time in humans.

Abbreviations
5-HTTLPR: Highly polymorphic region; CNS: Central Nervous System; CNV: Contingent negative variation; COMT enzyme: Enzyme catechol-o-methyltransferase; DAT: The dopamine transporter; fEP: Face identity perception; GABA: Gamma-aminobutyric acid; GAD: Glutamic acid decarboxylase; GWAS: Genome-wide association study; KD: Knockdown; MAF: Minor allele frequency; mRNA: Messenger RNA; PI: Peak interval; PSE: Point of subjective equality; RT: Response time; SCN: Suprachiasmatic nucleus; SET: Scalar Expectancy Theory; SNpc: Substantia nigra pars compacta; SNPs: Single nucleotide polymorphisms; SOA: Stimulus onset asynchrony; VNTRs: Numbers of tandem repeat variations; WT: Wild type

Authors' contributions
VM, TO, JB, GRP, DG, PR, BV and ST designed the study concept. Studies considered eligible for inclusion were read in full and their suitability for inclusion was determined independently by six reviewers (VM, AG, VL, FM, KR, and VC). CA, MO, VHB, and JB read and finalized the manuscript. All authors read and approved the final manuscript.

Authors' information

VM, TO, AG and VL are researchers of the Neuro-innovation Technology &
Brain Mapping Laboratory, Federal University of Piauí, Parnaíba, Brazil, and
Genetics and Molecular Biology Laboratory, Federal University of Piauí, Par-
naíba, Brazil.
JB, KR, FM, VC, and CA are researchers of the Neuro-innovation Technology &
Brain Mapping Laboratory, Federal University of Piauí, Parnaíba, Brazil.
GRP is a professor and mentor in the Master and PhD programs at Federal
University of Piauí. He is a head of the Genetics and Molecular Biology
Laboratory.
BV and PR are professors at the Federal University of Rio de Janeiro, and
Brain Mapping and Sensory Motor Integration Laboratory, Institute of
Psychiatry of Federal University of Rio de Janeiro, Brazil.
MO is professor of Master's Program in Local Development and Health
Sciences Applied Program on University Center Augusto Motta - UNISUAM,
Rio de Janeiro, Brazil.
DG is an adjunct professor of Biology at Camden County College,
Blackwood, New Jersey, USA.
VHB is professor at the Federal University of Piauí. Mentor in the Master
program at Federal University of Piauí. He is a head of the Brain Mapping
and Functionality Laboratory.
ST is professor at the Federal University of Piauí. Mentor in the Master and
PhD. programs at Federal University of Piauí. He is a head of the Neuro-
innovation Technology & Brain Mapping Laboratory.

Competing interests

The authors declare that they have no competing interests.

Author details

[1]Neuro-innovation Technology & Brain Mapping Laboratory, Federal
University of Piauí, Av. São Sebastião n° 2819 – Nossa Sra. de Fátima –,
Parnaíba, PI CEP 64202-020, Brazil. [2]Genetics and Molecular Biology
Laboratory, Federal University of Piauí, Parnaíba, Brazil. [3]The Northeast
Biotechnology Network (RENORBIO), Federal University of Piauí, Teresina,
Brazil. [4]Brain Mapping and Sensory Motor Integration Laboratory, Federal
University of Rio de Janeiro, Rio de Janeiro, Brazil. [5]Master's Program in Local
Development Program, University Center Augusto Motta - UNISUAM, Rio de
Janeiro, Brazil and Health Sciences Applied - Vassouras University, Rio de
Janeiro, Brazil. [6]Brain Mapping and Functionality Laboratory, Federal
University of Piauí, Parnaíba, Brazil. [7]Department of Biology, Camden County
College, Blackwood, NJ, USA.

References

1. Balci F, Ludvig EA, Abner R, Zhuang X, Poon P, Brunner D. Motivational effects on interval timing in dopamine transporter (DAT) knockdown mice. Brain Res. 2010;1325(14):89–99.
2. Herai T, Mogi K. Perception of temporal duration affected by automatic and controlled movements. Conscious Cogn. 2014;29:23–35.
3. Merchant H, Harrington DL, Meck WH. Neural basis of the perception and estimation of time. Annu Rev Neurosci. 2013;36:313–36.
4. Zhang L, Ptáček LJ, Fu YH. Diversity of human clock genotypes and consequences. Prog Mol Biol Transl Sci. 2013;119:51–81.
5. Matthews WJ, Meck WH. Time perception: the bad news and the good. Wiley Interdiscip Rev Cogn Sci. 2014;5(4):429–46.
6. Bartholomew AJ, Meck WH, Cirulli ET. Analysis of genetic and non-genetic factors influencing timing and time perception. PLoS One. 2015;10(12): e0143873.
7. Balci F, Wiener M, Cavdaroğlu B, Branch CH. Epistasis effects of dopamine genes on interval timing and reward magnitude in humans. Neuropsychologia. 2013;51(2):293–308.
8. Meck WH, Cheng RK, MacDonald CJ, Gainetdinov RR, Caron MG, Cevik MÖ. Gene-dose dependent effects of methamphetamine on interval timing in dopamine-transporter knockout mice. Neuropharmacology. 2012;62(3): 1221–9.
9. Zilles D, Meyer J, Schneider-Axmann T, Ekawardhani S, Gruber E, Falkai P, Gruber O. Genetic polymorphisms of 5-HTT and DAT but not COMT differentially affect verbal and visuospatial working memory functioning. Eur Arch Psychiatry Clin Neurosci. 2012;262(8):667–76.
10. Fallgatter AJ, Herrmann MJ, Roemmler J, Ehlis AC, Wagener A, Heidrich A, Ortega G, Zeng Y, Lesch KP. Allelic variation of serotonin transporter function modulates the brain electrical response for error processing. Neuropsychopharmacology. 2004;29(8):1506–11.
11. Green AE, Munafò MR, DeYoung CG, Fossella JA, Fan J, Gray JR. Using genetic data in cognitive neuroscience: from growing pains to genuine insights. Nat Rev Neurosci. 2008;9(9):710–20.
12. Cirulli ET, Kasperavičiūte D, Attix DK, Need AC, Ge D, Gibson G, Goldstein DB. Common genetic variation and performance on standardized cognitive tests. Eur J Hum Genet. 2010;18(7):815–20.
13. Sysoeva OV, Tonevitsky AG, Wackermann J. Genetic determinants of time perception mediated by the serotonergic system. PLoS One. 2010;5(9): e12650.
14. Rammsayer TH. Effects of body core temperature and brain dopamine activity on timing processes in humans. Biol Psychol. 1997;46(2):169–92.
15. Teixeira S, Machado S, Paes F, Velasques B, Silva JG, Sanfim AL, Minc D, Anghinah R, Menegaldo LL, Salama M, Cagy M, Nardi AE, Pöppel E, Bao Y, Szelag E, Ribeiro P, Arias-Carrión O. Time perception distortion in neuropsychiatric and neurological disorders. CNS Neurol Disord Drug Targets. 2013;12:567–82.
16. Allman MJ, Teki S, Griffiths TD, Meck WH. Properties of the internal clock: first-and second-order principles of subjective time. Annu Rev Psychol. 2014; 65:743–71.
17. Fontes R, Ribeiro J, Gupta DS, Machado D, Lopes-Júnior F, Magalhães F, Bastos VH, Rocha K, Marinho V, Lima G, Velasques B, Ribeiro P, Orsini M, Pessoa B, Leite MA, Teixeira S. Time perception mechanisms at central nervous system. Neurol Int. 2016;8(1):5939.
18. Jones CRG, Jahanshahi M. Dopamine modulates Striato-frontal functioning during temporal processing. Front Integr Neurosci. 2011;5:70.
19. Bender S, Rellum T, Freitag C, Resch F, Rietschel M, Treutlein J, Jennen-Steinmetz C, Brandeis D, Banaschewski T, Laucht M. Time-resolved influences of functional DAT1 and COMT variants on visual perception and post-processing. PLoS One. 2012;7(7):e41552.
20. Maksimov M, Vaht M, Murd C, Harro J, Bachmann T. Brain dopaminergic system related genetic variability interacts with target/mask timing in metacontrast masking. Neuropsychologia. 2015;71:112–8.
21. Wiener M, Lohoff FW, Coslett HB. Double dissociation of dopamine genes and timing in humans. J Cogn Neurosci. 2011;23:2811–21.
22. Wiener M, Lee YS, Lohoff FW, Coslett HB. Individual differences in the morphometry and activation of time perception networks are influenced by dopamine genotype. Neuroimage. 2014;89:10–22.
23. Drew MR, Simpson EH, Kellendonk C, Herzberg WG, Lipatova O, Fairhurst S, Kandel ER, Malapani C, Balsam PD. Transient overexpression of striatal D2 receptors impairs operant motivation and interval timing. J Neurosci. 2007; 27:7731–9.
24. Hildebrandt A, Kiy A, Reuter M, Sommer W, Wilhelm O. Face and emotion expression processing and the serotonin transporter polymorphism 5-HTTLPR/rs22531. Genes Brain Behav. 2016;15(5):453–64.
25. Price JS, Strong J, Eliassen J, McQueeny T, Miller M, Padula CB, Shear P, Lisdahl K. Serotonin transporter gene moderates associations between mood, memory, and hippocampal volume. Behav Brain Res. 2013;242: 158–65.
26. Schürks M, Frahnow A, Diener HC, Kurth T, Rosskopf D, Grabe HJ. Bi-allelic and tri-allelic 5-HTTLPR polymorphisms and triptan non-response in a cluster headache. J Headache Pain. 2014;21(15):46.
27. Beevers CG, Gibb BE, McGeary JE, Miller IW. Serotonin transporter genetic variation and biased attention for emotional word stimuli among psychiatric inpatients. J Abnorm Psychol. 2007;116(1):208–12.
28. Heinz A, Braus DF, Smolka MN, Wrase J, Puls I, Hermann D, Klein S, Grüsser SM, Flor H, Schumann G, Mann K, Büchel C. Amygdala prefrontal coupling depends on a genetic variation of the serotonin transporter. Nat Neurosci. 2005;8:20–1.
29. Anderson DE, Bell TA, Awh E. Polymorphisms in the 5-HTTLPR gene mediate storage capacity of visual working memory. J Cogn Neurosci. 2012; 24(5):1069–76.
30. Crişan LG, Pana S, Vulturar R, Heilman RM, Szekely R, Druga B, Dragoş N, Miu AC. Genetic contributions of the serotonin transporter to social learning of fear and economic decision making. Soc Cogn Affect Neurosci. 2009;4(4):399–408.

31. Lochner C, Hemmings S, Seedat S, Kinnear C, Schoeman R, Annerbrink K, Olsson M, Eriksson E, Moolman-Smook J, Allgulander C, Stein DJ. Genetics and personality traits in patients with social anxiety disorder: a case-control study in South Africa. Eur Neuropsychopharmacol. 2007;17(5):321–7.

32. Sysoeva OV, Maluchenko NV, Timofeeva MA, Portnova GV, Kulikova MA, Tonevitsky AG, Ivanitsky AM. Aggression and 5HTT polymorphism in females: a study of synchronized swimming and control groups. Int J Psychophysiol. 2009;72(2):173–8.

33. Seripa D, Pilotto A, Paroni G, Fontana A, D'Onofrio G, Gravina C, Urbano M, Cascavilla L, Paris F, Panza F, Padovani A, Pilotto A. Role of the serotonin transporter gene locus in the response to SSRI treatment of major depressive disorder in late life. J Psychopharmacol. 2015;29(5):623–33.

34. Nomura M, Kaneko M, Okuma Y, Nomura J, Kusumi I, Koyama T, Nomura Y. Involvement of serotonin transporter gene polymorphisms (5-HTT) in impulsive behavior in the Japanese population. PLoS One. 2015;10(3):e0119743.

35. Althaus M, Groen Y, Wijers AA, Mulder LJ, Minderaa RB, Kema IP, Dijck JD, Hartman CA, Hoekstra PJ. Differential effects of 5-HTTLPR and DRD2/ANKK1 polymorphisms on electrocortical measures of error and feedback processing in children. Clin Neurophysiol. 2009;120:93–107.

36. Burt SA, Mikolajewski AJ. Preliminary evidence that specific candidate genes are associated with adolescent-onset antisocial behavior. Aggress Behav. 2008;34(4):437–45.

37. Bekinschtein P, Renner MC, Gonzalez MC, Weisstaub N. Role of medial prefrontal cortex serotonin 2A receptors in the control of retrieval of recognition memory in rats. J Neurosci. 2013;33(40):15716–25.

38. Polesskaya OO, Sokolov BP. Differential expression of the "C" and "T" alleles of the 5-HT2A receptor gene in the temporal cortex of normal individuals and schizophrenics. J Neurosci Res. 2002;67(6):812–22.

39. Chun MM. Visual working memory as visual attention sustained over time. Neuropsychologia. 2011;49:1407–9.

40. Moreau AW, Amar M, Le Roux N, Morel N, Fossier P. Serotoninergic fine-tuning of the excitation-inhibition balance in rat visual cortical networks. Cereb Cortex. 2010;20(2):456–67.

41. Goldman N, Glei DA, Lin YH, Weinstein M. The serotonin transporter polymorphism (5-HTTLPR): allelic variation and links with depressive symptoms. Depress Anxiety. 2010;27(3):260–9.

42. Kometer M, Schmidt A, Jäncke L, Vollenweider FX. Activation of serotonin 2A receptors underlies the psilocybin-induced effects on α oscillations, N170 visual-evoked potentials, and visual hallucinations. J Neurosci. 2013;33(25):10544–51.

43. Addyman C, Rocha S, Mareschal D. Mapping the origins of time: scalar errors in infant time estimation. Dev Psychol. 2014;30:a0037108.

44. Drew MR, Fairhurst S, Malapani C, Horvitz JC, Balsam PD. Effects of dopamine antagonists on the timing of two intervals. Pharmacol Biochem Behav. 2003;75(1):9–15.

45. Richter A, Richter S, Barman A, Soch J, Klein M, Assmann A, Libeau C, Behnisch G, Wüstenberg T, Seidenbecher CI, Schott BH. Motivational salience and genetic variability of dopamine D2 receptor expression interact in the modulation of interference processing. Front Hum Neurosci. 2013;5(7):250.

46. Pan YQ, Qiao L, Xue XD, Fu JH. Association between ANKK1 (rs1800497) polymorphism of DRD2 gene and attention deficit hyperactivity disorder: a meta-analysis. Neurosci Lett. 2015;590(17):101–5.

47. Shih MC, Hoexter MQ, Andrade LA, Bressan RA. Parkinson's disease and dopamine transporter neuroimaging: a critical review. Sao Paulo Med J. 2006;124(3):168–75.

48. Greenwood TA, Badner JA, Byerley W, Keck PE, McElroy SL, Remick RA, Dessa Sadovnick A, Kelsoe JR. Heritability and linkage analysis of personality in bipolar disorder. J Affect Disord. 2013;151(2):748–55.

49. Fehér Á, Juhász A, Pákáski M, Kálmán J, Janka Z. Association between the 9 repeat allele of the dopamine transporter 40bp variable tandem repeat polymorphism and Alzheimer's disease. Psychiatry Res. 2014;220(1–2):730–1.

50. Maitra S, Sarkar K, Ghosh P, Karmakar A, Bhattacharjee A, Sinha S, Mukhopadhyay K. Potential contribution of dopaminergic gene variants in ADHD core traits and co-morbidity: a study on eastern Indian probands. Cell Mol Neurobiol. 2014;34(4):549–64.

51. Faraone SV, Spencer TJ, Madras BK, Zhang-James Y, Biederman J. Functional effects of dopamine transporter gene genotypes on in vivo dopamine transporter functioning: a meta-analysis. Mol Psychiatry. 2014;19:880–9.

52. Franke B, Hoogman M, Arias Vasquez A, Heister JG, Savelkoul PJ, Naber M, Scheffer H, Kiemeney LA, Kan CC, Kooij JJ, Buitelaar JK. Association of the dopamine transporter (SLC6A3/DAT1) gene 9–6 haplotype with adult ADHD. Am J Med Genet B Neuropsychiatr Genet. 2008;147B(8):1576–9.

53. Kanai R, Lloyd H, Bueti D, Walsh V. Modality-independent role of the primary auditory cortex in time estimation. Exp Brain Res. 2011;209(3):465–71.

54. Barzman D, Geise C, Lin P. Review of the genetic basis of emotion dysregulation in children and adolescents. World J Psychiatry. 2015;5(1):112–7.

55. Liu L, Cheng J, Su Y, Ji N, Gao Q, Li H, Yang L, Sun L, Qian Q, Wang Y. Deficiency of Sustained Attention in ADHD and Its Potential Genetic Contributor MAOA. J Atten Disord. 2018;22(9):878–85.

56. Wang LJ, Lee SY, Chen SL, Chang YH, Chen PS, Huang SY, Tzeng NS, Chen KC, Lee IH, Wang TY, Yang YK, Lu RB. A potential interaction between COMT and MTHFR genetic variants in Han Chinese patients with bipolar II disorder. Sci Rep. 2015;5(6):8813.

57. Rammsayer TH. On dopaminergic modulation of temporal information processing. Biol Psychol. 1993;36:209–22.

58. Agostino PV, Cheng RK. Contributions of dopaminergic signaling to timing accuracy and precision. Current Opinion in Behavioral Sciences. 2016;8:153–60.

59. Valenzuela FJ, Vera J, Venegas C, Muñoz S, Oyarce S, Muñoz K, Lagunas C. Evidences of polymorphism associated with circadian system and risk of pathologies: a review of the literature. Int J Endocrinol. 2016;2016:2746909.

60. Hu Y, Shmygelska A, Tran D, Eriksson N, Tung JY, Hinds DA. GWAS of 89,283 individuals identifies genetic variants associated with self-reporting of being a morning person. Nat Commun. 2016;7:10448.

61. Karthikeyan R, Marimuthu G, Ramasubramanian C, Arunachal G, BaHammam AS, Spence DW, Cardinali DP, Brown GM, Pandi-Perumal SR. Association of Per3 length polymorphism with bipolar I disorder and schizophrenia. Neuropsychiatr Dis Treat. 2014;10:2325–30.

62. Ofte HK, Tronvik E, Alstadhaug KB. Lack of association between a cluster headache and PER3 clock gene polymorphism. J Headache Pain. 2015;17:18.

63. Ozburn AR, Purohit K, Parekh PK, Kaplan GN, Falcon E, Mukherjee S, Cates HM, McClung CA. Functional implications of the CLOCK 3111T/C single-nucleotide polymorphism. Front Psychiatry. 2016;7:67.

64. Karatsoreos IN. Links between Circadian Rhythms and Psychiatric Disease. Front Behav Neurosci. 2014;8:162.

65. Agostino PV, Golombek DA, Meck WH. Unwinding the molecular basis of interval and circadian timing. Front Integr Neurosci. 2011;5:64.

66. Späti J, Aritake S, Meyer AH, Kitamura S, Hida A, Higuchi S, Moriguchi Y, Mishima K. Modeling circadian and sleep-homeostatic effects on short-term interval timing. Front Integr Neurosci. 2015;9:15.

67. Golombek DA, Bussi IL, Agostino PV. Minutes, days and years: molecular interactions among different scales of biological timing. Philos Trans R Soc Lond Ser B Biol Sci. 2014;369(1637):20120465.

68. Wilsmore BR, Grunstein RR, Fransen M, Woodward M, Norton R, Ameratunga S. Sleep habits, insomnia, and daytime sleepiness in a large and healthy community-based sample of new Zealanders. J Clin Sleep Med. 2013;9(6):559–66.

69. Wang H, Chen HOS. Association of clock gene polymorphism with insulin resistance in hypertension: a case-control study. J Hypertens. 2016;34:33–9.

70. Li J, Huang C, Lan Y, Wang Y. A cross-sectional study on the relationships among the polymorphism of period2 gene, work stress, and insomnia. Sleep Breath. 2015;19(4):1399–406.

71. Song HM, Cho CH, Lee HJ, Moon JH, Kang SG, Yoon HK, Park YM, Kim L. Association of CLOCK, ARNTL, PER2, and GNB3 polymorphisms with diurnal preference in a Korean population. Chronobiol Int. 2016;33(10):1455–63.

72. Agostino PV, do Nascimento M, Bussi IL, Eguía MC, Golombek DA. Circadian modulation of interval timing in mice. Brain Res. 2011;1370:154–63.

73. Kuriyama K, Uchiyama M, Suzuki H, Tagaya H, Ozaki A, Aritake S, Shibui K, Xin T, Lan L, Kamei Y, Takahashi K. Diurnal fluctuation of time perception under 30-h sustained wakefulness. Neurosci Res. 2005;53(2):123–8.

74. Bussi IL, Levín G, Golombek DA, Agostino PV. Involvement of dopamine signaling in the circadian modulation of interval timing. Eur J Neurosci. 2014;40(1):2299–310.

75. Tucci V, Buhusi CV, Gallistel R, Meck WH. Towards an integrated understanding of the biology of timing. Philos Trans R Soc Lond Ser B Biol Sci. 2014;369(1637):20120470.

76. Valomon A, Holst SC, Bachmann V, Viola AU, Schmidt C, Zürcher J, Berger W, Cajochen C, Landolt HP. Genetic polymorphisms of DAT1 and COMT differentially associate with actigraphy-derived sleep-wake cycles in young adults. Chronobiol Int. 2014;31(5):705–14.

77. Terhune DB, Russo S, Near J, Stagg CJ, Cohen KR. GABA predicts time perception. J Neurosci. 2014;34(12):4364–70.

78. Tsang SY, Zhong S, Mei L, Chen J, Ng SK, Pun FW, Zhao C, Jing B, Chark R, Guo J, Tan Y, Li L, Wang C, Chew SH, Xue H. Social cognitive role of schizophrenia candidate gene GABRB2. PLoS One. 2013;8(4):e62322.

79. DeWoskin D, Myung J, Belle MD, Piggins HD, Takumi T, Forger DB. Distinct roles for GABA across multiple timescales in mammalian circadian timekeeping. Proc Natl Acad Sci U S A. 2015;112(29):E3911–9.

80. Block RA, Grondin S. Timing and time perception: a selective review and commentary on recent reviews. Front Psychol. 2014;5:648.

81. Gupta DS. Processing of sub- and supra-second intervals in the primate brain results from the calibration of neuronal oscillators via sensory, motor, and feedback processes. Front Psychol. 2014;5:816.

82. Gupta DS, Chen L. 2016. Brain oscillations in perception, timing and action. Current Opinion in Behavioral Sciences. 2016;8:161–6.

83. Kononowicz TW, Van Wassenhove V. In search of oscillatory traces of the internal clock. Front Psychol. 2016;7:224.

84. Chen Y, Huang X. Modulation of alpha and Beta oscillations during an n-back task with varying temporal memory load. Front Psychol. 2015;6:2031.

85. Lacey MG, Gooding-Williams G, Prokic EJ, Yamawaki N, Hall SD, Stanford IM, Woodhall GL. Spike firing and IPSPs in layer V pyramidal neurons during beta oscillations in rat primary motor cortex (M1) in vitro. PLoS One. 2014;9: e85109.

86. Kraja AT, Borecki IB, Province MA. Microsatellite linkage analysis, single-nucleotide polymorphisms, and haplotype associations with ECB21 in the COGA data. BMC Genet. 2005;6(1):S94.

87. Kononowicz TW, van Rijn H. Decoupling interval timing and climbing neural activity: a dissociation between CNV and N1P2 amplitudes. J Neurosci. 2014; 34:2931–9.

88. Buzsáki G, Wang XJ. Mechanisms of gamma oscillations. Annu Rev Neurosci. 2012;35:203–25.

89. van Loon AM, Scholte HS, van Gaal S, van der Hoort BJ, Lamme VA. GABAA agonist reduces visual awareness: a masking-EEG experiment. J Cogn Neurosci. 2012;24:965–74.

90. Giersch A, Herzog MH. Lorazepam strongly prolongs visual information processing. Neuropsychopharmacology. 2004;29:1386–94.

91. Heaney CF, Kinney JW. Role of GABA(B) receptors in learning and memory and neurological disorders. Neurosci Biobehav Rev. 2016;63:1–28.

92. Oblak A, Gibbs TT, Blatt GJ. Reduced serotonin receptor subtypes in a limbic and a neocortical region in autism. Autism Res. 2013;6(6):571–83.

93. Unschuld PG, Ising M, Specht M, Erhardt A, Ripke S, Heck A, Kloiber S, Straub V, Brueckl T, Müller-Myhsok B, Holsboer F, Binder EB. Polymorphisms in the GAD2 gene-region are associated with susceptibility for unipolar depression and with a risk factor for anxiety disorders. Am J Med Genet B Neuropsychiatr Genet. 2009;150B(8): 1100–9.

94. Sadeghi NG, Pariyadath V, Apte S, Eagleman DM, Cook EP. Neural correlates of subsecond time distortion in the middle temporal area of visual cortex. J Cogn Neurosci. 2011;23:3829–40.

95. Mayo JP, Sommer MA. Neuronal correlates of visual time perception at brief timescales. Proc Natl Acad Sci U.S.A. 2013;110:1506–11.

96. Eagleman DM, Pariyadath V. Is subjective duration a signature of coding efficiency? Philos Trans R Soc B. 2009;364:1841–51.

97. Watson TD, Petrakis IL, Edgecombe J, Perrino A, Krystal JH, Mathalon DH. Modulation of the cortical processing of novel and target stimuli by drugs affecting glutamate and GABA neurotransmission. Int J Neuropsychopharmacol. 2009;12:357–70.

98. Muthukumaraswamy SD, Edden RA, Jones DK, Swettenham JB, Singh KD. Resting GABA concentration predicts peak gamma frequency and fMRI amplitude in response to visual stimulation. Proc Natl Acad Sci U.S.A. 2009; 106:8356–61.

99. Yizhar O, Fenno LE, Prigge M, Schneider F, Davidson TJ, O'Shea DJ, Sohal VS, Goshen I, Finkelstein J, Paz JT, Stehfest K, Fudim R, Ramakrishnan C, Huguenard JR, Hegemann P, Deisseroth K. Neocortical excitation/inhibition balance in information processing and social dysfunction. Nature. 2011;477: 171–8.

100. Kondo HM, Kitagawa N, Kitamura MS, Koizumi A, Nomura M, Kashino M. Separability and commonality of auditory and visual bistable perception. Cereb Cortex. 2012;22(8):1915–22.

101. Berryhill ME, Jones KT. tDCS selectively improves working memory in older adults with more education. Neurosci Lett. 2012;521:148–51.

102. Stelzel C, Basten U, Montag C, Reuter M, Fiebach CJ. Frontostriatal involvement in task switching depends on genetic differences in D2 receptor density. J Neurosci. 2010;30(42):14205–12.

5

Tumor xenograft animal models for esophageal squamous cell carcinoma

Nikki P. Lee*(ID), Chung Man Chan, Lai Nar Tung, Hector K. Wang and Simon Law

Abstract

Esophageal squamous cell carcinoma (ESCC) is the predominant subtype of esophageal cancer worldwide and highly prevalent in less developed regions. Management of ESCC is challenging and involves multimodal treatments. Patient prognosis is generally poor especially for those diagnosed in advanced disease stage. One factor contributing to this clinical dismal is the incomplete understanding of disease mechanism, for which this situation is further compounded by the presence of other limiting factors for disease diagnosis, patient prognosis and treatments. Tumor xenograft animal models including subcutaneous tumor xenograft model, orthotopic tumor xenograft model and patient-derived tumor xenograft model are vital tools for ESCC research. Establishment of tumor xenograft models involves the implantation of human ESCC cells/xenografts/tissues into immunodeficient animals, in which mice are most commonly used. Different tumor xenograft models have their own advantages and limitations, and these features serve as key factors to determine the use of these models at different stages of research. Apart from their routine use on basic research to understand disease mechanism of ESCC, tumor xenograft models are actively employed for undertaking preclinical drug screening project and biomedical imaging research.

Keywords: Subcutaneous tumor xenograft, Orthotopic tumor xenograft, Patient-derived tumor xenograft, ESCC

Background
Esophageal squamous cell carcinoma (ESCC) and its management

Cancer is a life-threatening disease causing about 8 million deaths annually worldwide. Esophageal cancer ranks sixth on the list of top most common causes of cancer-related deaths, contributing approximately half a million deaths each year (GLOBOCAN 2012). Among different subtypes of esophageal cancer, ESCC is the predominant histological type and is highly prevalent in less developed areas especially certain regions in Asia and Africa. Multimodality treatment is offered to ESCC patients. Early stage patients with resectable tumors are treated with upfront tumor resection, while advanced patients on the other hand are first treated with chemotherapy/chemoradiation for tumor downstaging before surgical resection [1, 2]. Although this pre-surgery neoadjuvant treatment can achieve excellent response in subgroups of patients who are sensitive to chemotherapy/

chemoradiation, about one-third of patients still exhibit only partial and suboptimal response. Even for responders of chemotherapy/chemoradiation, some of them may develop resistance in the later course of the treatment period. For those patients whose tumors are unresectable, and when the tumor is refractory to chemotherapy or radiotherapy, no effective treatment is available [3]. To provide more treatment options for patients not amendable by current therapies, new treatment approaches are proposed and evaluated in on-going clinical trials for their anti-tumor efficacies. Even with all these evolving and newly emerged treatment modalities, complete cure of disease is still difficult. In view of this, new treatments are urgently needed.

The use of tumor xenograft animal models for preclinical research

The main purpose of developing tumor xenograft animal models for research is to bridge basic and clinical research and to supplement the use of in vitro model systems [4]. Tumor xenograft animal models provide a more sophisticated platform to study the process of

* Correspondence: nikkilee@hku.hk
Department of Surgery, The University of Hong Kong, Faculty of Medicine Building, 21 Sassoon Road, Pokfulam, Hong Kong

tumorigenesis in an in vivo setting. This platform allows us to have a better understanding on the involvement of certain oncogenes or tumor suppressors in tumor development by uncovering their related signaling pathways and disease mechanisms [5]. Besides, the use of these models can provide us a research tool for preclinical drug response evaluation by determining the anti-tumor efficacies in addition to the drug toxicity, pharmacokinetics and pharmacodynamics [6]. Apart from drug response evaluation, these models can also facilitate biomedical imaging research by providing a model system for testing the usefulness and practicality on new tumor detection methods or reagents.

Mice are the most commonly used animals for tumor xenograft models because of several key advantageous features, such as the presence of comparable genome size with humans, short reproductive cycle, large litter size, low maintenance cost and ease of manipulation [5]. Different mouse strains in unique immunodeficiency backgrounds are used in cancer research, and these include athymic nude mice, SCID mice and NOD/SCID mice (SCID mice with an extra level of immunodeficiency). Among these strains, NOD/SCID mice demonstrate the best immunodeficiency due to the absence or defect in nearly all types of immune cells (B cells, T cells, dendritic cells, macrophages and natural killer cells), followed by SCID mice lacking B cells and T cells and then athymic nude mice without T cells [7]. Due to their various levels of immunodeficiency, different strains are considered for use for different research purposes. Taking into accounts the cost and features of different strains, athymic nude and SCID mice are preferably used for implanting human tumor cell lines, while SCID and NOD/SCID mice are rather used for the transplantation of human tumors.

Commonly used tumor xenograft animal models for ESCC research

Three types of tumor xenograft animal models for ESCC research are developed by implanting ESCC cells/xenografts or patient tumors in immunodeficient animals, namely subcutaneous, orthotopic and patient-derived tumor xenograft model (Fig. 1). Each of them has its own strengths and weaknesses in terms of model features (Table 1), establishment methods (Table 2) and preclinical utilities (Table 3), which place them in a unique position for early stage, mid stage or late stage research [8, 9].

Subcutaneous tumor xenograft model
Subcutaneous tumor xenograft model is a classical animal model for ESCC research. This model is established by implanting ESCC cells/xenografts under the skin of the immunodeficient animals to develop subcutaneous

tumors. The procedure of establishing subcutaneous tumor is technically simple as it only involves needle injection of ESCC cells or direct implantation of ESCC xenografts under the skin of animals. The growth of subcutaneous tumors can be performed non-invasively by using an electronic caliper to measure the palpable tumors. These technical procedures of tumor establishment and monitoring can maintain the reproducibility and effectiveness (both time and cost) of this model. Despite these advantages, this model suffers certain limitations as it does not fully represent the clinical situation. For instance, this model associates reduced tumor heterogeneity as in most scenarios homogeneous ESCC cell lines are used as the source material. Besides, subcutaneous tumors do not grow in their native tumor microenvironment and this makes them not suitable for the study of tumor-stromal interactions. With such strengths and weaknesses [8], this model is mainly used in early stage research to study the biology and mechanism of ESCC tumorigenesis.

Accumulating reports have revealed the mileage of applying subcutaneous tumor xenograft model for early stage research by using it to study tumor properties of ESCC-related molecules and their associated disease mechanisms. Overexpression of microRNA-340, a microRNA downregulated in ESCC tumors, in EC9706 ESCC cells inhibited the growth properties of these cells in a subcutaneous tumor xenograft model. The effect of this microRNA on ESCC was mediated in part via its effect on a protein transferase PSAT1, which was identified in the same study as a direct target of microRNA-340 [10]. Another study demonstrated faster growth of subcutaneous tumors derived from KYSE-30 ESCC cells with overexpression of a matrix metalloproteinase MMP1 when compared to the control cells. In addition, these MMP1-overexpressing ESCC cells also exhibited metastatic potentials. The ability of MMP1 to promote tumor progression and metastasis was concordantly revealed to be due to its stimulating effect on a tumorigenic pathway involving PI3K and AKT [11]. A separate report also utilized subcutaneous tumor xenograft model to reveal cellular retinoic acid binding protein 2 (CRABP2) as a tumor suppressor by showing slower growth rate of subcutaneous tumors derived from EC109 ESCC cells overexpressing CRABP2 when compared to the control experimental group [12]. These studies collectively signify the usefulness of this model on studying ESCC-related molecules and their related mechanisms in ESCC.

Apart from the use of subcutaneous tumor xenograft model for tumor biology study, attempts have been made for using this model to investigate the anti-tumor efficacies of new treatment methods or compounds/drugs for treating ESCC. Subcutaneous tumor-bearing

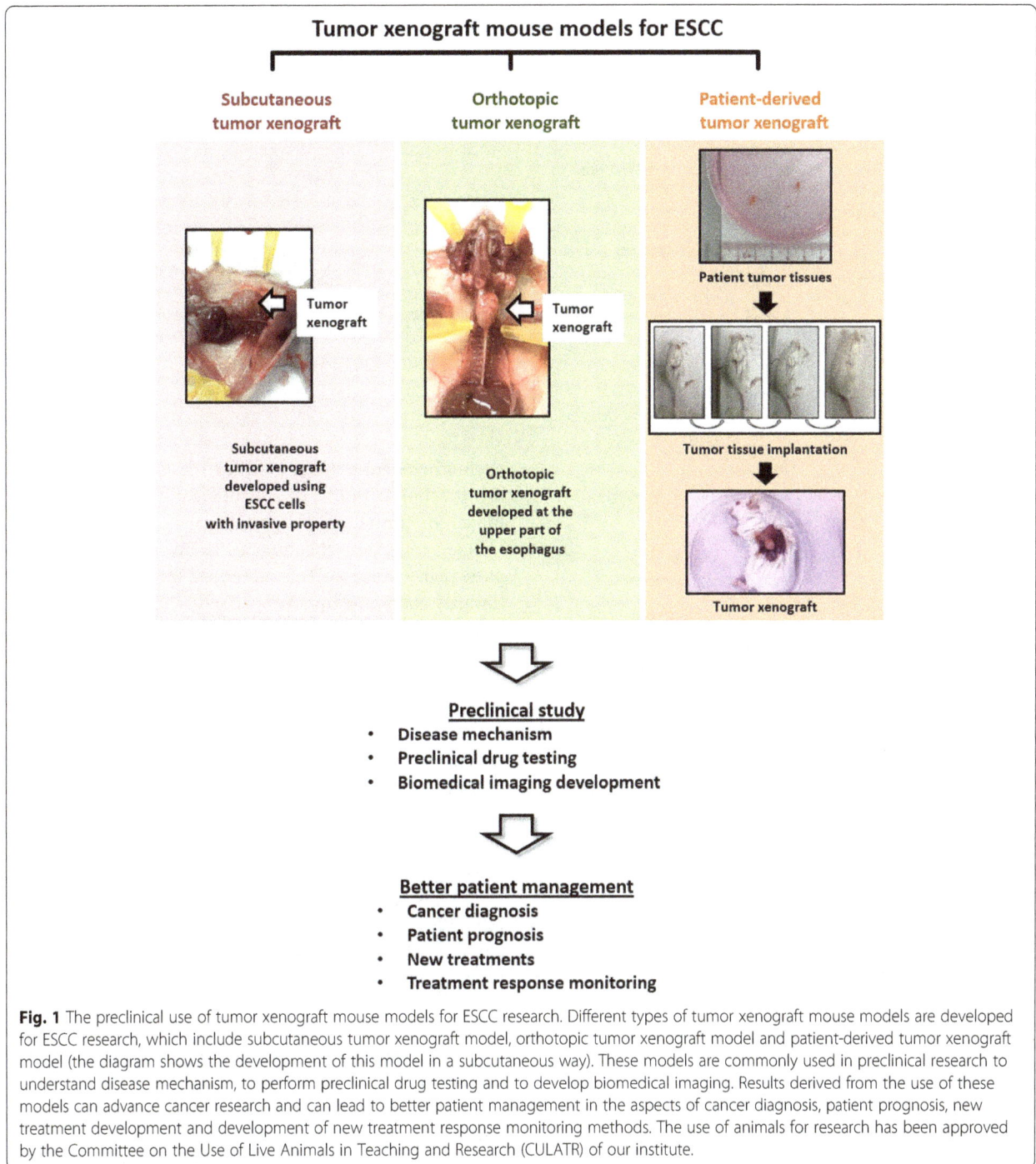

Fig. 1 The preclinical use of tumor xenograft mouse models for ESCC research. Different types of tumor xenograft mouse models are developed for ESCC research, which include subcutaneous tumor xenograft model, orthotopic tumor xenograft model and patient-derived tumor xenograft model (the diagram shows the development of this model in a subcutaneous way). These models are commonly used in preclinical research to understand disease mechanism, to perform preclinical drug testing and to develop biomedical imaging. Results derived from the use of these models can advance cancer research and can lead to better patient management in the aspects of cancer diagnosis, patient prognosis, new treatment development and development of new treatment response monitoring methods. The use of animals for research has been approved by the Committee on the Use of Live Animals in Teaching and Research (CULATR) of our institute.

mice were subjected to treatment to induce the expression of an ESCC prognostic marker microRNA-375 and smaller tumor size was obtained at the end of the experiment when compared to control experiment [13]. Apart from the routine use to examine new treatment methods, this model was also applied to investigate the anti-tumor efficacies of new compounds/drugs for counteracting ESCC, such as temsirolimus currently used for renal cell carcinoma patients [14]. Besides its utility on anti-tumorigenecity testing, this model can be applied to examine the chemo-sensitizing effects of test compounds. Treatment of subcutaneous tumor-bearing animals with Ginsenoside Rg3, an ingredient extracted from ginseng, provided evidence demonstrating the sensitizing effects of this compound to two chemotherapeutic drugs paclitaxel and cisplatin commonly used for ESCC patients [15]. More recently, a novel oxygen carrier YQ23 was shown to exert chemo-sensitizing effects

Table 1 Key features of tumor xenograft models for ESCC research

Tumor xenograft models	Key features
Subcutaneous	*Advantages*
	• easy to establish
	• low cost
	• palpable tumor for easy tumor size measurement
	Limitation
	• incorrect tumor microenvironment
Orthotopic	*Advantage*
	• correct tumor microenvironment
	Limitations
	• technique demanding
	• high cost
	• specialized imaging systems required for tumor size measurement
Patient-derived	*Advantage*
	• high resemblance to patient tumor
	Limitations
	• long latency period
	• limited engraftment rate
	• high cost
	• use of patient specimen

This table lists the key features of different tumor xenograft models for ESCC research based on comprehensive reviews on tumor xenograft models for cancer research [8, 35]

Table 3 Uses of different tumor xenograft models for preclinical drug testing for ESCC

Tumor xenograft models	Test compounds/drugs	References
Subcutaneous	Temsirolimus	[14]
Subcutaneous	YQ23 alone or combined with cisplatin or 5-fluorouracil	[16]
Subcutaneous	Ginsenoside Rg3 alone or combined with paclitaxel and cisplatin	[15]
Subcutaneous	Afatinib	[39]
Orthotopic	Temsirolimus	[14]
Patient-derived	Lapatinib alone and in combination with 5-fluorouracil or oxaliplatin	[25]
Patient-derived	Cisplatin and 5-fluorouracil	[26]
Patient-derived	Trastuzumab	[27]

chemotherapeutic drugs used for ESCC have highlighted the preclinical utility of subcutaneous tumor xenograft model for compound/drug testing.

Taken together, subcutaneous tumor xenograft models particularly those well characterized for their sensitivities towards chemotherapeutics currently used for ESCC are valuable research tools for studying tumor biology and disease mechanisms of ESCC in an in vivo setting and for performing preclinical anti-tumor efficacy studies (Table 3).

selectively on chemo-resistant subcutaneous SLMT-1 ESCC xenografts, but not chemo-sensitive HKESC-2 ESCC xenografts, in treatment plans using cisplatin or 5-fluorouracil, which are also traditional chemotherapeutic drugs used for ESCC patients [16]. The above studies examining the anti-tumor efficacies of test compounds/drugs alone or in combination with common

Orthotopic tumor xenograft model

Orthotopic tumor xenograft model is an alternate animal cancer model used for ESCC research. This model is established by implanting ESCC cells/xenografts in the esophagus of the immunodeficient animals to develop orthotopic tumors. The procedure of establishing orthotopic tumors is more technically demanding when compared to those needed for establishing subcutaneous tumors, as it requires small animal surgery and/or anesthesia. Two main approaches are employed to implant ESCC cells/xenografts in the animal esophagus, for which they differ at the site of tumor implantation. One method implants ESCC cells/xenografts in the upper region of the esophagus [17, 18], while the other implants ESCC cells/xenografts in the lower end of the esophagus at the abdominal region near the gastroesophageal junction [19–22]. Recently, we have also reported the survival comparison between animals with orthotopic tumor developed at the upper esophageal region and the lower region, and found that those with tumor at the abdominal region have better survival [23]. Although it is more time and labor intensive to establish orthotopic tumors, this model can accommodate the study of tumor growth in a correct tumor microenvironment as in the clinical situation and enable the study of tumor-stromal interactions [8]. However, it also suffers

Table 2 Technical details for establishing ESCC tumor xenograft models

Tumor xenograft model	Technical details	References
Subcutaneous	Starting material: human ESCC cell line	[36, 37]
	Injected cell number: 2×10^6	
	Mouse strain: nude, SCID, NOD/SCID	
	Cell injection site: flank	
Orthotopic	Starting material: Human ESCC cell line	[23]
	Mouse strain: nude	
	Tumor development site: cervical and abdominal esophagus	
Patient-derived	Starting material: Human ESCC tumor tissue	[37, 38]
	Mouse strain: NOD/SCID	
	Tumor implantation method: subcutaneous	

This table shows some examples from representative publications and does not mean to be inclusive

from the same limitation as the subcutaneous model by using ESCC cell lines as the source materials for tumor establishment. Another major disadvantage of this model is the need to use specialized imaging methods, e.g. the in vivo imaging system coupled with the use of bio-luminescent technology [19, 20, 22], to monitor tumor growth. Despite these limitations, the strengths of this model make it a valuable animal model for use in mid to late stage research.

Although orthotopic tumor xenograft model offers superior advantages in comparing with the subcutaneous model, its use remains restricted due to the above mentioned limitations. Despite these shortcomings, an expanding number of reports have exemplified the application of this model for studying ESCC tumorigenesis and for performing preclinical anti-tumorigenecity testing. When this model was used to reveal the tumor suppressing effect of a transmembrane protease DESC1, slower tumor growth rate was observed with the use of DESC1-expressing KYSE-150 ESCC cells when compared to those using control cells [22]. In an independent study using this model to examine the tumor phenotype of a tumor-related protein kinase AKT, an obvious tumor-suppressing effect was found associated with the knockdown of AKT, such that a reduced growth rate of orthotopic tumors was readily detected [19]. Aside its use to study tumor growth, this model can be applied to investigate the mechanism of tumor invasion. A comprehensive study pointed out the involvement of a cell surface molecule CD44H on tumor invasion based on the invasive patterns observed between orthotopic tumors derived from T.T ESCC cells and the invasive counterpart T.T-1 ESCC cells. T.T-1 ESCC cell line expressed high level of CD44H and was derived from tumor cells isolated from cervical lymph node in a T.T ESCC cells-derived orthotopic tumor xenograft model [17]. On top of its use to study tumor growth and invasion, this model is capable to assess the effects of test compounds on post-treatment survivals. A prolonged survival was observed in orthotopic ESCC tumor-bearing animals after treatment with an mTOR inhibitor temsirolimus, for which this inhibitor is currently used for renal cell carcinoma [14].

Generally, orthotopic tumor xenograft model supplements the regular use of subcutaneous model for the study of ESCC by providing a correct tumor microenvironment. In addition, this model functions as an indispensable tool in preclinical research for examining the anti-tumor effects of test compounds/drugs (Table 3).

Patient-derived tumor xenograft model

Patient-derived tumor xenograft model is a more advanced animal cancer model than the above mentioned models for ESCC research. This model is established with the use of ESCC tumors resected from patients to develop tumor xenografts in immunodeficient animals. The patient tumors can be implanted subcutaneously or orthotopically. Depending on the tumor implantation site, this model also retains certain features as the subcutaneous and orthotopic tumor xenograft models. Remarkably, tumor xenografts derived from patient tumors have preserved genetic, histological and phenotypic properties as the donor tumors. Since the stromal and cell components of the patient-derived tumor xenografts are maintained as in the donor tumors, the use of this model can exclude the disadvantages associated with the use of homogeneous tumor cell lines. Despite these advantages, this model inevitably suffers from several limitations [5, 7, 8]. The model establishment requires the use of resected patient tumors, for which some basic research laboratories may not have access to this specimen source. Besides, the engraftment rates of the patient tumors to form tumor xenografts are suboptimal and vary depending on a number of factors, such as tumor types, tumor implantation sites, mouse strains, tumor features and patient features [7]. Even for a patient tumor that can be successfully engrafted, it requires a long latency period to grow into a tumor xenograft and sometimes this process can last for as long as 6 months. Therefore, the above limitations have made the tumor establishment process a high cost and labor intensive procedure. Despite these downsides, this model is gradually replacing other animal cancer models to be used in mid and late stage research and is especially beneficial for the preclinical evaluation of anti-tumor efficacies of new compounds/drugs. Indeed, this model is sometimes referred to "clinical trials in a mouse" due to its superior power to predict clinical response of test compounds/drugs due to the high resemblance between tumor xenografts and donor tumors [8].

Considering all the pros and cons, patient-derived tumor xenograft model can provide us a research platform not only for studying the disease mechanisms of ESCC but can also facilitate preclinical drug screening. For the latter application, this model is more preferably used than the subcutaneous and orthotopic models due to its high clinical relevance, which supports its use on evaluating the anti-tumor efficacies of new compounds/drugs. In this area, individual research teams have established their own collections of patient-derived tumor xenograft models with preserved tumor heterogeneity for screening drugs or drug combinations for ESCC [24–27] (Table 4).

The patient-derived tumor xenograft models with well characterized molecular deregulations commonly found in ESCC can be used as a tool for testing currently used drugs for their new uses on ESCC. This process is important as it can research for new drugs for patients

Table 4 Collections of patient-derived tumor xenograft models for ESCC

Number of established models	Characterized deregulations	References
37	EGFR, K-ras, B-raf and PIK3CA mutation HER2 expression	[26]
25	HER2 expression and amplification	[27]
5	EGFR, K-ras, B-raf and PIK3CA mutation HER2 expression and amplification	[27]

Abbreviations used: *EGFR* epidermal growth factor receptor, *HER2* human epidermal growth factor receptor 2 *PIK3CA* phosphatidylinositol-4,5-bisphosphate 3-kinase catalytic subunit alpha

who are resistant to current drug treatments. Cisplatin and 5-fluorouracil are two chemotherapeutic drugs used for ESCC, however not all patients have good drug responses. To have a better understanding on the drug mechanism, Zhang et al. established a panel of patient-derived tumor xenograft models and well characterized them for common genetic aberrations frequently detected in ESCC, such as HER2 expression and mutations of EGFR (epidermal growth factor receptor), K-ras, B-raf and PIK3CA (phosphatidylinositol-4,5-bisphosphate 3-kinase catalytic subunit alpha). Using a panel of xenografts with well characterized HER2 and PIK3CA status to examine the treatment effect of cisplatin and 5-fluorouracil, tumor xenografts negative for HER2 and carrying wild-type PIK3CA were more sensitive to such treatment when comparing to HER2-positive xenografts irrespective of the mutation status of PIK3CA [26]. Results derived from this study have revealed the link between tumor genetic compositions and chemotherapeutic drug responses.

Apart from the use of patient-derived tumor xenograft models with defined genetic compositions for testing conventional chemotherapeutic drugs, these models have been used to examine the anti-tumor efficacies of drugs that are not clinically used for ESCC, such as trastuzumab and lapatinib. Testing the effect of trastuzumab on patient-derived tumor xenografts revealed HER2-positive ESCC was responsive to such treatment, but not for those carrying concurrent PIK3CA mutation. Further treatment of these HER2-positive and PIK3CA-mutated tumor xenografts with AKT inhibitor AZD5363 subsequently rendered the xenografts to be responsive to trastuzumab treatment again [27]. Another study examined the sensitizing effect of lapatinib on chemotherapeutic drugs oxaliplatin or 5-fluorouracil using a patient-derived tumor xenograft model. Combined treatment of lapatinib with 5-fluorouracil led to a more potent growth inhibitory effect than lapatinib alone or its combined treatment with oxaliplatin [25]. These studies have clearly presented the usefulness of these models for preclinical drug testing. Importantly, such testing on tumor xenografts with defined genetic backgrounds can facilitate the development of precision medicine by selecting drug treatment based on the genetic deregulations of the tumors.

Patient-derived tumor xenograft models can mimic the genetic diversity and composition of the clinical settings due to the high histological and pathological relevance between donor tumors and the established tumor xenografts. These earlier studies have put forth the preclinical application of these models for evaluating the anti-tumor efficacies of different drugs/compounds (Table 3). Derived results can also provide solid evidences supporting the use of new drugs/compounds for treatment of ESCC. Such preclinical test therefore forms a vital platform prior to clinical trials.

Conclusions
Conclusions and future perspectives
Tumor xenograft animal models remain indispensable tools for biomedical research and provide a fundamental platform for preclinical drug screening. Mainly, three broad types of tumor xenograft models, i.e. subcutaneous, orthotopic and patient-derived, are available and routinely used for ESCC research. Although these models are established in immunodeficient animals using human ESCC cells/xenografts/tissues, each of them indeed associate distinct advantages and disadvantages. The unique features of each model support its respective use in different stages of research. However, care must be taken when analyzing the results derived from different tumor xenograft studies as certain variables can affect the result interpretation and reproducibility. These variables can be tumor implantation sites, tumor properties, tumor origins and several others [6]. To expedite the utility of tumor xenograft models for preclinical drug testing, extra efforts should be dedicated to define fully the treatment sensitivities of ESCC cells/xenografts/tissues used for establishing tumor xenografts, such that the established xenografts can be used to represent specific clinical conditions. In addition, such characterized models can also provide a working platform to examine the treatment-sensitizing effects of test compounds/drugs.

Aside the above applications, tumor xenograft models can also be used to address new challenges on biomedical imaging. New imaging modalities such as optical coherence tomography can be examined and validated in various tumor xenograft models for their utility to detect tumors. Specifically for optical coherence tomography, the incorporation of contrast agent can enhance the detection capability on tumors and even for detecting early stage tumors [28]. Active research is devoted in this area for ESCC research. Initial attempt has been made to deploy the capacity of optical coherence tomography to reveal various layers of the mouse esophageal wall in a high resolution manner [29]. Such effort has launched the research towards this direction by further examining the image contrast-enhancing effects associated with contrast agents like nanoparticles [30]. In all, tumor xenograft models provide an ideal and versatile platform for ESCC research and can facilitate the research on tumor biology, preclinical drug testing and possibly biomedical imaging.

Although tumor xenograft models developed in immunodeficient mice are widely used in cancer research due to their low cost, the use of this animal type is suffered from the lack of immunity. Therefore, they have limited use in research that requires an intact immune system. Alternatively, this limitation can be addressed with the use of humanized mice, for which these mice are generated with a human immune system [31, 32]. The use of humanized mice can further enhance the clinical relevance of the patient-derived tumor xenograft model and is particularly useful to conduct immunotherapy study [31, 33, 34]. Another type of animal model that is gaining wide spread use is genetically engineered mice model that are generated by transgenic technologies [31, 33]. Together, these two additional types of animal models can be utilized in parallel to the tumor xenograft models to further enhance result interpretation and clinical relevance of the study.

Abbreviations
CRABP2: Cellular retinoic acid binding protein 2; EGFR: Epidermal growth factor receptor; ESCC: Esophageal squamous cell carcinoma; PIK3CA: Phosphatidylinositol-4,5-bisphosphate 3-kinase catalytic subunit alpha

Acknowledgements
We would like to acknowledge the technical assistance from Kin Tak Chan on the animal work presented in this study. This study was supported in part by Theme-based Research Scheme (T42-103/16-N) of the Research Grants Council.

Funding
This study was supported in part by Theme-based Research Scheme (T42–103/16-N) of the Research Grants Council.

Authors' contributions
NPL, LNT, SL wrote and commented on the manuscript; CMC, LNT, HKW performed the experiments; all authors read and approved the final manuscript.

Competing interests
Not applicable.

References
1. Tong DK, Law S, Kwong DL, Wei WI, Ng RW, Wong KH. Current management of cervical esophageal cancer. World J Surg. 2011;35(3):600–7.
2. Cools-Lartigue J, Spicer J, Ferri LE. Current status of management of malignant disease: current management of esophageal cancer. J Gastrointest Surg. 2015;19(5):964–72.
3. Saeki H, Nakashima Y, Zaitsu Y, Tsuda Y, Kasagi Y, Ando K, et al. Current status of and perspectives regarding neoadjuvant chemoradiotherapy for locally advanced esophageal squamous cell carcinoma. Surg Today. 2016;46(3):261–7.
4. Cekanova M, Rathore K. Animal models and therapeutic molecular targets of cancer: utility and limitations. Drug Des Devel Ther. 2014;8:1911–21.
5. Khaled WT, Liu P. Cancer mouse models: past, present and future. Semin Cell Dev Biol. 2014;27:54–60.
6. Kelland LR. Of mice and men: values and liabilities of the athymic nude mouse model in anticancer drug development. Eur J Cancer. 2004;40(6):827–36.
7. Cho SY, Kang W, Han JY, Min S, Kang J, Lee A, et al. An integrative approach to precision Cancer medicine using patient-derived xenografts. Mol Cells. 2016;39(2):77–86.
8. Ruggeri BA, Camp F, Miknyoczki S. Animal models of disease: pre-clinical animal models of cancer and their applications and utility in drug discovery. Biochem Pharmacol. 2014;87(1):150–61.
9. Nair DV, Reddy AG. Laboratory animal models for esophageal cancer. Vet World. 2016;9(11):1229–32.
10. Yan S, Jiang H, Fang S, Yin F, Wang Z, Jia Y, et al. MicroRNA-340 inhibits esophageal Cancer cell growth and invasion by targeting phosphoserine aminotransferase 1. Cell Physiol Biochem. 2015;37(1):375–86.
11. Liu M, Hu Y, Zhang MF, Luo KJ, Xie XY, Wen J, et al. MMP1 promotes tumor growth and metastasis in esophageal squamous cell carcinoma. Cancer Lett. 2016;377(1):97–104.
12. Yang Q, Wang R, Xiao W, Sun F, Yuan H, Pan Q. Cellular retinoic acid binding protein 2 is strikingly downregulated in human esophageal squamous cell carcinoma and functions as a tumor suppressor. PLoS One. 2016;11(2):e0148381.
13. Isozaki Y, Hoshino I, Akutsu Y, Hanari N, Mori M, Nishimori T, et al. Usefulness of microRNA-375 as a prognostic and therapeutic tool in esophageal squamous cell carcinoma. Int J Oncol. 2015;46(3):1059–66.
14. Nishikawa T, Takaoka M, Ohara T, Tomono Y, Hao H, Bao X, et al. Antiproliferative effect of a novel mTOR inhibitor temsirolimus contributes to the prolonged survival of orthotopic esophageal cancer-bearing mice. Cancer Biol Ther. 2013;14(3):230–6.
15. Chang L, Huo B, Lv Y, Wang Y, Liu W. Ginsenoside Rg3 enhances the inhibitory effects of chemotherapy on esophageal squamous cell carcinoma in mice. Mol Clin Oncol. 2014;2(6):1043–6.
16. Lee NP, Chan KT, Choi MY, Lam HY, Tung LN, Tzang FC, et al. Oxygen carrier YQ23 can enhance the chemotherapeutic drug responses of chemoresistant esophageal tumor xenografts. Cancer Chemother Pharmacol. 2015;76(6):1199–207.
17. Hori T, Yamashita Y, Ohira M, Matsumura Y, Muguruma K, Hirakawa K. A novel orthotopic implantation model of human esophageal carcinoma in nude rats: CD44H mediates cancer cell invasion in vitro and in vivo. Int J Cancer. 2001;92(4):489–96.
18. Ohara T, Takaoka M, Sakurama K, Nagaishi K, Takeda H, Shirakawa Y, et al. The establishment of a new mouse model with orthotopic esophageal cancer showing the esophageal stricture. Cancer Lett. 2010;293(2):207–12.
19. Ip JC, Ko JM, Yu VZ, Chan KW, Lam AK, Law S, et al. A versatile orthotopic nude mouse model for study of esophageal squamous cell carcinoma. Biomed Res Int. 2015;2015:910715.
20. Song S, Chang D, Cui Y, Hu J, Gong M, Ma K, et al. New orthotopic implantation model of human esophageal squamous cell carcinoma in athymic nude mice. Thorac Cancer. 2014;5(5):417–24.
21. Hu T, Qi H, Li P, Zhao G, Ma Y, Hao Q, et al. Comparison of GFP-expressing Imageable mouse models of human esophageal squamous cell carcinoma established in various anatomical sites. Anticancer Res. 2015;35(9):4655 63.

22. Ng HY, Ko JM, Yu VZ, Ip JC, Dai W, Cal S, et al. DESC1, a novel tumor suppressor, sensitizes cells to apoptosis by downregulating the EGFR/AKT pathway in esophageal squamous cell carcinoma. Int J Cancer. 2016;138(12):2940–51.

23. Tung LN, Song S, Chan KT, Choi MY, Lam HY, Chan CM, et al. Preclinical Study of Novel Curcumin Analogue SSC-5 Using Orthotopic Tumor Xenograft Model for Esophageal Squamous Cell Carcinoma. Cancer Res Treat. 2018:in press.

24. Jiang Y, Wu Q, Yang X, Zhao J, Jin Y, Li K, et al. A method for establishing a patient-derived xenograft model to explore new therapeutic strategies for esophageal squamous cell carcinoma. Oncol Rep. 2016;35(2):785–92.

25. Hou W, Qin X, Zhu X, Fei M, Liu P, Liu L, et al. Lapatinib inhibits the growth of esophageal squamous cell carcinoma and synergistically interacts with 5-fluorouracil in patient-derived xenograft models. Oncol Rep. 2013;30(2):707–14.

26. Zhang J, Jiang D, Li X, Lv J, Xie L, Zheng L, et al. Establishment and characterization of esophageal squamous cell carcinoma patient-derived xenograft mouse models for preclinical drug discovery. Lab Investig. 2014;94(8):917–26.

27. Wu X, Zhang J, Zhen R, Lv J, Zheng L, Su X, et al. Trastuzumab anti-tumor efficacy in patient-derived esophageal squamous cell carcinoma xenograft (PDECX) mouse models. J Transl Med. 2012;10:180.

28. Kim CS, Wilder-Smith P, Ahn YC, Liaw LH, Chen Z, Kwon YJ. Enhanced detection of early-stage oral cancer in vivo by optical coherence tomography using multimodal delivery of gold nanoparticles. J Biomed Opt. 2009;14(3):034008.

29. Xu J, Yu L, Wei X, Wang X, Chui PC, Chan KT, et al. Simultaneous dual-band optical coherence tomography for endoscopic applications. J Biomed Opt. 2014;19(12):126007.

30. Au KM, Lu Z, Matcher SJ, Armes SP. Polypyrrole nanoparticles: a potential optical coherence tomography contrast agent for cancer imaging. Adv Mater. 2011;23(48):5792–5.

31. Choi Y, Lee S, Kim K, Kim SH, Chung YJ, Lee C. Studying cancer immunotherapy using patient-derived xenografts (PDXs) in humanized mice. Exp Mol Med. 2018;50(8):99.

32. Morton JJ, Bird G, Refaeli Y, Jimeno A. Humanized mouse xenograft models: narrowing the tumor-microenvironment gap. Cancer Res. 2016;76(21):6153–8.

33. Lampreht Tratar U, Horvat S, Cemazar M. Transgenic mouse models in Cancer research. Front Oncol. 2018;8:268.

34. Wege AK. Humanized mouse models for the preclinical assessment of Cancer immunotherapy. BioDrugs. 2018;32(3):245–66.

35. Jung J, Seol HS, Chang S. The generation and application of patient-derived xenograft model for Cancer research. Cancer Res Treat. 2018;50(1):1–10.

36. Harada E, Serada S, Fujimoto M, Takahashi Y, Takahashi T, Hara H, et al. Glypican-1 targeted antibody-based therapy induces preclinical antitumor activity against esophageal squamous cell carcinoma. Oncotarget. 2017;8(15):24741–52.

37. Sugase T, Takahashi T, Serada S, Nakatsuka R, Fujimoto M, Ohkawara T, et al. Suppressor of cytokine signaling-1 gene therapy induces potent antitumor effect in patient-derived esophageal squamous cell carcinoma xenograft mice. Int J Cancer. 2017;140(11):2608–21.

38. Zou J, Liu Y, Wang J, Liu Z, Lu Z, Chen Z, et al. Establishment and genomic characterizations of patient-derived esophageal squamous cell carcinoma xenograft models using biopsies for treatment optimization. J Transl Med. 2018;16(1):15.

39. Wong CH, Ma BB, Hui CW, Tao Q, Chan AT. Preclinical evaluation of afatinib (BIBW2992) in esophageal squamous cell carcinoma (ESCC). Am J Cancer Res. 2015;5(12):3588–99.

MARCKS and MARCKS-like proteins in development and regeneration

Mohamed El Amri[1], Una Fitzgerald[2] and Gerhard Schlosser[1,3]* (iD)

Abstract

Background: The Myristoylated Alanine-Rich C-kinase Substrate (MARCKS) and MARCKS-like protein 1 (MARCKSL1) have a wide range of functions, ranging from roles in embryonic development to adult brain plasticity and the inflammatory response. Recently, both proteins have also been identified as important players in regeneration. Upon phosphorylation by protein kinase C (PKC) or calcium-dependent calmodulin-binding, MARCKS and MARCKSL1 translocate from the membrane into the cytosol, modulating cytoskeletal actin dynamics and vesicular trafficking and activating various signal transduction pathways. As a consequence, the two proteins are involved in the regulation of cell migration, secretion, proliferation and differentiation in many different tissues.

Main body: Throughout vertebrate development, MARCKS and MARCKSL1 are widely expressed in tissues derived from all germ layers, with particularly strong expression in the nervous system. They have been implicated in the regulation of gastrulation, myogenesis, brain development, and other developmental processes. Mice carrying loss of function mutations in either *Marcks* or *Marcksl1* genes die shortly after birth due to multiple deficiencies including detrimental neural tube closure defects. In adult vertebrates, MARCKS and MARCKL1 continue to be important for multiple regenerative processes including peripheral nerve, appendage, and tail regeneration, making them promising targets for regenerative medicine.

Conclusion: This review briefly summarizes the molecular interactions and cellular functions of MARCKS and MARCKSL1 proteins and outlines their vital roles in development and regeneration.

Keywords: MARCKS, MARCKS-like protein, Development, Regeneration, Cell migration

Background

The Myristoylated Alanine Rich C-Kinase Substrate (MARCKS) is a ubiquitous, highly conserved protein among vertebrates, which is essential for postnatal survival [1], and has been widely studied for its functions in the brain and nervous system. Being highly expressed in nervous tissue, particularly during early development but persisting in the adult, it plays numerous roles related to brain growth, neuronal migration, neurite outgrowth, neurotransmitter release, and synaptic plasticity (reviewed in [2]). In addition, the protein has been implicated in the regulation of other developmental events, including gastrulation [3], myogenesis [4], and vasculogenesis [5].

MARCKS protein has become established as a key regulator of many molecular interactions, such as those involving the dynamic actin cytoskeleton or membrane phosphoinositides (reviewed in [2, 6–8]). Many of the molecular characteristics of MARCKS are also shared by MARCKS-related proteins, including proteins with significant homology in the effector domain such as MARCKS-like protein 1 (MARCKSL1) and other proteins that have similar biochemical functions and localisation patterns, such as growth associated protein 43 (GAP43) and cytoskeletal-associated protein 23 (CAP23) [9]. Whereas GAP43 and CAP23 have long been shown to play important roles in neural regeneration [10, 11], only recently have MARCKS and MARCKSL1 been implicated in regeneration of neural and other tissues [12–14]. This review focuses on the emerging roles of MARCKS and MARCKS-like proteins in development

* Correspondence: gerhard.schlosser@nuigalway.ie
[1]Centre for Research in Medical Devices (CÚRAM), National University of Ireland, Galway, Biomedical Sciences Building, Newcastle Road, Galway, Ireland
[3]School of Natural Sciences and Regenerative Medicine Institute (REMEDI), National University of Ireland, Galway, Biomedical Sciences Building, Newcastle Road, Galway, Ireland
Full list of author information is available at the end of the article

and regeneration and explores possible mechanisms underlying their function.

Main text

Domain structures and molecular properties

MARCKS is an abundant, rod-shaped protein of 35 kDa [15], with three highly conserved functional domains [2, 16] (Fig. 1a). In the centre of the protein, the effector domain (ED) is rich in positively charged lysine residues, while multiple serine residues make it susceptible to phosphorylation by protein kinase C (PKC), or other protein kinases such as Rho kinase (ROCK) [2, 15, 17, 18]. Adjacent to the ED are two highly conserved regions. The first is the MARCKS Homology 2 (MH2) domain [19]. The second conserved region is the N-terminal domain containing a myristoylation site, which undergoes a reversible co-translational attachment of myristic acid to its N-terminal glycine residue [20]. In its non-phosphorylated state, the positively-charged ED attaches to the negatively charged cytosolic face of the plasma membrane [2] (Fig. 1b). As a result, the N-terminal myristoylation site reversibly inserts into

the plasma membrane, serving as a lipid anchor for the protein [21, 22]. Once the ED is phosphorylated, it loses its affinity for the plasma membrane, shifting MARCKS back into the cytoplasm [2] (Fig. 1b). This translocation, termed the 'electrostatic switch' [22], can also be achieved through increased Ca^{2+} levels, which enable calmodulin to bind to the ED of MARCKS [23] (Fig. 1b).

MARCKS-like protein 1 (MARCKSL1), also known as MARCKS-like protein (MLP), MARCKS-related protein (MRP), Brain Protein F52, or MacMARCKS, shares strong homology and functionality with MARCKS [24]. The 20 kDa protein has a very similar ED to that of MARCKS, which also binds F-actin, Ca^{2+}/calmodulin, and acidic phospholipids. In addition, MARCKSL1 contains the same N-terminal myristoylation consensus sequence found in MARCKS [25]. However, it is important to note that MARCKSL1 has a lower alanine content than MARCKS, resulting in potential functional differences, and a distinct distribution pattern in the brain [24].

Depending on their phosphorylation state, MARCKS or MARCKSL1 have been shown to engage in a number of different molecular interactions. First, when the ED of

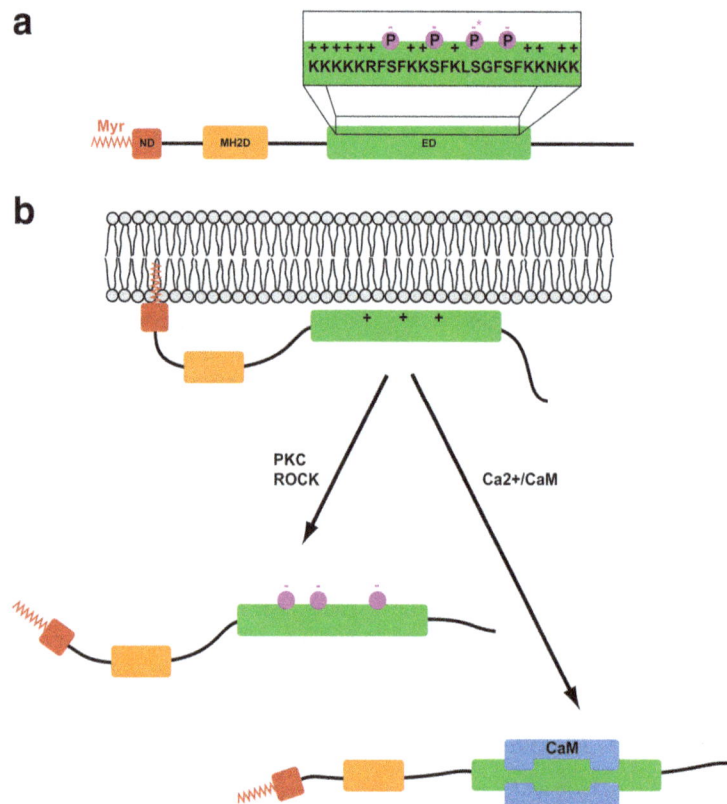

Fig. 1 MARCKS protein structure and electrostatic switch. **a** MARCKS protein has three protein domains, the N-Terminal domain (ND), which can be myristoylated (Myr), an MH2 domain (MH2D) and an effector domain (ED). The ED (amino acids 152–176 in human MARCKS) is magnified in the inset showing that it is highly positively charged and has 4 potential phosphorylation sites, one of which (asterisk) is poorly phosphorylated. **b** In the unphosphorylated state and in the absence of Calcium-calmodulin (CaM) binding, MARCKS is tethered to the membrane but becomes released into the cytosol when phosphorylated by protein kinase C (PKC) or Rho kinase (ROCK) or after Calcium-CaM binding. Modified from [8]

MARCKS is unphosphorylated and attached to the plasma membrane, it achieves cross-linking of actin filaments by directly binding to filamentous (F) actin [26, 27] (Fig. 2a). In addition, MARCKS can promote the polymerisation of actin [28]. In a similar way, MARCKSL1 bundles and stabilises F-actin upon phosphorylation, increasing filopodium dynamics [29]. These direct interactions with the cytoskeleton have been implicated in the regulation of cell migration in various developmental contexts (see below) as well as in the regulation of mucin secretion in the human bronchial epithelium. The latter process, which is dysregulated in asthma and other respiratory diseases, involves the dephosphorylation of cytoplasmic MARCKS, promoting its interaction with both F-actin and membrane bound proteins of secretory vesicles and resulting in increased mucin secretion [30, 31].

The electrostatic switch mechanism of MARCKS and MARCKSL1 also has important consequences for their ability to interact with phosphatidylinositol 4,5-bisphosphate (PIP$_2$) [7, 32, 33]. PIP$_2$ is a membrane component, with numerous cellular functions, including second messenger generation and membrane-anchoring of various proteins, including kinases and proteins with MARCKS-like domains [34, 35]. PIP$_2$ is either selectively hydrolysed by phospholipase C (PLC), producing inositol triphosphate (IP$_3$) and diacylglycerol (DAG) [36], or is further phosphorylated by phosphoinositide 3-kinase (PI3K) to form PIP$_3$. These three products act as second messengers in many eukaryotic signal transduction cascades. For example, DAG activates several PKC isozymes, stimulating the phosphorylation of select proteins by PKC. On the other hand, IP$_3$ regulates the cytoplasmic concentration of Ca^{2+} by gating a Ca^{2+} channel in the endoplasmic reticulum. Furthermore, IP$_3$ functions as a rate-limiting substrate in the synthesis of additional inositol polyphosphates, which can stimulate various protein kinases, transcription,

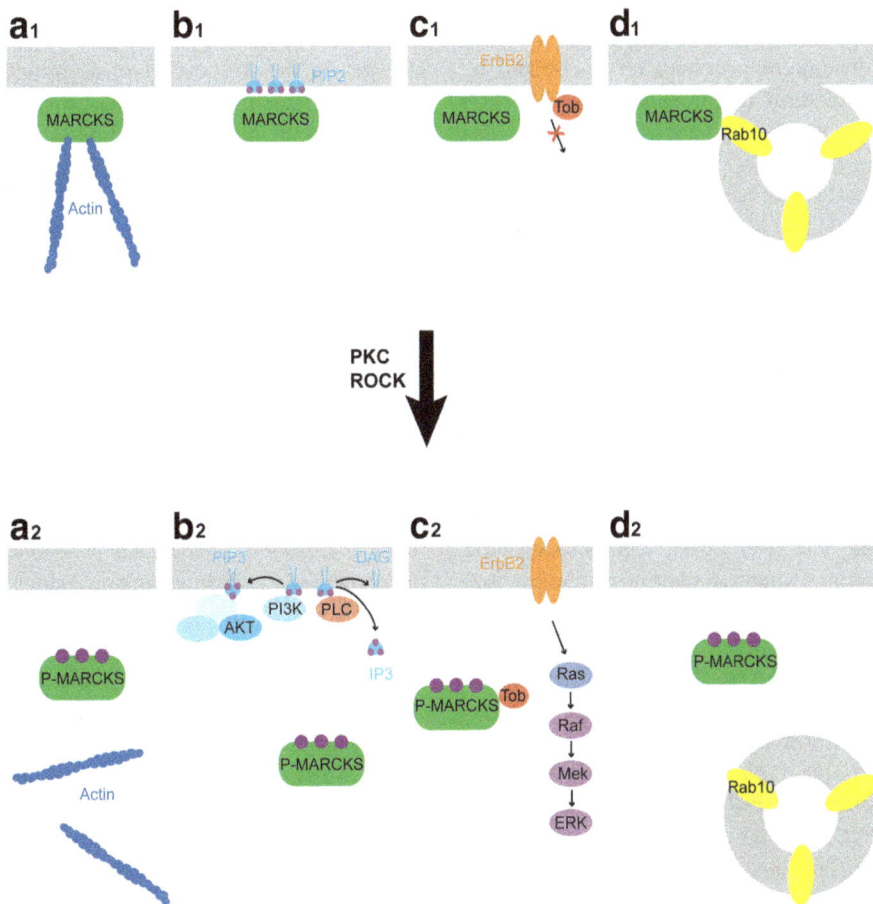

Fig. 2 Molecular interactions of MARCKS. Role of membrane-tethered, unphosphorylated MARCKS (a_1–d_1) is compared with its cytosolic, phosphorylated form (a_2–d_2). Membranes are depicted in grey; phosphorylation is indicated by purple circles. **a** Direct actin binding of unphosphorylated MARCKS. **b** PIP$_2$ sequestration of unphosphorylated MARCKS; upon phosphorylation of MARCKS, PIP$_2$ becomes accessible to PLC and PI3K. **c** Phosphorylated MARCKS binds to Tob resulting in activation of ErbB2 signalling. **d** Unphosphorylated MARCKS binds to Rab10 promoting exocytosis of vesicles. See text for details

and mRNA processing events [36–38]. PIP$_3$, finally, is involved in activating the AKT signalling pathway with a plethora of diverse functions [39].

It has been recurrently shown that membrane-bound MARCKS can isolate and sequester PIP$_2$ within specific membrane micro-domains, or "lipid rafts", for participation in later signal transduction events, suggesting that it can modulate PIP$_2$-dependent cellular processes by controlling the spatial availability of the phospholipid for enzymes such as PLC and PI3K [34, 40–42] (Fig. 2b). While PIP$_2$ is critical for the activity and localisation of several membrane associated proteins, including focal adhesion kinase (FAK) [34, 35] many of the PIP$_2$-dependent processes that MARCKS modulates remain currently unknown. However, PIP$_2$ sequestration by MARCKS and related proteins has been shown to promote axon outgrowth [43]. While the mechanism is not completely resolved, it has been proposed that unmasked PIP$_2$ interacts with and inhibits proteins promoting actin dynamics (e.g. gelsolin, cofilin, profilin), thereby indirectly stabilizing the cortical actin cytoskeleton. After sequestration of PIP$_2$ by MARCKS, these proteins are released and now promote cell motility [43].

A further PIP$_2$-dependent process that is affected by MARCKS is the activation of phospholipase D (PLD) [7, 44, 45], which is involved in cytoskeletal actin dynamics, membrane trafficking, cell migration, and mitosis [46–51]. Since PIP$_2$ is required for PLD activation, it has been proposed that MARCKS-mediated PLD activation results from the phosphorylation-induced release of PIP$_2$ [7]. PLD acts by hydrolysing phosphatidylcholine (PC), producing choline and phosphatidic acid (PA), which serve as second messengers in many signal transduction cascades [52, 53]. For instance, PA is known to play a significant role in actin stress fibre formation [54, 55], vesicular trafficking [56], cell proliferation [57, 58], neurite outgrowth [59], and MAP-kinase activation [60]. In addition, PA can also be converted into DAG and lysophosphatidic acid (LPA) [61], a potent signalling molecule with functions such as neurite retraction [62] and cell proliferation [63].

In addition to its PIP$_2$-dependent modulation of various signalling pathways, MARCKS affects other signalling pathways by different mechanisms. As an example, following phosphorylation by PKC, MARCKS activates an ErbB2-mediated signal pathway, by binding to the anti-proliferative negative cell-cycle regulator Transducer of ErbB2 (TOB2), thereby decreasing its affinity to ErbB2 [64] (Fig. 2c). This in turn, promotes cell proliferation and maintenance of normal radial glial identity [65]. In addition, the exogenous overexpression of ErbB2 induces mature astrocytes to become radial glial progenitors in the adult mouse brain, promoting both neurogenesis and targeted neuronal migration

[66]. Furthermore, MARCKS has been associated with polysialic acid (PSA), which influences neural differentiation, migration [67] and axonal commissure formation [68–70]. When PSA is added to neural cell adhesion molecules (NCAMs) as a post-translational modification, it co-localises with MARCKS in the plasma membrane, stimulating neurite outgrowth [71]. Moreover, MARCKS has recently been shown to modulate Netrin-1 - Deleted in Colorectal Cancer (DCC) signalling by disrupting the localisation patterns of two of its subcellular mediators, proto-oncogene tyrosine-kinase SRC and FAK. As a result, axonal navigation in the corpus callosum becomes aberrant during a crucial phase of mouse brain development [72].

The apical localisation of MARCKS in ependymal and radial glial cells [73, 74] and the displacement of cell-polarity proteins such as aPKC, PAR3, CDC42, as well as β-catenin, prominin, and N-cadherin in *Marcks$^{-/-}$* mouse embryos [73], suggest that MARCKS is also able to interact with membrane-associated proteins related to cell polarity and anchor them apically, although evidence for direct protein-protein interactions is currently lacking. However, radial glial cell polarity is perturbed in *Marcks$^{-/-}$* embryos, resulting in reduced proliferation, changes in the proportion of asymmetric cell divisions, and displacement of radial glia cells, which can act both as neural progenitor cells and as pro-migratory scaffolds for neurons in the developing cortex [2, 73]. In addition, MARCKS may also affect cell polarity via PIP$_2$-dependent mechanisms [73, 75–77].

Finally, MARCKS has been shown to interact with various vesicular proteins. Direct interactions with Rab10 in plasmalemmal precursor vesicles (PPVs) provide membranes to outgrowing axons when the ED is not phosphorylated [78] (Fig. 2d). Interactions with other vesicle associated proteins such as synapsin [79] or various chaperones [31] have been described and may contribute to the role of MARCKS for secretion of mucin, neurotransmitters, as well as inflammatory cytokines [31, 80–83]. MARCKS probably affects secretion by several distinct mechanisms, since the unphosphorylated form of the protein promotes mucin secretion [30, 31], while the phosphorylated form promotes neurotransmitter release and gut peptide secretion [80, 81].

In summary, MARCKS interacts with numerous molecular pathways. Much less is known about MARCKSL1, but the overall consequences of its interactions appear to be similar to MARCKS. Most notably, MARCKS affects cytoskeletal rearrangements, various signalling pathways, and vesicular trafficking. As a consequence, the protein affects predominantly cellular processes relying on these pathways during development or in the adult such as cell migration, secretion and phagocytosis, and cell proliferation and differentiation. Cell migration is affected not only by MARCKS' capacity for direct actin binding but also by multiple downstream effects of PIP_2 sequestration [26, 27, 43, 44]. Secretion and phagocytosis likewise appear to be modulated by several MARCKS interacting factors [31, 78, 79]. Finally, cell proliferation and differentiation are modulated by MARCKS' interaction with various signalling pathways, as well as possibly its interactions with cell polarity proteins [64, 73, 84].

A large body of evidence indicates that the electrostatic switch mechanism between membrane bound (unphosphorylated) and cytosolic (phosphorylated or CaM-bound) MARCKS plays a crucial role in the regulation of each of these processes. However, there is conflicting evidence for the precise role of membrane bound versus cytosolic MARCKS. As discussed above, secretion appears to be promoted by unphosphorylated, membrane bound MARCKS in some contexts [30, 31] but by phosphorylated, cytosolic MARCKS in other contexts [80, 81]. Similarly, unphosphorylated, membrane bound MARCKS or MARCKSL1 have been shown to promote lamellipodium formation, axon outgrowth and cell motility in neurons and cancer cells in some studies [29, 43, 85–87], whereas phosphorylated, cytosolic MARCKS has been shown to promote cell motility in other studies [88–92]. Moreover, neither phosphorylation of the ED nor myristoylation of MARCKS are necessary for normal gross brain morphology in a transgenic line of mice overexpressing MARCKS [93–95], whereas myristoylation, but not phosphorylation, of MARCKS is required for radial glial polarity and localisation [73].

While some of these apparently paradoxical findings may be due to context-dependent interactions of MARCKS with different binding partners, others may reflect the dynamic requirement of both phosphorylated and unphosphorylated forms of MARCKS. Indeed, phosphorylation of MARCKS in migrating muscle precursors and neutrophils has been shown to be transient, followed by rapid dephosphorylation. While the phosphorylated form permits initial adhesion, the dephosphorylated form of MARCKS supports later stages of cell spreading [96, 97].

Role of MARCKS and MARCKSL1 in development

MARCKS and MARCKSL1 are expressed almost ubiquitously during vertebrate development, from early developmental stages and onwards, although there are some differences in MARCKS and MARCKSL1 expression patterns between species, developmental stages, tissues, and the phosphorylation state of the proteins. MARCKS and MARCKSL1 mRNA were shown to be maternally supplied in anamniotes and continue to be expressed throughout cleavage and gastrulation [16, 98, 99]. After neurulation, expression of MARCKS and MARCKSL1 is upregulated in the central (CNS) and peripheral nervous system (PNS) of all vertebrates, but continues to be expressed in many mesodermal and endodermal tissues [16, 24, 98–102]. During embryonic development of the CNS, MARCKS is first upregulated in the neuroepithelial cells of the emergent neural tube [100], before localising into the apical membranes of ventricular-zone neural progenitor cells (NPCs) [73, 103]. Subsequently, it is found particularly enriched in axons and dendrites [104, 105].

The nearly ubiquitous expression pattern of MARCKS and MARCKSL1 suggests that they play a vital role during vertebrate development and this is supported by many functional studies. For example, five gene-knockout studies in mice have shown that MARCKS and MARCKSL1 are both required for embryogenesis [1, 24, 100, 106, 107]. According to these reports, the absence of MARCKS and MARCKSL1 interfered with neural tube closure, leading to spina bifida and exencephaly, which resulted in perinatal lethality [108]. In addition, the disruption of the *Marcks* gene led to severe neuromuscular defects and decreased body size in mice [1, 73, 93, 100]. Other neural embryonic defects included agenesis of forebrain commissures (e.g. the corpus callosum), neuronal ectopia, and abnormal retinal/cortical laminations [1, 100].

Additional functional studies in frog and zebrafish have shown that MARCKS plays an important role during early embryonic events such as gastrulation [3]. For example, by blocking MARCKS protein synthesis in *Xenopus* embryos using antisense morpholino oligonucleotides (MO), Ioka et al. reported impaired convergent extension movements due to cytoskeletal deregulation [3]. In zebrafish embryos, blocking the two MARCKS paralogs *marcksa* and *marksb* also resulted in gross phenotypic defects, including severely curved and truncated tails, gill-formation abnormalities, skeletal muscle deformities, and an abnormal brain architecture [16].

The neural abnormalities observed in MARCKS mutants strongly suggest that MARCKS has multiple roles in the developing nervous system. For example, it maintains normal radial glial cell polarity and cell adhesion in the neocortex during brain development [73]. Since mice with mutant non-myristoylatable MARCKS [94] were only partially rescued from severe cranial defects and perinatal death in comparison with mice lacking MARCKS PKC-phosphorylation sites [109], it can be speculated that the function of radial glial cells depends on MARCKS myristoylation rather than phosphorylation [73]. Similarly, in another study, a phosphorylation deficient mutant form of MARCKS protein was able to rescue CNS defects observed in $Marcks^{-/-}$ knockout mice, suggesting that phosphorylation of MARCKS is not essential for CNS development [93].

However, another study suggests that the phosphorylation status of MARCKS plays a significant role in spinal cord development. In this study, Garrett et al. conditionally blocked the γ-Protocadherin allele Pcdh-γ, creating high levels of PKC that phosphorylated MARCKS [110]. As a result, dendrite complexity and arborisation were drastically reduced, having severe implications on CNS development. To confirm these results, dendrite abnormalities were rescued by blocking PKC, PLC, and FAK, the latter of which binds to γ-Protocadherins.

Moreover, MARCKS has been implicated in the regulation of neuronal migration and axon outgrowth during PNS and CNS development by modulating growth cone adhesion [85, 111] and the dynamics of the actin cytoskeleton [29, 43]. The latter results in the stimulation of lamellipodia formation and neurite outgrowth by dephosphorylated MARCKS [29, 86, 112].

MARCKS and MARCKSL1 are also implicated in cell adhesion and migration of neural crest cells (NCCs). NCCs are a group of transient migratory cells that originate from the neural tube during embryogenesis and give rise to a variety of different cell types, including sensory neurons and glial cells of the PNS, cranial cartilage, and bone [113, 114]. It has been suggested that migrating-precursor cells of the PNS that originate from NCCs express a significantly higher amount of MARCKS in chick embryos [102]. In addition, mice lacking MARCKSL1 have been shown to have impaired NCC migration, contributing to severe abnormalities including exencephaly and neural-tube defects [107]. For future experiments, it would be interesting to trace the behaviour and fate of MARCKS and MARCKSL1 in NCCs using cell-adhesion and cell-migration assays to further elucidate their role in development and regeneration.

In addition, MARCKS and MARCKSL1 are also involved in modulating migration during development of many other tissues. For example, by reversibly blocking MARCKS-translocation and myoblast-fusion in chick embryos, Kim et al. found that PKC-controlled MARCKS translocation is a prerequisite for myoblast fusion, a key cellular event that shapes the formation, fusion, and repair of embryonic muscle cells [4, 109, 115]. Moreover, MARCKS regulates vascular endothelial cell migration by influencing insulin-dependent signalling to PIP$_2$, which in turn affects actin assembly and cellular development in the vascular endothelium [5]. MARCKS has also been shown to play a critical role in angiotensin-II signalling, which directly influences endothelial cell motility [116].

As a whole, the role of MARCKS in cell migration, secretion, proliferation and differentiation appears common to a diverse array of developmental functions, and continues to be important in several adult tissues. For example, as discussed above, adult MARCKS plays an important role in mucin secretion in the airways [30]. Moreover, in the mature nervous system, MARCKS and MARCKSL1 serve a variety of functions, including the promotion of neurotransmitter release and gut peptide secretion [80, 81], as well as a role in synaptic plasticity and learning and memory, possibly due to their ability to promote dendritic spine maintenance [2, 105, 117]. In addition, MARCKS and MARCKSL1 play important roles in the immune system, where they promote migration of inflammatory cells and the secretion of cytokines as discussed in more detail below. Dysregulation of MARCKS or MARCKSL1 has also been implicated in many different cancers, where they affect tumorigenesis, metastasis and angiogenesis [8, 118].

Role of MARCKS and MARCKSL1 in regeneration

There is strong evidence for a role of the proteins GAP43 and CAP23 in regeneration in both the PNS and CNS [10, 11, 119–123]. These two proteins are structurally and mechanistically related PKC substrates that share numerous functions including PIP$_2$- and- actin cytoskeletal regulation with MARCKS [9, 43, 124]. Based on these similarities, the trio of GAP43, MARCKS and CAP23 is commonly referred to as GMC proteins.

For example, GAP43 and CAP23 are highly expressed in mouse motor nerves during regeneration [120, 125] and play a critical role in regulating nerve sprouting [124, 126]. They have also been implicated in the regeneration of axons in the dorsal root ganglia and sciatic nerves [43, 127], olfactory epithelia [128], retinal ganglion cells [129], and the cerebral cortex [130]. Co-expression of these two proteins triggers a 60-fold increase in dorsal root ganglion axon regeneration after spinal cord injury in mice [131]. In the cerebellum, overexpression of GAP43 induces axonal sprouting [132, 133], while downregulation of GAP43 by RNAi interferes with axonal regrowth after injury [134].

In contrast to other GMC proteins, MARCKS and MARCKSL1 have only recently emerged as potentially important players during the regenerative process. In 2000, McNamara et al. showed that MARCKS expression, like GAP43, is significantly upregulated in regenerating neurons after facial axonal lesions in rats [12]. Both proteins are also highly expressed during neurite outgrowth of dorsal root ganglia and superior cervical ganglia [123]. Furthermore, MARCKS is highly upregulated during optic nerve regeneration [135] and during axonal sprouting after brain stroke [126], suggesting that MARCKS, like GAP43 and CAP23, may play an important role in axon outgrowth during regeneration in both PNS and CNS, although disappointingly, functional studies confirming this are still lacking. Outside of the nervous system, MARCKS has also been shown to be upregulated during lens regeneration [136] and during cardiac tissue regeneration following infarction [137], while MARCKSL1 is elevated during lungfish fin regeneration [14]. Using qPCR analysis on the fin blastema, a collection of relatively undifferentiated and proliferating cells capable of regeneration, it was shown that lungfish *Marcksl1* reaches its highest level of expression 1 day post amputation, returning to basal levels at 3 weeks post-amputation [14].

A recent publication by Sugiura et al. now suggests a different and more pervasive role for MARCKSL1 in regeneration, by demonstrating that extracellularly released axolotl MARCKS-like protein (AxMLP) is responsible for inducing the early proliferative response in axolotl tail and limb regeneration [13]. Using a variety of experimental strategies, these researchers identified AxMLP as an extracellular factor that is strongly associated with cell proliferation and blastemal length. For instance, in-vivo knock-down studies revealed that AxMLP is necessary for the elevated levels of cell proliferation following injury, while immunohistochemical analysis of AxMLP distribution in epidermal and spinal cord tissues showed that the protein is mostly cytoplasmic in uninjured tissue, before translocating to the membrane following injury in accordance with its proposed extracellular secretion.

Today, the mechanisms of AxMLP extracellular release remain currently unknown. Confirmation and elucidation of the mode of MARCKSL1 secretion promises to provide novel insights into unconventional protein secretion mechanisms since it does not contain a signal peptide. In addition, secretion of MARCKS or MARCKSL1 so far has only been reported in the highly regenerative axolotl but has not been found in other vertebrates, raising the possibility that secretion of these proteins may be linked to their ability to promote regeneration.

Taken together with previous observations, this study suggests that MARCKS and MARCKSL1 play important roles during regeneration. While the underlying molecular mechanisms are still unresolved, insights from molecular and developmental studies suggest some candidate pathways, which will be discussed in the following sections. As summarized above, MARCKS and MARCKSL1 have important roles in the development of multiple tissues, but they have also been shown to be important in the inflammatory response to injury. This suggests that MARCKS and MARCKSL1 may potentially affect the regenerative response in two very different but not mutually exclusive ways. First, by promoting the regenerative process in the injured tissue itself and second, by modulating the inflammatory response.

Potential direct roles in the injured tissue

The first response to limb- or tail amputation in species capable of regeneration is the formation of a blastema, involving the migration of cells, followed by cell-cycle re-entry and blastemal-cell proliferation. These cellular mechanisms, including migration, proliferation, and differentiation, are known to be conserved amongst most species after injury [138]. MARCKS and MARCKSL1 have been implicated in many of the processes underlying blastema formation, suggesting that they may play multiple roles during this process. First, MARCKS has been shown to promote proliferation, by activating the ErbB2-mediated signal pathway or by interacting with cell polarity proteins [64, 73]. As mentioned previously, ErbB2 overexpression has also been shown to induce astrocytes to dedifferentiate and revert to a progenitor state [66] and similar processes would be required during blastema formation.

Second, MARCKS has been shown to induce cellular migration, which is another critical component of regeneration [139–141]. As discussed above, MARCKS influences cell migration by a multitude of mechanisms, including its interactions with actin, PIP_2 sequestration, and the activation of various signalling pathways. In addition, MARCKS has been shown to mediate the effects of the noncanonical Wnt pathway on cortical actin dynamics during the formation of lamellipodia- and filopodia-like protrusions [3]. This pathway has been shown to promote regeneration in *Xenopus* and zebrafish, and is necessary for axolotl appendage regeneration [142]. The established role of MARCKS in promoting axon outgrowth via its effect on cell adhesion and actin dynamics may also contribute to neural regeneration.

Potential indirect roles in modulating inflammation

The process of inflammation also plays a critical role in the regeneration of injured tissue through a variety of highly conserved pathways. Although severe inflammation typically inhibits regeneration, a moderate and well-regulated inflammatory response may actually be required for the initiation of regeneration [143–145]. Depending on the injury site and organism, cells such as macrophages and neutrophils that infiltrate the wound and secrete cytokines are characteristic of the inflammatory response [139, 144, 146–150]. Macrophages, which are necessary for salamander limb regeneration [151, 152], are known to functionally depend on MARCKS and MARCKSL1.

The importance of MARCKS and MARCKSL1 in inflammation is well established. MARCKSL1 was initially termed 'MacMARCKS' due to its high level of expression in macrophages [153], and up to date, numerous studies have associated MARCKS and MARCKSL1 with normal macrophage function [154, 155]. For instance, both MARCKS and MARCKSL1 are implicated in macrophage transmigration [156] through a process involving phosphorylation, actin binding, and cytosol translocation [90]. During the inflammatory response, MARCKS has also been shown to act as a major regulator of human neutrophil migration and adhesion [88], also promoting neutrophil secretion of inflammatory cytokines [82, 83, 157, 158].

Finally, MARCKS upregulation is associated with microglial activation and neuroinflammation after CNS injuries [159]. Interestingly, although the mechanisms of microglial activation during axonal regeneration remain disputable [160, 161], studies suggest that amyloid beta might be responsible for promoting microglial activation by stimulating PKC and MAPK to phosphorylate MARCKS [162].

Conclusions

Over the past three decades, major advances in research have identified MARCKS and MARCKSL1 as key players during developmental and regenerative processes. These include brain, kidney, blood-vessel, and muscle development, as well as appendage regeneration. However, while numerous molecular interactions of MARCKS-related molecules, such as their interactions with the actin cytoskeleton and membrane phosphoinositides have been unravelled, their respective role for various developmental and regenerative processes is very poorly understood. Moreover, these multifaceted molecules probably contribute to development and regeneration by additional mechanisms which remain yet to be characterised.

For example, the phosphorylation-site domain (ED) in MARCKS is homologous to a region in diacylglycerol kinase zeta (DGKζ), which has been shown to bind to and modulate the function of retinoblastoma protein (Rb) [163–165]. Rb is implicated in cell cycle regulation and has been shown to be important for cell cycle re-entry of newt myotubes [166–168], but whether this function is MARCKS or MARCKSL1 dependent has not been investigated yet. The ED also acts as a nuclear localisation signal, suggesting that MARCKS may have unrecognized functions in the nucleus, including potential roles in the modulation of gene expression and of nuclear PIP_2 localisation [169].

Retinoic acid (RA) is another factor which has been shown to affect MARCKS function in rat hippocampal cells, where it leads to its translocation from the membrane to the cytosol [170]. As a metabolite of vitamin A, RA plays a significant role in numerous regenerative processes such as nerve, auditory hair cell, fin/limb and lung regeneration [171–177], but whether any of these effects depend on MARCKS remains yet to be explored. Finally, the demonstration that AxMLP acts as a secreted factor in axolotl limb regeneration suggests additional and hitherto unknown modes of action.

Therefore, further research is required to assess the precise mechanisms by which MARCKS and MARCKSL1 contribute to development and regeneration, providing professionals with the molecular tools that will help them design new therapies for illnesses such as asthma, cancer, and spinal cord injury [8, 131, 178].

Abbreviations

aPKC: Atypical protein kinase C; AxMLP: Axolotl MLP; CAP23: Cytoskeletal associated protein 23; DAG: Diacylglycerol; DGKζ: Diacylglycerol kinase zeta; ED: Effector domain; FAK: Focal adhesion kinase; GAP43: Growth associated protein 43; hpa: Hours post-amputation; IP3: Inositol triphosphate; LPA: Lysophosphatidic acid; MARCKS: Myristoylated alanine-rich C-kinase substrate; MARCKSL1: MARCKS-like 1; MH2: MARCKS homology 2; MLP: MARCKS-like protein; MO: Morpholino oligonucleotides; MRP: MARCKS-related protein; NCAM: Neural cell adhesion molecule; NCCs: Neural crest cells; NPCs: Neural progenitor cells; PA: Phosphatidic acid; PAR3: Partitioning defective 3; PC: Phosphatidylcholine; PI3K: Phosphoinositide 3-kinase; PIP_2: Phosphatidylinositol 4,5-bisphosphate; PKC: Protein kinase C; PLC: Phospholipase C; PLD: Phospholipase D; PPVs: Plasmalemmal precursor vesicles; PSA: Polysialic acid; RA: Retinoic acid; Rb: Retinoblastoma protein; ROCK: Rho kinase; TOB2: Transducer of ErbB2

Funding

This work was supported in part by the Hardiman Research Scholarship from NUI Galway.

Authors' contributions

MEA and GS have written the manuscript and UF has contributed to its revision. All authors have made contributions to the conception and design of this review and have reviewed the manuscript.

Competing interests

The authors declare that they have no competing interests.

Author details

[1]Centre for Research in Medical Devices (CÚRAM), National University of Ireland, Galway, Biomedical Sciences Building, Newcastle Road, Galway, Ireland. [2]Galway Neuroscience Centre, School of Natural Sciences, Biomedical Sciences Building, National University of Ireland, Newcastle Road, Galway, Ireland. [3]School of Natural Sciences and Regenerative Medicine Institute (REMEDI), National University of Ireland, Galway, Biomedical Sciences Building, Newcastle Road, Galway, Ireland.

References

1. Stumpo DJ, Bock CB, Tuttle JS, Blackshear PJ. MARCKS deficiency in mice leads to abnormal brain development and perinatal death. Proc Natl Acad Sci U S A. 1995;92(4):944–8.
2. Brudvig JJ, Weimer JM. X MARCKS the spot: myristoylated alanine-rich C kinase substrate in neuronal function and disease. Front Cell Neurosci. 2015;9:407.
3. Iioka H, Ueno N, Kinoshita N. Essential role of MARCKS in cortical actin dynamics during gastrulation movements. J Cell Biol. 2004;164(2):169–74.
4. Kim SS, Kim JH, Kim HS, Park DE, Chung CH. Involvement of the theta-type protein kinase C in translocation of myristoylated alanine-rich C kinase substrate (MARCKS) during myogenesis of chick embryonic myoblasts. Biochem J. 2000;347(Pt 1):139–46.
5. Kalwa H, Michel T. The MARCKS protein plays a critical role in phosphatidylinositol 4,5-bisphosphate metabolism and directed cell movement in vascular endothelial cells. J Biol Chem. 2011;286(3):2320–30.
6. Arbuzova A, Schmitz AA, Vergeres G. Cross-talk unfolded: MARCKS proteins. Biochem J. 2002;362(Pt 1):1–12.
7. Sundaram M, Cook HW, Byers DM. The MARCKS family of phospholipid binding proteins: regulation of phospholipase D and other cellular components. Biochem Cell Biol. 2004;82(1):191–200.
8. Fong LWR, Yang DC, Chen C-H. Myristoylated alanine-rich C kinase substrate (MARCKS): a multirole signaling protein in cancers. Cancer Metastasis Rev. 2017;36(4):737–47.

9. Wiederkehr A, Staple J, Caroni P. The motility-associated proteins GAP-43, MARCKS, and CAP-23 share unique targeting and surface activity-inducing properties. Exp Cell Res. 1997;236(1):103–16.

10. Skene JP. Axonal growth-associated proteins. Annu Rev Neurosci. 1989; 12(1):127–56.

11. Holahan MR. A shift from a pivotal to supporting role for the growth-associated protein (GAP-43) in the coordination of axonal structural and functional plasticity. Front Cell Neurosci. 2017;11:266.

12. McNamara R, Jiang Y, Streit W, Lenox R. Facial motor neuron regeneration induces a unique spatial and temporal pattern of myristoylated alanine-rich C kinase substrate expression. Neuroscience. 2000;97(3):581–9.

13. Sugiura T, Wang H, Barsacchi R, Simon A, Tanaka EM. MARCKS-like protein is an initiating molecule in axolotl appendage regeneration. Nature. 2016; 531(7593):237–40.

14. Nogueira AF, Costa CM, Lorena J, Moreira RN, Frota-Lima GN, Furtado C, Robinson M, Amemiya CT, Darnet S, Schneider I. Tetrapod limb and sarcopterygian fin regeneration share a core genetic programme. Nat Commun. 2016;7:13364.

15. Ramsden JJ. MARCKS: a case of molecular exaptation? Int J Biochem Cell Biol. 2000;32(5):475–9.

16. Ott LE, McDowell ZT, Turner PM, Law JM, Adler KB, Yoder JA, Jones SL. Two myristoylated alanine-rich C-kinase substrate (MARCKS) paralogs are required for normal development in zebrafish. Anat Rec (Hoboken). 2011; 294(9):1511–24.

17. Ikenoya M, Hidaka H, Hosoya T, Suzuki M, Yamamoto N, Sasaki Y. Inhibition of rho-kinase-induced myristoylated alanine-rich C kinase substrate (MARCKS) phosphorylation in human neuronal cells by H-1152, a novel and specific rho-kinase inhibitor. J Neurochem. 2002;81(1):9–16.

18. Nagumo H, Ikenoya M, Sakurada K, Furuya K, Ikuhara T, Hiraoka H, Sasaki Y. Rho-associated kinase phosphorylates MARCKS in human neuronal cells. Biochem Biophys Res Commun. 2001;280(3):605–9.

19. Toledo A, Zolessi FR, Arruti C. A novel effect of MARCKS phosphorylation by activated PKC: the dephosphorylation of its serine 25 in chick neuroblasts. PLoS One. 2013;8(4):e62863.

20. Manenti S, Sorokine O, Van Dorsselaer A, Taniguchi H. Demyristoylation of the major substrate of protein kinase C (MARCKS) by the cytoplasmic fraction of brain synaptosomes. J Biol Chem. 1994;269(11): 8309–13.

21. Kim J, Blackshear PJ, Johnson JD, McLaughlin S. Phosphorylation reverses the membrane association of peptides that correspond to the basic domains of MARCKS and neuromodulin. Biophys J. 1994;67(1):227–37.

22. McLaughlin S, Aderem A. The myristoyl-electrostatic switch: a modulator of reversible protein-membrane interactions. Trends Biochem Sci. 1995;20(7):272–6.

23. Kim J, Shishido T, Jiang X, Aderem A, McLaughlin S. Phosphorylation, high ionic strength, and calmodulin reverse the binding of MARCKS to phospholipid vesicles. J Biol Chem. 1994;269(45):28214–9.

24. Stumpo DJ, Eddy RL, Haley LL, Sait S, Shows TB, Lai WS, Young WS, Speer MC, Dehejia A, Polymeropoulos M. Promoter sequence, expression, and fine chromosomal mapping of the human gene (MLP) encoding the MARCKS-like protein: Identification of neighboring and linked polymorphic loci forMLPandMACSand use in the evaluation of human neural tube defects. Genomics. 1998;49(2):253–64.

25. Umekage T, Kato K. A mouse brain cDNA encodes a novel protein with the protein kinase C phosphorylation site domain common to MARCKS. FEBS Lett. 1991;286(1–2):147–51.

26. Hartwig JH, Thelen M, Rosen A, Janmey PA, Nairn AC, Aderem A. MARCKS is an actin filament crosslinking protein regulated by protein kinase C and calcium-calmodulin. Nature. 1992;356(6370):618–22.

27. Yarmola EG, Edison AS, Lenox RH, Bubb MR. Actin filament cross-linking by MARCKS: characterization of two actin-binding sites within the phosphorylation site domain. J Biol Chem. 2001;276(25):22351–8.

28. Wohnsland F, Schmitz AA, Steinmetz MO, Aebi U, Vergères G. Interaction between actin and the effector peptide of MARCKS-related protein IDENTIFICATION OF FUNCTIONAL AMINO ACID SEGMENTS. J Biol Chem. 2000;275(27):20873–9.

29. Bjorkblom B, Padzik A, Mohammad H, Westerlund N, Komulainen E, Hollos P, Parviainen L, Papageorgiou AC, Iljin K, Kallioniemi O, Kallajoki M, Courtney MJ, Magard M, James P, Coffey ET. C-Jun N-terminal kinase phosphorylation of MARCKSL1 determines actin stability and migration in neurons and in cancer cells. Mol Cell Biol. 2012;32(17):3513–26.

30. Li Y, Martin LD, Spizz G, Adler KB. MARCKS protein is a key molecule regulating mucin secretion by human airway epithelial cells in vitro. J Biol Chem. 2001;276(44):40982–90.

31. Park J, Fang S, Crews AL, Lin KW, Adler KB. MARCKS regulation of mucin secretion by airway epithelium in vitro: interaction with chaperones. Am J Respir Cell Mol Biol. 2008;39(1):68–76.

32. Wang J, Arbuzova A, Hangyás-Mihályné G, McLaughlin S. The effector domain of myristoylated alanine-rich C kinase substrate binds strongly to phosphatidylinositol 4, 5-bisphosphate. J Biol Chem. 2001;276(7): 5012–9.

33. Ziemba BP, Burke JE, Masson G, Williams RL, Falke JJ. Regulation of PI3K by PKC and MARCKS: single-molecule analysis of a reconstituted signaling pathway. Biophys J. 2016;110(8):1811–25.

34. McLaughlin S, Wang J, Gambhir A, Murray D. PIP2 and proteins: interactions, organization, and information flow. Annu Rev Biophys Biomol Struct. 2002;31(1):151–75.

35. Goni GM, Epifano C, Boskovic J, Camacho-Artacho M, Zhou J, Bronowska A, Martin MT, Eck MJ, Kremer L, Grater F, Gervasio FL, Perez-Moreno M, Lietha D. Phosphatidylinositol 4,5-bisphosphate triggers activation of focal adhesion kinase by inducing clustering and conformational changes. Proc Natl Acad Sci U S A. 2014;111(31):E3177–86.

36. Essen LO, Perisic O, Katan M, Wu Y, Roberts MF, Williams RL. Structural mapping of the catalytic mechanism for a mammalian phosphoinositide-specific phospholipase C. Biochemistry. 1997;36(7):1704–18.

37. Suh PG, Park JI, Manzoli L, Cocco L, Peak JC, Katan M, Fukami K, Kataoka T, Yun S, Ryu SH. Multiple roles of phosphoinositide-specific phospholipase C isozymes. BMB Rep. 2008;41(6):415–34.

38. Kadamur G, Ross EM. Mammalian phospholipase C. Annu Rev Physiol. 2013;75:127–54.

39. Manning BD, Toker AAKT. PKB signaling: navigating the network. Cell. 2017;169(3):381–405.

40. Gambhir A, Hangyás-Mihályné G, Zaitseva I, Cafiso DS, Wang J, Murray D, Pentyala SN, Smith SO, McLaughlin S. Electrostatic sequestration of PIP2 on phospholipid membranes by basic/aromatic regions of proteins. Biophys J. 2004;86(4):2188–207.

41. McLaughlin S, Murray D. Plasma membrane phosphoinositide organization by protein electrostatics. Nature. 2005;438(7068):605.

42. Gamper N, Shapiro MS. Target-specific PIP2 signalling: how might it work? J Physiol. 2007;582(3):967–75.

43. Laux T, Fukami K, Thelen M, Golub T, Frey D, Caroni P. GAP43, MARCKS, and CAP23 modulate PI(4,5)P(2) at plasmalemmal rafts, and regulate cell cortex actin dynamics through a common mechanism. J Cell Biol. 2000;149(7):1455–72.

44. Morash SC, Rose SD, Byers DM, Ridgway ND, Cook HW. Overexpression of myristoylated alanine-rich C-kinase substrate enhances activation of phospholipase D by protein kinase C in SK-N-MC human neuroblastoma cells. Biochem J. 1998;332(Pt 2):321–7.

45. Morash SC, Byers DM, Cook HW. Activation of phospholipase D by PKC and GTPγS in human neuroblastoma cells overexpressing MARCKS. Biochim. Biophys. Acta Mol. Cell Biol. Lipids. 2000;1487(2):177–89.

46. Cockcroft S, Phospholipase D. Regulation by GTPases and protein kinase C and physiological relevance. Prog Lipid Res. 1996;35(4):345–70.

47. Gomez-Cambronero J, Keire P, Phospholipase D. A novel major player in signal transduction. Cell Signal. 1998;10(6):387–97.

48. Frohman MA, Sung T-C, Morris AJ. Mammalian phospholipase D structure and regulation. Biochim. Biophys. Acta Mol. Cell Biol. Lipids. 1999;1439(2):175–86.

49. Exton J. Regulation of phospholipase D. Biochim. Biophys. Acta Mol. Cell Biol. Lipids. 1999;1439(2):121–33.

50. Exton JH. Regulation of phospholipase D. FEBS Lett. 2002;531(1):58–61.

51. Foster DA, Xu L. Phospholipase D in cell proliferation and Cancer11National Cancer institute, and the institutional support from the research centers in minority institutions (RCMI) program of the NIH. Mol Cancer Res. 2003;1(11): 789–800.

52. Brown HA, Thomas PG, Lindsley CW. Targeting phospholipase D in cancer, infection and neurodegenerative disorders. Nat Rev Drug Discov. 2017;16(5):351.

53. Selvy PE, Lavieri RR, Lindsley CW, Brown HA. Phospholipase D: enzymology, functionality, and chemical modulation. Chem Rev. 2011;111(10):6064–119.

54. Kam Y, Exton JH. Phospholipase D activity is required for actin stress fiber formation in fibroblasts. Mol Cell Biol. 2001;21(12):4055–66.

55. Cross MJ, Roberts S, Ridley AJ, Hodgkin MN, Stewart A, Claesson-Welsh L, Wakelam MJ. Stimulation of actin stress fibre formation mediated by activation of phospholipase D. Curr Biol. 1996;6(5):588–97.

56. Roth MG. Molecular mechanisms of PLD function in membrane traffic. Traffic. 2008;9(8):1233–9.

57. Joseph T, Bryant A, Frankel P, Wooden R, Kerkhoff E, Rapp UR, Foster DA. Phospholipase D overcomes cell cycle arrest induced by high-intensity Raf signaling. Oncogene. 2002;21(22):3651.

58. Zhang W, Wang C, Qin C, Wood T, Olafsdottir G, Welti R, Wang X. The oleate-stimulated phospholipase D, PLDdelta, and phosphatidic acid decrease H2O2-induced cell death in Arabidopsis. Plant Cell. 2003;15(10): 2285–95.

59. Zhang Y, Huang P, Du G, Kanaho Y, Frohman MA, Tsirka SE. Increased expression of two phospholipase D isoforms during experimentally induced hippocampal mossy fiber outgrowth. Glia. 2004;46(1):74–83.

60. Rizzo MA, Shome K, Vasudevan C, Stolz DB, Sung T-C, Frohman MA, Watkins SC, Romero G. Phospholipase D and its product, phosphatidic acid, mediate agonist-dependent raf-1 translocation to the plasma membrane and the activation of the mitogen-activated protein kinase pathway. J Biol Chem. 1999;274(2):1131–9.

61. Lin M-E, Herr DR, Chun J. Lysophosphatidic acid (LPA) receptors: signaling properties and disease relevance. Prostaglandins Other Lipid Mediat. 2010;91(3–4):130–8.

62. Nishizuka Y. Intracellular signaling by hydrolysis of phospholipids and activation of protein kinase C. Science. 1992;258(5082):607–14.

63. Moolenaar WH. Lysophosphatidic acid, a multifunctional phospholipid messenger. J Biol Chem. 1995;270(22):12949–52.

64. Cho SJ, La M-h, Ahn JK, Meadows GG, Joe CO. Tob-mediated cross-talk between MARCKS phosphorylation and ErbB-2 activation. Biochem Biophys Res Commun. 2001;283(2):273–7.

65. Anton E, Marchionni M, Lee K, Rakic P. Role of GGF/neuregulin signaling in interactions between migrating neurons and radial glia in the developing cerebral cortex. Development. 1997;124(18):3501–10.

66. Ghashghaei H, Weimer JM, Schmid RS, Yokota Y, McCarthy KD, Popko B, Anton E. Reinduction of ErbB2 in astrocytes promotes radial glial progenitor identity in adult cerebral cortex. Genes Dev. 2007;21(24):3258–71.

67. Angata K, Huckaby V, Ranscht B, Terskikh A, Marth JD, Fukuda M. Polysialic acid-directed migration and differentiation of neural precursors are essential for mouse brain development. Mol Cell Biol. 2007;27(19):6659–68.

68. Zhang H, Miller RH, Rutishauser U. Polysialic acid is required for optimal growth of axons on a neuronal substrate. J Neurosci. 1992;12(8):3107–14.

69. Marx M, Rutishauser U, Bastmeyer M. Dual function of polysialic acid during zebrafish central nervous system development. Development. 2001;128(24): 4949–58.

70. Langhauser M, Ustinova J, Rivera-Milla E, Ivannikov D, Seidl C, Slomka C, Finne J, Yoshihara Y, Bastmeyer M, Bentrop J. Ncam1a and Ncam1b: two carriers of polysialic acid with different functions in the developing zebrafish nervous system. Glycobiology. 2011;22(2):196–209.

71. Theis T, Mishra B, von der Ohe M, Loers G, Prondzynski M, Pless O, Blackshear PJ, Schachner M, Kleene R. Functional role of the interaction between polysialic acid and myristoylated alanine-rich C kinase substrate at the plasma membrane. J Biol Chem. 2013;288(9):6726–42.

72. Brudvig JJ, Cain JT, Schmidt-Grimminger GG, Stumpo DJ, Roux KJ, Blackshear PJ, Weimer JM. MARCKS is necessary for netrin-DCC signaling and Corpus callosum formation. Mol Neurobiol. 2018; https://doi.org/10. 1007/s12035-018-0990-3.

73. Weimer JM, Yokota Y, Stanco A, Stumpo DJ, Blackshear PJ, Anton ES. MARCKS modulates radial progenitor placement, proliferation and organization in the developing cerebral cortex. Development. 2009;136(17):2965–75.

74. Muthusamy N, Sommerville LJ, Moeser AJ, Stumpo DJ, Sannes P, Adler K, Blackshear PJ, Weimer JM, Ghashghaei HT. MARCKS-dependent mucin clearance and lipid metabolism in ependymal cells are required for maintenance of forebrain homeostasis during aging. Aging Cell. 2015;14(5): 764–73.

75. Janetopoulos C, Devreotes P. Phosphoinositide signaling plays a key role in cytokinesis. J Cell Biol. 2006;174(4):485–90.

76. Marín-Vicente C, Nicolás FE, Gómez-Fernández JC, Corbalán-García S. The PtdIns (4, 5) P2 ligand itself influences the localization of PKCα in the plasma membrane of intact living cells. J Mol Biol. 2008;377(4):1038–52.

77. Martin-Belmonte F, Mostov K. Phosphoinositides control epithelial development. Cell Cycle. 2007;6(16):1957–61.

78. Xu X-H, Deng C-Y, Liu Y, He M, Peng J, Wang T, Yuan L, Zheng Z-S, Blackshear PJ, Luo Z-G. MARCKS regulates membrane targeting of Rab10 vesicles to promote axon development. Cell Res. 2014;24(5):576.

79. Mizutani A, Tokumitsu H, Hidaka H. Acidic calmodulin binding protein, ACAMP-81, is MARCKS protein interacting with synapsin I. Biochem Biophys Res Commun. 1992;182(3):1395–401.

80. Li J, O'Connor KL, Greeley GH, Blackshear PJ, Townsend CM, Evers BM. Myristoylated alanine-rich C kinase substrate-mediated neurotensin release via protein kinase C-δ downstream of the rho/ROK pathway. J Biol Chem. 2005;280(9):8351–7.

81. Park J, Fang S, Adler KB. Regulation of airway mucin secretion by MARCKS protein involves the chaperones heat shock protein 70 and cysteine string protein. Proc Am Thorac Soc. 2006;3(6):493.

82. Takashi S, Park J, Fang S, Koyama S, Parikh I, Adler KBA. Peptide against the N-terminus of myristoylated alanine-rich C kinase substrate inhibits degranulation of human leukocytes in vitro. Am J Respir Cell Mol Biol. 2006;34(6):647–52.

83. Damera G, Jester WF, Jiang M, Zhao H, Fogle HW, Mittelman M, Haczku A, Murphy E, Parikh I, Panettieri RA Jr. Inhibition of myristoylated alanine-rich C kinase substrate (MARCKS) protein inhibits ozone-induced airway neutrophilia and inflammation. Exp Lung Res. 2010;36(2):75–84.

84. Zhao J, Izumi T, Nunomura K, Satoh S, Watanabe S. MARCKS-like protein, a membrane protein identified for its expression in developing neural retina, plays a role in regulating retinal cell proliferation. Biochem J. 2007;408(1): 51–9.

85. Gatlin JC, Estrada-Bernal A, Sanford SD, Pfenninger KH. Myristoylated, alanine-rich C-kinase substrate phosphorylation regulates growth cone adhesion and pathfinding. Mol Biol Cell. 2006;17(12):5115–30.

86. Shiraishi M, Tanabe A, Saito N, Sasaki Y. Unphosphorylated MARCKS is involved in neurite initiation induced by insulin-like growth factor-I in SH-SY5Y cells. J Cell Physiol. 2006;209(3):1029–38.

87. Yu D, Makkar G, Dong T, Strickland DK, Sarkar R, Monahan TS. MARCKS signaling differentially regulates vascular smooth muscle and endothelial cell proliferation through a KIS-, p27kip1- dependent mechanism. PLoS One. 2015;10(11):e0141397.

88. Eckert RE, Neuder LE, Park J, Adler KB, Jones SL. Myristoylated alanine-rich C-kinase substrate (MARCKS) protein regulation of human neutrophil migration. Am J Respir Cell Mol Biol. 2010;42(5):586–94.

89. Chen X, Rotenberg SA. PhosphoMARCKS drives motility of mouse melanoma cells. Cell Signal. 2010;22(7):1097–103.

90. Green TD, Park J, Yin Q, Fang S, Crews AL, Jones SL, Adler KB. Directed migration of mouse macrophages in vitro involves myristoylated alanine-rich C-kinase substrate (MARCKS) protein. J Leukoc Biol. 2012;92(3):633–9.

91. Sheats MK, Sung EJ, Adler KB, Jones SL. In vitro neutrophil migration requires protein kinase C-Delta (delta-PKC)-mediated Myristoylated alanine-rich C-kinase substrate (MARCKS) phosphorylation. Inflammation. 2015;38(3): 1126–41.

92. Yu D, Makkar G, Strickland DK, Blanpied TA, Stumpo DJ, Blackshear PJ, Sarkar R, Monahan TS. Myristoylated alanine-rich protein kinase substrate (MARCKS) regulates small GTPase Rac1 and Cdc42 activity and is a critical mediator of vascular smooth muscle cell migration in intimal hyperplasia formation. J Am Heart Assoc. 2015;4(10):e002255.

93. Scarlett CO, Blackshear PJ. Neuroanatomical development in the absence of PKC phosphorylation of the myristoylated alanine-rich C-kinase substrate (MARCKS) protein. Brain Res Dev Brain Res. 2003;144(1):25–42.

94. Swierczynski SL, Siddhanti SR, Tuttle JS, Blackshear PJ. Nonmyristoylated MARCKS complements some but not all of the developmental defects associated with MARCKS deficiency in mice. Dev Biol. 1996;179(1):135–47.

95. Kim HS, Swierczynski SL, Tuttle JS, Lai WS, Blackshear PJ. Transgenic complementation of MARCKS deficiency with a nonmyristoylatable, pseudo-phosphorylated form of MARCKS: evidence for simultaneous positive and dominant-negative effects on central nervous system development. Dev Biol. 1998;200(2):146–57.

96. Disatnik MH, Boutet SC, Pacio W, Chan AY, Ross LB, Lee CH, Rando TA. The bi-directional translocation of MARCKS between membrane and cytosol regulates integrin-mediated muscle cell spreading. J Cell Sci. 2004;117 (Pt 19):4469–79.

97. Sheats MK, Pescosolido KC, Hefner EM, Sung EJ, Adler KB, Jones SL. Myristoylated alanine rich C kinase substrate (MARCKS) is essential to beta2-integrin dependent responses of equine neutrophils. Vet Immunol Immunopathol. 2014;160(3–4):167–76.

98. Shi Y, Sullivan SK, Pitterle DM, Kennington EA, Graff JM, Blackshear PJ. Mechanisms of MARCKS gene activation during Xenopus development. J Biol Chem. 1997;272(46):29290–300.

99. Zhao H, Cao Y, Grunz H. Isolation and characterization of a Xenopus gene (XMLP) encoding a MARCKS-like protein. Int J Dev Biol. 2001;45(7):817–26.

100. Blackshear PJ, Lai WS, Tuttle JS, Stumpo DJ, Kennington E, Nairn AC, Sulik KK. Developmental expression of MARCKS and protein kinase C in mice in relation to the exencephaly resulting from MARCKS deficiency. Brain Res Dev Brain Res. 1996;96(1–2):62–75.

101. Zolessi FR, Arruti C. Sustained phosphorylation of MARCKS in differentiating neurogenic regions during chick embryo development. Brain Res Dev Brain Res. 2001;130(2):257–67.

102. Ruiz-Perera LM, Arruti C, Zolessi FR. Early phosphorylation of MARCKS at Ser25 in migrating precursor cells and differentiating peripheral neurons. Neurosci Lett. 2013;544:5–9.

103. McNamara RK, Wees EA, Lenox RH. Differential subcellular redistribution of protein kinase C isozymes in the rat hippocampus induced by kainic acid. J Neurochem. 1999;72(4):1735–43.

104. Wees E, McNamara R, Meberg P, Kuhn T, Lenox R. The PKC substrate MARCKS is enriched in neuronal growth cones and developmentally regulated in the rat hippocampus. Soc Neurosci Abs. 1998;24:537.

105. Calabrese B, Halpain S. Essential role for the PKC target MARCKS in maintaining dendritic spine morphology. Neuron. 2005;48(1):77–90.

106. Wu M, Chen DF, Sasaoka T, Tonegawa S. Neural tube defects and abnormal brain development in F52-deficient mice. Proc Natl Acad Sci. 1996;93(5):2110–5.

107. Chen J, Chang S, Duncan SA, Okano HJ, Fishell G, Aderem A. Disruption of the MacMARCKS gene prevents cranial neural tube closure and results in anencephaly. Proc Natl Acad Sci. 1996;93(13):6275–9.

108. Fleming A, Copp AJ. A genetic risk factor for mouse neural tube defects: defining the embryonic basis. Hum Mol Genet. 2000;9(4):575–81.

109. Kim SS, Kim JH, Lee SH, Chung SS, Bang OS, Park D, Chung CH. Involvement of protein phosphatase-1-mediated MARCKS translocation in myogenic differentiation of embryonic muscle cells. J Cell Sci. 2002;115(Pt 12):2465–73.

110. Garrett AM, Schreiner D, Lobas MA, Weiner JA. γ-protocadherins control cortical dendrite arborization by regulating the activity of a FAK/PKC/MARCKS signaling pathway. Neuron. 2012;74(2):269–76.

111. Sosa LJ, Malter JS, Hu J, Bustos Plonka F, Oksdath M, Nieto Guil AF, Quiroga S, Pfenninger KH. Protein interacting with NIMA (never in mitosis a)-1 regulates axonal growth cone adhesion and spreading through myristoylated alanine-rich C kinase substrate isomerization. J Neurochem. 2016;137(5):744–55.

112. Yamaguchi H, Shiraishi M, Fukami K, Tanabe A, Ikeda-Matsuo Y, Naito Y, Sasaki Y. MARCKS regulates lamellipodia formation induced by IGF-I via association with PIP2 and beta-actin at membrane microdomains. J Cell Physiol. 2009;220(3):748–55.

113. Cordero DR, Brugmann S, Chu Y, Bajpai R, Jame M, Helms JA. Cranial neural crest cells on the move: their roles in craniofacial development. Am J Med Genet A. 2011;155A(2):270–9.

114. Martik ML, Bronner ME. Regulatory logic underlying diversification of the neural crest. Trends Genet. 2017;33(10):715–27.

115. Rochlin K, Yu S, Roy S, Baylies MK. Myoblast fusion: when it takes more to make one. Dev Biol. 2010;341(1):66–83.

116. Kalwa H, Sartoretto JL, Sartoretto SM, Michel T. Angiotensin-II and MARCKS: a hydrogen peroxide- and RAC1-dependent signaling pathway in vascular endothelium. J Biol Chem. 2012;287(34):29147–58.

117. Trovo L, Ahmed T, Callaerts-Vegh Z, Buzzi A, Bagni C, Chuah M, Vandendriessche T, D'Hooge R, Balschun D, Dotti CG. Low hippocampal PI(4,5)P(2) contributes to reduced cognition in old mice as a result of loss of MARCKS. Nat Neurosci. 2013;16(4):449–55.

118. Finlayson AE, Freeman KW. A cell motility screen reveals role for MARCKS-related protein in adherens junction formation and tumorigenesis. PLoS One. 2009;4(11):e7833.

119. Zhang Y, Bo X, Schoepfer R, Holtmaat AJ, Verhaagen J, Emson PC, Lieberman AR, Anderson PN. Growth-associated protein GAP-43 and L1 act synergistically to promote regenerative growth of Purkinje cell axons in vivo. Proc Natl Acad Sci U S A. 2005;102(41):14883–8.

120. Mason MR, Lieberman A, Grenningloh G, Anderson P. Transcriptional upregulation of SCG10 and CAP-23 is correlated with regeneration of the axons of peripheral and central neurons in vivo. Mol Cell Neurosci. 2002;20(4):595–615.

121. Makwana M, Raivich G. Molecular mechanisms in successful peripheral regeneration. FEBS J. 2005;272(11):2628–38.

122. Verhaagen J, Van Hooff C, Edwards P, De Graan P, Oestreicher A, Schotman P, Jennekens F, Gispen W. The kinase C substrate protein B-50 and axonal regeneration. Brain Res Bull. 1986;17(6):737–41.

123. Szpara ML, Vranizan K, Tai YC, Goodman CS, Speed TP, Ngai J. Analysis of gene expression during neurite outgrowth and regeneration. BMC Neurosci. 2007;8(1):100.

124. Frey D, Laux T, Xu L, Schneider C, Caroni P. Shared and unique roles of CAP23 and GAP43 in actin regulation, neurite outgrowth, and anatomical plasticity. J Cell Biol. 2000;149(7):1443–54.

125. Caroni P, Aigner L, Schneider C. Intrinsic neuronal determinants locally regulate extrasynaptic and synaptic growth at the adult neuromuscular junction. J Cell Biol. 1997;136(3):679–92.

126. Carmichael ST, Archibeque I, Luke L, Nolan T, Momiy J, Li S. Growth-associated gene expression after stroke: evidence for a growth-promoting region in peri-infarct cortex. Exp Neurol. 2005;193(2):291–311.

127. Van der Zee C, Nielander HB, Vos JP, da Silva SL, Verhaagen J, Oestreicher AB, Schrama LH, Schotman P, Gispen WH. Expression of growth-associated protein B-50 (GAP43) in dorsal root ganglia and sciatic nerve during regenerative sprouting. J Neurosci. 1989;9(10):3505–12.

128. Pellier-Monnin V, Astic L, Bichet S, Riederer BM, Grenningloh G. Expression of SCG10 and stathmin proteins in the rat olfactory system during development and axonal regeneration. J Comp Neurol. 2001;433(2):239–54.

129. Doster SK, Lozano AM, Aguayo AJ, Willard MB. Expression of the growth-associated protein GAP-43 in adult rat retinal ganglion cells following axon injury. Neuron. 1991;6(4):635–47.

130. Mason M, Lieberman A, Anderson P. Corticospinal neurons up-regulate a range of growth-associated genes following intracortical, but not spinal, axotomy. Eur J Neurosci. 2003;18(4):789–802.

131. Bomze HM, Bulsara KR, Iskandar BJ, Caroni P, Skene JP. Spinal axon regeneration evoked by replacing two growth cone proteins in adult neurons. Nat Neurosci. 2001;4(1):38.

132. Aigner L, Arber S, Kapfhammer JP, Laux T, Schneider C, Botteri F, Brenner HR, Caroni P. Overexpression of the neural growth-associated protein GAP-43 induces nerve sprouting in the adult nervous system of transgenic mice. Cell. 1995;83(2):269–78.

133. Buffo A, Holtmaat AJ, Savio T, Verbeek JS, Oberdick J, Oestreicher AB, Gispen WH, Verhaagen J, Rossi F, Strata P. Targeted overexpression of the neurite growth-associated protein B-50/GAP-43 in cerebellar Purkinje cells induces sprouting after axotomy but not axon regeneration into growth-permissive transplants. J Neurosci. 1997;17(22):8778–91.

134. Allegra Mascaro AL, Cesare P, Sacconi L, Grasselli G, Mandolesi G, Maco B, Knott GW, Huang L, De Paola V, Strata P, Pavone FS. In vivo single branch axotomy induces GAP-43-dependent sprouting and synaptic remodeling in cerebellar cortex. Proc Natl Acad Sci U S A. 2013;110(26):10824–9.

135. Veldman MB, Bemben MA, Thompson RC, Goldman D. Gene expression analysis of zebrafish retinal ganglion cells during optic nerve regeneration identifies KLF6a and KLF7a as important regulators of axon regeneration. Dev Biol. 2007;312(2):596–612.

136. Sousounis K, Bhavsar R, Looso M, Kruger M, Beebe J, Braun T, Tsonis PA. Molecular signatures that correlate with induction of lens regeneration in newts: lessons from proteomic analysis. Hum Genomics. 2014;8:22.

137. Bock-Marquette I, Shrivastava S, Pipes GT, Thatcher JE, Blystone A, Shelton JM, Galindo CL, Melegh B, Srivastava D, Olson EN. Thymosin β4 mediated PKC activation is essential to initiate the embryonic coronary developmental program and epicardial progenitor cell activation in adult mice in vivo. J Mol Cell Cardiol. 2009;46(5):728–38.

138. Gurtner GC, Callaghan MJ, Longaker MT. Progress and potential for regenerative medicine. Annu Rev Med. 2007;58:299–312.

139. Gurtner GC, Werner S, Barrandon Y, Longaker MT. Wound repair and regeneration. Nature. 2008;453(7193):314.

140. Friedl P, Gilmour D. Collective cell migration in morphogenesis, regeneration and cancer. Nat Rev Mol Cell Biol. 2009;10(7):445.

141. Ridley AJ, Schwartz MA, Burridge K, Firtel RA, Ginsberg MH, Borisy G, Parsons JT, Horwitz AR. Cell migration: integrating signals from front to back. Science. 2003;302(5651):1704–9.

142. Kawakami Y, Esteban CR, Raya M, Kawakami H, Martí M, Dubova I, Belmonte JCI. Wnt/β-catenin signaling regulates vertebrate limb regeneration. Genes Dev. 2006;20(23):3232–7.

143. Donnelly DJ, Popovich PG. Inflammation and its role in neuroprotection, axonal regeneration and functional recovery after spinal cord injury. Exp Neurol. 2008;209(2):378–88.

144. Mescher AL, Neff AW, King MW. Inflammation and immunity in organ regeneration. Dev. Comp. Immunol. 2017;66:98–110.

145. Eming SA, Wynn TA, Martin P. Inflammation and metabolism in tissue repair and regeneration. Science. 2017;356(6342):1026–30.

146. Guo Q, Li S, Liang Y, Zhang Y, Zhang J, Wen C, Lin S, Wang H, Su B. Effects of C3 deficiency on inflammation and regeneration following spinal cord injury in mice. Neurosci Lett. 2010;485(1):32–6.

147. Karin M, Clevers H. Reparative inflammation takes charge of tissue regeneration. Nature. 2016;529(7586):307.

148. Silburt J, Lipsman N, Aubert I. Disrupting the blood–brain barrier with focused ultrasound: perspectives on inflammation and regeneration. Proc Natl Acad Sci. 2017;114(33):E6735–6.

149. Cooper PR, Takahashi Y, Graham LW, Simon S, Imazato S, Smith AJ. Inflammation–regeneration interplay in the dentine–pulp complex. J Dent. 2010;38(9):687–97.

150. Forn-Cuní G, Varela M, Pereiro P, Novoa B, Figueras A. Conserved gene regulation during acute inflammation between zebrafish and mammals. Sci Rep. 2017;7:41905.

151. Godwin JW, Pinto AR, Rosenthal NA. Macrophages are required for adult salamander limb regeneration. Proc Natl Acad Sci. 2013;110(23):9415–20.

152. Tanaka EM. The molecular and cellular choreography of appendage regeneration. Cell. 2016;165(7):1598–608.

153. Li J, Aderem A. MacMARCKS, a novel member of the MARCKS family of protein kinase C substrates. Cell. 1992;70(5):791–801.

154. Carballo E, Pitterle DM, Stumpo DJ, Sperling RT, Blackshear PJ. Phagocytic and macropinocytic activity in MARCKS-deficient macrophages and fibroblasts. Am J Phys Cell Phys. 1999;277(1):C163–73.

155. Zhou X, Li J. Macrophage-enriched myristoylated alanine-rich C kinase substrate and its phosphorylation is required for the phorbol ester-stimulated diffusion of β2 integrin molecules. J Biol Chem. 2000;275(26):20217–22.

156. Chun K-R, Bae EM, Kim J-K, Suk K, Lee W-H. Suppression of the lipopolysaccharide-induced expression of MARCKS-related protein (MRP) affects transmigration in activated RAW264. 7 cells. Cell Immunol. 2009;256(1):92–8.

157. Li J, D'annibale-Tolhurst MA, Adler KB, Fang S, Yin Q, Birkenheuer AJ, Levy MG, Jones SL, Sung EJ, Hawkins EC, Yoder JA, Nordone SK. A myristoylated alanine-rich C kinase substrate-related peptide suppresses cytokine mRNA and protein expression in LPS-activated canine neutrophils. Am J Respir Cell Mol Biol. 2013;48(3):314–21.

158. Lee SM, Suk K, Lee WH. Myristoylated alanine-rich C kinase substrate (MARCKS) regulates the expression of proinflammatory cytokines in macrophages through activation of p38/JNK MAPK and NF-kappaB. Cell Immunol. 2015;296(2):115–21.

159. Eun SY, Kim EH, Kang KS, Kim HJ, Jo SA, Kim SJ, Jo SH, Kim SJ, Blackshear PJ, Kim J. Cell type-specific upregulation of myristoylated alanine-rich C kinase substrate and protein kinase C-alpha, −beta I, −beta II, and -delta in microglia following kainic acid-induced seizures. Exp Mol Med. 2006;38(3):310–9.

160. Shokouhi BN, Wong BZ, Siddiqui S, Lieberman AR, Campbell G, Tohyama K, Anderson PN. Microglial responses around intrinsic CNS neurons are correlated with axonal regeneration. BMC Neurosci. 2010;11(1):13.

161. Kitayama M, Ueno M, Itakura T, Yamashita T. Activated microglia inhibit axonal growth through RGMa. PLoS One. 2011;6(9):e25234.

162. Hasegawa H, Nakai M, Tanimukai S, Taniguchi T, Terashima A, Kawamata T, Fukunaga K, Miyamoto E, Misaki K, Mukai H, Tanaka C. Microglial signaling by amyloid beta protein through mitogen-activated protein kinase mediating phosphorylation of MARCKS. Neuroreport. 2001;12(11):2567–71.

163. Topham MK, Bunting M, Zimmerman GA, McIntyre TM, Blackshear PJ, Prescott SM. Protein kinase C regulates the nuclear localization of diacylglycerol kinase-ζ. Nature. 1998;394(6694):697.

164. Luo B, Prescott SM, Topham MK. Protein kinase Cα phosphorylates and negatively regulates diacylglycerol kinase ζ. J Biol Chem. 2003; 278(41):39542–7.

165. Los AP, de Widt J, Topham MK, van Blitterswijk WJ, Divecha N. Protein kinase C inhibits binding of diacylglycerol kinase-ζ to the retinoblastoma protein. Biochimica et Biophysica Acta (BBA)-molecular. Cell Res. 2007;1773(3):352–7.

166. Tanaka EM, Gann AA, Gates PB, Brockes JP. Newt myotubes reenter the cell cycle by phosphorylation of the retinoblastoma protein. J Cell Biol. 1997; 136(1):155–65.

167. Sage J, Miller AL, Pérez-Mancera PA, Wysocki JM, Jacks T. Acute mutation of retinoblastoma gene function is sufficient for cell cycle re-entry. Nature. 2003;424(6945):223.

168. Weber T, Corbett MK, Chow LM, Valentine MB, Baker SJ, Zuo J. Rapid cell-cycle reentry and cell death after acute inactivation of the retinoblastoma gene product in postnatal cochlear hair cells. Proc Natl Acad Sci. 2008; 105(2):781–5.

169. Rohrbach TD, Shah N, Jackson WP, Feeney EV, Scanlon S, Gish R, Khodadadi R, Hyde SO, Hicks PH, Anderson JC, Jarboe JS, Willey CD. The effector domain of MARCKS is a nuclear localization signal that regulates cellular PIP2 levels and nuclear PIP2 localization. PLoS One. 2015;10(10):e0140870.

170. Wang L, Watson DG, Lenox RH. Myristoylation alters retinoic acid-induced down-regulation of MARCKS in immortalized hippocampal cells. Biochem Biophys Res Commun. 2000;276(1):183–8.

171. Maden M. Retinoic acid in the development, regeneration and maintenance of the nervous system. Nat Rev Neurosci. 2007;8(10):755.

172. Lefebvre PP, Malgrange B, Staecker H, Moonen G, Van De Water TR. Retinoic acid stimulates regeneration of mammalian auditory hair cells. Science. 1993;260(5108):692–5.

173. Maden M. Vitamin a and pattern formation in the regenerating limb. Nature. 1982;295(5851):672.

174. Maden M, Hind M. Retinoic acid, a regeneration-inducing molecule. Dev Dyn. 2003;226(2):237–44.

175. White JA, Boffa MB, Jones B, Petkovich M. A zebrafish retinoic acid receptor expressed in the regenerating caudal fin. Development. 1994;120(7):1861–72.

176. Wehner D, Weidinger G. Signaling networks organizing regenerative growth of the zebrafish fin. Trends Genet. 2015;31(6):336–43.

177. Chang JT, Lehtinen MK, Sive H. Zebrafish cerebrospinal fluid mediates cell survival through a retinoid signaling pathway. Dev. Neurobiol. 2016;76(1):75–92.

178. Singer M, Martin LD, Vargaftig BB, Park J, Gruber AD, Li Y, Adler KB. A MARCKS-related peptide blocks mucus hypersecretion in a mouse model of asthma. Nat Med. 2004;10(2):193.

Toward population specific and personalized treatment of *Helicobacter pylori* infection

Jyh-Ming Liou[1,2*†], Po-Yueh Chen[3†], Yu-Ting Kuo[1,2], Ming-Shiang Wu[1,2*†] and for the Taiwan Gastrointestinal Disease and Helicobacter Consortium

Abstract

In the face of rising prevalence of antibiotic resistance, susceptibility testing to provide personalized treatment is recommended prior to eradication therapy for *Helicobacter pylori* (*H. pylori*). Yet, population specific treatment according to the local prevalence of antibiotic resistance may be an alternative if susceptibility testing is not available. In this article, we reviewed the global prevalence of primary antibiotic resistance and the efficacies of commonly used regimens in antibiotic susceptible and resistance strains. We then constructed a model to predict the efficacies of these regimens and proposed an algorithm to choose the optimal first-line and rescue therapies according to the prevalence of antibiotic resistance. Clarithromycin-based therapy (triple, sequential, concomitant, and hybrid therapies) for 14 days remains the treatment of choice in regions with low clarithromycin resistance (≤15%) and bismuth quadruple therapy may be an alternative therapy. In regions with high clarithromycin resistance (> 15%), bismuth quadruple therapy is the treatment of choice and non-bismuth quadruple therapy may be an alternative. Either levofloxacin-based therapy or bismuth quadruple therapy may be used as second-line rescue therapy for patients fail after clarithromycin-based therapies, whereas levofloxacin-based therapy may be used for patients fail after bismuth quadruple therapy. Susceptibility testing or genotypic resistance should be determined after two or more eradication failures. However, empirical therapy according to prior medication history to avoid the empirical reuse of levofloxacin and clarithromycin may be an acceptable alternative after consideration of cost, patient preference, and accessibility. Rifabutin-based therapy for 14 days may serve as the fourth-line therapy. New antibiotics specific for *H. pylori* are highly anticipated.

Keywords: *H. pylori*, Resistance, Eradication, First-line, Rescue, Precision medicine, Gastric cancer

Background

Helicobacter pylori (*H. pylori*) infection is a causal factor of peptic ulcer disease, gastric cancer (adenocarcinoma) and mucosal associated lymphoid tissue lymphoma [1]. Eradication of *H. pylori* may reduce the recurrence rate of peptic ulcer and may reduce the risk of gastric cancer [1–3]. However, the efficacy of standard triple therapy containing a proton pump inhibitor (PPI), clarithromycin, with amoxicillin or metronidazole has been declining in many countries [4, 5]. Factors that might lead to treatment failure include the presence of antibiotic resistance, lack of good compliance, inadequate treatment length, and inadequate suppression of gastric acid secretion [6, 7]. Of these, the presence of antibiotic resistance is the most important factor [6, 7]. Therefore, the best strategy to increase the eradication rate is to provide individualized treatment according to antibiotic susceptibility testing (personalized treatment) [8]. However, endoscopy with biopsy and culture for *H. pylori* are costly and time consuming (2–4 weeks). Besides, the successful rate of culture and susceptibility testing ranges from 75 to 90% [9, 10]. Therefore, susceptibility testing guided therapy is not widely applicable for the first-line therapy and is not easily accessible even for

* Correspondence: jyhmingliou@gmail.coml; mingshiang@ntu.edu.tw
†Jyh-Ming Liou, Po-Yueh Chen and Ming-Shiang Wu contributed equally to this work.
[1]Division of Gastroenterology and Hepatology, Department of Internal Medicine, National Taiwan University Hospital, Taipei, Taiwan
Full list of author information is available at the end of the article

refractory *H. pylori* infection [11, 12]. Development of less invasive and less costly tests, such as genotyping of antibiotic resistance genes using gastric biopsy, gastric juice or fecal samples might be an alternative [10]. Yet, the accuracies of these tests using fecal samples are still less than perfect. Another strategy is to choose the best regimen for a population according to the prevalence of antibiotic resistance (population specific treatment) [13–16]. The efficacy of a regimen for *H. pylori* eradication can be predicted as long as its efficacies in susceptible and resistant strains and the prevalence of antibiotic resistance in the population are known [17, 18]. Therefore, we reviewed the global prevalence of antibiotic resistance and the efficacies of different regimens in antibiotic susceptible and resistant strains and constructed prediction models to predict the efficacies of these regimens in regions with different prevalence of antibiotic resistance in this article. Finally, we proposed an algorithm to choose the optimal first-line and rescue therapies according to the prevalence of antibiotic resistance.

Updated prevalence of primary antibiotic resistance worldwide [19–24]

The prevalence of primary antibiotic resistance varies from country to country and changes with time. The updated global prevalence of antibiotic resistance was as follows (Fig. 1).

Clarithromycin resistance

The overall prevalence of primary clarithromycin resistance was 10% (95% CI 4–16) in America's region [22], 17% (95% CI 15–18) in Asia-Pacific [5], and 18% (95% CI 16–20) in Europe [22]. However, there were trends of rising clarithromycin resistance in these regions. The pooled resistance rates of clarithromycin resistance after 2011 were 21% (95% CI 18–25%) in Asia-Pacific, 20% (95% CI 12–28%) in America, and 28% (95% CI 25–31%) in Europe, as shown in Table 1. In Asia-Pacific region [5], clarithromycin resistance was higher than 15% in 13 countries: Bangladesh, China, India, Iran, Japan, Nepal, New Zealand, Pakistan, Saudi Arabia, Singapore, South Korea, Turkey, and Vietnam. In contrast, frequency of resistance was less than 15% in eight countries: Bhutan, Indonesia, Laos, Malaysia, Myanmar, Russia (data were specifically from eastern Russia), Taiwan, and Thailand (Fig. 1).

Metronidazole resistance

The overall prevalence of primary clarithromycin resistance was 23% (95% CI 2–44) in Americas [22], 32%

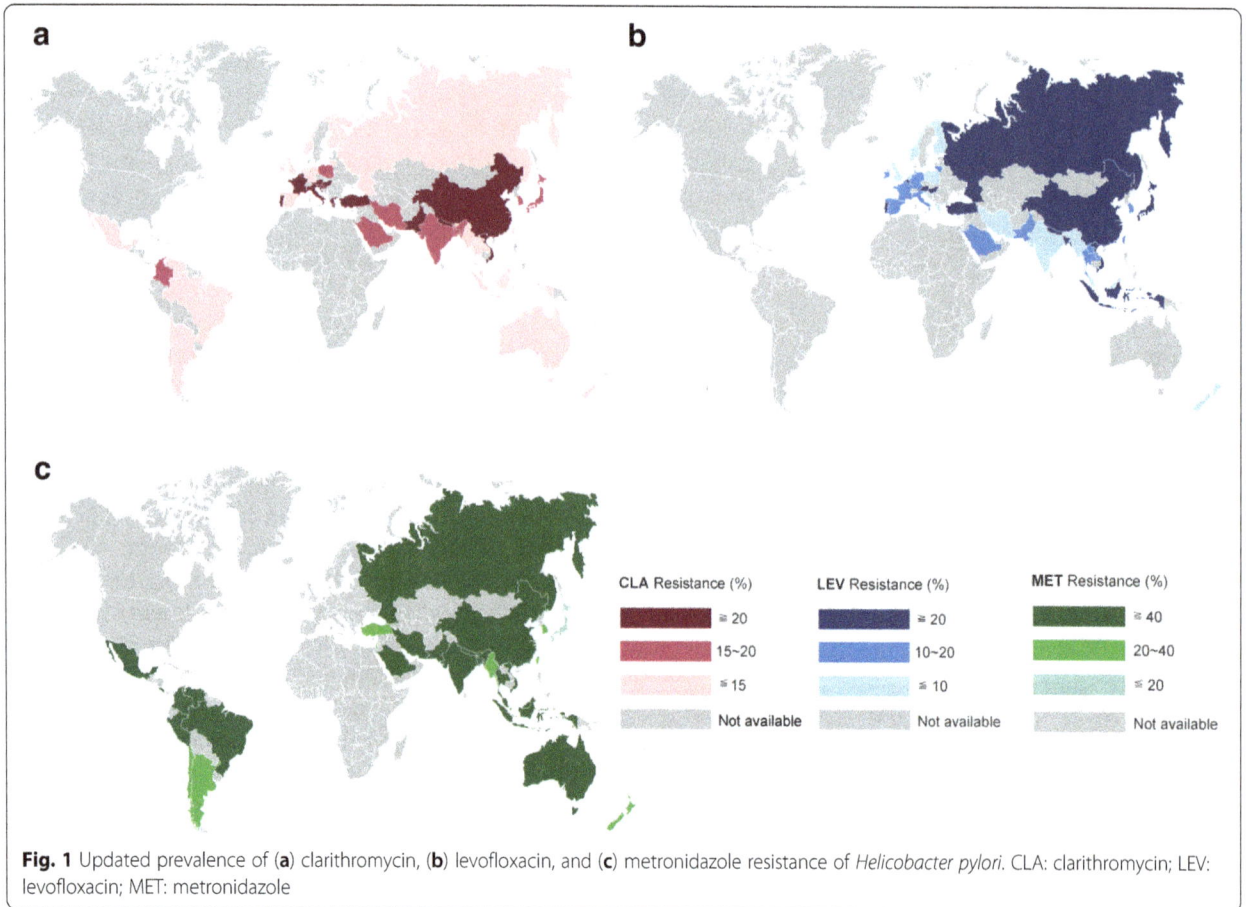

Fig. 1 Updated prevalence of (**a**) clarithromycin, (**b**) levofloxacin, and (**c**) metronidazole resistance of *Helicobacter pylori*. CLA: clarithromycin; LEV: levofloxacin; MET: metronidazole

Table 1 Prevalence of primary antibiotic resistance of *H pylori* by time period, stratified by WHO region

WHO region	Prevalence of primary resistance		
	Clarithromycin	Metronidazole	Levofloxacin
Americas region [23]			
2006–2008	11 (3–19)	26 (10–42)	N/A
2009–2011	9 (2–15)	21 (13–33)	11 (5–16)
2012–2016	20 (12–28)	29 (0–59)	19 (5–16)
European region [23]			
2006–2008	28 (24–32)	38 (33–43)	15 (12–18)
2009–2011	23 (20–27)	33 (25–40)	13 (9–17)
2012–2016	28 (25–31)	46 (34–58)	12 (8–15)
Asia-Pacific region [5]			
2006–2010	19 (16–23)	50 (44–56)	17 (13–21)
2011–2015	21 (18–25)	45 (39–48)	27 (21–34)

WHO world health organization

(95% CI 27–36) in Europe [22], and 44% (95% CI 39–48) in Asia-Pacific [5]. Although there were no remarkable changes in metronidazole resistance over time compared to clarithromycin, the pooled prevalence of primary metronidazole resistance after 2011 was greater 25% in these regions (Table 1). According to data for 2006–15 in Asia-Pacific, metronidazole resistance was higher than 40% in most countries, except Japan, Myanmar, South Korea, Taiwan, and Turkey [5].

Levofloxacin resistance

The overall prevalence of primary levofloxacin resistance was 11% (95% CI 9–13) in Europe [22], 15% (95% CI 5–16) in Americas [22], and 18% (95% CI 15–22) in Asia-Pacific [5]. Prevalence of resistance to levofloxacin in America and Asia-Pacific rose significantly over time during the period investigated. The pooled prevalence of primary levofloxacin resistance after 2011 was 19% (95% CI 5–16%) in America, 12% (95% CI 8–15%) in Europe, and 27% (95% CI 21–34%) in Asia-Pacific (Table 1). In Asia-Pacific regions, resistance to levofloxacin increased over time in all included countries, except in Iran. The levofloxacin resistance rates were significantly higher in Eastern Asia (including China, Hong Kong, Japan, South Korea, and Taiwan) than in western Asia (including Israel, Saudi Arabia, and Turkey) and southeastern Asia (including Indonesia, Laos, Malaysia, Myanmar, Singapore, Thailand, and Vietnam) [5]. Megraud et al. [19] and Liou et al. [21] showed that fluoroquinolone resistance correlated with consumption of fluoroquinolones in Europe and Taiwan, respectively. The global consumption of fluoroquinolones has significantly increased since 2000 [23], which might be explained by the recommendation in 2004 guidelines to use

fluoroquinolone monotherapy as an alternative first-line therapy for community-acquired pneumonia [24].

Amoxicillin resistance

The overall prevalence of primary amoxicillin resistance was 0% (95% CI 0–0) in Europe [22], 3% (95% CI 2–4) in Asia-Pacific [5], and 10% (95% CI 2–19) in Americas [22]. The trend in amoxicillin resistance was only available in Asia-Pacific region and country-specific data showed no remarkable changes in resistance over time [5]. Although amoxicillin resistance was uncommon in the Asia-Pacific region, resistance to amoxicillin was higher than 10% in Pakistan and India.

Tetracycline resistance

The overall prevalence of primary tetracycline resistance was 0% (95% CI 0–0) in Europe, [23] 4% (95% CI 2–5) in Asia-Pacific [5], and 4% (95% CI 1–11) in Americas [22]. The trend in tetracycline resistance was only available in Asia-Pacific region and no remarkable changes over time [5]. The prevalence of resistance to tetracycline was < 10% in all countries, except Pakistan and India, where tetracycline resistance was higher than 10%.

Strategies to improve the efficacy of first-line therapy

The dosages and frequencies of PPI, bismuth, and antibiotics of the commonly used regimens are shown in Table 2. There are several strategies to improve the efficacy of first-line therapy, including extending the length of treatment to 14 days, the use of vonoprazan or higher dosage of PPI, the use of four drug regimens (bismuth quadruple therapy, concomitant therapy, sequential therapy, or hybrid therapy), susceptibility testing (or genotypic resistance) guided therapy, and supplementation with probiotics (Table 3) [25–39].

Extending the treatment length of triple therapy to 14 days

Clarithromycin-based triple therapy remains one of the treatment options in countries where the prevalence of clarithromycin resistance is lower than 15% [13–16, 25]. A Cochrane meta-analysis of 59 randomized trials showed that the efficacy of triple therapy may be increased by extending its treatment length from 7 days to 10 days (75.7% vs 79.9%, RR 0.80, 95% CI 0.72 to 0.89), from 7 or 14 days (72.9% vs 81.9%, RR 0.66, 95% CI 0.60 to 0.74), or from 10 days to 14 days (78.5% vs 84.4%, RR 0.72, 95% CI 0.58 to 0.90) [26]. Therefore, extending the treatment length of triple therapy to 14 days is recommended in several international consensus reports [13–16, 25].

Table 2 Regimens commonly used for *H. pylori* eradication

First-line Regimens	Dosing and frequencies
Clarithromycin triple therapy	A PPI bid, clarithromycin 500 mg bid, and amoxicillin 1 g bid or metronidazole 500 mg bid for 7–14 days
Bismuth quadruple therapy	A PPI bid, bismuth qid, tetracycline 500 mg qid, and metronidazole 500 mg tid for 7–14 days
Sequential therapy	A PPI bid plus amoxicillin 500 mg bid for 5–7 days, followed by a PPI bid plus clarithromycin 500 mg bid and metronidazole 500 mg bid for another 5–7 days
Concomitant therapy	A PPI bid plus amoxicillin 500 mg bid, clarithromycin 500 mg bid and metronidazole 500 mg bid for 7–14 days
Hybrid therapy	A PPI bid plus amoxicillin 500 mg bid for 5–7 days, followed by a PPI bid plus amoxicillin 500 mg bid, clarithromycin 500 mg bid and metronidazole 500 mg bid for another 5–7 days
Second-line/ third regimens	
Levofloxacin triple therapy	A PPI bid, levofloxacin 500 mg qd, and amoxicillin 1 g bid for 10–14 days
Levofloxacin sequential therapy	A PPI bid plus amoxicillin 500 mg bid for 7 days, followed by a PPI bid plus levofloxacin 250 mg bid and metronidazole 500 mg bid for another 7 days
Levofloxacin concomitant therapy	A PPI bid plus amoxicillin 500 mg bid, levofloxacin 250 mg bid and metronidazole 500 mg bid for 7–14 days
Bismuth quadruple therapy	A PPI bid, bismuth qid, tetracycline 500 mg qid, and metronidazole 500 mg tid for 7–14 days
Fourth-line regimen	
Rifabutin triple therapy	A PPI bid, rifabutin 150 mg bid, and amoxicillin 1 g bid for 14 days

Dosage of proton pump inhibitors (PPI): omeprazole 20 mg, lansoprazole 30 mg, esomeprazole 20 mg, pantoprazole 40 mg, rabeprazole 20 mg

Use of higher dosage of PPI or vonoprazan

The minimum inhibitory concentrations (MICs) of amoxicillin, clarithromycin, and levofloxacin are higher in acidic environment [7, 9]. Therefore, increasing the gastric pH values through the use of higher dosage of PPI may increase the efficacy of eradication therapy for *H. pylori* [7]. The standard dosages of PPI used for *H. pylori* eradication were omeprazole 20 mg, esomeprazole 20 mg, pantoprazole 40 mg, lansoprazole 30 mg, and rabeprazole 20 mg given twice daily. Meta-analysis of 6

Table 3 Strategies to improve the efficacy of first-line therapy

Strategy for improvement	Supporting evidence
Extending the treatment length of triple therapy to 14 days	Meta-analysis of 59 randomized trials showed that triple therapy for 14 days is more effective than triple therapy given for 7 or 10 days [26].
Use of higher dosage of PPI or vonoprazan	Meta-analysis of 6 randomized trials showed that the use of higher dosage of PPI may increase the eradication rate. Two randomized trials showed that vonoprazan-based triple therapy was superior to standard dose PPI-based triple therapy, particularly for clarithromycin resistant strains [30–32].
Use of four drug regimen	
Bismuth quadruple therapy	Randomized trials showed that bismuth quadruple therapy was superior to triple therapy in regions with high clarithromycin resistance (> 15%) [29, 33, 35].
Concomitant therapy	Meta-analysis of randomized trials showed that concomitant therapy given for 5 or 10 days was superior to 5- or 7- or 10-day PAC based triple therapy, but was not superior to 14-day triple therapy. A non-randomized trial showed that 14-day concomitant therapy was superior to 14-day triple therapy [29, 34, 38, 39].
Sequential therapy	Meta-analysis of randomized trials showed that 10-day sequential therapy was superior to triple therapy for 10 days or less, but was not superior to 14-day triple therapy. Meta-analysis of 4 randomized trials showed that 14-day sequential therapy was superior to 14-day triple therapy [27, 28, 33].
Hybrid therapy	A randomized trial showed that 14-day hybrid therapy was superior to 14-day triple therapy. Another randomized trial showed that 12-day reverse hybrid therapy was superior to 12-day triple therapy [37].
Susceptibility testing guided therapy	Meta-analysis of randomized trials showed that susceptibility testing guided therapy was superior to empirical triple therapy given for 7 or 10 days [8].
Supplementation with probiotics	Meta-analysis of randomized trials showed that supplementation with probiotics may reduce the adverse effects and increase the efficacy of triple therapy [40–43].

PPI proton pump inhibitor

randomized trials ($N = 1703$) showed that the use of higher dosage of PPI may increase the eradication rate of standard triple therapy [30, 31]. However, only two trials compared the same PPI of different dosage [30, 31]. Vonoprazan, a potassium-competitive acid blocker (P-CAB), is a novel gastric acid secretion suppressant. A randomized trial showed that vonoprazan-based triple therapy is superior to lansoprazole-based triple therapy in Japan, especially for clarithromycin resistant strains [32]. It's efficacy against clarithromycin resistant strains has been confirmed in several retrospective or prospective non-randomized studies in Japan. However, the finding needs to be validated in more trials outside Japan.

Use of four drug regimen

Clarithromycin based triple therapy is not recommended in countries where the prevalence of clarithromycin resistance is higher than 15% in international consensus reports [13–16, 25]. Bismuth quadruple therapy or non-bismuth quadruple therapies (concomitant therapy, sequential therapy, hybrid therapy) are recommended in these regions [13–16, 25, 27–29, 33–37]. Recent meta-analysis of randomized trials showed that 14-day sequential therapy, but not 10-day sequential therapy, was superior to 14-day triple therapy [13]. A recent randomized trial showed that 14-day sequential therapy was not inferior to 10-day bismuth quadruple therapy [33]. Therefore, extending the treatment length of sequential therapy to 14 days is recommended [27–29, 33]. Our recent systematic review and meta-analysis showed that concomitant therapy for 5, 7 or 10 days was superior to triple therapy for 7 or 10 days, but was not superior to 14-day triple therapy [38]. A non-randomized trial showed that 14-day concomitant therapy was superior to 14-day triple therapy [39]. Therefore, the treatment length of concomitant therapy is 14 days in several international consensus reports [13–16]. Although the Maastricht V and the Toronto Consensus recommended that bismuth quadruple therapy should be given for 14 days, the evidence level supporting the recommendation is low [13, 14]. Our recent trials showed that bismuth quadruple therapy given for 10 days was superior to 14-day triple therapy and its efficacy was greater than 90% in Taiwan [36]. Therefore, 10-day bismuth quadruple therapy is an acceptable regimen in Taiwan.

Susceptibility testing guided therapy

Meta-analysis of 9 randomized trials including 1958 subjects showed that susceptibility testing guided therapy was more effective than empirical triple therapy for 7 or 10 days in the first-line treatment of H. pylori infection [8]. However, most of these trials randomize patients after endoscopy and/or culture which is not similar to that in clinical practice because patients might decline endoscopy, the yield rate of culture is only 70–90%, and the accuracy of susceptibility testing is not 100% [8]. Besides, whether susceptibility testing guided therapy is superior to 14-day triple therapy or bismuth quadruple therapy are still unknown.

Supplementation with probiotics

A recent meta-analysis showed that probiotics may induce a significant reduction in delta values of urea breath test than placebo (8.61% with a 95%CI: 5.88–11.34, vs 0.19% for placebo, $P < 0.001$) [40]. However, only about 10–15% of H. pylori infection was eradicated with probiotic monotherapy [40]. Earlier studies showed that supplementation of probiotics may increase the eradication rate of triple therapy, probably through the alleviation of adverse effects of triple therapy [41]. However, more recent meta-analysis of 21 randomized control trials showed that standard therapy plus probiotics may reduce the frequency of adverse effect compared to standard therapy with or without a placebo, but does not increase the eradication rate of standard therapy [42]. Yet, another meta-analysis of randomized trial showed that adjunctive use of some multi-strain probiotics may increase the eradication rate and reduce the risk of adverse events but not all mixtures were effective [43]. Therefore, routine supplementation of probiotics is not recommended in the Toronto and the Asean Consensus Reports considering the controversial results and the cost [14, 15].

Efficacies of different eradication regimens in susceptible and resistant strains

The efficacies of six commonly used regimens in susceptible and resistant strains in the first-line treatment of H. pylori infection were reviewed in this article. Pooled analyses of efficacies of the six different regimens in antibiotic susceptible and resistant strains according to the length of treatment were shown in Table 4 and in Additional file 1: Tables S1-S6 [8–30, 33–38]. Except for 5-day concomitant therapy and 7-day bismuth quadruple therapy, the eradication rates of the other regimens were greater than 90% in clarithromycin susceptible strains (Table 4). However, the efficacy of levofloxacin triple therapy was only 87.5% in the first-line therapy, even for levofloxacin susceptible strains. The efficacies of triple therapy, sequential therapy, concomitant therapy, and hybrid therapy were significantly lower in clarithromycin resistant strains, especially when the treatment length were 10 days or less (Table 4). The efficacies of bismuth quadruple therapy were not affected by clarithromycin resistance. However, the efficacy of bismuth quadruple therapy was affected by metronidazole resistance when it was given for 7 days.

Table 4 Eradication rate in susceptible and resistant strains[a]
[8–30, 33–38]

	Clarithromycin susceptible	Clarithromycin resistant
Triple therapy: PPI-amoxicillin-clarithromycin		
7 days	88.5% (2428/2744)	25.8% (121/469)
10 days	90.8% (267/294)	44% (37/84)
14 days	89.6% (841/939)	43.3% (55/127)
Sequential therapy		
10 days	91% (1470/1616)	65% (225/346)
14 days	98.1% (304/310)	72.2% (26/36)
Concomitant therapy		
5 days	84.4% (76/90)	50% (2/4)
7 days	96.3% (181/188)	83.3% (20/24)
10 days	94.5% (598/633)	80.5% (120/149)
Hybrid therapy		
10–14 days	96.8% (418/432)	81.8% (117/143)
Bismuth quadruple therapy		
7 days	87.2% (321/368)	87.2% (321/368)
10 days	93.9% (512/545)	91.4% (139/152)
14 days	96.9% (94/97)	92.3% (12/13)
Bismuth quadruple therapy	Metronidazole susceptible	Metronidazole resistant
7 days	92% (252/274)	73.4% (69/94)
10 days	94.3% (764/810)	89.8% (397/442)
14 days	96.1% (99/103)	93.2% (41/44)
	Levofloxacin susceptible	Levofloxacin resistant
Triple therapy: PPI-amoxicillin-levofloxacin	81.8% (189/231)	33.3% (10/30)

PPI proton pump inhibitor
[a]detailed data shown in supplementary materials

Prediction of different regimens in regions with different prevalence of antibiotic resistance

The efficacy of a regimen which contains antibiotic A (drug A) and antibiotic B (drug B) in a region can be predicted if the prevalence of antibiotic resistance in that region and the efficacy of this regimen in susceptible and resistant strains are known [17, 18] . Assuming the prevalence of antibiotic resistance for drug A and drug B are p and q, respectively, the prevalence of dual drug resistance and dual susceptible strains would be p*q and (1-p)*(1-q), respectively. Therefore, the estimated eradication rate of that regimen would be 【ER_{SS}* (1-p)*(1-q)】 + 【ER_{SR}* (1-p)*q】 + 【ER_{RS} *P*(1-q)】 + 【ER_{RR}* P*q】, where ER_{SS}, ER_{SR}, ER_{RS}, and ER_{RR} are eradication rates in dual susceptible, susceptible to drug A but resistant to drug B, resistant to drug A but susceptible to drug B, and dual resistant strains, respectively. Based on this prediction model and the efficacies

of different regimens in antibiotic susceptible and resistant strains, the efficacies of these regimens in regions with different prevalence of antibiotic resistance can be predicted, as shown in Fig. 2. For example, the predicted efficacy of 7-day standard triple therapy according to the prevalence of clarithromycin resistance would be 0.885(1-p) + 0.258p (p is the prevalence of clarithromycin resistance). Comparing to other regimens, the eradication rates of 7-day, 10-day, 14-day triple therapy and 5-day concomitant therapy would be lower than 80% in regions where the prevalence of clarithromycin resistance is higher than 20% (Fig. 2). Among these regimens, the efficacy of bismuth quadruple therapy would remain higher than 90% in regions with high prevalence of primary clarithromycin resistance (Fig. 2). The efficacies of metronidazole-containing regimens, including sequential therapy, concomitant therapy, hybrid therapy and bismuth quadruple therapy were also affected by metronidazole resistance, but the effect size was relatively smaller (Fig. 2). The efficacy of levofloxacin triple therapy for treatment-naïve patients would be lower than 80% when the levofloxacin-resistant rate higher than 15%.

Based on the Hp-normogram in Fig. 2, bismuth quadruple therapy and non-bismuth quadruple therapy (14-day sequential therapy, 14-day concomitant therapy, and 14-day hybrid therapy) are the preferred regimens for the first-line treatment of H. pylori infection in regions with higher prevalence of clarithromycin resistance. Standard triple therapy given for 14 day may still be an option in regions where the prevalence of clarithromycin resistance is lower than 15%. Levofloxacin triple therapy is not recommended in the first- line treatment of H. pylori infection due to its low efficacy.

Second-line therapy
After failure of one eradication therapy, the choice of second-line eradication regimen can be empirical or guided by susceptibility testing [13–16, 25]. A recent meta-analysis of 4 randomized trials failed to show the superiority of susceptibility testing guided therapy over empirical therapy in the second-line therapy, probably attributed to the small sample size and the heterogeneity among the trials [8]. Therefore, the majority of these patients were treated empirically in clinical practice. Antibiotics used in previous eradication therapy are important and helpful to guide the second-line rescue therapy (Fig. 3). The Taiwan Consensus Report recommended the avoidance of empirical reuse of clarithromycin and levofloxacin without susceptibility testing because the secondary resistance rates of clarithromycin and levofloxacin are high for patients who fail after clarithromycin-based and levofloxacin-based therapies, respectively [25]. Bismuth quadruple therapy and

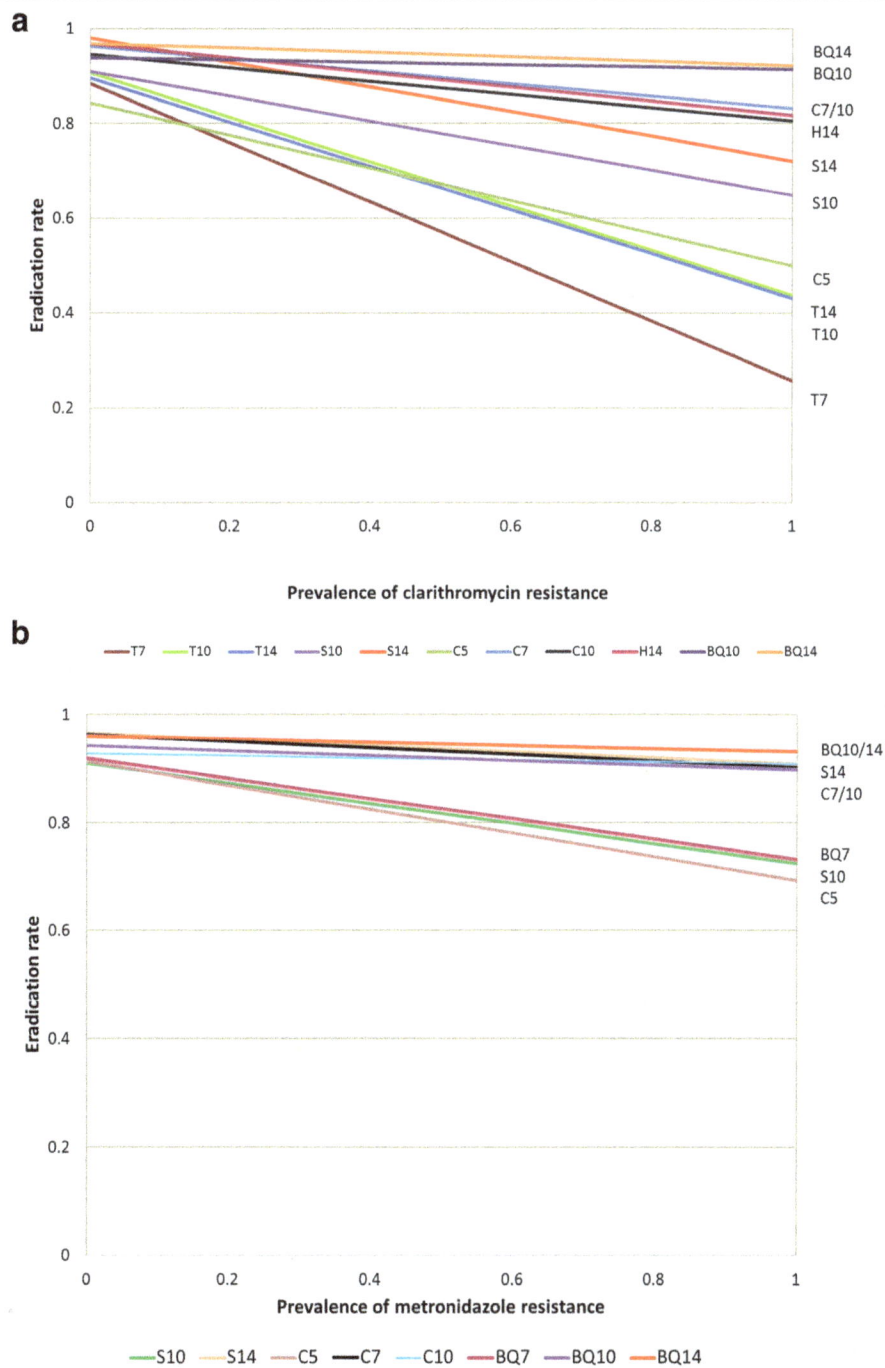

Fig. 2 Predicted efficacies of different regimens according to prevalence of (**a**) clarithromycin resistance and (**b**) metronidazole resistance. T7: triple therapy for 7 days; T10: triple therapy for 10 days; T14: triple therapy for 14 days; S10: sequential therapy for 10 days; S14: sequential therapy for 14 days; C5: concomitant therapy for 5 days; C7: concomitant therapy for 7 days; C10: concomitant therapy for 10 days; H14: hybrid therapy for 14 days; BQ10: bismuth quadruple therapy for 10 days; BQ14: bismuth quadruple therapy for 14 days

levofloxacin based therapy are the most commonly used second-line rescue regimens for patients who fail after clarithromycin-based therapies [13–16, 25]. An earlier systematic review and meta-analysis showed similar efficacies of levofloxacin triple therapy and bismuth quadruple therapy in the second-line therapy [44]. However, the frequency of adverse effects was higher for bismuth quadruple therapy than levofloxacin triple therapy [44]. Yet, the prevalence of levofloxacin resistance is rising in recent years in many parts of the world [5, 19–22]. Therefore, Chen et al. found that the efficacy of levofloxacin triple therapy was only 74% in the second-line

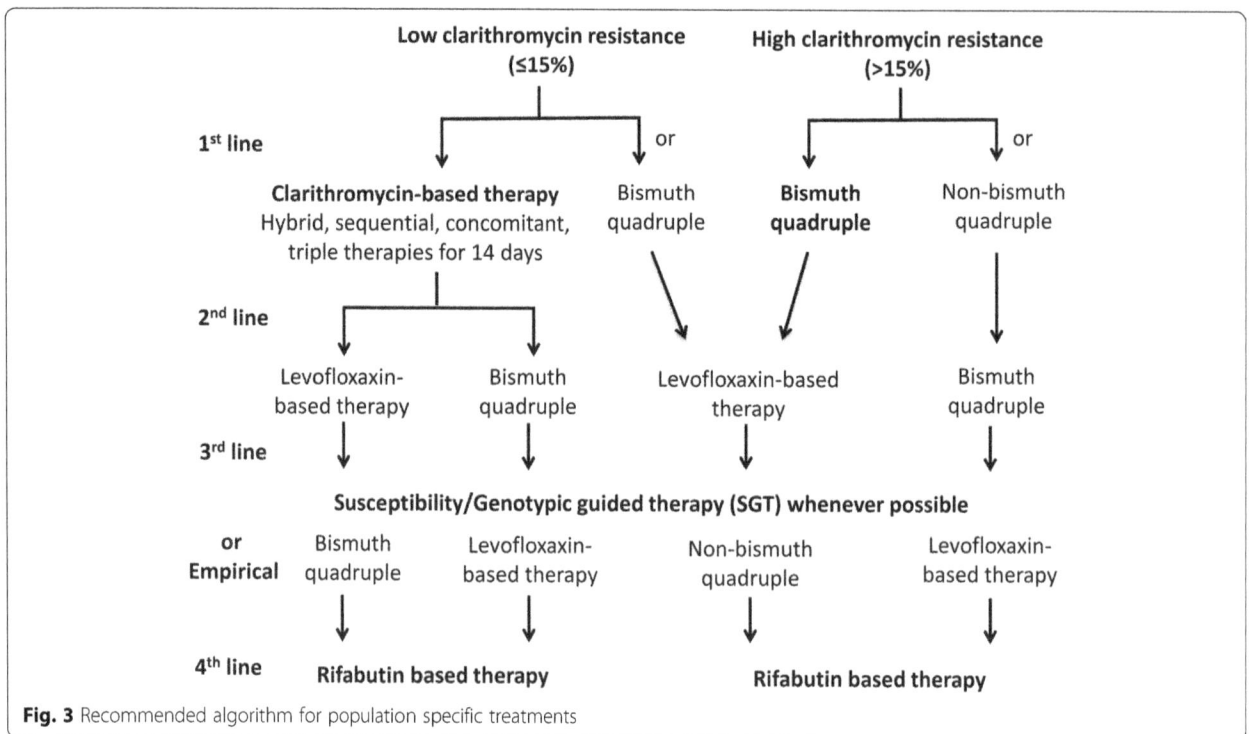

Fig. 3 Recommended algorithm for population specific treatments

therapy in a recent systematic review and meta-analysis [45]. Liou et al. further showed that levofloxacin sequential therapy for 10 days was superior to levofloxacin triple therapy for 10 days in the second-line treatment in Taiwan [46, 47]. Levofloxacin concomitant therapy given for 5 days has been shown to be similarly effective as levofloxacin sequential therapy for 10 days in the first-line therapy, but its efficacy in the second-line therapy remains unknown [48]. In another randomized trial in Taiwan, Hsu et al. showed that modified bismuth quadruple therapy containing bismuth, a PPI, tetracycline, and levofloxacin for 10 days was superior to levofloxacin triple therapy for 10 days in the second-line therapy [49]. Non-bismuth quadruple therapy (preferably concomitant therapy) may be a second-line rescue therapy for patients who fail after bismuth quadruple therapy, but the level of evidence is low for this recommendation [13–16].

Treatment of refractory *H. pylori* infection

Refractory *H. pylori* infection is defined as failure after two or more eradication therapies. Earlier Maastricht Consensus Reports recommended that susceptibility testing should be done after failure of two eradication therapies whenever possible [50] . However, susceptibility testing for *H. pylori* is not widely available because of it is costly (endoscopy required), time consuming (2–4 weeks) and the successful culture rate varies from 70 to 90%. Besides, the reported efficacies of susceptibility testing guided therapy were not satisfactory, ranging from 36 to 91% in some published retrospective or

prospective case series [11, 12]. Therefore, the majority of patients are treated empirically in routine clinical practice. Bismuth quadruple therapy and levofloxacin-based therapy are commonly used as third-line rescue therapy, whereas rifabutin-based therapy is usually reserved as fourth-line rescue therapy [13–16, 25]. Bismuth quadruple therapy may be used as the third-line rescue therapy for patients fail after clarithromycin-based therapy and levofloxacin-based therapy in previous eradication therapies [13–16]. Levofloxacin-based therapy may be used as the third-line rescue therapy for patients fail after clarithromycin-based therapy and bismuth quadruple therapy. 23S rRNA mutations and gyrase A mutations correlate well with clarithromycin and levofloxacin resistance, respectively [10]. Our previous pilot trial showed that genotypic resistance guided therapy may achieve 80% eradication rate in the third line treatment [51]. Therefore, we further conducted a multicenter randomized trial to compare the efficacies of genotypic resistance guided therapy vs. empirical therapy for refractory *H. pylori* infection [52]. We found that *H. pylori* was eradicated in 160/205 patients receiving genotypic resistance-guided therapy (78%) and 148/205 patients receiving empirical therapy 72.2% ($P = 0.170$) [52]. This is the first randomized trial to show that properly designed empirical therapy is an acceptable alternative to genotypic resistance-guided therapy for eradication of refractory *H. pylori* infection after consideration of cost, patient preference, and accessibility [52]. However, further studies are warranted to compare the efficacy of susceptibility testing guided therapy to genotypic resistance guided therapy or empirical therapy according to medication history.

Conclusion

The rising prevalence of primary clarithromycin and levofloxacin resistance of *H. pylori* is a global problem. However, the prevalence of antibiotic resistance varies greatly in different countries and regions. We proposed an algorithm to choose the optimal first-line and rescue therapies according to the prevalence of antibiotic resistance in this article (Fig. 3). Clarithromycin-based therapy (triple, sequential, concomitant, and hybrid therapies) given for 14 days remains the treatment of choice in regions with low clarithromycin resistance (≤15%). Bismuth quadruple therapy may be an alternative therapy in this region. In regions with high clarithromycin resistance (> 15%), bismuth quadruple therapy is the treatment of choice. Non-bismuth quadruple therapy may be an alternative if the prevalence of dual clarithromycin and metronidazole resistance is lower than 10%. Either levofloxacin-based therapy or bismuth quadruple therapy may be used as second-line rescue therapy for patients fail after clarithromycin-based therapies, whereas levofloxacin-based therapy may be used for patients fail after bismuth quadruple therapy. Susceptibility testing or genotypic resistance should be determined after two or more eradication failures. However, empirical therapy according to prior medication history to avoid the empirical reuse of levofloxacin and clarithromycin may be an acceptable alternative after consideration of cost, patient preference, and accessibility. Rifabutin-based therapy given for 14 days may be used as the fourth-line rescue therapy. New antibiotics specific for *H. pylori* are highly anticipated.

Additional file

Additional file 1: Table S1–1. Efficacy of 7-day triple therapy in the first line treatment of the individual studies. **Table S1–2**. Efficacy of 10-day triple therapy in the first line treatment of the individual studies. **Table S1–3**. Efficacy of 14-day triple therapy in the first line treatment of the individual studies. **Table S2–1**. Efficacy of 10-day sequential therapy in the first line treatment of the individual studies. **Table S2–2**. Efficacy of 14-day sequential therapy in the first line treatment of the individual studies. **Table S3–1**. Efficacy of 5-day or less concomitant therapy in the first line treatment of the individual studies. **Table S3–2**. Efficacy of 7-day concomitant therapy in the first line treatment of the individual studies. **Table S3–3**. Efficacy of 10-day concomitant therapy in the first line treatment of the individual studies. **Table S3–4**. Efficacy of 14-day concomitant therapy in the first line treatment of the individual studies. **Table S4**. Efficacy of 10–14 day hybrid therapy in the first line treatment of the individual studies. **Table S5–1**. Efficacy of 7-day or less bismuth quadruple therapy in the first line treatment of the individual studies. **Table S5–2**. Efficacy of 10-day bismuth quadruple therapy in the first line treatment of the individual studies. **Table S5–3**. Efficacy of 14-day bismuth quadruple therapy in the first line treatment of the individual studies. **Table S6**. Efficacy of Levofloxacin triple therapy in the first line treatment of the individual studies. (DOCX 221 kb)

Abbreviations
BQ10: Bismuth quadruple therapy for 10 days; BQ14: Bismuth quadruple therapy for 14 days; C10: Concomitant therapy for 10 days; C5: Concomitant therapy for 5 days; C7: Concomitant therapy for 7 days; CIs: Confidence intervals; CLA: Clarithromycin; *H. pylori*: Helicobacter pylori; H14: Hybrid therapy for 14 days; LEV: Levofloxacin; MET: Metronidazole; PPI: Proton pump inhibitor; S10: Sequential therapy for 10 days; S14: Sequential therapy for 14 days; T10: Triple therapy for 10 days; T14: Triple therapy for 14 days.; T7: Triple therapy for 7 days

Acknowledgements
The authors would like to express their special thanks to the staff of the Eighth Core Lab, Department of Medical Research, National Taiwan University Hospital for their technological support.
Taiwan Gastrointestinal Disease and Helicobacter Consortium investigators. Steering committee of The Taiwan Gastrointestinal Disease and Helicobacter Consortium: Jyh-Ming Liou (Taipei), Yi-Chia Lee (Taipei), Mei-Jyh Chen (Taipei), Jaw-Town Lin (Taipei), Chun-Ying Wu (Taipei), Jeng-Yih Wu (Kaohsiung), Ching-Chow Chen (Taipei), Chun-Hung Lin (Taipei), Yu-Ren Fang (Yun-Lin), Ming-Jong Bair (Taitung), Jiing-Chyuan Luo (Taipei), and Ming-Shiang Wu (Taipei). Others investigators of the Taiwan Helicobacter Consortium in this study: Tsu-Yao Cheng (Taipei), Ping-Huei Tseng (Taipei), Han-Mo Chiu (Taipei), Chun-Chao Chang (Taipei), Chien-Chun Yu (Yun-Lin), Min-Chin Chiu (Yun-Lin),Yen-Nien Chen (Hsinchu), Wen-Hao Hu (Hsinchu), Chu-Kuang Chou (Chia-Yi), Chi-Ming Tai (Kaohsiung), Ching-Tai Lee (Kaohsiung), Wen-Lun Wang (Kaohsiung), and Wen-Shiung Chang (Taipei).

Funding
This work was financially supported by the "Center of Precision Medicine" from The Featured Areas Research Center Program within the framework of the Higher Education Sprout Project by the Ministry of Education (MOE) in Taiwan (Grant Number: NTU- 107 L9014–1), the Ministry of Science and Technology, Executive Yuan, ROC, Taiwan (Grant Number: TCTC-TR2 106–2321-B-002-025 and MOST 107–3017-F-002-002), the Ministry of Health and Welfare of Taiwan (Grant Number: MOHW106-TDU-B-211–113002,MOHW107-TDU-B-211–123002), and National Taiwan University Hospital (Grant Number: NTUH 104-P05, NTUH 106-P06). The funding source had no role in study design, data collection, analysis or interpretation, report writing or the decision to submit this paper for publication.

Authors' contributions
The study was conceived by JML with input from PYC, YTK, and MSW. JML, PYC, and YTK drafted the article which was critically revised by JML and MSW. All authors commented on drafts and approved the final version. All authors participated in the decision to submit for publication.

Competing interests
The authors declare that they have no competing interests.

Author details
[1]Division of Gastroenterology and Hepatology, Department of Internal Medicine, National Taiwan University Hospital, Taipei, Taiwan. [2]Department of Internal Medicine, College of Medicine, National Taiwan University, No. 7, Chung-Shan S. Road, Taipei, Taiwan. [3]Division of Gastroenterology and Hepatology, Department of Internal medicine, Chia-Yi Christian Hospital, Chia-Yi, Taiwan.

References

1. Suerbaum S, Michetti P. *Helicobacter pylori* infection. N Engl J Med. 2002; 347(15):1175–86.
2. Lee YC, Chiang TH, Chou CK, Tu YK, Liao WC, Wu MS, et al. Association between *Helicobacter pylori* eradication and gastric Cancer incidence: a systematic review and meta-analysis. Gastroenterology 2016;150(5):1113–1124 e5.
3. Chen LT, Lin JT, Tai JJ, Chen GH, Yeh HZ, Yang SS, et al. Long-term results of anti-*Helicobacter pylori* therapy in early-stage gastric high-grade transformed MALT lymphoma. J Natl Cancer Inst. 2005;97(18):1345–53.
4. Graham DY. *Helicobacter pylori* update: gastric cancer, reliable therapy, and possible benefits. Gastroenterology. 2015;148(4):719–31. e3
5. Kuo YT, Liou JM, El-Omar EM, Wu JY, Leow AHR, Goh KL, et al. Primary antibiotic resistance in *Helicobacter pylori* in the Asia-Pacific region: a systematic review and meta-analysis. Lancet Gastroenterol Hepatol. 2017; 2(10):707–15.
6. Megraud F. *H pylori* antibiotic resistance: prevalence, importance, and advances in testing. Gut. 2004;53(9):1374–84.
7. Vakil N, Megraud F. Eradication therapy for *Helicobacter pylori*. Gastroenterology. 2007;133(3):985–1001.
8. Lopez-Gongora S, Puig I, Calvet X, Villoria A, Baylina M, Munoz N, et al. Systematic review and meta-analysis: susceptibility-guided versus empirical antibiotic treatment for *Helicobacter pylori* infection. J Antimicrob Chemother. 2015;70(9):2447–55.
9. Megraud F, Lehours P. *Helicobacter pylori* detection and antimicrobial susceptibility testing. Clin Microbiol Rev. 2007;20(2):280–322.
10. Liou JM, Chang CY, Sheng WH, Wang YC, Chen MJ, Lee YC, et al. Genotypic resistance in *Helicobacter pylori* strains correlates with susceptibility test and treatment outcomes after levofloxacin- and clarithromycin-based therapies. Antimicrob Agents Chemother. 2011;55(3):1123–9.
11. Gisbert JP. "rescue" regimens after *Helicobacter pylori* treatment failure. World J Gastroenterol. 2008;14(35):5385–402.
12. Puig I, Lopez-Gongora S, Calvet X, Villoria A, Baylina M, Sanchez-Delgado J, et al. Systematic review: third-line susceptibility-guided treatment for *Helicobacter pylori* infection. Therap Adv Gastroenterol. 2016;9(4):437–48.
13. Malfertheiner P, Megraud F, O'Morain CA, Gisbert JP, Kuipers EJ, Axon AT, et al. Management of *Helicobacter pylori* infection-the Maastricht V/Florence consensus report. Gut. 2017;66(1):6–30.
14. Fallone CA, Chiba N, van Zanten SV, Fischbach L, Gisbert JP, Hunt RH, et al. The Toronto consensus for the treatment of *Helicobacter pylori* infection in adults. Gastroenterology. 2016;151(1):51–69 e14.
15. Mahachai V, Vilaichone RK, Pittayanon R, Rojborwonwitaya J, Leelakusolvong S, Maneerattanaporn M, et al. *Helicobacter pylori* management in ASEAN: the Bangkok consensus report. J Gastroenterol Hepatol. 2018;33(1):37–56.
16. Chey WD, Leontiadis GI, Howden CW, Moss SF. ACG clinical guideline: treatment of *Helicobacter pylori* infection. Am J Gastroenterol. 2017;112(2): 212–39.
17. Liou JM, Wu MS, Lin JT. Treatment of *Helicobacter pylori* infection: where are we now? J Gastroenterol Hepatol. 2016;31(12):1918–26.
18. Graham DY. Hp-normogram (normo-graham) for assessing the outcome of *H. pylori* therapy: effect of resistance, duration, and CYP2C19 genotype. Helicobacter. 2016;21(2):85–90.
19. Megraud F, Coenen S, Versporten A, Kist M, Lopez-Brea M, Hirschl AM, et al. *Helicobacter pylori* resistance to antibiotics in Europe and its relationship to antibiotic consumption. Gut. 2013;62(1):34–42.
20. Camargo MC, Garcia A, Riquelme A, Otero W, Camargo CA, Hernandez-Garcia T, et al. The problem of *Helicobacter pylori* resistance to antibiotics: a systematic review in Latin America. Am J Gastroenterol. 2014;109(4):485–95.
21. Liou JM, Chang CY, Chen MJ, Chen CC, Fang YJ, Lee JY, et al. The primary resistance of *Helicobacter pylori* in Taiwan after the National Policy to restrict antibiotic consumption and its relation to virulence factors-a Nationwide study. PLoS One. 2015;10(5):e0124199.
22. Savoldi A, Carrara E, Graham Prof DY, Conti M, Tacconelli E. Prevalence of antibiotic resistance in *Helicobacter pylori*: a systematic review and meta-analysis in World Health Organization regions. Gastroenterology. 2018. Jul 7; https://doi.org/10.1053/j.gastro.2018.07.007.
23. Van Boeckel TP, Gandra S, Ashok A, Caudron Q, Grenfell BT, Levin SA, et al. Global antibiotic consumption 2000 to 2010: an analysis of national pharmaceutical sales data. Lancet Infect Dis. 2014;14(8):742–50.
24. Niederman MS. Review of treatment guidelines for community-acquired pneumonia. Am J Med. 2004;117(Suppl 3A):51S–7S.
25. Sheu BS, Wu MS, Chiu CT, Lo JC, Wu DC, Liou JM, et al. Consensus on the clinical management, screening-to-treat, and surveillance of *Helicobacter pylori* infection to improve gastric cancer control on a nationwide scale. Helicobacter. 2017;22(3) https://doi.org/10.1111/hel.12368.
26. Yuan Y, Ford AC, Khan KJ, Gisbert JP, Forman D, Leontiadis GI, et al. Optimum duration of regimens for *Helicobacter pylori* eradication. Cochrane Database Syst Rev. 2013;12:CD008337.
27. Liou JM, Chen CC, Chen MJ, Chen CC, Chang CY, Fang YJ, et al. Sequential versus triple therapy for the first-line treatment of *Helicobacter pylori*: a multicentre, open-label, randomised trial. Lancet. 2013;381(9862):205–13.
28. Liou JM, Chen CC, Lee YC, Chang CY, Wu JY, Bair MJ, et al. Systematic review with meta-analysis: 10- or 14-day sequential therapy vs. 14-day triple therapy in the first line treatment of *Helicobacter pylori* infection. Aliment Pharmacol Ther. 2016;43(4):470–81.
29. Liou JM, Chen CC, Chang CY, Chen MJ, Chen CC, Fang YJ, et al. Sequential therapy for 10 days versus triple therapy for 14 days in the eradication of *Helicobacter pylori* in the community and hospital populations: a randomised trial. Gut. 2016;65(11):1784–92.
30. Villoria A, Garcia P, Calvet X, Gisbert JP, Vergara M. Meta-analysis: high-dose proton pump inhibitors vs. standard dose in triple therapy for *Helicobacter pylori* eradication. Aliment Pharmacol Ther. 2008;28(7):868–77.
31. McNicholl AG, Linares PM, Nyssen OP, Calvet X, Gisbert JP. Meta-analysis: esomeprazole or rabeprazole vs. first-generation pump inhibitors in the treatment of *Helicobacter pylori* infection. Aliment Pharmacol Ther. 2012; 36(5):414–25.
32. Murakami K, Sakurai Y, Shiino M, Funao N, Nishimura A, Asaka M. Vonoprazan, a novel potassium-competitive acid blocker, as a component of first-line and second-line triple therapy for *Helicobacter pylori* eradication: a phase III, randomised, double-blind study. Gut. 2016;65(9):1439–46.
33. Liou JM, Chen CC, Fang YJ, Chen PY, Chang CY, Chou CK, et al. 14 day sequential therapy versus 10 day bismuth quadruple therapy containing high-dose esomeprazole in the first-line and second-line treatment of *Helicobacter pylori*: a multicentre, non-inferiority, randomized trial. J Antimicrob Chemother. 2018; https://doi.org/10.1093/jac/dky183. [Epub ahead of print]
34. Wu DC, Hsu PI, Wu JY, Opekun AR, Kuo CH, Wu IC, et al. Sequential and concomitant therapy with four drugs is equally effective for eradication of *H pylori* infection. Clin Gastroenterol Hepatol. 2010;8(1):36–41 e1.
35. Venerito M, Krieger T, Ecker T, Leandro G, Malfertheiner P. Meta-analysis of bismuth quadruple therapy versus clarithromycin triple therapy for empiric primary treatment of *Helicobacter pylori* infection. Digestion. 2013;88(1):33–45.
36. Liou JM, Fang YJ, Chen CC, Bair MJ, Chang CY, Lee YC, et al. Concomitant, bismuth quadruple, and 14-day triple therapy in the first-line treatment of *Helicobacter pylori*: a multicentre, open-label, randomised trial. Lancet. 2016; 388(10058):2355–65.
37. Hsu PI, Lin PC, Graham DY. Hybrid therapy for helicobacter pylori infection: a systemic review and meta-analysis. World J Gastroenterol. 2015;21(45): 12954–62.
38. Chen MJ CC, Chen YN, Chen CC, Fang YJ, Lin JT, Wu MS, Liou JM. Systematic review with meta-analysis: concomitant therapy versus triple therapy for the first-line treatment of *Helicobacter pylori* infection. Am J Gastroenterol 2018;(in press).
39. Molina-Infante J, Lucendo AJ, Angueira T, Rodriguez-Tellez M, Perez-Aisa A, Balboa A, et al. Optimised empiric triple and concomitant therapy for *Helicobacter pylori* eradication in clinical practice: the OPTRICON study. Aliment Pharmacol Ther. 2015;41(6):581–9.
40. Losurdo G, Cubisino R, Barone M, Principi M, Leandro G, Ierardi E, et al. Probiotic monotherapy and *Helicobacter pylori* eradication: a systematic review with pooled-data analysis. World J Gastroenterol. 2018;24(1):139–49.
41. Dang Y, Reinhardt JD, Zhou X, Zhang G. The effect of probiotics supplementation on *Helicobacter pylori* eradication rates and side effects during eradication therapy: a meta-analysis. PLoS One. 2014;9(11):e111030.
42. Lu C, Sang J, He H, Wan X, Lin Y, Li L, et al. Probiotic supplementation does not improve eradication rate of *Helicobacter pylori* infection compared to placebo based on standard therapy: a meta-analysis. Sci Rep. 2016;6:23522.
43. McFarland LV, Huang Y, Wang L, Malfertheiner P. Systematic review and meta-analysis: multi-strain probiotics as adjunct therapy for *Helicobacter pylori* eradication and prevention of adverse events. United European Gastroenterol J. 2016;4(4):546–61.

44. Saad RJ, Schoenfeld P, Kim HM, Chey WD. Levofloxacin-based triple therapy versus bismuth-based quadruple therapy for persistent *Helicobacter pylori* infection: a meta-analysis. Am J Gastroenterol. 2006;101(3):488–96.
45. Chen PY, Wu MS, Chen CY, Bair MJ, Chou CK, Lin JT, et al. Systematic review with meta-analysis: the efficacy of levofloxacin triple therapy as the first- or second-line treatments of *Helicobacter pylori* infection. Aliment Pharmacol Ther. 2016;44(5):427–37.
46. Liou JM, Chen CC, Chen MJ, Chang CY, Fang YJ, Lee JY, et al. Empirical modified sequential therapy containing levofloxacin and high-dose esomeprazole in second-line therapy for *Helicobacter pylori* infection: a multicentre clinical trial. J Antimicrob Chemother. 2011;66(8):1847–52.
47. Liou JM, Bair MJ, Chen CC, Lee YC, Chen MJ, Chen CC, et al. Levofloxacin sequential therapy vs levofloxacin triple therapy in the second-line treatment of *Helicobacter pylori*: a randomized trial. Am J Gastroenterol. 2016;111(3):381–7.
48. Federico A, Nardone G, Gravina AG, Iovene MR, Miranda A, Compare D, et al. Efficacy of 5-day levofloxacin-containing concomitant therapy in eradication of *Helicobacter pylori* infection. Gastroenterology. 2012;143(1):55–61 e1. quize e13–4
49. Hsu PI, Tsai FW, Kao SS, Hsu WH, Cheng JS, Peng NJ, et al. Ten-day quadruple therapy comprising proton pump inhibitor, bismuth, tetracycline, and levofloxacin is more effective than standard levofloxacin triple therapy in the second-line treatment of *Helicobacter pylori* infection: a randomized controlled trial. Am J Gastroenterol. 2017;112(9):1374–81.
50. Malfertheiner P, Megraud F, O'Morain CA, Atherton J, Axon AT, Bazzoli F, et al. Management of *Helicobacter pylori* infection--the Maastricht IV/ Florence consensus report. Gut. 2012;61(5):646–64.
51. Liou JM, Chen CC, Chang CY, Chen MJ, Fang YJ, Lee JY, et al. Efficacy of genotypic resistance-guided sequential therapy in the third-line treatment of refractory *Helicobacter pylori* infection: a multicentre clinical trial. J Antimicrob Chemother. 2013;68(2):450–6.
52. Liou JM, Chen PY, Luo JC, Lee JY, Chen CC, Fang YJ, et al. Efficacies of genotypic resistance-guided vs empirical therapy for refractory *Helicobacter pylori* infection. Gastroenterology. 2018;

8

B cell subset alteration and the expression of tissue homing molecules in dengue infected patients

Kovit Pattanapanyasat[1], Ladawan Khowawisetsut[2], Ampaiwan Chuansumrit[3], Kulkanya Chokephaibulkit[4], Kanchana Tangnararatchakit[3], Nopporn Apiwattanakul[3], Chonnamet Techasaensiri[3], Premrutai Thitilertdecha[1,5], Tipaporn Sae-Ung[6] and Nattawat Onlamoon[1,5]* iD

Abstract

Background: B cells play an essential role during dengue viral infection. While a major expansion of antibody secreting cells (ASCs) was observed, the importance of these increased frequencies of ASCs remains unclear. The alteration of B cell subsets may result from the expression of tissue specific homing molecules leading to their mobilization and distribution to different target organs during acute dengue viral infection.

Methods: In this study, whole blood samples were obtained from thirty pediatric dengue-infected patients and ten healthy children and then stained with fluorochrome-conjugated monoclonal antibodies against CD3, CD14, CD19, CD20, CD21, CD27, CD38, CD45, CD138 and homing molecules of interest before analyzed by polychromatic flow cytometry. B cell subsets were characterized throughout acute infection period.

Results: Data shows that there were no detectable differences in frequencies of resting, activated and tissue memory cells, whereas the frequency of ASCs was significantly increased and associated with the lower frequency of naïve cells. These results were found from patients with both dengue fever and dengue hemorrhagic fever, suggesting that such change or alteration of B cells was not associated with disease severity. Moreover, several homing molecules (e.g., CXCR3 and CCR2) were found in ASCs, indicating that ASCs may distribute to inflamed tissues and various organs.

Conclusions: Findings from this study provide insight into B cell subset distribution. Furthermore, organ mobilization according to homing molecule expression on different B cell subsets during the course of dengue viral infection also suggests they are distributed to inflamed tissues and various organs.

Keywords: Antibody secreting cells, Trafficking molecules, Severity, Dengue

Background

Varied clinical outcomes are one of the hallmarks of dengue viral infection. The outcomes range from asymptomatic infection to infection that can result in mild fever (dengue fever or DF) or severe hemorrhagic fever (dengue hemorrhagic fever or DHF) and dengue shock syndrome (DSS) [1]. The major characteristic symptoms of DSS are hemorrhagic phenomenon (e.g., petechiae, mild mucous membrane or skin bleeding) and shock [2, 3]. The dengue virus results in 50–100 million infections leading to 500,000 hospitalizations and > 20,000 fatal cases per year worldwide as estimated by the World Health Organization (WHO) [4–6]. The dengue virus is transmitted primarily by a bite from an infected female mosquito, *Aedes aegypti*. The infection by dengue virus occurs in humans of all ages. Although a marked increase in a number of adult with severe dengue was also observed in countries such as Taiwan, Singapore and Sri Lanka, the highest rates of

* Correspondence: nattawat.onl@mahidol.ac.th
[1]Biomedical Research Incubator Unit, Research Group and Research Network Division, Research Department, Faculty of Medicine Siriraj Hospital, Mahidol University, Bangkok, Thailand
[5]Research group in Immunobiology and Therapeutic Sciences, Faculty of Medicine Siriraj Hospital, Mahidol University, 2 Wanglang Road, Bangkoknoi, Bangkok 10700, Thailand
Full list of author information is available at the end of the article

severe dengue occur in children from some countries such as Thailand and Viet Nam [7].

There are four serotypes of dengue including DENV-1, DENV-2, DENV-3 and DENV-4 [8] that express both serotype unique and cross reactive epitopes. After primary DENV infection, recovered patients generate potent antibody responses that to a large extent cross react with the 4 serotypes. However, homologous reinfection does not occur and whether antibodies are responsible for this protection is not fully known. Patients that are re-infected with the different serotype (heterologous) not only remain susceptible to infection with the heterologous dengue virus but in select cases show an increased susceptibility to developing a severe form of the disease termed dengue hemorrhagic fever (DHF) and dengue shock syndrome (DSS). While still considered controversial, the phenomenon is termed antibody mediated enhancement (ADE) [9–12].

B cells have been shown to play a major role during infection with dengue viruses highlighted by the recent observation of a significantly high number of plasmablast/plasma cells that appear during acute dengue infection [13–16]. Activation of B cells through dengue-specific B cell receptor (BCR) has been reasoned to induce B cell proliferation and differentiation into effector plasma cells or long lived memory B cells [17]. The antibody secreting cells (ASCs), which is refer to a combination of both plasmablasts and plasma cells, produced antibodies which have an important role not only in the protection against subsequent exposure [18] but can also lead to an increase in the risk of infection in some cases [19].

The objectives of the present study were to characterize in detail changes in the B cell subpopulations and plasmablasts/plasma cells during acute dengue infection and to identify alterations in the expression of trafficking molecules by the different B cell subsets. It was reasoned that the identification of unique set of homing markers by cells in these patients with the severe forms of the disease may provide clues to the pathogenic mechanisms that distinguish asymptomatic from DHF/DSS. The results of this study are the basis of this report.

Methods
Study population and sample collection
In this study, 30 dengue infected children and 10 healthy, age-matched children were recruited from the Faculty of Medicine Siriraj Hospital and Faculty of Medicine Ramathibodi Hospital, Mahidol University, Bangkok, Thailand. The patients were categorized into dengue fever (DF), dengue hemorrhagic fever (DHF) based on the 1997 WHO classification of dengue infection which has been currently acceptable for clinical practice in Thailand. Information about patient cohort is detailed in Table 1 while the clinical features of patients are also shown in Table 2.

Table 1 Summary of study subjects

Characteristic	DF	DHF	Healthy individuals
Total number of samples	10	20	10
Number of males/number of females	3/7	6/14	5/5
Age (year)	5–14	5–19	10–19
Number of patients infected with dengue virus serotype:			
1	5	4	–
2	1	3	–
3	4	9	–
4	–	2	–
1 / 2	–	1	–
1 / 4	–	1	–

The blood samples were collected aseptically by venipuncture into a sterile 3.2% sodium citrate blood collection tube and immediately transported to the laboratory and stored at room temperature (RT) until ready for flow cytometric analyses.

Monoclonal antibodies and reagents
Fluorochrome-conjugated monoclonal antibodies against a variety of cell surface molecules using for the phenotypic characterization of B cell subsets included anti-CD3 conjugated with phycoerythrin-cyanine 7 (PE-Cy7), anti-CD14 conjugated with allophycocyanin- cyanine 7 (APC-Cy7), anti-CD19 conjugated with brilliant violet 510 (BV510), anti-CD20 conjugated with alexa fluor 700 (A700), anti-CD21 conjugated with allophycocyanin (APC), anti-CD27 conjugated with brilliant violet 605 (BV605), anti-CD38 conjugated with brilliant violet 421 (BV421), anti-CD45 conjugated with peridinin chlorophyll protein (PerCP), anti-CD138 conjugated with fluorescein isothiocyanate (FITC). PE-conjugated monoclonal antibodies against a variety of cell surface specific homing molecule that have previously been reported to facilitate the migration of cells to different tissues or organs were utilized and included antibodies against CCR2, CCR7, CCR9, CCR10, CD29, CD62L, CD103, CD122, CD132, CD137, CXCR3, CD278, β7 integrin and CXCR4.

Immunofluorescent staining and flow cytometric analysis
Aliquots of whole blood samples in a volume of 100 μL were stained with a pre-determined optimal concentration of a cocktail of fluorochrome-conjugated monoclonal antibodies against cell surface molecules. These included CD3, CD14, CD19, CD20, CD21, CD27, CD38, CD45, and CD138. Each aliquot was then stained with, either CCR2, CCR7, CCR9, CCR10, CD29, CD62L, CD103, CD122, CD132, CD137, CXCR3, CD278, β7 integrin or CXCR4. The stained samples were incubated for 15 min in the dark at RT. After incubation, 2 mL of 1X FACS lysing solution was added to each tube and the

Table 2 Clinical feature of dengue infected patients

Patient ID	Category	Clinical feature
V001	DF	No evidence of leakage.
V002	DF	Hematocrit rising 14%, evidence of pleural effusion not noted.
V003	DF	Hematocrit rising 10%, evidence of pleural effusion not noted.
V004	DF	No evidence of leakage.
V005	DF	No evidence of leakage.
V006	DF	No evidence of leakage, hypermenorrhea.
V007	DF	Hematocrit rising 8% (from 37 to 40%).
V008	DF	No evidence of leakage.
V009	DF	No evidence of leakage.
V010	DF	No evidence of leakage.
V011	DHF I	No bleeding, there was evidence of hemoconcentration, right pleural effusion by physical examination and chest X-ray.
V012	DHF I	Decrease breath sounds in the right lung but negative chest X-ray, hemoconcentration from 38 to 43%.
V013	DHF I	Hematocrit rising 14%, evidence of pleural effusion not noted.
V014	DHF I	Evidence of minimal right pleural effusion.
V015	DHF I	Minimal right pleural effusion, decrease breath sound right lung.
V016	DHF I	Mild dehydration and hypokalemia.
V017	DHF I	Mild dehydration
V018	DHF I	Moderated dehydration.
V019	DHF I	Hyponatremia with mild dehydration.
V020	DHF I	Mild dehydration
V021	DHF I	Mild dehydration
V022	DHF I	Right pleural effusion.
V023	DHF I	Mild dehydration
V024	DHF II	Hematocrit rising from 35 to 42%, lowest Hematocrit being 32.8%, epistaxis, chest X-ray with right pleural effusion.
V025	DHF II	Right pleural effusion.
V026	DHF III	Narrow pulse pressure, hemoconcentration, chest X-ray with right pleural effusion.
V027	DHF III	Evidence of hypotension but not profound shock.
V028	DHF III	Hemoconcentration and hypotension, underlying disease of b-thalassemia, pleural effusion from physical examination and chest X-ray.
V029	DHF III	Hemoconcentration, hypoalbuminemia, vaginal bleeding, epistaxis, narrow pulse pressure, chest X-ray with pleural effusion.
V030	DHF III	Hypokalemia.

tubes incubated for 10 min in the dark at RT to lyse red blood cells. The samples were then washed in phosphate buffered saline (PBS). The supernatant fluid was discarded and the stained cells were re-suspended in 300 μL of PBS. Stained samples were stored at 2 °C to 8 °C until ready for analysis (less than 8 h after blood collection). The stained samples were analyzed on an LSRFortessa flow cytometer by using FACSDiva software (BD Bioscience, San Jose, CA). Data analysis was performed using FlowJo software (Tree Star, Ashland, OR).

Statistical analysis
GraphPad Prism 5.0 (GraphPad software) was used for statistical analysis. Mann-Whitney U test and 1-way ANOVA followed by Bonferroni's multiple comparisons test were used for unpaired analysis for comparisons among the groups of data sets. The data for each comparative analysis was calculated as mean ± SD. P-values < 0.05 were considered statistically significant.

Results
Identification of changes in B cell subsets during acute dengue infection
We first sought out to characterize changes in B cell subsets, in the blood samples from patients with acute DENV infection, to establish a foundation for our studies aimed at defining the tissue and organ homing molecules on these subsets. The overarching rationale for this study was that knowledge of the homing patterns of the subsets may help distinguish the severe forms of dengue. The gating strategy utilized for the identification of B cell subsets is illustrated in Fig. 1. As noted, the gated population of CD19 and CD20 expressing lymphoid cells was utilized as a marker for total B cells. The differential expression of CD21, CD27, CD38 and CD138 by the gated population of CD19+/CD20+ B cells was then utilized to distinguish the B cells into 6 subpopulations. The CD21+CD27- subset was identified as naïve B cells and CD21+CD27+ was considered as resting memory B cells, while CD21-CD27- was considered as tissue memory B cells. The CD21-CD27+ subset was further analyzed based on the expression of CD27 and CD38 to distinguish activated memory B cells from ASCs. The activated memory B cells were identified as cells expressing CD21-CD27+CD38-/low and the ASCs were identified as cells that were CD21-CD27+CD38high. The ASC populations, in turn, were further distinguished into plasmablasts that were identified based as cells expressing CD27highCD38highCD138- whereas plasma cells were identified based on the expression of CD27highCD38highCD138+ .

The frequencies of B cell subpopulations in samples (n = 30) from dengue patients were compared with samples from healthy individuals (n = 10). As seen in Fig. 2, the samples from the dengue patients showed a lower percentage of the naïve B cell subset and a high percentage of ASC populations as compared with the control samples. When further identifying ASC subsets into

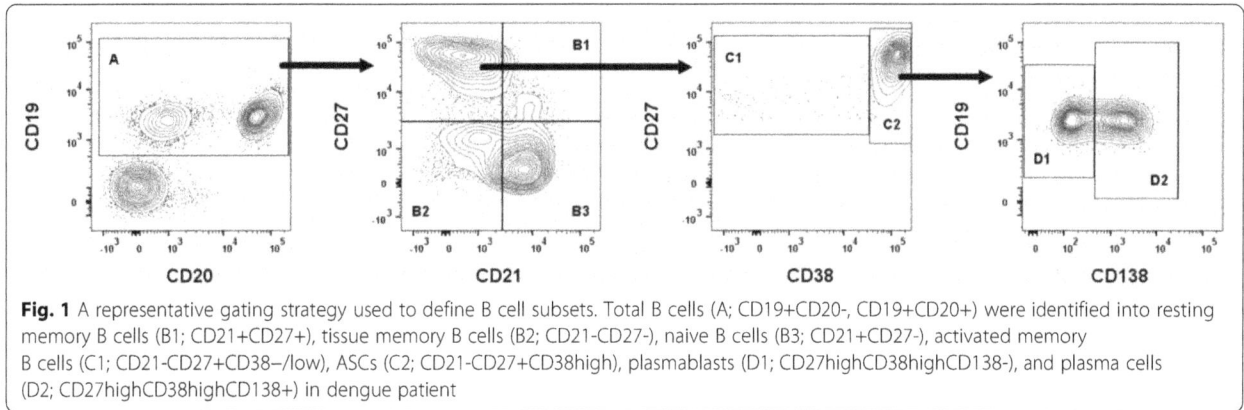

Fig. 1 A representative gating strategy used to define B cell subsets. Total B cells (A; CD19+CD20-, CD19+CD20+) were identified into resting memory B cells (B1; CD21+CD27+), tissue memory B cells (B2; CD21-CD27-), naive B cells (B3; CD21+CD27-), activated memory B cells (C1; CD21-CD27+CD38-/low), ASCs (C2; CD21-CD27+CD38high), plasmablasts (D1; CD27highCD38highCD138-), and plasma cells (D2; CD27highCD38highCD138+) in dengue patient

plasmablasts and plasma cells, both of them from the dengue patients still showed significantly higher percentages when compared to healthy individuals. These changes are consistent with our previous reports of changes in subsets of B cells during acute dengue infection [15]. The other B cell subsets including resting memory, tissue memory and activated memory were presented in low frequencies and there were no significant differences in these subsets between samples from the dengue patients and controls. We next analyzed these data in efforts to determine if the degree of changes in the B cell subsets noted were correlated with the severity of DENV infection in these patients. Interestingly, no significant difference in any B cell subpopulations were noted in samples from DF and DHF patients (data not shown).

Kinetics of different B cell subsets during acute DENV infection

Since significant changes of B cell subsets occur during acute dengue infection, it was reasoned that the frequency of each B cell subset may differ based on the kinetics of infection. To address this issue, the results of the B cell subsets were compared in relation to day of defervescence (D0) which was defined as the date when the fever dropped below 37.5 °C and remained so for 48 h. The day prior to defervescence was defined as day minus 1 (D-1) whereas the day after defervescence was defined as day plus 1 (D+1). The kinetics of B cell subsets in samples from day D-2 to +3 of defervescence were thus examined. Since the evaluated data from each patient was not complete for the entire period, the data from each available time point were pooled and the number

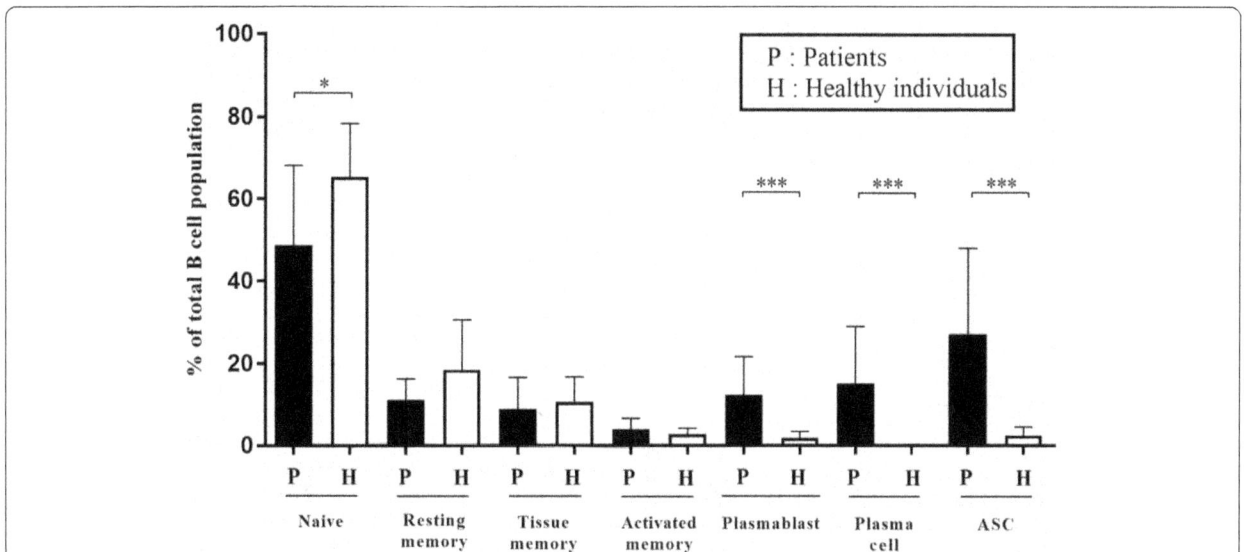

Fig. 2 Comparisons of B cell subsets during acute DENV infections. High level of ASCs was observed in dengue infected patients. Significantly lower frequencies of naïve and resting memory B cells were observed in patients when compare with healthy individuals (*p < 0.05, by Mann-Whitney U test). Significantly higher frequencies of plasmablasts/plasma cells or ASCs were observed in patients when compare with healthy individuals (***p ≤ 0.0005, by Mann-Whitney U test), whereas activated memory and tissue memory B cells were not significantly different when compare between patients with dengue and healthy individuals

of patients that were evaluated on each time point was indicated. As seen in Fig. 3, there appeared to be a gradual decrease in the average percentage of naïve B cells at D-2 to +3 giving values of 61.8%, 50.3%, 47.2%, 41.2%, 37.8% and 51.0%, respectively. The average percentage of resting memory B cells at D-2 to D+3 while not statistically significant showed a trend towards an increase with values of 9.4%, 10.3%, 10.5%, 12.2%, 11.3% and 15.3%, respectively. On the other hand, there was clearly a significant decrease in the frequencies of tissue memory B cells from D-2 to +3 with values of average percentage of 10.7%, 11.7%, 8.1%, 6.9%, 6.7% and 3.4%, respectively. The average percentages of activated memory B cells at D-2 to +3 did not show an appreciable change. When the data for the frequencies of ASCs were analyzed, the average percentages of plasmablasts at D–2 to +3 were 6.2%, 14.1%, 12.7%, 12.6%, 18.9% and 11.8%, respectively, whereas the average percentages of plasma cells at D-2 to +3 were 11.6%, 8.7%, 17.7%, 21.8%, 23.1% and 14.5%, respectively. Thus, a significant increase in the frequency of ASCs as a function of time was noted for these subsets.

We also determined whether there was any difference between B cell subset responses based on the phases of disease. Three different phases were identified including the febrile phase (D-2 and D-1), the defervescence phase (D0 and D+1) and the afebrile phase (D+2 and D+3) as shown in Table 3. We found that there was a gradual decrease in the average frequency of naïve B cells with values of 53.3%, 44.6% and 41.8% associated with the febrile, defervescence and afebrile phases, respectively. While the average percentage of resting memory and activated B cells did not show significant changes based on the phases of the diseases, the average percentage of tissue memory B cells associated with febrile, defervescence phase and afebrile phases gave values of 11.4%, 7.6% and 5.7%, respectively, denoting a significant decrease as a function of disease phase. The average percentages of plasmablasts and plasma cells also progressively increased from the febrile phase and defervescence phase to the afebrile phase with values of 12.0%, 12.7% and 16.9% for the plasmablasts and 9.5%, 19.5% and 20.7%, respectively for the plasma cells. The results for the levels of the other subsets showed no difference in any phase of infection. Moreover, analyses of these data based on the different phases did not show any difference based on the severity (DF versus DHF/DSS) of DENV infection.

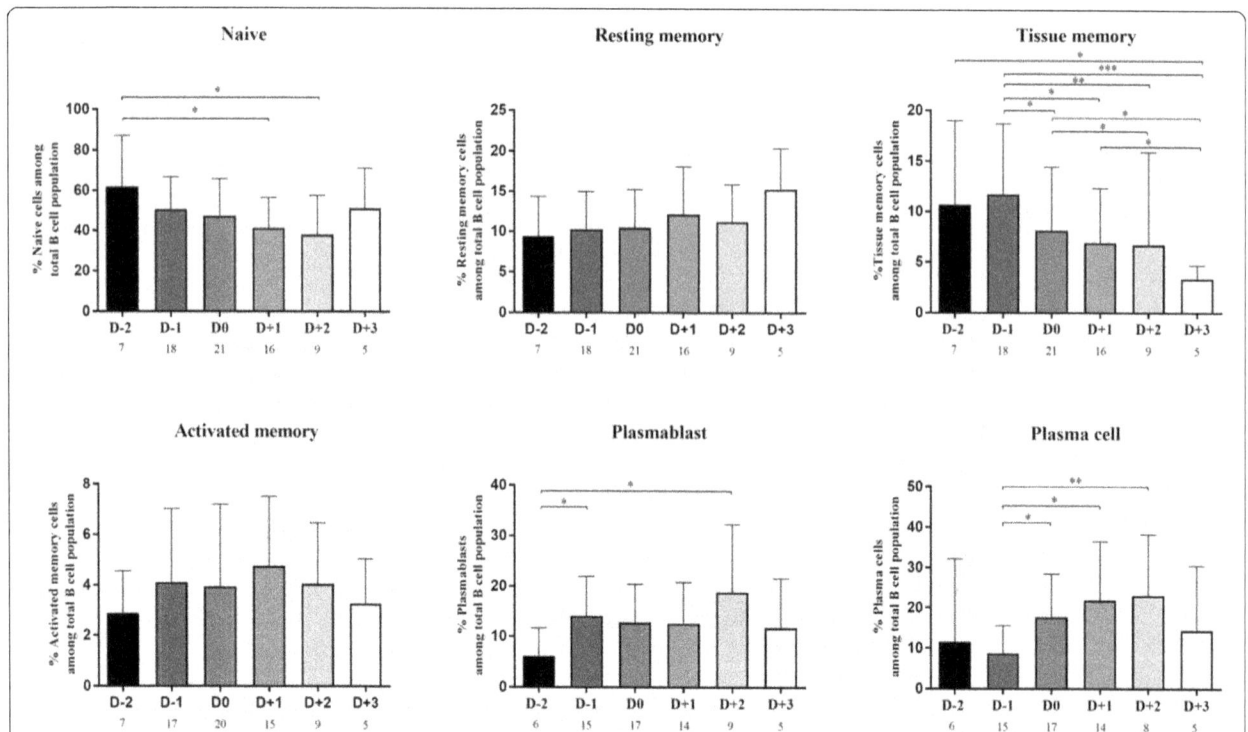

Fig. 3 Percentage of B cell subsets at different time points during acute DENV infection. Values (n) indicate numbers of patients for each time point. The percentage of naïve and tissue memory B cells had started decreasing from D-2 and D-1 to D+2 and D+3, respectively, whereas plasma cells started to increase from D-1 and to D+2. Other subsets of B cell including resting memory, activated memory and plasmablast showed no specific pattern. Only tissue memory showed significantly lower frequencies at D+2 and D+3 when compare with D-1 (*p < 0.05, ** p < 0.005 and ***p ≤ 0.0005 by Mann-Whitney U test)

Table 3 Comparison of B cell subsets between different phases during acute infection

Acute infection phases	Frequency (%)					
	Naïve B cells	Resting memory B cells	Tissue memory B cells	Activated memory B cells	Plasmablasts	Plasma cells
Febrile (D-2 and D-1)	52.7 ± 19.9*	9.9 ± 4.4	11.0 ± 7.0*,**	3.8 ± 2.8	12.6 ± 8.2	10.1 ± 11.8*,**
Defervescense (D0 and D+1)	44.4 ± 18.2	12.1 ± 5.3	7.5 ± 6.3***	4.4 ± 3.2	12.0 ± 8.1	19.3 ± 12.8
Afebrile (D+2 and D+3)	43.4 ± 21.4	13.7 ± 4.9	5.8 ± 9.2	3.6 ± 1.9	15.0 ± 13.6	18.5 ± 16.5

Results are showed as mean percentages ± standard deviation. *indicates $p < 0.05$ when compare to defervescence phase, **indicates $p < 0.05$ when compare to afebrile phase and ***indicates $p < 0.05$ when compare between defervescence and afebrile phase

Comparative analysis of the tissue/organ homing molecule expression on B cell subsets

The precise mechanisms that lead to DHF/DSS in a subset of dengue infected patients has been a subject of intense investigation by a number of laboratories for quite some time and remains to be defined. We hypothesized that an examination of cell surface molecules that promote the trafficking of B cells to specific tissue/organs may provide clues as to the site at which the host immune response is focused during acute infection. We thus selected to study cell surface molecules that promote cells to traffic to the skin (CCR10), gut tissues (β7, CCR9 and CD103 or αEβ7), lymph nodes (CCR7, CD62L), lung (CD278), central nervous system (CD29), bone marrow (CXCR4, CD122, CD132, CD137) and/or inflamed tissues (CXCR3, CCR2). We studied the expression of these homing markers on different B cell subsets in blood samples from healthy subjects ($n = 8$) and dengue infected patients ($n = 9$). A summary of the data on these markers on the various B cell subsets in samples from dengue patients as compared with healthy subjects are illustrated in Fig. 4.

While significant differences in the frequencies of subsets that express a variety of these markers was noted, it was reasoned that a focus on those markers that were increased in samples from dengue infected patients as compared with healthy controls would be more informative to begin with than those that decreased with the prejudice that such increases would suggest increased trafficking to the specific tissue/organ. What appears clear is that the most notable increases in homing markers appeared to be expressed by plasmablasts and plasma cells from the dengue infected patients as compare with healthy controls. Thus, significant increases were noted in the frequencies of plasmablasts and plasma cells from dengue patients that expressed CCR9 (homing to the small intestine), CCR7 and CD62L (lymph node homing), CXCR4 (bone marrow homing) and markers such as CXCR3 and CCR2 that are associated with homing to inflammatory sites. These findings suggest that there is a greater degree of mobilization of the plasmablasts and plasma cells to the small intestine, lymph nodes and the bone marrow that serve as sites where the inflammatory response to dengue is apparently occurring. Increased frequencies of tissue memory B cells that expressed CCR7 and activated memory B cells that expressed CXCR4 and CCR2 were also noted but the significance of these findings remain unclear. In contrast, significant decreases in the frequencies of naïve B cells that expressed CCR9 and CD62L and resting memory B cells that expressed CCR9, CCR7 and CXCR3 as well as activated memory B cells that expressed CD62L in blood samples from the dengue infected patient as compared with healthy controls were also noted. The significance of such decreases in dengue infected patients is not clear at present.

The expression of homing molecules were also compared between different B cell populations that were observed in dengue infected patients. When compared to naïve B cells, lower frequencies of plasmablasts and plasma cells that expressed β7 ($p = 0.0224$ and 0.0003, respectively) and CCR7 ($p < 0.0001$) were observed. The frequency of plasma cells that expressed CCR7 was also lower than resting memory B cells ($p = 0.0154$). In contrast, higher frequencies of plasmablasts and plasma cells that expressed CD62L were observed when compared to tissue memory ($p < 0.0001$) and activated memory ($p = 0.0060$ and 0.0044, respectively) B cells. Frequencies of plasmablasts and plasma cells that expressed CXCR3 and CCR2 were also higher than naïve, resting memory and tissue memory B cells ($p < 0.001$). Moreover, higher frequencies of plasmablasts and plasma cells that expressed CCR2 were observed when compared to activated memory B cells ($p = 0.0160$ and 0.0063, respectively). Significant changes in the frequencies of activated memory B cells that express homing molecules were also observed. When compared to naïve B cells, lower frequencies of activate memory B cells that expressed β7 ($p < 0.0001$) and CCR7 ($p = 0.0010$) were observed. In addition, when compared to activated memory B cells, lower frequencies of naïve, resting memory and tissue memory B cells that expressed CD29 ($p = 0.0003$, 0.0011 and 0.0126, respectively), CXCR3 ($p < 0.0001$) and CCR2 ($p = 0.0008$, 0.0017 and 0.0072, respectively) were observed. Frequencies of activated memory B cells that express CD137 were also higher than naïve ($p = 0.0088$) and resting memory ($p = 0.0197$) B cells. Taken together, the results showed that B cell populations with activated

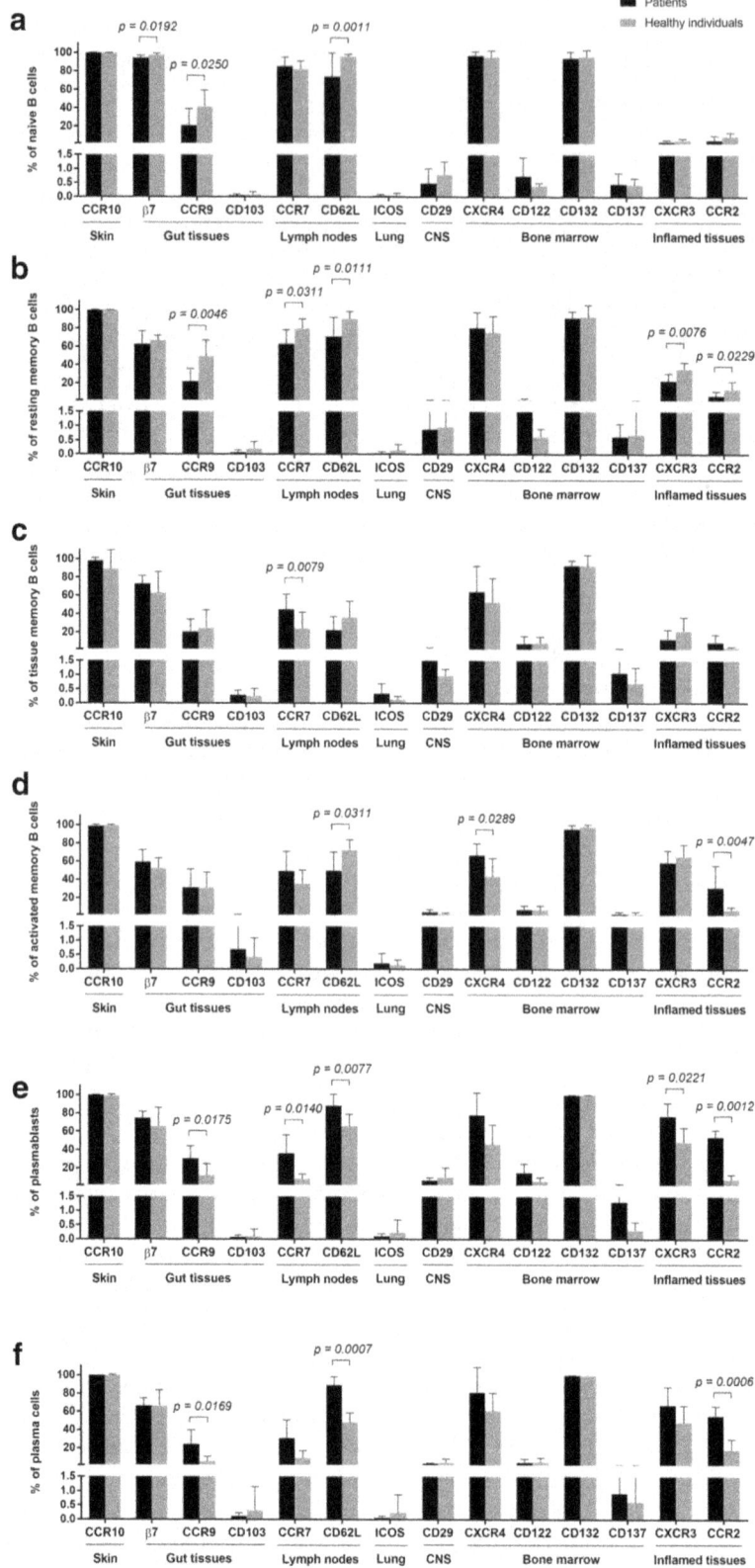

Fig. 4 (See legend on next page.)

(See figure on previous page.)

Fig. 4 Comparison of specific organ homing molecules of B cell subsets. Frequencies of B cell subsets including (**a**) naïve B cells, (**b**) resting memory B cells, (**c**) tissue memory B cells, (**d**) activated memory T cells, (**e**) plasmablasts and (**f**) plasma cells, were observed for their specific expressions to different organs; skin (CCR10), gut tissues (β7, CCR9, and CD103), lymph nodes (CCR7 and CD62L), lung (ICOS), CNS (CD29), bone marrow (CXCR4, CD122, CD132, and CD137), and inflamed tissues (CXCR3 and CCR2). Changes in frequencies of B cell subpopulations expressing individual marker were compared between dengue-infected patients and healthy donors. Significant differences are indicated when p-values < 0.05 by 1-way ANOVA followed by Bonferroni's multiple comparisons test

phenotype (activated memory B cells, plasmablasts and plasma cells) had higher ability to mobilized to inflamed tissues than cells in resting stage (naïve, resting memory and tissue memory B cells).

Discussion

Several studies have previously documented the findings that dengue virus infection results in marked increases in B cells, especially plasmablasts, plasma cells or antibody-secreting cells (ASCs) [14–16, 20]. The results reported herein confirm these previous findings. While there is a reason to suspect that healthy individuals living in dengue endemic areas might have high or equal level of activated B cells when compare to acute infected patients as a result of previous exposure or an inapparent dengue infection, low levels of plamablasts, plasma cells and activated memory B cells in healthy subjects as observed in this study suggests that dengue exposure must reach a certain threshold in order to induce B cell responses. The natural infection might be required to maintain sufficient levels of antigen exposure as suggested by a study showing that a long term dengue immune memory after vaccination with a chimeric tetravalent DENV vaccine appears relatively low when compare to individuals with a history of natural infection [21]. As reported earlier, the activated B cells proliferate and differentiate into substantial numbers of antibody-secreting cells to produce soluble antibodies against a wide variety of dengue viral epitopes, some of which specifically recognize and neutralize the dengue virus [14, 22]. Amongst these antibodies are also antibodies that are potentially involved in the enhancement of severe disease including DHF or DSS in secondary infection or re-infection with the different type of the dengue virus [23]. Therefore, during acute dengue infection, a large number of plasmablasts, plasma cells or ASC are produced in response to invading foreign pathogens. Moreover, our study also shows that there is a decrease in the frequencies of naïve B cells in dengue infected patients, which is consistent with a previous report of dengue patients in northeast Brazil that showed the decreased proportion of naïve and resting memory B cells [20]. Their study also showed that B cells in individuals with severe secondary DENV infection were induced to undergo apoptosis by the expression of the pro-apoptotic marker CD95 or Fas receptor (FasR). Thus apoptotic cell death may be promoted through the engagement of the CD95/CD95L or FasR/

FasL pathway [20, 24–26]. These data suggest that decreased naïve and resting memory B cells in patients maybe secondary to apoptosis that is induced by dengue virus [27, 28].

Several reports on B cell subsets during dengue infection have been published. One such report showed interestingly that the frequencies of plasmablast were significantly higher in patients following secondary DF and complicated dengue fever (DFC) infection than during primary dengue infection [20]. A study of pediatric dengue patients in Nicaragua reported that the frequencies of plasmablasts/plasma cells was not significantly different in samples from DF as compared with patients with DHF/DSS [16] that is similar to the results of the studies we report herein. Other studies conducted on dengue patients in Brazil and Singapore studied the kinetics of the plasmablast response and reported that peak plasmablast were observed between days 4–7 of dengue symptoms [14, 20]. Similarly, a report of dengue patients in Thailand found that peak plasmablasts were observed in dengue patients at day 6 or 7 after onset of symptoms [15]. While these data showed plasmablast response at different days after the beginning of fever symptom, our study observed the kinetics of B cell subsets at D-2 to +3 of defervescence. We found that while the frequencies of plasma cells and ASCs were low during the febrile phase (D-2 or –1), these frequencies gradually increased during the afebrile phase (D+2 or +3). In contrast, naïve and tissue memory B cells showed high numbers during the febrile phase (D-2 or –1) that gradually decreased during the afebrile phase (D+2 or +3). Other subsets of B cell including resting memory, activated memory and plamablasts showed similar levels at different time points of infection. Therefore, our results suggest that in the early stage of infection, naïve and tissue memory B cells encounter dengue virus and become activated. These activated B cells develop into plasmablasts/plasma cells or ASCs to produce antibodies which are then specifically eliminated during the late stages of infection. However, comparisons of B cell subset responses in patients with DF and DHF at different time points of infection showed that none of the changes in B cell subsets were associated with the severity of infection. Interestingly, while both plasmablasts and plasma cells contribute to a pool of ASCs, the kinetic levels of these 2 populations are differences as plasmablasts relatively maintain their levels whereas plasma cells decline in a later period. Data indicate that blood circulating plasmablasts derived from activated memory B cells whereas it developmental fate to become either short-lived plasmablasts or long-lived plasma cells remain unclear [29]. However, the decline in plasma cell level suggested the migration of these blood circulating plasma cells to their survival niches such as bone marrow which is crucial for the generation of long-lived plasma cells [30]. It is also unclear how these ASCs contribute to the maintenance of dengue-specific antibody in the serum especially in people from endemic area that may have a repeat exposure to the dengue virus.

B cells play an important role in adaptive immune system by secretion of antigen specific antibodies that contribute to protection and response against the invading pathogens. During the course of infection, effector B cells are mobilized to different organs or tissues in response to chemokine gradients that are generated by cells at sites of infection. The type of cells within a given infected tissue synthesize distinct set of chemokines and the effector cells expressing the receptor for the chemokine set up a pattern of migration that leads to the trafficking of cells to the site of infection. The migration of effector B cells into the infected areas thus mainly depends on adhesion molecules, homing receptors and chemokines. To understand B cell responses in different location, it is important to determine homing markers expressed on B cells, locations that these homing markers guide B cell to go to and the function of B cells at the site of infection. Therefore, we examined homing molecules that express on different B cell subsets that may lead to the migration of these B cells to different tissues or organs where they are optimally suited to deal with particular type of infections. We thus included the analysis of different homing markers that included CCR10 (home to skin) [31, 32], β7 integrin, CCR9 and CD103 (home to gut tissue) [33–35], CCR7, CD62L (home to lymph nodes) [36, 37], CD278 (home to lung) [38], CD29 (home to the central nervous system) [39], CXCR4, CD122, CD132, and CD137 (home to bone marrow) [40–42], CXCR3 and CCR2 (home to inflamed tissues) [43, 44].

While low expression levels of ICOS and CD29 indicated that none of these B cell subsets mobilize to lung and central nervous system, it may be possible that these 2 markers as well as CD103 are not suitable for being used as an organ target marker for B cells. In contrast, some homing markers changed significantly during the course of dengue viral infection. Decreased levels of β7, CCR9, CCR7, CD62L, CXCR3 and CCR2 were observed in naïve and resting memory B cells. It indicated that the migrations of these B cell subsets to gut tissue, lymph nodes and inflamed tissues were reduced during dengue infection. The expression of CD62L on activated

memory B cells was also obviously decreased whereas the expressions of CXCR4 and CCR2 were increased. It indicated that the migration of activated memory B cells to lymph node was reduced while their mobilization to bone marrow and inflamed tissues was elevated during dengue infection. Therefore, it might be possible that some activated memory B cells are denied re-entry into the lymph node and migrate into peripheral tissues sites of infection as well as bone marrow while they differentiated into plasmablasts/plasma cells.

In this study, an increased level of CCR7 was observed in tissue memory B cells. It indicated that the migration of these cells to lymph node was raised during dengue infection and their presence may be important in controlling immune response in lymph node. Although the function of this B cell subset is not well defined, tissue memory B cells (also called atypical memory B cells) present high-level expression of multiple inhibitory receptors on the cell surface. This expression results in B cell exhaustion. Therefore, this B cell subset proliferates and differentiates poorly in response to Ag-stimulated B cell [45, 46].

Since a marked increase of ASCs was observed during acute infection of dengue virus, the information on ASCs mobilization is important to understand B cell response during the course of disease. The results demonstrated that plasmablasts and plasma cells showed similar expression pattern for most homing molecules. While predominant frequencies of CD62L expression were observed on plasmablasts and plasma cells, remarkable higher frequencies of CCR7expression were also observed on both plasmablasts and plasma cells in dengue patients when compared with healthy individuals. However, the CCR7 expression levels in plasmablasts and plasma cells still lower than those observed in naïve and resting memory B cells. In contrast, high expression levels of CXCR4 were observed in both populations although no significant difference was observed when compared to healthy individuals. It indicated that down-regulation of CCR7 and up-regulation of CXCR4 may promote these subsets to leave from LNs and migrate to bone marrow. This observation was supported by a study showed that down-regulation of CCR7 on plasma cells can reduced the responsiveness to the B and T cell zone chemokine in lymph node whereas an increase chemotactic sensitivity to the CXCR4 ligand can promote the mobilization to bone marrow [47].

Previous study reported that CCR9 is mainly function in IgA-ASCs migrating to the small intestine during infection with rotavirus [48]. Interestingly, the expression levels of CCR9, on plasmablasts and plasma cells were increased during dengue infection. It indicated the potential migration of plasmablasts and plasma cells to gut tissues. Some evidence showed that dengue infection induced intestinal mucosal injury as demonstrated by increased serum levels of intestinal fatty acid binding protein which were used as a specific marker for mucosal injury [49]. Moreover, dengue infection in a mouse model revealed that inoculation of immune complexes formed with serotype cross-reactive antibodies resulted in increased vascular permeability in the small intestine [50]. Taken together, the potential migration of CCR9 expressing plasmablasts to the gut tissues may promote the formation of immune complexes which leads to severe small intestinal pathology. More interestingly, plasmablasts and plasma cells had significantly higher frequencies of CXCR3 and CCR2 expression in dengue patients than healthy individuals. They also showed highest frequencies when compared to other B cell subsets. It might be possible that high expressions of CXCR3 and CCR2 in both populations guide these effector cells to the inflamed areas. A previous study showed that CXCR3 and its ligands play a crucial role in the elimination and inflammatory responses to invading virus by leading plasmablasts or plasma cells to inflamed tissues [51]. CCR2 is also essential during monocytes transmigrate to inflamed tissues [44]. Interaction between CCR2 and its CC-chemokine ligand recruits monocytes to sites of infection and these monocytes can participate in the initial inflammatory response by producing tumor necrosis factor (TNF) and chemokines [44].

Therefore, it might be possible that elevation of these homing markers during infection promote plasmablasts and plasma cells or ASCs into those specific sites which might involve in protection or pathogenesis of dengue infection. Taken together, these data are very useful for our understanding of B cell subset distributions and organ mobilization based on the expression of homing molecules on different B cell subsets during the course of dengue viral infection.

Conclusions

This study highlights the alteration of B cell subsets including naïve, resting, activated, and tissue memory cells as well as antibody secreting cells (ASCs) in pediatric dengue-infected patients during acute infection. The study found that the frequency of naïve B cells was markedly low, whereas that of ASCs was significantly increased. Moreover, results suggest that the change was not related to disease severity. It is also interesting to discover that the massively increased numbers of ASCs during acute infection expressed tissue homing markers, such as CXCR3 and CCR2, suggesting that these ASCs may distribute to inflamed tissues and various organs. Our findings, therefore, are very useful for better understanding of B cell subset distribution and organ mobilization according to homing molecule expression on different B cell subsets during the course of dengue viral infection.

Acknowledgements
The authors gratefully acknowledge the kind co-operation of the dengue infected patients. We thank the primary care physicians and nurses who worked hard in providing us important clinical supports for this study. We also would like to express our gratitude to Prof. Dr. Aftab A. Ansari for his valuable comments on this study.

Funding
This work was supported by The National Institute of Health/ National Institute of Allergy and Infectious Diseases [grant number R01AI099385]; The Thailand Research Fund Distinguished Research Professor Grant [grant number DPG5980001] to KP; Siriraj Graduate Thesis Scholarship to TS; and Chalermphrakiat Grant from Faculty of Medicine Siriraj Hospital to LK, PT and NO.

Authors' contributions
KP: research idea formation and supervision; LK: performed the experiment and data analysis; AC, KC, KT, NA, and CT: patient recruitment and diagnosis; PT: data analysis and manuscript editing; TS: performed the experiment and data analysis; NO: research idea formation, research monitoring, and manuscript writing. All authors read and approved the final manuscript.

Competing interests
The authors declare that they have no competing interest.

Author details
[1]Biomedical Research Incubator Unit, Research Group and Research Network Division, Research Department, Faculty of Medicine Siriraj Hospital, Mahidol University, Bangkok, Thailand. [2]Department of Parasitology, Faculty of Medicine Siriraj Hospital, Mahidol University, Bangkok, Thailand. [3]Department of Pediatrics, Faculty of Medicine Ramathibodi Hospital, Mahidol University, Bangkok, Thailand. [4]Department of Pediatrics, Faculty of Medicine Siriraj Hospital, Mahidol University, Bangkok, Thailand. [5]Research group in Immunobiology and Therapeutic Sciences, Faculty of Medicine Siriraj Hospital, Mahidol University, 2 Wanglang Road, Bangkoknoi, Bangkok 10700, Thailand. [6]Master of Science program in Immunology, Department of Immunology, Faculty of Medicine Siriraj Hospital, Mahidol University, Bangkok, Thailand.

References
1. Bhamarapravati N, Tuchinda P, Boonyapaknavik V. Pathology of Thailand haemorrhagic fever: a study of 100 autopsy cases. Ann Trop Med Parasitol. 1967;61(4):500–10.
2. Eram S, Setyabudi Y, Sadono TI, Sutrisno DS, Gubler DJ, Sulianti Saroso J. Epidemic dengue hemorrhagic fever in rural Indonesia. II. Clinical studies. Am J Trop Med Hyg. 1979;28(4):711–6.
3. Gubler DJ. Dengue and dengue hemorrhagic fever. Clin Microbiol Rev. 1998;11(3):480–96.
4. Guzman MG, Halstead SB, Artsob H, et al. Dengue: a continuing global threat. Nat Rev Microbiol. 2010;8(12 Suppl):S7–16.
5. Alen MM, De Burghgraeve T, Kaptein SJ, Balzarini J, Neyts J, Schols D. Broad antiviral activity of carbohydrate-binding agents against the four serotypes of dengue virus in monocyte-derived dendritic cells. PLoS One. 2011;6(6):e21658.
6. Simmons CP, Farrar JJ, Nguyen v V, Wills B. Dengue. N Engl J Med. 2012; 366(15):1423–32.
7. Pinheiro FP, Corber SJ. Global situation of dengue and dengue haemorrhagic fever, and its emergence in the Americas. World Health Stat Q. 1997;50(3–4):161–9.
8. Gibbons RV, Vaughn DW. Dengue: an escalating problem. BMJ. 2002; 324(7353):1563–6.
9. Roehrig JT. Antigenic structure of flavivirus proteins. Adv Virus Res. 2003;59: 141–75.

10. Rothman AL. Immunology and immunopathogenesis of dengue disease. Adv Virus Res. 2003;60:397–419.

11. Flipse J, Wilschut J, Smit JM. Molecular mechanisms involved in antibody-dependent enhancement of dengue virus infection in humans. Traffic. 2013; 14(1):25–35.

12. Halstead S. Dengue antibody-dependent enhancement: knowns and unknowns. Microbiol Spec. 2014;2(6). https://doi.org/10.1128/microbiolspec.AID-0022-2014.

13. Jampangern W, Vongthoung K, Jittmittraphap A, et al. Characterization of atypical lymphocytes and immunophenotypes of lymphocytes in patients with dengue virus infection. Asian Pac J Allergy Immunol. 2007;25(1):27–36.

14. Balakrishnan T, Bela-Ong DB, Toh YX, et al. Dengue virus activates polyreactive, natural IgG B cells after primary and secondary infection. PLoS One. 2011;6(12):e29430.

15. Wrammert J, Onlamoon N, Akondy RS, et al. Rapid and massive virus-specific plasmablast responses during acute dengue virus infection in humans. J Virol. 2012;86(6):2911–8.

16. Zompi S, Montoya M, Pohl MO, Balmaseda A, Harris E. Dominant cross-reactive B cell response during secondary acute dengue virus infection in humans. PLoS Negl Trop Dis. 2012;6(3):e1568.

17. Dal Porto JM, Gauld SB, Merrell KT, Mills D, Pugh-Bernard AE, Cambier J. B cell antigen receptor signaling 101. Mol Immunol. 2004;41(6–7):599–613.

18. Sabin AB. Research on dengue during world war II. Am J Trop Med Hyg. 1952;1(1):30–50.

19. Littaua R, Kurane I, Ennis FA. Human IgG fc receptor II mediates antibody-dependent enhancement of dengue virus infection. J Immunol. 1990;144(8): 3183–6.

20. Garcia-Bates TM, Cordeiro MT, Nascimento EJ, et al. Association between magnitude of the virus-specific plasmablast response and disease severity in dengue patients. J Immunol. 2013;190(1):80–7.

21. Velumani S, Toh YX, Balasingam S, et al. Low antibody titers 5 years after vaccination with the CYD-TDV dengue vaccine in both pre-immune and naive vaccinees. Hum Vaccin Immunother. 2016;12(5):1265–73.

22. Correa AR, Berbel AC, Papa MP, Morais AT, Pecanha LM, Arruda LB. Dengue virus directly stimulates polyclonal B cell activation. PLoS One. 2015;10(12): e0143391.

23. Whitehead SS, Blaney JE, Durbin AP, Murphy BR. Prospects for a dengue virus vaccine. Nat Rev Microbiol. 2007;5(7):518–28.

24. Lechner H, Amort M, Steger MM, Maczek C, Grubeck-Loebenstein B. Regulation of CD95 (APO-1) expression and the induction of apoptosis in human T cells: changes in old age. Int Arch Allergy Immunol. 1996;110(3):238–43.

25. Myint KS, Endy TP, Mongkolsirichaikul D, et al. Cellular immune activation in children with acute dengue virus infections is modulated by apoptosis. J Infect Dis. 2006;194(5):600–7.

26. Mongkolsapaya J, Dejnirattisai W, Xu XN, et al. Original antigenic sin and apoptosis in the pathogenesis of dengue hemorrhagic fever. Nat Med. 2003;9(7):921–7.

27. Chen TH, Tang P, Yang CF, et al. Antioxidant defense is one of the mechanisms by which mosquito cells survive dengue 2 viral infection. Virology. 2011;410(2):410–7.

28. Morchang A, Panaampon J, Suttitheptumrong A, et al. Role of cathepsin B in dengue virus-mediated apoptosis. Biochem Biophys Res Commun. 2013; 438(1):20–5.

29. Fink K. Origin and function of circulating plasmablasts during acute viral infections. Front Immunol. 2012;3:78.

30. Radbruch A, Muehlinghaus G, Luger EO, et al. Competence and competition: the challenge of becoming a long-lived plasma cell. Nat Rev Immunol. 2006;6(10):741–50.

31. Homey B, Wang W, Soto H, et al. Cutting edge: the orphan chemokine receptor G protein-coupled receptor-2 (GPR-2, CCR10) binds the skin-associated chemokine CCL27 (CTACK/ALP/ILC). J Immunol. 2000;164(7):3465–70.

32. Egbuniwe IU, Karagiannis SN, Nestle FO, Lacy KE. Revisiting the role of B cells in skin immune surveillance. Trends Immunol. 2015;36(2):102–11.

33. Mora JR, Iwata M, Eksteen B, et al. Generation of gut-homing IgA-secreting B cells by intestinal dendritic cells. Science. 2006;314(5802):1157–60.

34. Brenan M, Rees DJ. Sequence analysis of rat integrin alpha E1 and alpha E2 subunits: tissue expression reveals phenotypic similarities between intraepithelial lymphocytes and dendritic cells in lymph. Eur J Immunol. 1997;27(11):3070–9.

35. Vossenkamper A, Blair PA, Safinia N, et al. A role for gut-associated lymphoid tissue in shaping the human B cell repertoire. J Exp Med. 2013; 210(9):1665–74.

36. Park C, Hwang IY, Sinha RK, Kamenyeva O, Davis MD, Kehrl JH. Lymph node B lymphocyte trafficking is constrained by anatomy and highly dependent upon chemoattractant desensitization. Blood. 2012;119(4):978–89.

37. Kansas GS, Ley K, Munro JM, Tedder TF. Regulation of leukocyte rolling and adhesion to high endothelial venules through the cytoplasmic domain of L-selectin. J Exp Med. 1993;177(3):833–8.

38. Sakthivel P, Grunewald J, Eklund A, Bruder D, Wahlstrom J. Pulmonary sarcoidosis is associated with high-level inducible co-stimulator (ICOS) expression on lung regulatory T cells--possible implications for the ICOS/ICOS-ligand axis in disease course and resolution. Clin Exp Immunol. 2016; 183(2):294–306.

39. Graus-Porta D, Blaess S, Senften M, et al. Beta1-class integrins regulate the development of laminae and folia in the cerebral and cerebellar cortex. Neuron. 2001;31(3):367–79.

40. Eash KJ, Greenbaum AM, Gopalan PK, Link DC. CXCR2 and CXCR4 antagonistically regulate neutrophil trafficking from murine bone marrow. J Clin Invest. 2010;120(7):2423–31.

41. Herndler-Brandstetter D, Landgraf K, Jenewein B, et al. Human bone marrow hosts polyfunctional memory CD4+ and CD8+ T cells with close contact to IL-15-producing cells. J Immunol. 2011;186(12):6965–71.

42. Zhao S, Xing Y, Natkunam Y. Use of CD137 ligand expression in the detection of small B-cell lymphomas involving the bone marrow. Hum Pathol. 2014;45(5):1024–30.

43. Muehlinghaus G, Cigliano L, Huehn S, et al. Regulation of CXCR3 and CXCR4 expression during terminal differentiation of memory B cells into plasma cells. Blood. 2005;105(10):3965–71.

44. Tsou CL, Peters W, Si Y, et al. Critical roles for CCR2 and MCP-3 in monocyte mobilization from bone marrow and recruitment to inflammatory sites. J Clin Invest. 2007;117(4):902–9.

45. Kardava L, Moir S, Wang W, et al. Attenuation of HIV-associated human B cell exhaustion by siRNA downregulation of inhibitory receptors. J Clin Invest. 2011;121(7):2614–24.

46. Moir S, Ho J, Malaspina A, et al. Evidence for HIV-associated B cell exhaustion in a dysfunctional memory B cell compartment in HIV-infected viremic individuals. J Exp Med. 2008;205(8):1797–805.

47. Hargreaves DC, Hyman PL, Lu TT, et al. A coordinated change in chemokine responsiveness guides plasma cell movements. J Exp Med. 2001;194(1):45–56.

48. Feng N, Jaimes MC, Lazarus NH, et al. Redundant role of chemokines CCL25/TECK and CCL28/MEC in IgA+ plasmablast recruitment to the intestinal lamina propria after rotavirus infection. J Immunol. 2006;176(10): 5749–59.

49. Vejchapipat P, Theamboonlers A, Chongsrisawat V, Poovorawan Y. An evidence of intestinal mucosal injury in dengue infection. Southeast Asian J Trop Med Public Health. 2006;37(1):79–82.

50. Watanabe S, Chan KW, Wang J, Rivino L, Lok SM, Vasudevan SG. Dengue virus infection with highly neutralizing levels of cross-reactive antibodies causes acute lethal small intestinal pathology without a high level of viremia in mice. J Virol. 2015;89(11):5847–61.

51. Hauser AE, Debes GF, Arce S, et al. Chemotactic responsiveness toward ligands for CXCR3 and CXCR4 is regulated on plasma blasts during the time course of a memory immune response. J Immunol. 2002;169(3):1277–82.

9

Visceral pain: gut microbiota, a new hope?

Matteo M Pusceddu[*] and Melanie G Gareau[*] (ID)

Abstract

Background: Visceral pain is a complex and heterogeneous disorder, which can range from the mild discomfort of indigestion to the agonizing pain of renal colic. Regulation of visceral pain involves the spinal cord as well as higher order brain structures. Recent findings have linked the microbiota to gastrointestinal disorders characterized by abdominal pain suggesting the ability of microbes to modulate visceral hypersensitivity and nociception to pain.

Main body: In this review we describe the neuroanatomical basis of visceral pain signaling and the existing evidence of its manipulation exerted by the gut microbiota. We included an updated overview of the potential therapeutic effects of dietary intervention, specifically probiotics and prebiotics, in alleviating hypersensitivity to visceral pain stimuli.

Conclusions: The gut microbiota dramatically impacts normal visceral pain sensation and affects the mechanisms mediating visceral nociception. Furthermore, manipulation of the gut microbiota using prebiotics and probiotics plays a potential role in the regulation of visceral pain disorders.

Keywords: Microbiota-gut-brain axis, Microbiome, Visceral pain, Probiotics, Prebiotics, FGID, IBS, Colitis

Background

The increasing burden of visceral pain disorders has generated a growing interest by researchers and clinicians in studying the origins of pain from internal organs. Visceral pain is a complex and heterogeneous disorder which can range from the mild discomfort of indigestion to the agonizing pain of renal colic, typically disproportionately affecting more women than men [5, 10]. The most prevalent forms of visceral pain are categorized as functional gastrointestinal disorders (FGID) such as irritable bowel syndrome (IBS), which exceeds US$ 40 billion in medical costs and affects an estimated 10–15% of the US and European populations [62, 71]. Visceral pain disorders exert a tremendous pressure on the health care system and are associated with psychological distress, sleep disorders and sexual dysfunction, negatively impacting overall patient quality of life [35]. Moreover, both ageing and gender affect the progression of visceral pathology and pain, with IBS reported twice as frequently in women than in men [7].

The mechanisms involved in the perception of gastrointestinal pain and discomfort are complex. Stretch, inflammation, ischemia, pH, bacterial products, immune mediators, and neurotransmitters have all been associated with visceral pain [67]. Nociceptors, expressing transient receptor potential (TRP) at the nerve terminations, sense painful stimuli and project signals onto spinal nociceptive neurons located in the lateral neck of the dorsal horn of the spinal cord, which convey information to supraspinal centers (Fig. 1). Here, the signal reaches several brain areas such as thalamus, hypothalamus, limbic system and cortex, which in concert code the afferent information and generate an efferent signal back to the periphery [9]. Thus, the descending pathways modulate neuronal activity exerting either an inhibitory or a facilitatory effect on the sensation of pain. However, repeated or chronic nociceptors' activation, due to chronic release of inflammatory mediators and pain signals following tissue injury, can lead to sensitization of the receptors and unpredictable bouts of visceral pain [32, 76]. For instance, substance P, serotonin, acetylcholine, prostaglandin 2, histamine, and cytokines are some of the mediators thought to play a role in the regulation of pain stimuli [76]. As alterations in the perception and maintenance of this type of pain involves multiple factors, making it challenging and often unsatisfactory in the choice and the development of adequate treatment options.

* Correspondence: mpusceddu@ucdavis.edu; mgareau@ucdavis.edu
Department of Anatomy, Physiology and Cell Biology, School of Veterinary Medicine, University of California Davis, One Shield Avenue, Davis, CA, USA

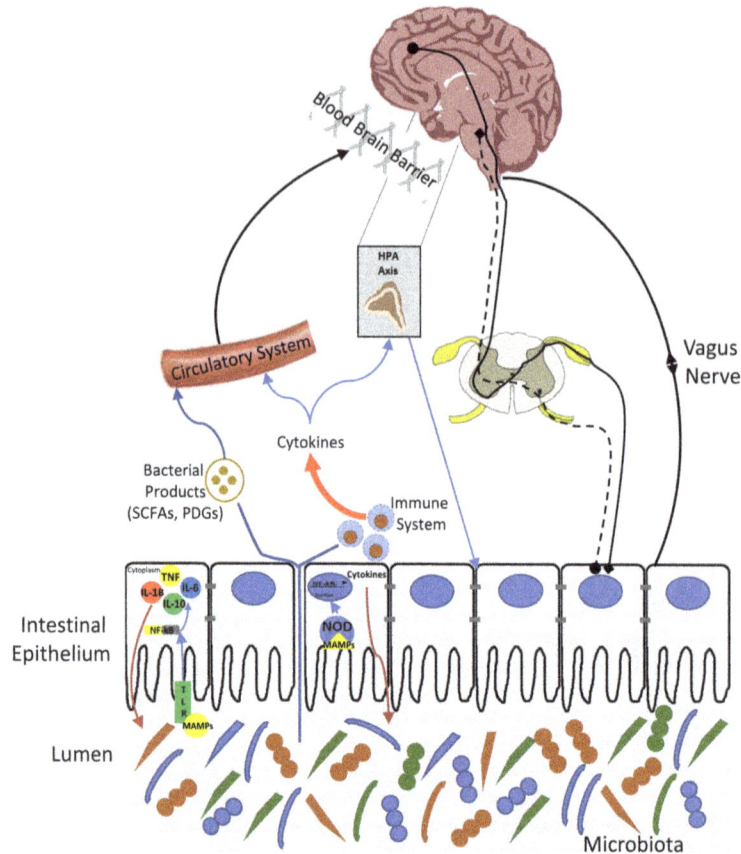

Fig. 1 Gut microbiota-host interaction. Schematic representing the different ways of interaction between the microbiota and host. Painful stimuli sensed by nociceptors expressed at the nerve terminations project signals onto spinal nociceptive neurons located in the lateral neck of the dorsal horn of the spinal cord, which convey information to supraspinal centers. Here, the signal reaches several brain areas such as the thalamus, hypothalamus, limbic system, and cortex, which in concert code the afferent information and generate an efferent signal back to the periphery. The microbiota, which resides in the lumen of the gastrointestinal tract, can influence several factors involved in pain perception and its signaling such as the vagus nerve, cytokine production, corticosterone secretion, short chain fatty acids (SCFAs), and microbial metabolite release

The microbiota has emerged as a novel target for the treatment of visceral pain. A correlation between visceral pain disorders, such as IBS, and microbial dysbiosis has been demonstrated in patients [19, 21]. Further evidence supports the role of bacterial, viral, and parasitic infections in triggering IBS symptoms. A recent systematic review and meta-analysis of 45 studies, comprising 21,421 individuals with enteritis, showed that the development of IBS was increased more than 10% up to at least 12 months post-infection. Moreover, the risk of IBS was found to be 4-fold higher than in individuals who did not have infectious enteritis, although heterogeneity among the studies were found. The increased risk of developing IBS was seen predominantly in women, as well as in individuals treated with antibiotics during the enteritis. [42]. Of interest, the improvement of visceral hypersensitivity through the use of certain beneficial probiotics and prebiotics has been recently proposed [26]. Moreover, significant enthusiasm has been generated following the potential benefits exerted by fecal material transplantation having been observed in patients with visceral pain [37, 59]. Therefore, the role of the intestinal microbiota has emerged as an essential player in the development of future therapeutic approaches for visceral pain.

Gut microbiota development

The gut microbiome comprises more than 1000 species and 7000 strains dominated mainly by bacteria, but also includes viruses, protozoa, archaea and fungi [46]. This ecosystem occupies different niches in the human body, interacting with most, if not all, organs of the host throughout the lifespan. As first proposed by Tissier [73], colonization of the gut was assumed to commence at birth, making the human placenta an excellent sterile compartment for the growing offspring. However, the detection of a shared microbial signature between the placenta, amniotic fluid, and meconium suggests a direct maternal to infant transfer of microbiomes that starts in utero [43]. This maternal imprinting of the infant microbiota is then strengthened by breastfeeding during the first weeks of life giving shape to a much more complex microbiota in the offspring composed mostly by the genera Lactobacillus, Staphylococcus, Enterococcus, and Bifidobacterium [52]. The switch from breast milk to the introduction of solid food makes the microbiome gradually more complex, culminating in a more mature gut microbiota by 3 years of age [57]. Starting in the early stages of life, the microbiome establishes a long evolutionary symbiosis with the host, which influences essentially all organs, systems, as well as their functionality. For instance, the formation of a more mature microbiota early in life coincides with the development of the immune system, suggesting the microbiota is responsible for the priming of the immune system [4, 31].

From the gut, the microbiota can communicate with the central nervous system (CNS) forming a complex crosstalk between the gut, its microbiome, and the brain known as the microbiota-gut-brain (MGB) axis [17]. This bidirectional communication between the gut microbiota and the brain is believed to participate in the regulation of gastrointestinal homeostasis and affect CNS function including mood, cognition, and pain perception. The mechanisms by which the gut microbiota interacts with the host will be discussed thoroughly in this review article.

Gut microbiota and its interaction with the host

The gastrointestinal (GI) tract is the most heavily colonized organ of the human body, which hosts an increasing microbial concentration from 10^1 to 10^3 cells up to 10^{11}–10^{12} cells per gram of fecal contents in the stomach and in the colon, respectively [36]. Here the microbiota is recognized by the host by specific receptors expressed on different cells of the innate immune system, such as macrophages, neutrophils, NK cells, dendritic cells and intestinal epithelial cells. Specifically, microbe- or pathogen-associated molecular patterns (MAMPs or PAMPs), such as lipopolysaccharide (LPS) and peptidoglycans (PGN), are sensed by pattern recognition receptors (PRRs), including Toll-Like receptors (TLRs) and NOD-like receptors which are expressed on the host cell surface or in the cytosolic compartment of numerous cell types including immune cells [51]. The activation of PRRs triggers an enzymatic cascade leading to the synthesis and release of proinflammatory cytokines. In a chronically inflamed host, the integrity of the intestinal mucosal barrier is impaired facilitating bacterial infiltration across the gut and the migration of diverse bacterial antigens from the underlying lamina propria systemically via the blood. Therefore, following inflammation, a combination of cytokines and bacterial products, such as peptidoglycans and LPS, circulate into the blood, reaching several distant organs and systems including the CNS and the blood brain barrier (BBB). Whether cytokines can cross the BBB or not still needs to be clarified. However, evidence reveals that cytokines can influence brain areas and their functionality, suggesting a correlation exists between brain cytokines levels and psychiatric symptoms (including perception of pain), known as cytokine-induced sickness behavior [78]. Moreover, the heightened inflammatory tone induced by a leaky gut is also responsible for the activation of the hypothalamic-pituitary-adrenal (HPA) axis and consequently the release of corticosterone, the most potent stress hormone. This highlights the importance of the microbiota in influencing the neuroendocrine system [15]. Recent evidence indicates PGN can translocate into the brain and be sensed by PRRs within the CNS. [3]. Moreover, microglial control of astrocytes and CNS inflammation can be modulated by metabolites of dietary tryptophan produced by commensal bacteria, suggesting a novel signaling pathway that mediates the communication between the gut microbiota and the brain [65]. Other microbial products, specifically short chain fatty acids (SCFAs), can enter the blood and exert an effect centrally, influencing memory and cognition through epigenetic mechanisms [24, 45]. Furthermore, the microbiota is believed to influence function and metabolism of enteroendocrine cells, inducing the expression of several peptides, such as glucagon-like peptides (GLP) and peptide YY (PYY), which are known to control energy homeostasis, glucose metabolism, gut barrier function, and metabolic inflammation [8]. The microbiota is also capable of regulating the synthesis and release of several neurotransmitters in the GI tract. Microbial dependent-serotonin (5-HT) biosynthesis has emerged as a critical player, due to its implication in colonic function and GI disorders [34, 77]. For instance, lower mucosal 5-HT content, tryptophan hydroxylase (TPH) 1, and serotonin reuptake transporter (SERT) expression levels have been reported in some studies involving IBS patients [13, 25, 38]. Furthermore, exposure to selective serotonin reuptake inhibitor (SSRIs) in some cases have been shown to ameliorate IBS symptoms, such as enhanced orocecal transit and increased colonic motility [11, 72]. Moreover, the antagonism of specific 5-HT receptors abundantly expressed in the gut, such as 5-HT$_3$, has been shown to reduce visceral pain, slow colonic transit, and enhance small intestinal absorption [6]. Despite this evidence, the role of 5-HT signaling in the gut remains confusing and controversial, therefore further research is warranted [48]. In addition to 5-HT, the neurotransmitters γ-aminobutyric acid (GABA), dopamine (DA) and acetylcholine (ACh) are also synthesized in the lumen of the intestine by the microbiota and these neurotransmitters are believed to communicate with the brain via the vagus nerve [47]. It is also believed that the microbiota communicates with the CNS through the enteric nervous system (ENS) via vagal parasympathetic and sympathetic tracts [55]. A schematic representing the pathways of interaction between the microbiota and host is shown in Fig. 1.

Visceral pain: Microbiota & Preclinical Studies

In recent years, preclinical studies have shed light on the role played by the microbiota in visceral pain. Studies using germ free mice (GF; mice raised without any exposure to microorganisms), have shown the commensal microbiota is necessary for development of an adequate pain sensitivity [2], which is blunted in response to several stimuli including bacterial LPS and interleukin (IL)-1β in GF mice [12]. Reestablishment of a normal microbiota through microbial transfer from conventional to GF mice has demonstrated that the microbiota is necessary for the restoration of normal excitability of gut sensory neurons [49]. Of note, fecal transplant from IBS patients reproduced certain features characteristics of IBS in GF mice, including hypersensitivity to colorectal distension, [14]. In another study, GF rats inoculated with the microbiota from patients with IBS developed abnormal gut fermentation mostly characterized by increased H2 excretion and sulfide production, [14] which have been reported in IBS [41, 69]. GF rodents represent a valuable tool for the investigation of visceral pain and related pathologies arising from intestinal dysbiosis.

Probiotics in animal models

As an alternative to a GF state, chronic antibiotic administration is also used as a model to deplete the gut microbiota. Antibiotics can alter the innate mucosal immune system and attenuate visceral pain-related responses provoked by intracolonic capsaicin and intraperitoneal acetic acid administration in mice [1]. However, exposure to antibiotics during early life can also increase visceral sensitivity in adult rats, suggesting that alterations of the microbiota induced in specific time windows of life are crucial to the development of a sensitivity to pain [53].

Probiotics, bacteria that can confer beneficial effects onto the host following consumptionhave demonstrated improvements in animal models of visceral hypersensitivity. Despite these highly interesting findings, the mechanisms involved in mediating these benefits remain unkown [29] (Table 1). Live luminal administration of *Lactobacillus reuteri* (DSM 17938) and its conditioned medium dose-dependently reduced jejunal spinal nerve firing evoked by distension or capsaicin, with 80% of this response blocked by a specific transient receptor potential cation channel subfamily V member 1 (TRPV1) channel antagonist or in TRPV1 knockout mice [58]. *Lactobacillus acidophilus*-mediated analgesic effects function in the gut similarly to the effects of morphine, inducing upregulation of both opioid and cannabinoid receptors in rodents [66]. *Lactobacillus paracasei* administration blunted antibiotic-induced visceral sensitivity to colorectal distension (CRD) and increased substance P levels in the mice colon [74]. Interestingly, exposure to chronic stress has been used as a valuable rodent model of IBS and visceral sensitivity, suggesting the MGB axis serves as an important regulator of visceral pain. For instance, the neonatal maternal

Table 1 Effects of prebiotics and probiotics in preclinical studies

Animals	Treatment	Length of treatment	Outcomes	References
Adult male Swiss Webster	Live luminal *Lactobacillus reuteri* (DSM 17938)	9 days	DSM ↓ capsaicin-evoked (1) firing of spinal nerve action potentials and (2) Ca^{2+} increase in DRG neurons.	[58]
Sprague Dawley rats	*Lactobacillus acidophilus*	15 days	*L. acidophilus* ↑MOR1 and CB2 expression in intestinal epithelial cells restoring normal perception of visceral pain.	[66]
Female NIH Swiss mice and Balb/c mice	*Lactobacillus paracasei* (NCC2461)	10 days	*L. paracasei* ↓antibiotic-induced CRD hypersensitivity and SP immunolabelling in the myenteric plexus.	[74]
Sprague Dawley rats	*Lactobacillus rhamnosus and Lactobacillus helveticus*	15 days	Probiotics ↓ MS-induced CRD hypersensitivity, plasma CORT levels and short-circuit current in the gut.	[27]
Sprague Dawley rats	*Lactobacillus paracasei*	15 days	*L. paracasei* ↓ MS-induced CRD hypersensitivity.	[23]
Wistar rats	VSL#3	60 days	VSL#3 reversed MS-induced CRD hypersensitivity and alterations of i.e. TPH1, CCL2, NOS3, NTRK1, IL-10, TRPV4, gene expression levels.	[18]
C57BL/6 mice	*Lactobacillus rhamnosus and Lactobacillus helveticus*	15 days	Probiotics prevented c. rodentium-induced epithelial cell hyperplasia and reduction in cell proliferation as well as transcription of IL-10 and FOXP3.	[64]

Abbreviations: MOR1 Opioid Receptor Mu, *CB2* Cannabinoid Receptor, *CRD* colorectal distension, *MS* maternal separation, *CORT* corticosterone, *TPH1* Tryptophan hydroxylase, *CCL2* C-C Motif Chemokine Ligand, *NOS3* nitric oxide synthase, *NTRK1* Neurotrophic Receptor Tyrosine Kinase, *IL-10* interleukin, *TRPV4* Transient Receptor Potential Cation Channel Subfamily V Member 4, *FOXP3* Forkhead Box P3

separation (MS) paradigm, which consists of separating murine pups from their mothers for 3 h per day for at least 10 days, induces several alterations related to visceral pain such as hypersensitivity to CRD, increased gut permeability, activation of the immune system, increased hypothalamic pituitary adrenal (HPA) axis activation and altered intestinal microbial composition [28, 54, 60, 70]. In this regard, a specific probiotics cocktail made of *L. helveticus* and *L. rhamnosus* reduced both macromolecular and paracellular permeability in MS [27]. The same probiotics treatment also ameliorated the MS-induced gut functional abnormalities and bacterial adhesion/penetration into the mucosa and blunted the HPA axis response [27]. *L. paracasei* and VSL#3, (composed of *B. longum, B. infantis, B. breve, L. acidophilus, L. casei, L. bulgaricus, L. plantarum*, and *Streptococcus salivarius*), were also able to reverse MS-induced hyperalgesia and allodynia during CRD and restored normal gut permeability [18, 23]. Moreover, VSL#3 was found to modulate the serotonergic system, specifically TPH1 expression levels, which is typically altered in IBS. VSL#3 was also shown to reduce gut permeability through upregulation of specific tight junction proteins (occluding, ZO-1) in a rat model of IBS induced by chronic intracolonic instillation of 4% acetic acid [16]. Similarly, both *L. helveticus* and *L. rhamnosus* administration were shown to restore the function of the intestinal barrier and increased the levels of tight junction proteins in two different animal models of colitis [44, 64].

Visceral pain: Microbiota & Clinical Studies

Intestinal dysbiosis has also been reported in individuals suffering from visceral pain, including IBS patients, making the microbiota itself a novel target for treatment [29, 61]. A reduction in the levels of Bifidobacterium, Lactobacillus [68] as well as alterations in the Firmicutes:Bacteroidetes ratio, which represent the most abundant phylum bacteria found within the human gut microbiome [63], have been identified in IBS patients. VSL#3 treatment has been shown to be effective in five small different randomized control trials (RCT) in IBS patients that fulfilled the Rome II or Rome III criteria. At least 6 weeks of VSL#3 treatment were necessary to observe improvements in symptomatology, such as reduced abdominal pain/discomfort, or improved abdominal bloating/gassiness, when compared to placebo [33, 39, 40, 50, 63]. A larger study involving 362 women with IBS demonstrated efficacy of *B. infantis* in reducing pain, bloating and improving bowel movements after 4 weeks of treatment compared to placebo [75]. Similarly, *L. rhamnosus* [30] and *L. plantarum* [20] both showed amelioration in abdominal pain and bloating together with reduced visceral pain in two different large RCT studies in IBS patients. *Escherichia coli* DSM 17252 has also showed improvements in 298 IBS patients compared to placebo. After 8 weeks of treatment, both abdominal pain and general pain scores were significantly ameliorated in the IBS group provided with probiotics [22]. One study showed beneficial effects of the prebiotic fructoligosaccharides (FOS) in patients affected by minor functional bowel disorders (FBD; Rome II criteria). After 6 weeks of treatment, 105 FBD patients showed reduced incidence and intensity of gastrointestinal symptoms over placebo [56]. Taken together, these studies highlight the potential for beneficial probiotics for the treatment of visceral pain.

The paucity of information coming from the accumulated clinical evidence to date limits our understanding on the efficacy of both prebiotics and probiotics in visceral pain (Table 2). Limitations are mostly due to inconsistencies within the studies, types of probiotics provided, length of the treatment and different types of pain disorders being treated. Nonetheless, the data to date suggests potential benefits exerted by specific probiotics and prebiotics in patients with visceral pain.

Table 2 Effects of prebiotics and probiotics in clinical studies

Participants	Treatment	Length of Trial	Outcomes	References
50 IBS children, Rome II criteria.	*Lactobacillus* GG vs placebo.	6 weeks	LGG ↓ incidence abdominal distention.	[50]
48 IBS patients, Rome II criteria.	VSL#3 vs placebo.	4 and 8 weeks	↓ flatulence and colonic transit.	[39]
30 Rome III FC patients; 30 controls.	VSL#3 vs placebo.	2 weeks	VSL#3 ↑complete spontaneous bowel movements.	[40]
59 IBS children.	VSL#3 vs placebo.	6 weeks	VSL#3 ↓ abdominal pain/discomfort, and bloating/gassiness.	[33]
104 children diagnosed with FAPD, IBS or FD.	*Lactobacillus* GG vs placebo.	4 weeks.	LGG treatment moderately improved abdominal pain.	[30]
105 FBD patients.	sc-FOS vs placebo.	6 weeks	sc-FOS ↓ intensity of digestive disorder symptoms ↑ quality of life, ↑ discomfort scores.	[56]

Abbreviations: FBD Functional Bowel Disorders, FAPD Functional Abdominal Pain Disorders, FD Functional Dyspepsia, sc-FOS short-chain Fructo-oligosaccharides

Conclusions

Increasing evidence strongly indicates that the gut microbiota plays a pivotal role in the regulation of visceral pain. Its association with autonomic and emotional reactions and visceral function makes the gut microbiota an appealing target for novel pharmacological strategies against visceral pain in FGIDs, including IBS. Despite this, whether the microbiota is driving the abnormalities found in visceral pain and related pathologies remains to be resolved. Moreover, our knowledge on the crosstalk between the gut and brain and the mechanisms by which the microbiota could alleviate visceral pain is still in its early infancy. The provocative preclinical evidence on the influence of the microbiota in the regulation of visceral pain seems promising but still need to be confirmed clinically. Even though growing clinical research has found alleviation in the symptomatology of visceral pain after microbial manipulation with both prebiotics and probiotics, many lack power. Further studies with greater numbers of patients showing consistent results are warranted. Finally, whether fecal transplantation could be considered as a viable therapeutic option to modify the microbiota for benefit in visceral pain still needs to be confirmed.

Abbreviations

5-HT: Serotonin; ACh: Acetylcholine; BBB: Blood brain barrier; CNS: Central nervous system; DA: Dopamine; ENS: Enteric nervous system; FBD: Functional bowel disorder; FGID: Functional gastrointestinal disease; GABA: Gamma-Aminobutyric acid; GF: Germ-free; GI: Gastrointestinal; GLP: Glucagon like peptide; HPA: Hypothalamic-pituitary-adrenal axis; IBS: Irritable bowel syndrome; IL: Interleukin; LPS: Lipopolysaccharide; MAMP: Microbial associated molecular pattern; MGB: Microbiota-gut-brain; MS: Maternal separation; PAMP: Pathogen associated molecular pattern; PGN: Peptidoglycan; PRR: Pattern recognition receptor; PYY: Peptide YY; RCT: Randomized control trial; SCFA: Short chain fatty acids; SERT: Serotonin reuptake transporter; SSRI: Serotonin selective reuptake inhibitor; TLR: Toll-like receptor; TPH: Tryptophan hydroxylase; TRP: Transient receptor potential; TRPV1: Transient receptor potential cation channel subfamily V member 1; ZO-1: Zonnula occuldens

Funding

Research was supported by NIH 1R01AT009365–01 (MGG), NIH 5R21MH108154–01 (MGG).

Authors' contributions

MMP & MGG wrote the manuscript. Both authors read and approved the final manuscript.

Competing interests

The authors declare that they have no competing interests.

References

1. Aguilera M, Cerda-Cuellar M, Martinez V. Antibiotic-induced dysbiosis alters host-bacterial interactions and leads to colonic sensory and motor changes in mice. Gut Microbes. 2015;6(1):10–23.

2. Amaral FA, Sachs D, Costa VV, Fagundes CT, Cisalpino D, Cunha TM, Ferreira SH, Cunha FQ, Silva TA, Nicoli JR, Vieira LQ, Souza DG, Teixeira MM. Commensal microbiota is fundamental for the development of inflammatory pain. Proc Natl Acad Sci U S A. 2008;105(6):2193–7.

3. Arentsen T, Qian Y, Gkotzis S, Femenia T, Wang T, Udekwu K, Forssberg H, Diaz Heijtz R. The bacterial peptidoglycan-sensing molecule Pglyrp2 modulates brain development and behavior. Mol Psychiatry. 2017;22(2):257–66.

4. Belkaid Y, Hand TW. Role of the microbiota in immunity and inflammation. Cell. 2014;157(1):121–41.

5. Cain KC, Jarrett ME, Burr RL, Rosen S, Hertig VL, Heitkemper MM. Gender differences in gastrointestinal, psychological, and somatic symptoms in irritable bowel syndrome. Dig Dis Sci. 2009;54(7):1542–9.

6. Camilleri M. Serotonergic modulation of visceral sensation: lower gut. Gut. 2002;51(Suppl 1):i81–6.

7. Canavan C, West J, Card T. The epidemiology of irritable bowel syndrome. Clin Epidemiol. 2014;6:71–80.

8. Cani PD, Everard A, Duparc T. Gut microbiota, enteroendocrine functions and metabolism. Curr Opin Pharmacol. 2013;13(6):935–40.

9. Chang L. Brain responses to visceral and somatic stimuli in irritable bowel syndrome: a central nervous system disorder? Gastroenterol Clin N Am. 2005;34(2):271–9.

10. Chang L, Heitkemper MM. Gender differences in irritable bowel syndrome. Gastroenterology. 2002;123(5):1686–701.

11. Chial HJ, Camilleri M, Burton D, Thomforde G, Olden KW, Stephens D. Selective effects of serotonergic psychoactive agents on gastrointestinal functions in health. Am J Physiol Gastrointest Liver Physiol. 2003;284(1):G130–7.

12. Chichlowski M, Rudolph C. Visceral pain and gastrointestinal microbiome. J Neurogastroenterol Motil. 2015;21(2):172–81.

13. Coates MD, Mahoney CR, Linden DR, Sampson JE, Chen J, Blaszyk H, Crowell MD, Sharkey KA, Gershon MD, Mawe GM, Moses PL. Molecular defects in mucosal serotonin content and decreased serotonin reuptake transporter in ulcerative colitis and irritable bowel syndrome. Gastroenterology. 2004;126(7):1657–64.

14. Crouzet L, Gaultier E, Del'Homme C, Cartier C, Delmas E, Dapoigny M, Fioramonti J, Bernalier-Donadille A. The hypersensitivity to colonic distension of IBS patients can be transferred to rats through their fecal microbiota. Neurogastroenterol Motil. 2013;25(4):e272–82.

15. Cussotto S, Sandhu KV, Dinan TG, Cryan JF. The neuroendocrinology of the microbiota-gut-brain Axis: a Behavioural perspective. Front Neuroendocrinol. 2018;51:80–101.

16. Dai C, Guandalini S, Zhao DH, Jiang M. Antinociceptive effect of VSL#3 on visceral hypersensitivity in a rat model of irritable bowel syndrome: a possible action through nitric oxide pathway and enhance barrier function. Mol Cell Biochem. 2012;362(1–2):43–53.

17. Dinan TG, Cryan JF. Gut-brain axis in 2016: brain-gut-microbiota axis - mood, metabolism and behaviour. Nat Rev Gastroenterol Hepatol. 2017;14(2):69–70.

18. Distrutti E, Cipriani S, Mencarelli A, Renga B, Fiorucci S. Probiotics VSL#3 protect against development of visceral pain in murine model of irritable bowel syndrome. PLoS One. 2013;8(5):e63893.

19. Distrutti E, Monaldi L, Ricci P, Fiorucci S. Gut microbiota role in irritable bowel syndrome: new therapeutic strategies. World J Gastroenterol. 2016;22(7):2219–41.

20. Ducrotte P, Sawant P, Jayanthi V. Clinical trial: lactobacillus plantarum 299v (DSM 9843) improves symptoms of irritable bowel syndrome. World J Gastroenterol. 2012;18(30):4012–8.

21. Dupont HL. Review article: evidence for the role of gut microbiota in irritable bowel syndrome and its potential influence on therapeutic targets. Aliment Pharmacol Ther. 2014;39(10):1033–42.

22. Enck P, Zimmermann K, Menke G, Klosterhalfen S. Randomized controlled treatment trial of irritable bowel syndrome with a probiotic E.-coli preparation (DSM17252) compared to placebo. Zeitschrift fur Gastroenterologie. 2014;52(1):64.

23. Eutamene H, Lamine F, Chabo C, Theodorou V, Rochat F, Bergonzelli GE, Corthesy-Theulaz I, Fioramonti J, Bueno L. Synergy between lactobacillus paracasei and its bacterial products to counteract stress-induced gut permeability and sensitivity increase in rats. J Nutr. 2007;137(8):1901–7.

24. Ferrante RJ, Kubilus JK, Lee J, Ryu H, Beesen A, Zucker B, Smith K, Kowall NW, Ratan RR, Luthi-Carter R, Hersch SM. Histone deacetylase inhibition by

sodium butyrate chemotherapy ameliorates the neurodegenerative phenotype in Huntington's disease mice. J Neurosci. 2003;23(28):9418–27.

25. Foley S, Garsed K, Singh G, Duroudier NP, Swan C, Hall IP, Zaitoun A, Bennett A, Marsden C, Holmes G, Walls A, Spiller RC. Impaired uptake of serotonin by platelets from patients with irritable bowel syndrome correlates with duodenal immune activation. Gastroenterology. 2011;140(5): 1434–1443 e1431.

26. Ford AC, Quigley EM, Lacy BE, Lembo AJ, Saito YA, Schiller LR, Soffer EE, Spiegel BM, Moayyedi P. Efficacy of prebiotics, probiotics, and synbiotics in irritable bowel syndrome and chronic idiopathic constipation: systematic review and meta-analysis. Am J Gastroenterol. 2014;109(10):1547–61 quiz 1546, 1562.

27. Gareau MG, Jury J, MacQueen G, Sherman PM, Perdue MH. Probiotic treatment of rat pups normalises corticosterone release and ameliorates colonic dysfunction induced by maternal separation. Gut. 2007;56(11): 1522–8.

28. Gareau MG, Jury J, Yang PC, MacQueen G, Perdue MH. Neonatal maternal separation causes colonic dysfunction in rat pups including impaired host resistance. Pediatr Res. 2006;59(1):83–8.

29. Gareau MG, Sherman PM, Walker WA. Probiotics and the gut microbiota in intestinal health and disease. Nat Rev Gastroenterol Hepatol. 2010; 7(9):503–14.

30. Gawronska A, Dziechciarz P, Horvath A, Szajewska H. A randomized double-blind placebo-controlled trial of lactobacillus GG for abdominal pain disorders in children. Aliment Pharmacol Ther. 2007;25(2):177–84.

31. Gensollen T, Iyer SS, Kasper DL, Blumberg RS. How colonization by microbiota in early life shapes the immune system. Science. 2016;352(6285): 539–44.

32. Greenwood-Van Meerveld B, Johnson AC. Stress-induced chronic visceral pain of gastrointestinal origin. Front Syst Neurosci. 2017;11:86.

33. Guandalini S, Magazzu G, Chiaro A, La Balestra V, Di Nardo G, Gopalan S, Sibal A, Romano C, Canani RB, Lionetti P, Setty M. VSL#3 improves symptoms in children with irritable bowel syndrome: a multicenter, randomized, placebo-controlled, double-blind, crossover study. J Pediatr Gastroenterol Nutr. 2010;51(1):24–30.

34. Hata T, Asano Y, Yoshihara K, Kimura-Todani T, Miyata N, Zhang XT, Takakura S, Aiba Y, Koga Y, Sudo N. Regulation of gut luminal serotonin by commensal microbiota in mice. PLoS One. 2017;12(7):e0180745.

35. Hungin AP, Whorwell PJ, Tack J, Mearin F. The prevalence, patterns and impact of irritable bowel syndrome: an international survey of 40,000 subjects. Aliment Pharmacol Ther. 2003;17(5):643–50.

36. Hyland NP, Cryan JF. Microbe-host interactions: influence of the gut microbiota on the enteric nervous system. Dev Biol. 2016;417(2):182–7.

37. Johnsen PH, Hilpusch F, Cavanagh JP, Leikanger IS, Kolstad C, Valle PC, Goll R. Faecal microbiota transplantation versus placebo for moderate-to-severe irritable bowel syndrome: a double-blind, randomised, placebo-controlled, parallel-group, single-Centre trial. Lancet Gastroenterol Hepatol. 2018;3(1): 17–24.

38. Kerckhoffs AP, ter Linde JJ, Akkermans LM, Samsom M. SERT and TPH-1 mRNA expression are reduced in irritable bowel syndrome patients regardless of visceral sensitivity state in large intestine. Am J Physiol Gastrointest Liver Physiol. 2012;302(9):G1053–60.

39. Kim HJ, Vazquez Roque MI, Camilleri M, Stephens D, Burton DD, Baxter K, Thomforde G, Zinsmeister AR. A randomized controlled trial of a probiotic combination VSL# 3 and placebo in irritable bowel syndrome with bloating. Neurogastroenterol Motil. 2005;17(5):687–96.

40. Kim SE, Choi SC, Park KS, Park MI, Shin JE, Lee TH, Jung KW, Koo HS, Myung SJ. Constipation research group of Korean Society of N. and motility. Change of fecal Flora and Effectiveness of the short-term VSL#3 probiotic treatment in patients with functional constipation. J Neurogastroenterol Motil. 2015;21(1):111–20.

41. King TS, Elia M, Hunter JO. Abnormal colonic fermentation in irritable bowel syndrome. Lancet. 1998;352(9135):1187–9.

42. Klem F, Wadhwa A, Prokop LJ, Sundt WJ, Farrugia G, Camilleri M, Singh S, Grover M. Prevalence, risk factors, and outcomes of irritable bowel syndrome after infectious enteritis: a systematic review and meta-analysis. Gastroenterology. 2017;152(5):1042–1054 e1041.

43. Kundu P, Blacher E, Elinav E, Pettersson S. Our gut microbiome: the evolving inner self. Cell. 2017;171(7):1481–93.

44. Laval L, Martin R, Natividad JN, Chain F, Miquel S, Desclee de Maredsous C, Capronnier S, Sokol H, Verdu EF, van Hylckama Vlieg JE, Bermudez-Humaran

LG, Smokvina T, Langella P. Lactobacillus rhamnosus CNCM I-3690 and the commensal bacterium Faecalibacterium prausnitzii A2-165 exhibit similar protective effects to induced barrier hyper-permeability in mice. Gut Microbes. 2015;6(1):1–9.

45. Levenson JM, O'Riordan KJ, Brown KD, Trinh MA, Molfese DL, Sweatt JD. Regulation of histone acetylation during memory formation in the hippocampus. J Biol Chem. 2004;279(39):40545–59.

46. Lloyd-Price J, Abu-Ali G, Huttenhower C. The healthy human microbiome. Genome Med. 2016;8(1):51.

47. Lyte M. Microbial endocrinology and the microbiota-gut-brain axis. Adv Exp Med Biol. 2014;817:3–24.

48. Mawe GM, Hoffman JM. Serotonin signalling in the gut--functions, dysfunctions and therapeutic targets. Nat Rev Gastroenterol Hepatol. 2013; 10(8):473–86.

49. McVey Neufeld KA, Mao YK, Bienenstock J, Foster JA, Kunze WA. The microbiome is essential for normal gut intrinsic primary afferent neuron excitability in the mouse. Neurogastroenterol Motil. 2013;25(2):183–e188.

50. Michail S, Kenche H. Gut microbiota is not modified by randomized, double-blind, placebo-controlled trial of VSL#3 in diarrhea-predominant irritable bowel syndrome. Probiotics Antimicrob Proteins. 2011;3(1):1–7.

51. Mogensen TH. Pathogen recognition and inflammatory signaling in innate immune defenses. Clin Microbiol Rev. 2009;22(2):240–73 Table of Contents.

52. Moles L, Gomez M, Heilig H, Bustos G, Fuentes S, de Vos W, Fernandez L, Rodriguez JM, Jimenez E. Bacterial diversity in meconium of preterm neonates and evolution of their fecal microbiota during the first month of life. PLoS One. 2013;8(6):e66986.

53. O'Mahony SM, Felice VD, Nally K, Savignac HM, Claesson MJ, Scully P, Woznicki J, Hyland NP, Shanahan F, Quigley EM, Marchesi JR, O'Toole PW, Dinan TG, Cryan JF. Disturbance of the gut microbiota in early-life selectively affects visceral pain in adulthood without impacting cognitive or anxiety-related behaviors in male rats. Neuroscience. 2014;277:885–901.

54. O'Mahony SM, Hyland NP, Dinan TG, Cryan JF. Maternal separation as a model of brain-gut axis dysfunction. Psychopharmacology. 2011;214(1):71–88.

55. Obata Y, Pachnis V. The effect of microbiota and the immune system on the development and Organization of the Enteric Nervous System. Gastroenterology. 2016;151(5):836–44.

56. Paineau D, Payen F, Panserieu S, Coulombier G, Sobaszek A, Lartigau I, Brabet M, Galmiche JP, Tripodi D, Sacher-Huvelin S, Chapalain V, Zourabichvili O, Respondek F, Wagner A, Bornet FR. The effects of regular consumption of short-chain fructo-oligosaccharides on digestive comfort of subjects with minor functional bowel disorders. Br J Nutr. 2008;99(2):311–8.

57. Palmer C, Bik EM, DiGiulio DB, Relman DA, Brown PO. Development of the human infant intestinal microbiota. PLoS Biol. 2007;5(7):e177.

58. Perez-Burgos A, Wang L, McVey Neufeld KA, Mao YK, Ahmadzai M, Janssen LJ, Stanisz AM, Bienenstock J, Kunze WA. The TRPV1 channel in rodents is a major target for antinociceptive effect of the probiotic lactobacillus reuteri DSM 17938. J Physiol. 2015;593(17):3943–57.

59. Pinn DM, Aroniadis OC, Brandt LJ. Is fecal microbiota transplantation the answer for irritable bowel syndrome? A single-center experience. Am J Gastroenterol. 2014;109(11):1831–2.

60. Pusceddu MM, El Aidy S, Crispie F, O'Sullivan O, Cotter P, Stanton C, Kelly P, Cryan JF, Dinan TG. N-3 polyunsaturated fatty acids (PUFAs) reverse the impact of early-life stress on the gut microbiota. PLoS One. 2015;10(10): e0139721.

61. Pusceddu MM, Murray K, Gareau MG. Targeting the microbiota, from irritable bowel syndrome to mood disorders: focus on probiotics and prebiotics. Curr Pathobiol Rep. 2018;6(1):1–13.

62. Quigley EM, Bytzer P, Jones R, Mearin F. Irritable bowel syndrome: the burden and unmet needs in Europe. Dig Liver Dis. 2006;38(10):717–23.

63. Rajilic-Stojanovic M, Biagi E, Heilig HG, Kajander K, Kekkonen RA, Tims S, de Vos WM. Global and deep molecular analysis of microbiota signatures in fecal samples from patients with irritable bowel syndrome. Gastroenterology. 2011;141(5):1792–801.

64. Rodrigues DM, Sousa AJ, Johnson-Henry KC, Sherman PM, Gareau MG. Probiotics are effective for the prevention and treatment of Citrobacter rodentium-induced colitis in mice. J Infect Dis. 2012;206(1):99–109.

65. Rothhammer V, Borucki DM, Tjon EC, Takenaka MC, Chao C-C, Ardura-Fabregat A, de Lima KA, Gutiérrez-Vázquez C, Hewson P, Staszewski O, Blain M, Healy L, Neziraj T, Borio M, Wheeler M, Dragin LL, Laplaud DA, Antel J, Alvarez JI, Prinz M, Quintana FJ. Microglial control of astrocytes in response to microbial metabolites. Nature. 2018;557(7707):724–8.

66. Rousseaux C, Thuru X, Gelot A, Barnich N, Neut C, Dubuquoy L, Dubuquoy C, Merour E, Geboes K, Chamaillard M, Ouwehand A, Leyer G, Carcano D, Colombel JF, Ardid D, Desreumaux P. Lactobacillus acidophilus modulates intestinal pain and induces opioid and cannabinoid receptors. Nat Med. 2007;13(1):35–7.

67. Sengupta JN. Visceral pain: the neurophysiological mechanism. Handb Exp Pharmacol. 2009;194:31–74.

68. Si JM, Yu YC, Fan YJ, Chen SJ. Intestinal microecology and quality of life in irritable bowel syndrome patients. World J Gastroenterol. 2004;10(12):1802–5.

69. SM OM, Dinan TG, Cryan JF. The gut microbiota as a key regulator of visceral pain. Pain. 2017;158(Suppl 1):S19–28.

70. Soderholm JD, Yates DA, Gareau MG, Yang PC, MacQueen G, Perdue MH. Neonatal maternal separation predisposes adult rats to colonic barrier dysfunction in response to mild stress. Am J Physiol Gastrointest Liver Physiol. 2002;283(6):G1257–63.

71. Soubieres A, Wilson P, Poullis A, Wilkins J, Rance M. Burden of irritable bowel syndrome in an increasingly cost-aware National Health Service. Frontline Gastroenterol. 2015;6(4):246–51.

72. Tack J, Broekaert D, Corsetti M, Fischler B, Janssens J. Influence of acute serotonin reuptake inhibition on colonic sensorimotor function in man. Aliment Pharmacol Ther. 2006;23(2):265–74.

73. Tissier H. Recherches sur la flore intestinale des nourrissons (état normal et pathologique), Méd.--Paris, 1900.

74. Verdu EF, Bercik P, Verma-Gandhu M, Huang XX, Blennerhassett P, Jackson W, Mao Y, Wang L, Rochat F, Collins SM. Specific probiotic therapy attenuates antibiotic induced visceral hypersensitivity in mice. Gut. 2006; 55(2):182–90.

75. Whorwell PJ, Altringer L, Morel J, Bond Y, Charbonneau D, O'Mahony L, Kiely B, Shanahan F, Quigley EM. Efficacy of an encapsulated probiotic Bifidobacterium infantis 35624 in women with irritable bowel syndrome. Am J Gastroenterol. 2006;101(7):1581–90.

76. Widgerow AD, Kalaria S. Pain mediators and wound healing--establishing the connection. Burns. 2012;38(7):951–9.

77. Yano JM, Yu K, Donaldson GP, Shastri GG, Ann P, Ma L, Nagler CR, Ismagilov RF, Mazmanian SK, Hsiao EY. Indigenous bacteria from the gut microbiota regulate host serotonin biosynthesis. Cell. 2015;161(2):264–76.

78. Yarlagadda A, Alfson E, Clayton AH. The blood brain barrier and the role of cytokines in neuropsychiatry. Psychiatry (Edgmont). 2009;6(11):18–22.

10

The human C-type lectin 18 is a potential biomarker in patients with chronic hepatitis B virus infection

Tsung-Yu Tsai[1,2], Cheng-Yuan Peng[2,3], Hwai-I Yang[4], Ya-Lang Huang[4], Mi-Hua Tao[5], Shin-Sheng Yuan[6], Hsueh-Chou Lai[2] and Shie-Liang Hsieh[4,7,8*] (iD)

Abstract

Background: Hepatitis B virus (HBV) infection is a common disease worldwide and is known to cause liver disease. C-type lectin 18 (CLEC18) is a novel secretory lectin highly expressed in human hepatocytes. Because the liver is the major target of HBV infection, we investigated whether the expression of CLEC18 can be used as a biomarker for HBV infection.

Methods: The expression level of CLEC18 in human liver chimeric mice with/without HBV infection was measured by quantitative real time polymerase chain reaction (qPCR) assay. Baseline plasma CLEC18 levels in 271 treatment-naive patients with chronic hepatitis B (CHB) undergoing nucleos(t)ide analogue (NUC) therapy and 35 healthy donors were measured by enzyme-linked immunosorbent assay, and the relationships to other clinical data were analyzed.

Results: The expression of CLEC18 was down-regulated in the human liver chimeric mice after HBV infection. Plasma CLEC18 levels were lower in the patients with CHB compared to the healthy donors and positively correlated with HBV DNA and HBsAg levels ($P < 0.05$). Multivariate Cox proportional hazard regression analysis identified a baseline plasma CLEC18 level of 320–2000 pg/mL to be an independent predictor of HBeAg loss (hazard ratio (HR): 2.077, $P = 0.0318$), seroconversion (HR: 2.041, $P = 0.0445$) and virological response (HR: 1.850, $P = 0.0184$) in 101 HBeAg-positive patients with CHB undergoing NUC therapy.

Conclusions: Plasma CLEC18 levels were correlated with the stage of HBV infection and could predict HBeAg loss and seroconversion in the patients with CHB undergoing NUC therapy.

Keywords: Hepatitis B virus, C-type lectin 18, HBeAg seroconversion

Background

Hepatitis B virus (HBV) infection is a global health problem. Current treatment options for hepatitis B e antigen (HBeAg)-positive HBV-infected patients include interferon therapy and nucleos(t)ide analogues (NUCs). HBeAg loss and seroconversion are defined as an intermediate therapeutic endpoint in HBeAg-positive patients [1, 2]. Evaluating the treatment outcome, the status of liver fibrosis is important for patients with chronic hepatitis B (CHB). Clinically, a decline in HBV DNA levels during treatment and high serum alanine aminotransferase (ALT) level can predict HBeAg loss and HBeAg seroconversion [3]. A liver biopsy is the gold standard method to assess the stage of liver fibrosis, although it has the disadvantage of a high complication rate. Noninvasive methods using biomarkers such as hepatitis B surface antigen (HBsAg), serum ALT levels [4], and scoring systems such as fibrosis-4 (FIB-4) and aspartate aminotransferase (AST) to platelet ratio index (APRI) have also been proposed [5, 6]. However, these methods have limitations as independent disease markers [7, 8]. In addition, other immune markers such as tumor necrosis factor-alpha (TNF-α), programmed cell death protein-1 (PD-1) [9] and serum markers such as apolipoprotein and haptoglobulin are not specific for HBV disease and

* Correspondence: edmond158162@gmail.com
[4]Genomics Research Center, Academia Sinica, 128, Academia Road, Sec. 2, Nankang District, Taipei 115, Taiwan
[7]Institute of Clinical Medicine, National Yang-Ming University, Taipei, Taiwan
Full list of author information is available at the end of the article

can easily be influenced by other diseases [8]. Biomarkers to assess the treatment outcome of HBV infection and liver fibrosis are still under development.

C-type lectin 18 (CLEC18) is a novel secretory C-type lectin, and we previously showed that CLEC18 is highly expressed in the liver. It is localized in the endoplasmic reticulum, Golgi apparatus, and endosomes, and it can be detected in human plasma by enzyme-linked immunosorbent assay (ELISA). CLEC18 is secreted into the culture supernatant of innate immune cells such as monocytes, dendritic cells and macrophages, which suggests that it is related to the function of the innate immune system [10].

HBV can weaken the host immune response without inducing a pattern recognition receptor (PRR)-mediated cytokine response [11, 12]. The mechanisms by which HBV attenuates Toll-like receptor (TLR)-mediated cytokine responses have been investigated [13], however an association between CLEC18 and HBV infection has yet to be elucidated.

The liver is the major target of HBV infection, and CLEC18 is highly expressed in the liver. Therefore, we hypothesized that the expression of CLEC18 would be influenced by HBV infection. The aim of this study was to investigate the expression of CLEC18 in the liver and its potential role as a biomarker for HBV infection.

Methods

Infection of human liver chimeric mice with HBV

Human liver chimeric mice were generated from Fah −/−/Rag2−/−/Il2rg−/− mice (FRG mice) with transplanted human hepatocytes (kindly provided by Dr. Mi-Hua Tao) [14–16]. Each human liver chimeric mouse was infected with HBV, produced by HBV transgenic mice using the hydrodynamic vein injection method as described previously [14]. In brief, 6-week-old FRG mice were intrasplenically transplanted with human hepatocytes (BD Biosciences, USA). HBV obtained from ICR/HBV transgenic mice was hydrodynamically injected into the FRG mice after 3–4 months of transplantation, as previously described [17]. The mice were then sacrificed at 10 and 26 weeks after HBV infection, and liver samples were collected for analysis.

CLEC18 detection in the human liver chimeric mice with/without HBV infection

Total ribonucleic acid (RNA) was extracted from liver tissues using Trizol according to the manufacturer's instructions (Invitrogen, USA). The RNA was subjected to reverse transcription using a RevertAid™ First Strand complementary DNA (cDNA) Synthesis Kit (Fermentas), and was then used as the template for polymerase chain reaction (PCR) amplification. CLEC18 cDNA levels in the liver tissue were quantified by real-time PCR using

hybridization probes (Roche Life Science, CH) with a thermocycler (LightCycler480°II, Roche, CH) as previously described [13].

Patients

We enrolled 271 treatment-naïve patients with CHB (101 positive and 170 negative for HBeAg) who received NUC treatment with indications according to the guidelines of the Asian Pacific Association for the Study of the Liver (APASL) at the Hepatology Clinic of China Medical University Hospital in Taichung, Taiwan from August 2005 to August 2016 [2]. The inclusion criteria were age ≥ 20 years and a history of HBsAg carriage for more than 6 months. The exclusion criteria were coinfection caused by other etiologies such as hepatitis C virus, hepatitis D virus, or human immunodeficiency virus; decompensated liver disease; other forms of liver disease; hepatocellular carcinoma at baseline; coexisting severe medical diseases or cancer; and the concurrent use of immunomodulatory drugs or corticosteroids. Among the 101 HBeAg-positive patients, 80 received entecavir, 17 received tenofovir, three received telbivudine, and one received lamivudine. Of these patients, 56 achieved HBeAg loss and 36 achieved HBeAg seroconversion. All of these patients received NUC therapy until the end of the follow-up period of this study, and none experienced viral resistance. Plasma was stored in − 80 ° C refrigerators. We also enrolled 35 healthy donors who volunteered for blood donation (17 men and 18 women, 14 aged > 40 years and 21 aged < 40 years). Healthy donors were defined as those who did not have any chronic diseases or cancer and had normal annual health examination reports, including ALT.

Laboratory examinations

Baseline plasma CLEC18 levels were measured retrospectively using our inhouse ELISA (being licensed to Biolegend) and ELISA from CUSABIO Life Science. We tested both ELISA kits with recombinant proteins and healthy donor sera. Both ELISA kits had a lower limit of detection of 0.078 ng/mL and correlated with each other well. Platelets, prothrombin time (PT), and serum levels of albumin, total bilirubin, creatinine, alpha-fetoprotein (AFP), ALT and serum HBV DNA were measured at baseline. HBeAg and anti-HBe antibodies (Architect i2000 assay; Abbott Diagnostics, Abbott Park, IL, USA) were detected before treatment in order to categorize the patients as being HBeAg positive or negative. HBeAg and anti-HBe antibodies were detected at baseline and every 3 months during treatment in the HBeAg-positive group. HBsAg levels were quantified retrospectively in the patients enrolled before September 2009 and prospectively in those enrolled thereafter using Abbott Architect HBsAg QT assays (dynamic range, 0.05–250 IU/mL) at baseline and annually thereafter. Serum HBV DNA levels were measured at baseline, 3, 6, and 12 months; and then every 6 months thereafter.. HBV genotyping was performed as previously described [18]. Liver fibrosis (F) was staged according to the METAVIR system [19]. Cirrhosis was defined by one of the following: 1) presence of cirrhosis-related complications such as ascites and esophageal or gastric varices; 2) ultrasonographic evidence of a nodular surface and coarse echotexture of the liver with ascites and/or splenomegaly; and 3) histology. Fatty liver was defined on the basis of repeated ultrasonographic findings with increased echogenicity in the liver. Liver biopsies in these patients were performed before NUC therapy.

Definition of cutoff values

We stratified the patients into three subgroups according to the values close to the cutoff values of baseline plasma CLEC18 (319.52 and 2015.08 pg/mL, risk estimate: 0.297) and HBsAg levels (2889.3–12,022.2 IU/mL, risk estimate: 0.366) which were associated with the highest rates of HBeAg loss in the patients with CHB receiving NUC therapy using classification and regression tree (CART) analysis (see Additional File 1). We defined the cutoff for age (40 years) and HBV DNA (8.3 $\log_{10}$ IU/mL) as the median of the 101 patients, and the cutoff for ALT (5× upper limit of normal (ULN)) according to a previous study [20]. The cutoff values for total bilirubin, PT, platelet, and AFP were based on normal values, and those for APRI and FIB-4 were based on previous reports [8, 9, 21].

Therapeutic endpoints

HBeAg loss was defined as the absence of serum HBeAg during NUC treatment, and HBeAg seroconversion was defined as HBeAg loss with the presence of anti-HBe antibodies. Virological response was defined as undetectable serum HBV DNA.

Statistical analysis

Continuous variables were compared between two groups using the Student's t-test (T), labeled as "T" in Table 1, and presented as the mean ± standard deviation (SD). Categorical variables were analyzed using the chi-squared test, labeled as "C" in Table 1. Linear regression analysis was used to identify factors associated with CLEC18 expression. Cox proportional hazard regression analysis was used to identify factors associated with HBeAg loss, seroconversion, and virological response. Logistic regression analysis was used to identify factors associated with liver pathological fibrosis stage. Kaplan-Meier analysis and the log-rank test were used to compare the cumulative incidence rates of HBeAg loss and seroconversion in subgroups of patients with

CHB. SAS version 9.4 (SAS Institute, Inc., Cary, NC, USA) and SPSS (IBM Corp. Released 2013, IBM SPSS Statistics for Windows, Version 22.0. Armonk, NY, USA) were used for statistical analyses. A two-sided P value of < 0.05 was considered to be statistically significant.

Results

Down-regulation of the expression of CLEC18 in the liver

The relative mRNA expression levels of human CLEC18 were dramatically down-regulated in the liver tissues of HBV-infected human liver chimeric mice at 10 and 26 weeks after infection compared to the non-infected controls. Mouse CLEC18 was not detected, indicating that the liver tissue collected was only human (Fig. 1). This finding suggested that HBV down-regulated the expression of CLEC18 in human hepatocytes.

Baseline patient characteristics

The baseline patient characteristics are presented in Table 1. In brief, the HBeAg-positive patients were significantly younger and had lower prevalence rates of genotype B infection and cirrhosis, a higher platelet count, and higher levels of ALT, HBV DNA, and HBsAg than the HBeAg-negative patients.

Decreased plasma CLEC18 levels in the patients with CHB

In order to understand the role of CLEC18 in different stages of CHB, we divided the patients with CHB into four groups according to the presence of HBeAg and HBV DNA levels. The mean plasma CLEC18 levels were 3106, 663, 281, 264, and 113 pg/mL in the healthy donors ($n = 35$), treatment-naïve HBeAg-positive CHB patients with HBV DNA > 2.0×10^7 IU/mL ($n = 101$), HBeAg-negative CHB patients with HBV DNA > 2.0×10^7 IU/mL ($n = 65$), DNA 2000–2.0×10^7 IU/mL ($n = 64$), and DNA < 2000 IU/mL ($n = 41$), respectively. The plasma CLEC18 level was significantly lower in each HBV-infected group compared to the healthy donors and in the HBeAg-negative group compared to HBeAg-positive group ($P < 0.05$–0.001) (Table 2). There were no significant changes in plasma CLEC18 levels with different viral loads in the HBeAg-negative patients.

Factors associated with plasma CLEC18 levels in the patients with CHB

We used univariate and multivariate linear regression analyses to identify factors associated with plasma CLEC18 levels in the patients with CHB (Table 3). Univariate analysis revealed that age was negatively associated with plasma CLEC18 levels, and that HBeAg positivity, HBsAg, HBV DNA, and ALT levels were positively associated with plasma CLEC18 levels. Multivariate analysis identified age to be a marginal independent factor associated with plasma CLEC18 levels.

Table 1 Baseline patient characteristics

Variables Mean ± SD or N (%)	Total (n = 271)	HBeAg-negative (n = 170)	HBeAg-positive (n = 101)	P Value
Age	47.39 ± 11.35	51.57 ± 10.45	40.37 ± 10.44	< 0.0001^T
Gender				0.6454^C
Man	187 (69.0)	119 (70.0)	68 (67.33)	
Woman	84 (31.0)	51 (30.0)	33 (32.67)	
Genotype				0.0003^C
B	166 (62.88)	118 (71.08)	48 (48.98)	
C	98 (37.12)	48 (28.92)	50 (51.02)	
HBsAg: $\log_{10}$ IU/mL	3.34 ± 0.84	3.04 ± 0.89	3.85 ± 0.66	< 0.0001^T
HBV DNA: $\log_{10}$ IU/mL	6.89 ± 2.16	5.91 ± 1.84	8.56 ± 0.93	< 0.0001^T
Cirrhosis				0.0028^C
No	182 (67.16)	103 (60.59)	79 (78.22)	
Yes	89 (32.84)	67 (39.41)	22 (21.78)	
Fatty liver				0.2510^C
No	133 (49.08)	88 (51.76)	45 (44.55)	
Yes	138 (50.92)	82 (48.42)	56 (55.45)	
Albumin: g/dL	4.07 ± 0.51	4.04 ± 0.54	4.10 ± 0.48	0.5446^T
ALT: IU/L	281.5 ± 411.2	210.8 ± 333.2	400.5 ± 472.3	0.0002^T
Total bilirubin: mg/dL	1.40 ± 1.34	1.32 ± 0.95	1.54 ± 1.54	0.7096^T
Platelet: × 10^3/μL	161.0 ± 60.73	149.4 ± 65.8	180.8 ± 58.1	0.0004^T
PT: seconds prolonged	1.71 ± 2.00	1.69 ± 1.73	1.86 ± 1.91	0.3551^T
Cr: mg/dL	0.88 ± 0.49	0.90 ± 0.61	0.86 ± 0.40	0.2857^T
AFP: ng/mL	25.31 ± 75.62	21.24 ± 44.57	32.17 ± 89.88	0.4094^T
Numbers of liver biopsy	164	105	59	
METAVIR Activity grade				0.5302^C
0,1	97 (59.15)	64 (60.95)	33 (55.93)	
2,3	67 (40.85)	41 (39.05)	26 (44.07)	
METAVIR Fibrosis stage				0.0949^C
0–2	91 (57.59)	52 (52.53)	39 (66.10)	
3,4	67 (42.41)	47 (47.47)	20 (33.90)	

T Student's T-test, *C* Chi-squared test

Role of plasma CLEC18 in the prediction of HBeAg loss and seroconversion in the patients with CHB receiving NUC treatment

The overall NUC treatment duration was 59.51 ± 3.21 months for the HBeAg-positive patients. The times to HBeAg loss and seroconversion were 37.69 ± 2.86 months and 45.61 ± 3.26 months, respectively. Among the 101 HBeAg-positive patients, 56 (55.44%) patients experienced HBeAg loss and 36 (35.64%) patients experienced HBeAg seroconversion during NUC treatment.

Univariate analysis identified that baseline ALT level > 5× ULN, AFP > 20 ng/mL, HBsAg level of 2900–12,000 IU/mL, and plasma CLEC18 level of 320–2000 pg/mL were significantly associated with HBeAg loss (Table 4), and that baseline ALT level > 5× ULN, AFP > 20 ng/mL, and plasma

CLEC18 level of 320–2000 pg/mL were significantly associated with HBeAg seroconversion (Table 5). Multivariate analysis identified that a baseline plasma CLEC18 level of 320–2000 pg/mL was an independent predictor of HBeAg loss (hazard ratio [HR]: 2.077, 95% confidence interval [CI]:1.066–4.046, P = 0.0318) and seroconversion (HR: 2.041, 95% CI: 1.018–4.092, P = 0.0445) in the patients with CHB receiving NUC therapy. Baseline HBsAg level could significantly predict HBeAg loss (Table 4).

The cumulative incidence rates of HBeAg loss and seroconversion in the patients with CHB undergoing NUC therapy with a baseline plasma CLEC18 level of 320–2000 pg/mL were significantly higher than those in the other patients (P < 0.001 and P = 0.002, respectively)

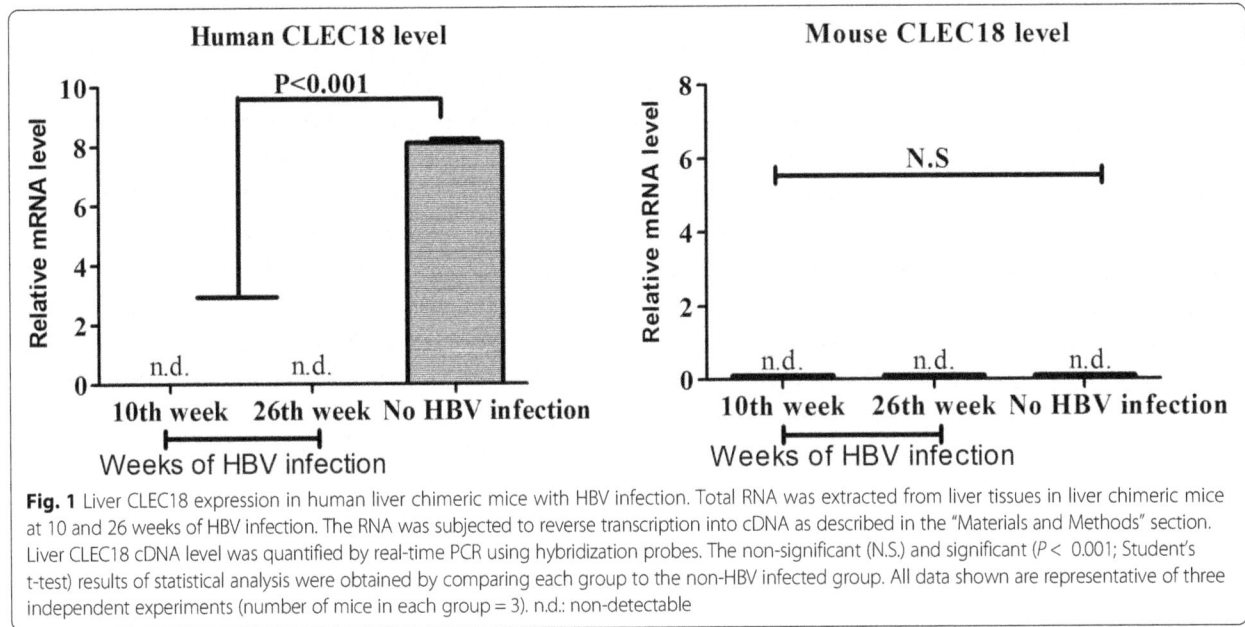

Fig. 1 Liver CLEC18 expression in human liver chimeric mice with HBV infection. Total RNA was extracted from liver tissues in liver chimeric mice at 10 and 26 weeks of HBV infection. The RNA was subjected to reverse transcription into cDNA as described in the "Materials and Methods" section. Liver CLEC18 cDNA level was quantified by real-time PCR using hybridization probes. The non-significant (N.S.) and significant ($P < 0.001$; Student's t-test) results of statistical analysis were obtained by comparing each group to the non-HBV infected group. All data shown are representative of three independent experiments (number of mice in each group = 3). n.d.: non-detectable

(Fig. 2a). The cumulative incidence of HBeAg loss but not HBeAg seroconversion in the patients with CHB undergoing NUC therapy with a baseline HBsAg level of 2900–12,000 IU/mL was significantly higher than that in the other patients ($P = 0.029$ and $P = 0.338$, respectively) (Fig. 2b).

Role of plasma CLEC18 in the prediction of virological response in the patients with CHB receiving NUC treatment

The overall NUC treatment duration was 61.68 ± 2.30 months for the HBeAg-negative patients. The times to virological response were 11.48 ± 0.86 months in the HBeAg-positive and 5.56 ± 0.37 months in the HBeAg-negative patients with CHB receiving NUC therapy. In the HBeAg-positive patients, univariate analysis identified that a baseline HBsAg level of 2900–12,000 IU/mL, HBV DNA level $< 8.3 \log_{10}$ IU/mL, ALT level $> 5\times$ ULN, and plasma CLEC18 level of 320–2000 pg/mL were significantly associated with virological response. Multivariate analysis identified that a baseline plasma CLEC18 level of 320–2000 pg/mL was an independent predictor of virological response

(HR: 1.850, 95% CI: 1.109–3.085, $P = 0.0184$) (Table 6). In the HBeAg-negative patients, no factor was significantly associated with virological response.

Correlation between plasma CLEC18 and baseline HBsAg levels

We analyzed the relationship between CLEC18 and HBsAg levels in the HBeAg-positive patients. CLEC18 and HBsAg levels had a low Spearman's correlation coefficient (data not shown). The correlation between categorized plasma CLEC18 levels (< 320, 320–2000 and > 2000 pg/mL) and categorized HBsAg levels (< 2900, 2900–12,000 and $> 12,000$ IU/mL) was not significant (see Additional File 2, $P = 0.2558$).

The association between plasma CLEC18 levels and liver fibrosis

Of the 271 enrolled patients with CHB, 172 received a liver biopsy. Univariate analysis identified that an age > 40 years, female sex, HBV genotype C, baseline HBsAg $< 3.0 \log_{10}$ IU/mL, HBV DNA $< 6 \log_{10}$ IU/mL, ALT $< 5\times$ ULN, platelet $< 150 \times 10^3$/uL were significantly

Table 2 Plasma CLEC18 levels in the patients with CHB

Group (viral load IU/mL)	Number of patients	CLEC18 level(Mean ± SD pg/mL)	P Value[1]	P Value[2]
Healthy donors	35	3106.06 ± 4708.13	–	–
HBeAg-positive ($> 2 \times 10^7$)	101	663.59 ± 1375.62	< 0.001	–
HBeAg-negative ($> 2 \times 10^7$)	65	281.68 ± 753.07	< 0.001	0.0196
HBeAg-negative ($2000-2 \times 10^7$)	64	264.68 ± 553.70	< 0.001	0.0106
HBeAg-negative (< 2000)	41	113. 28 ± 231.69	< 0.001	0.0057

P value[1]: Compared to healthy donors (Student's t-test)
P value[2]:Compared to HBeAg-positive($> 2 \times 10^7$) group (Student's t-test)

Table 3 Factors associated with CLEC18 levels in the patients with CHB

Variables	Univariate analysis				Multivariate analysis			
	Parameter Estimate	Standard Error	T Value	P Value	Parameter Estimate	Standard Error	T Value	P Value
Age	−18.41386	5.17495	−3.56	0.0004	−11.3821	6.1275	−1.86	0.0644
Sex: Man vs Woman	−25.76591	128.98391	−0.20	0.8418				
Genotype: C vs B	29.89732	126.53368	0.24	0.8134				
HBeAg: (+) vs (−)	428.94574	120.57574	3.56	0.0004	194.63847	162.600	1.20	0.2324
HBsAg $\log_{10}$ IU/mL	189.40927	67.77183	2.79	0.0056	20.737	91.28661	0.23	0.8205
HBV DNA $\log_{10}$ IU/mL	85.07892	27.25278	3.12	0.0020	25.6009	40.78698	0.63	0.5308
Cirrhosis: Yes vs No	− 142.57582	126.72962	−1.13	0.2616				
Fatty liver: Yes vs No	−38.09601	119.31101	−0.32	0.7497				
ALT: IU/L	0.30495	0.14451	2.11	0.0358	0.09404	0.16072	0.59	0.5590
Total bilirubin: mg/dL	−5.61291	45.41720	−0.12	0.9017				
Platelet: $\times 10^3$ /µL	1.16809	0.97747	1.20	0.2331				
PT: seconds prolonged	−19.80886	31.83170	−0.62	0.5343				
Cr: mg/dL	17.03954	124.23906	0.14	0.8910				
AFP: ng/mL	0.99144	0.79197	1.25	0.2117				
METAVIR Activity grade 2, 3 vs 0, 1	− 102.09187	167.92687	−0.61	0.5441				
METAVIR Fibrosis stage 3, 4 vs 0–2	− 303.34073	171.59770	−1.77	0.0791				

associated with METAVIR fibrosis stages 3 and 4, while CLEC18 showed borderline significance ($P = 0.0501$). Multivariate analysis revealed that a baseline plasma CLEC18 level of < 320 pg/mL was not significantly associated with METAVIR fibrosis stages 3 and 4 (see Additional File 3).

Discussion

This is the first study to investigate the expression, association and predictive value of CLEC18 in HBV infection. Because it is difficult to obtain liver tissue in patients with CHB, we analyzed the plasma levels of CLEC18 as an alternative.

Table 4 Factors associated with HBeAg loss in HBeAg-positive patients

Variables	Univariate analysis		Multivariate analysis	
	Hazard Ratio (95% CI)	P Value	Hazard Ratio (95% CI)	P Value
Age: ≥ 40 vs < 40 years old	0.693 (0.408–1.179)	0.1761		
Sex: Man vs Woman	1.103 (0.609–1.996)	0.7466		
Genotype: C vs B	1.118 (0.661–1.892)	0.6774		
Cirrhosis: Yes vs No	1.150 (0.617–2.144)	0.6591		
HBsAg: 2900–12,000 vs < 2900 or > 12,000 IU/mL	2.696 (1.555–4.673)	0.0004	2.108 (1.133–3.924)	0.0186
HBV DNA: ≥ 8.3 vs < 8.3 $\log_{10}$ IU/mL	0.938 (0.534–1.646)	0.8223		
ALT: ≥ 5 × vs < 5 × ULN	2.452 (1.433–4.195)	0.0011	2.055 (1.145–3.690)	0.0158
Total bilirubin: ≥ 1.2 vs < 1.2 mg/dL	1.622 (0.959–2.744)	0.0713		
PT: seconds prolonged	1.130 (0.995–1.282)	0.0592	1.140 (0.981–1.325)	0.0865
Platelet: ≥ 150 vs < 150 × 10^3/µL	1.551 (0.887–2.710)	0.1234		
AFP: ≥ 20 vs < 20 ng/mL	3.178 (1.732–5.829)	0.0002	2.583 (1.258–5.303)	0.0097
CLEC18: pg/mL	1.000 (0.999–1.000)	0.2708		
CLEC18: 320–2000 vs < 320 or > 2000 pg/mL	2.842 (1.637–4.933)	0.0002	2.077 (1.066–4.046)	0.0318

Table 5 Factors associated with HBeAg seroconversion in the HBeAg-positive patients

Variables	Univariate analysis		Multivariate analysis	
	Hazard Ratio (95% CI)	P Value	Hazard Ratio (95% CI)	P Value
Age: ≥ 40 vs < 40 years old	0.700 (0.363–1.351)	0.2878		
Sex: Man vs Woman	0.741 (0.370–1.485)	0.3984		
Genotype: C vs B	1.480 (0.756–2.898)	0.2525		
Cirrhosis: Yes vs No	1.133 (0.532–2.411)	0.7464		
HBsAg: 2900–12,000 vs < 2900 or > 12,000 IU/mL	1.754 (0.897–3.340)	0.1008		
HBV DNA: ≥ 8.3 vs < 8.3 $\log_{10}$ IU /mL	0.907 (0.453–1.815)	0.7832		
ALT: ≥ 5 × vs < 5 × ULN	3.115 (1.551–6.254)	0.0014	2.562 (1.241–5.288)	0.0110
Total bilirubin: ≥ 1.2 vs < 1.2 mg/dL	1.392 (0.723–2.682)	0.3228		
PT: seconds prolonged	1.114 (0.955–1.298)	0.1688		
Platelet: ≥ 150 vs < 150 × 10^3/μL	1.149 (0.565–2.336)	0.7021		
AFP: ≥ 20 vs < 20 ng/mL	2.388 (1.166–4.888)	0.0173	1.950 (0.927–4.103)	0.0783
CLEC18: pg/mL	1.000 (0.999–1.000)	0.3755		
CLEC18: 320–2000 vs < 320 or > 2000 pg/mL	2.609 (1.342–5.072)	0.0047	2.041 (1.018–4.092)	0.0445

Plasma CLEC18 decreases during HBV infection. The natural history of chronic HBV infection includes four distinct phases: an immune-tolerant phase, an immune clearance phase, an inactive or residual phase, and a reactivation phase [19]. In the immune-tolerant phase, the patients tend to be younger and have higher HBV DNA levels. As the patients become older, the disease progresses to the inactive phase, and the patients experience HBeAg loss and seroconversion with a decrease in HBV DNA replicative activity [22, 23]. We divided treatment-naïve patients with CHB undergoing NUC therapy into groups to mimic the disease progression of HBV infection. Interestingly, plasma CLEC18 levels were dramatically down-regulated in the patients with CHB (Table 2), suggesting that plasma CLEC18 levels are related to disease progression in HBV infection.

The baseline plasma CLEC18 levels were higher in the HBeAg-positive CHB patients than those in the HBeAg-negative CHB patients. Most of the HBeAg-negative CHB patients had low or even undetectable plasma CLEC18 levels, which precluded further evaluations of the associations with clinical features. The reason why the HBeAg-negative CHB patients exhibited low plasma CLEC18 levels is unknown, however it is possible that HBV infection down-regulates the expression of CLEC18 in the liver, and that long-term chronic infection with HBV results in lower plasma CLEC18 levels.

Previous studies have shown that HBV can attenuate the host immune response [10–12] such as by inhibiting TLR3-mediated cytokine response, which is correlated with the suppression of IFN-β and suppressed activation of IRF-3 and NF-kB [24]. We speculate that CLEC18 may play a role in regulating PRR-mediated cytokine

secretion or activating interferon-stimulating genes during viral infection. HBV blocks the expression of CLEC18, which may then result in attenuation of the host immune response. There were no significant correlations between baseline plasma CLEC18 and HBsAg levels, either in linear regression analysis or categorized correlation analysis. However, both may play a role in predicting HBeAg loss and/or seroconversion. The reason why we did not see a significant correlation between baseline plasma HBsAg and CLEC18 levels may be because most of the patients had low plasma CLEC18 levels, which precluded further statistical correlations with HBsAg levels in our study population. Further studies are needed to investigate whether plasma CLEC18 levels are correlated with HBsAg kinetics during NUC treatment. The mechanism by which HBV regulates the expression of CLEC18 during the disease course also remains to be elucidated.

Wang et al. reported that a high baseline HBsAg level (> 10,000 IU/mL) was associated with a lower rate of virological response, and that an on-treatment decline in HBsAg alone was not a good predictor of HBeAg loss and seroconversion in patients with CHB undergoing entecavir treatment [25]. Similar studies have reported that baseline HBsAg level alone or in combination with on-treatment declines in HBsAg, HBeAg, and HBV DNA levels can increase the predictive accuracy of HBeAg seroconversion [26]. However, none of these studies identified a clear cutoff value of HBsAg to predict treatment outcomes in patients receiving NUC treatment. Interestingly, we demonstrated that the subgroups of patients with a baseline HBsAg level of 2900–12,000 IU/mL had a higher likelihood of HBeAg loss

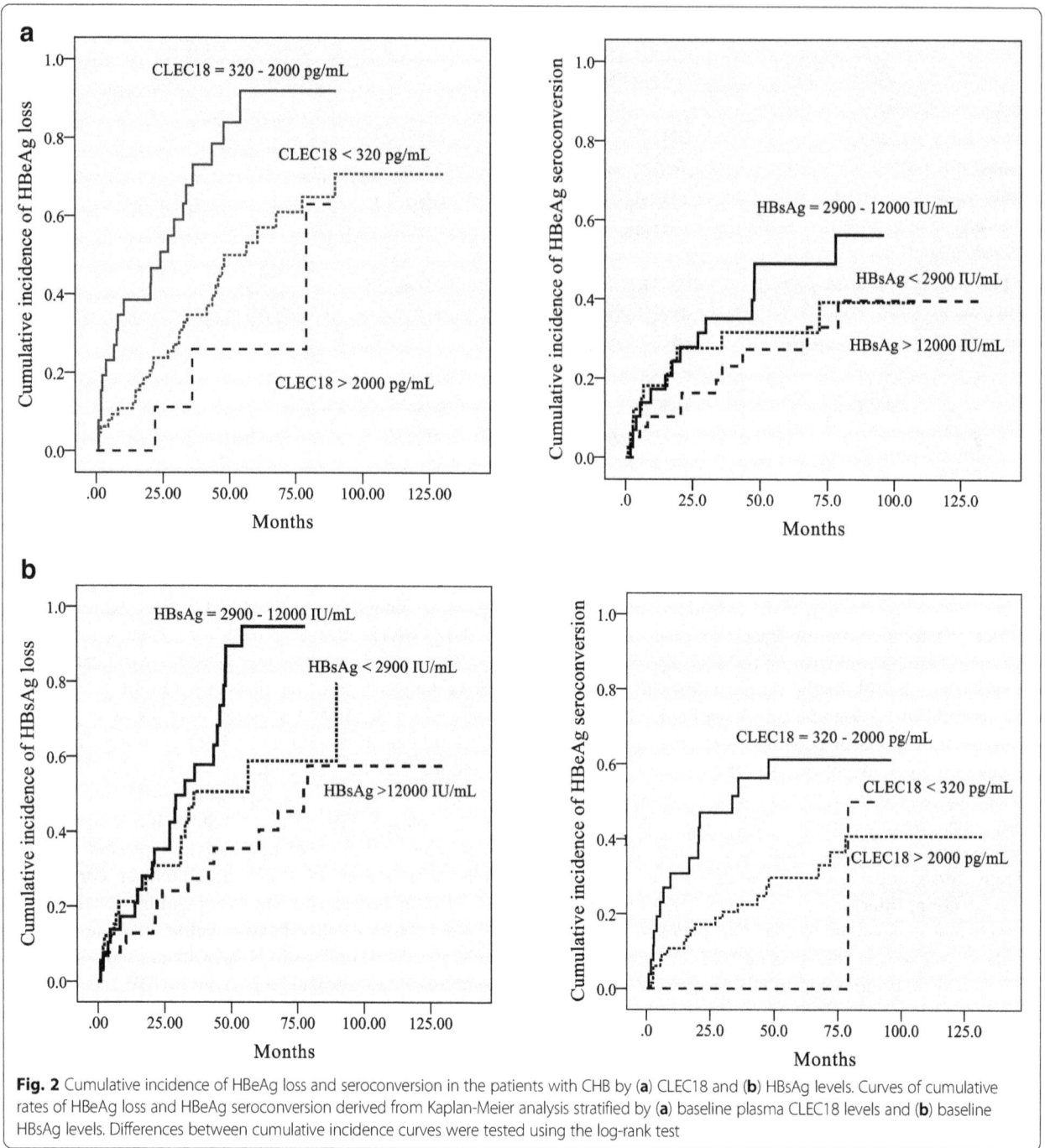

Fig. 2 Cumulative incidence of HBeAg loss and seroconversion in the patients with CHB by (**a**) CLEC18 and (**b**) HBsAg levels. Curves of cumulative rates of HBeAg loss and HBeAg seroconversion derived from Kaplan-Meier analysis stratified by (**a**) baseline plasma CLEC18 levels and (**b**) baseline HBsAg levels. Differences between cumulative incidence curves were tested using the log-rank test

and seroconversion. It is possible that the patients with CHB who had already achieved a low HBsAg level of < 2900 IU/mL and remained positive for HBeAg were less likely to lose HBeAg despite treatment, although the underlying immunological and virologic mechanisms remain to be determined. Patients with CHB with a high HBsAg level may have an impaired immune response to HBV owing to the inhibitory effect of viral antigens. The reason why the patients with a baseline HBsAg level of 2900–12,000 IU/mL and CLEC18 level of 320–2000 pg/

mL tended to achieve HBeAg loss remains unknown. We speculate that HBV regulates CLEC18 via an unknown pathway in HBeAg-positive CHB patients receiving NUC therapy. This interaction between HBV and CLEC18 may then result in the apparent concordance in the associations between HBsAg and CLEC18 levels and HBeAg loss during NUC therapy. Further investigations into the underlying mechanism are needed. Although a baseline HBsAg level of 2900–12,000 IU/mL was significantly associated with HBeAg loss, it was not significantly associated

Table 6 Factors associated with virological response in the HBeAg-positive patients

Variables	Univariate analysis		Multivariate analysis	
	Hazard Ratio (95% CI)	P Value	Hazard Ratio (95% CI)	P Value
Age: ≥ 40 vs < 40 years old	0.813 (0.544–1.215)	0.3125		
Sex: Man vs Woman	0.755 (0.488–1.166)	0.2045		
Genotype: C vs B	1.063 (0.707–1.598)	0.7691		
Cirrhosis: Yes vs No	1.257 (0.778–2.031)	0.3502		
HBsAg: 2900–12,000 vs < 2900 or > 12,000 IU/mL	1.698 (1.065–2.706)	0.0260	1.449 (0.890–2.359)	0.1359
HBV DNA: ≥ 8.3 vs < 8.3 $\log_{10}$ IU/mL	0.583 (0.378–0.899)	0.0147	0.395 (0.247–0.631)	0.0001
ALT: ≥ 5 × vs < 5 × ULN	1.909 (1.240–2.939)	0.0033	2.191 (1.373–3.496)	0.0010
Total bilirubin: ≥ 1.2 vs < 1.2 mg/dL	1.301 (0.861–1.967)	0.2115		
PT: seconds prolonged	1.015 (0.914–1.128)	0.7751		
Platelet: ≥ 150 vs < 150 × 10^3/μL	1.297 (0.831–2.025)	0.2525		
AFP: ≥ 20 vs < 20 ng/mL	1.230 (0.742–2.038)	0.4227		
CLEC18: pg/mL	1.000 (1.000–1.000)	0.9850		
CLEC18: 320–2000 vs < 320 or > 2000 pg/mL	1.979 (1.238–3.163)	0.0044	1.850 (1.109–3.085)	0.0184

with a virological response in the HBeAg-positive CHB patients receiving NUC therapy. The reason remains to be investigated.

Taken together, we propose that a range of baseline plasma HBsAg and CLEC18 levels is better than a single cutoff value to predict HBeAg loss and/or seroconversion in NUC-treated HBeAg-positive patients, and that a range of baseline plasma CLEC18 levels can predict a virological response in these patients.

Developing an accurate biomarker to allow for the early management of liver fibrosis is important. In the current study, a plasma CLEC18 level < 320 pg/mL was not significantly associated with liver fibrosis. Whether the level of CLEC18 in the liver reflects liver fibrosis is unknown. Although it was not possible to define liver fibrosis using CLEC18 as a single biomarker, whether CLEC18 can be used in combination with other biomarkers to predict liver fibrosis remains to be elucidated. Further studies are also needed to elucidate whether CLEC18 can be used as a biomarker for liver fibrosis.

There were two limitations to the present study. First, we focused on the prediction of treatment outcomes during NUC therapy, and patients who did not meet the criteria for receiving NUC therapy according to the APASL guidelines [2] were not enrolled, such as immune-tolerant patients (high HBV DNA > 2×10^7 IU/mL, normal ALT levels, HBeAg-positive) and inactive HBsAg carriers (HBsAg-positive, anti-HBe-positive with persistent normal serum ALT levels and HBV DNA < 2000 IU/mL). Further studies enrolling such subgroups of patients are warranted. Second, not all of the HBeAg-positive patients received the same treatment regimen. Nonetheless, the majority of the patients received potent NUCs, with 80

and 17 receiving entecavir and tenofovir, respectively, both of which are first-line therapy as recommended by the APASL guidelines [2].

Conclusion
Plasma CLEC18 levels were decreased in the patients with CHB and could predict HBeAg loss, seroconversion and virological response in the HBeAg-positive patients with CHB undergoing NUC therapy. Further studies are warranted to clarify the role of CLEC18 in CHB.

Abbreviations
AFP: Alpha-fetoprotein; ALT: Alanine aminotransferase; APASL: Asian Pacific Association for the Study of the Liver; APRI: AST to platelet ratio index; AST: Aspartate aminotransferase; CART: Classification and regression tree; cDNA: Complementary DNA; CHB: Chronic hepatitis B; CLEC18: C-type lectin 18; ELISA: Enzyme-linked immunosorbent assay; FIB-4: Fibrosis-4; FRG: Fah −/−/Rag2−/−/Il2rg−/−; HBeAg: Hepatitis B e antigen; HBsAg: Hepatitis B surface antigen; HBV: Hepatitis B virus infection; HR: Hazard ratio; NUC: Nucleos(t)ide analogue; PD-1: Programmed cell death protein-1; PRR: Pattern recognition receptor; PT: Prothrombin time; qPCR: Quantitative real time polymerase chain reaction; RNA: Ribonucleic acid; SD: Standard deviation; TLR: Toll-like receptor; TNF-α: Tumor necrosis factor-alpha; ULN: Upper limit of normal

Acknowledgements
We thank Dr. Ding-Shinn Chen for assistance with data analysis and interpretation. We thank Mi-Hua Tao for providing HBV-infected human liver FRG mice. We thank the Taiwan Mouse Clinic (NRPGM) for technical support in physiological metabolism experiments. We are also grateful to the technical services provided by the Transgenic Mouse Model Core Facility (NRPGM).

Funding
This work was supported by Academia Sinica and the Ministry of Science and Technology (MOST 106–2321-B-001-037, MOST 106–2320-B-001-023-MY3, MOST 105–2321-B-001-053, AS-105-TP-B08), and Summit and Thematic Research Projects.

Authors' contributions

TYT designed, performed, analyzed experiments, and wrote the manuscript. HIY data analysis and interpretation, YLH data analysis, MHT analyzed experiments, S-SY data analysis and interpretation, HCL data analysis. CYP and SLH designed, analyzed experiments, data interpretation, and drafted and revised the manuscript. All authors read and approved the final manuscript.

Competing interests

The authors declare that they have no competing interests.

Author details

[1]Ph.D. Program for Translational Medicine, China Medical University and Academia Sinica, Taichung and Taipei, Taiwan. [2]Division of Hepatogastroenterology, Department of Internal Medicine, China Medical University Hospital, 2, Yude St., North District, Taichung 404, Taiwan. [3]School of Medicine, China Medical University, Taichung, Taiwan. [4]Genomics Research Center, Academia Sinica, 128, Academia Road, Sec. 2, Nankang District, Taipei 115, Taiwan. [5]Institute of Biomedical Sciences, Academia Sinica, 128, Academia Road, Sec. 2, Nankang District, Taipei 115, Taiwan. [6]Institute of Statistical Sciences, Academia Sinica, 128, Academia Road, Sec. 2, Nankang District, Taipei 115, Taiwan. [7]Institute of Clinical Medicine, National Yang-Ming University, Taipei, Taiwan. [8]Department of Medical Research, Taipei Veterans General Hospital, Taipei, Taiwan.

References

1. European Association For The Study Of The L. EASL clinical practice guidelines: management of chronic hepatitis B virus infection. J Hepatol. 2012;57:167–85.
2. Liaw YF, Kao JH, Piratvisuth T, Chan HL, Chien RN, Liu CJ, et al. Asian-Pacific consensus statement on the management of chronic hepatitis B: a 2012 update. Hepatol Int. 2012;6:531–61.
3. Lok AS, McMahon BJ. Chronic hepatitis B: update 2009. Hepatology. 2009;50: 661–2.
4. Peng CY, Hsieh TC, Hsieh TY, Tseng KC, Lin CL, Su TH, et al. HBV-DNA level at 6 months of entecavir treatment predicts HBeAg loss in HBeAg-positive chronic hepatitis B patients. J Formos Med Assoc. 2015;114:308–13.
5. Sterling RK, Lissen E, Clumeck N, Sola R, Correa MC, Montaner J, et al. Development of a simple noninvasive index to predict significant fibrosis in patients with HIV/HCV coinfection. Hepatology. 2006;43:1317–25.
6. Lin ZH, Xin YN, Dong QJ, Wang Q, Jiang XJ, Zhan SH, et al. Performance of the aspartate aminotransferase-to-platelet ratio index for the staging of hepatitis C-related fibrosis: an updated meta-analysis. Hepatology. 2011;53: 726–36.
7. Enomoto M, Morikawa H, Tamori A, Kawada N. Noninvasive assessment of liver fibrosis in patients with chronic hepatitis B. World J Gastroenterol. 2014;20:12031–8.
8. Bonino F, Piratvisuth T, Brunetto MR, Liaw YF. Diagnostic markers of chronic hepatitis B infection and disease. Antivir Ther. 2010;15(3):35–44.
9. Zhang Z, Zhang JY, Wang LF, Wang FS. Immunopathogenesis and prognostic immune markers of chronic hepatitis B virus infection. J Gastroenterol Hepatol. 2012;27:223–30.
10. Huang YL, Pai FS, Tsou Y, Mon HC, Hsu TL, Wu CY, et al. Human CLEC18 gene cluster contains C-type lectins with differential glycan-binding specificity. J Biol Chem. 2015;290:21252–63.
11. Zoulim F, Luangsay S, Durantel D. Targeting innate immunity: a new step in the development of combination therapy for chronic hepatitis B. Gastroenterology. 2013;144:1342–4.
12. Chang J, Block TM, Guo JT. The innate immune response to hepatitis B virus infection: implications for pathogenesis and therapy. Antivir Res. 2012;96: 405–13.
13. Jiang M, Broering R, Trippler M, Poggenpohl L, Fiedler M, Gerken G, et al. Toll-like receptor-mediated immune responses are attenuated in the presence of high levels of hepatitis B virus surface antigen. J Viral Hepat. 2014;21:860–72.
14. Shih YM, Sun CP, Chou HH, Wu TH, Chen CC, Wu PY, et al. Combinatorial RNA interference therapy prevents selection of pre-existing HBV variants in human liver chimeric mice. Sci Rep. 2015;5:15259.
15. Azuma H, Paulk N, Ranade A, Dorrell C, Al-Dhalimy M, Ellis E, et al. Robust expansion of human hepatocytes in fah–/–/Rag2–/–/Il2rg–/– mice. Nat Biotechnol. 2007;25:903–10.
16. Bissig KD, Le TT, Woods NB, Verma IM. Repopulation of adult and neonatal mice with human hepatocytes: a chimeric animal model. Proc Natl Acad Sci U S A. 2007;104:20507–11.
17. Yang PL, Althage A, Chung J, Chisari FV. Hydrodynamic injection of viral DNA: a mouse model of acute hepatitis B virus infection. Proc Natl Acad Sci U S A. 2002;99:13825–30.
18. Peng CY, Lai HC, Su WP, et al. Early hepatitis B surface antigen decline predicts treatment response to entecavir in patients with chronic hepatitis B. Sci Rep. 2017;7:42879.
19. Intraobserver and interobserver variations in liver biopsy interpretation in patients with chronic hepatitis C. The French METAVIR cooperative study group. Hepatology. 1994;20:15–20.
20. Wang CC, Tseng KC, Peng CY, Hsieh TY, Lin CL, Su TH. Viral load and alanine aminotransferase correlate with serologic response in chronic hepatitis B patients treated with entecavir. J Gastroenterol Hepatol. 2013;28:46–50.
21. Chou R, Wasson N. Blood tests to diagnose fibrosis or cirrhosis in patients with chronic hepatitis C virus infection: a systematic review. Ann Intern Med. 2013;158:807–20.
22. Liaw YF, Chu CM. Hepatitis B virus infection. Lancet. 2009;373:582–92.
23. Hui CK, Leung N, Yuen ST, Zhang HY, Leung KW, Lu L, et al. Natural history and disease progression in Chinese chronic hepatitis B patients in immune-tolerant phase. Hepatology. 2007;46:395–401.
24. Wu J, Meng Z, Jiang M, Pei R, Trippler M, Broering R, et al. Hepatitis B virus suppresses toll-like receptor-mediated innate immune responses in murine parenchymal and nonparenchymal liver cells. Hepatology. 2009;49:1132–40.
25. Wang CC, Tseng TC, Wang PC, Lin HH, Kao JH. Baseline hepatitis B surface antigen quantitation can predict virologic response in entecavir-treated chronic hepatitis B patients. J Formos Med Assoc. 2014;113:786–93.
26. Li MH, Zhang L, Qu XJ, Lu Y, Shen G, Li ZZ, et al. The predictive value of baseline HBsAg level and early response for HBsAg loss in patients with HBeAg-positive chronic hepatitis B during pegylated interferon alpha-2a treatment. Biomed Environ Sci. 2017;30:177–84.

β-aminoisobutyric acid attenuates LPS-induced inflammation and insulin resistance in adipocytes through AMPK-mediated pathway

Tae Woo Jung[1,2], Hyung Sub Park[2], Geum Hee Choi[2], Daehwan Kim[2] and Taeseung Lee[2,3*] ⓘ

Abstract

Background: β-aminoisobutyric acid (BAIBA) is produced in skeletal muscle during exercise and has beneficial effects on obesity-related metabolic disorders such as diabetes and non-alcoholic fatty liver disease. Thus, it is supposed to prevent high fat diet (HFD)-induced inflammation and insulin resistance in adipose tissue though anti-inflammatory effects in obesity. Previous reports have also demonstrated strong anti-inflammatory effects of BAIBA.

Methods: We used BAIBA treated fully differentiated 3T3T-L1 mouse adipocytes to investigate the effects of exogenous BAIBA on inflammation and insulin signaling in adipocytes. Insulin signaling-mediated proteins and inflammation markers were measured by Western blot analysis. Secretion of pro-inflammatory cytokines were measured by ELISA. Lipid accumulation in differentiated 3 T3-L1 cells was stained by Oil red-O. Statistical analysis was performed by ANOVA and student's t test.

Results: BAIBA treatment suppressed adipogenesis assessed by adipogenic markers as well as lipid accumulation after full differentiation. We showed that BAIBA treatment stimulated AMP-activated protein kinase (AMPK) phosphorylation in a dose-dependent manner and lipopolysaccharide (LPS)-induced secretion of pro-inflammatory cytokines such as TNFα and MCP-1 was abrogated in BAIBA-treated 3 T3-L1 cells. Treatment of 3 T3-L1 cells with BAIBA reduced LPS-induced NFκB and IκB phosphorylation. Furthermore, BAIBA treatment ameliorated LPS-induced impairment of insulin signaling measured by IRS-1 and Akt phosphorylation and fatty acid oxidation. Suppression of AMPK by small interfering (si) RNA significantly restored these changes.

Conclusions: We demonstrated anti-inflammatory and anti-insulin resistance effects of BAIBA in differentiated 3 T3-L1 cells treated with LPS through AMPK-dependent signaling. These results provide evidence for the beneficial effects of BAIBA not only in liver and skeletal muscle cells but also in adipose tissue.

Keywords: BAIBA, AMPK, NFκB, Inflammation, Insulin resistance, Adipocyte

Background

Low-grade chronic adipose tissue inflammation and macrophage infiltration into adipose tissue are main characteristics of adipose tissue dysfunction in obesity [1, 2]. Abnormal secretion of pro-inflammatory cytokines by adipose tissue and macrophage infiltration results in the development of metabolic disorders such as insulin resistance and atherosclerosis [3].

Although regular exercise has beneficial effects on atherosclerosis in humans [4], the underlying mechanisms remain unclear. β-aminoisobutyric acid (BAIBA) is a natural catabolite of thymine that has been shown to attenuate obesity via stimulation of fatty acid oxidation and suppression of lipogenesis in animal models [5]. Recently, BAIBA was identified as a myokine released by skeletal muscle through a proliferator-activated receptor-gamma

* Correspondence: tslee@snubh.org
[2]Department of Surgery, Seoul National University Bundang Hospital, Seoul National University College of Medicine, 166 Gumi-ro, Bundang-gu, Seongnam 463-707, Korea
[3]Department of Surgery, Seoul National University College of Medicine, Seoul, Korea
Full list of author information is available at the end of the article

coactivator-1α (PGC-1α)-dependent pathway during physical activity. BAIBA stimulates the browning of white adipose tissue and fatty acid oxidation in the liver via a PPAR α-mediated pathway [6].

AMPK is an energy sensor that maintains cellular energy homeostasis [7] and inhibits the nuclear factor-κB (NFκB)-dependent inflammatory process [8]. AMPK activation by 5-aminoimidazole-4-carboximide ribonucleotide (AICAR) increases insulin sensitivity in various organs such as skeletal muscle [9], liver [10], and adipose tissue [11]. Jung et al. reported that BAIBA attenuated inflammation and insulin resistance in high fat diet (HFD)-fed mice, and that this effect was negated by siRNA-mediated suppression of AMPK [12]. BAIBA-mediated AMPK signaling has been reported to attenuate ER stress in response to hyperlipidemia, thereby ameliorating hepatic apoptosis [13]. Furthermore, BAIBA was shown to ameliorate renal fibrosis through suppression of a reactive oxygen species-mediated pathway [14]. Therefore, BAIBA-induced AMPK seems to play an important role in the pathogenesis of metabolic disorders.

Here, we investigated [5] the effect of BAIBA on LPS-induced inflammation and insulin resistance in differentiated 3 T3-L1 cells; [1] the mechanisms of BAIBA-mediated suppression of inflammation and insulin resistance through AMPK-mediated pathway.

Methods
Cell cultures, reagents, and antibodies
The mouse pre-adipocytes 3 T3-L1 (ATCC, Manassas, VA, USA) were cultured in Dulbecco's modified eagle medium (DMEM; Invitrogen, Carlsbad, CA, USA) supplemented with 10% fetal bovine serum (Invitrogen), 100 units/mL penicillin, and 100 μg/mL streptomycin (Invitrogen). Cells were cultured in a humidified atmosphere of 5% CO$_2$ at 37 °C. Differentiation was induced 48 h post confluence (day 2) by cultivation in culture medium supplemented with 1 μM insulin, 0.5 mM IBMX and 0.5 μg/ml dexamethansone for 2 days. After another 2 days in medium containing 1 μM insulin. Human primary adipocytes (Zenbio, Research Triangle Park, NC, USA) were fed with Omental Adipocyte Medium (Zenbio). Primary adipocytes were cultured in a humidified atmosphere containing 5% CO$_2$ at 37 °C pending uses. Differentiated 3 T3-L1 cells or human primary adipocytes were treated with 10 μg/ml LPS (Sigma, St Louis, MO, USA) and 0–30 μM BAIBA (Sigma) for 10 days. Differentiated 3 T3-L1 cells or human primary adipocytes were treated with 0–5 μM glimepiride (Sigma) [15] and 0–10 mM metformin (Sigma) [16] for 24 h. Human primary adipocytes were treated with 10 μM compound C (Sigma) for 24 h. Insulin (10 nM) was used to stimulate insulin signaling (insulin receptor

substrate (IRS-1) and Akt) for 3 min. Anti-phospho Akt (Ser473; 1:1000), anti-Akt (1:1000), anti-phospho AMPK (Thr172; 1:1000), anti-AMPK (1:2500), anti-phospho NFκBp65 (1:1000), anti- NFκBp65 (1:2500), anti-phospho IκB (1:1000), anti-IκB (1:1000), anti-phospho ACC (1:1000), anti-ACC (1:1000), and anti-adiponectin antibodies were purchased from Cell Signaling Technology (Beverly, MA, USA). Anti-CPT1 (1:2000) and anti-β-actin (1:5000) were obtained from Santa Cruz Biotechnology (Santa Cruz, CA, USA).

Western blot analysis
Differentiated 3 T3-L1 cells were harvested and proteins were extracted with lysis buffer (PRO-PREP; Intron Biotechnology, Seoul, Republic of Korea) for 60 min at 4 °C. Protein samples (30 μg) were subjected to 12% SDS-PAGE, transferred to a nitrocellulose membrane (Amersham Bioscience, Westborough, MA, USA), and probed with the indicated primary antibodies followed by secondary antibodies conjugated with horseradish peroxidase (Santa Cruz Biotechnology). The signals were detected using enhanced chemiluminescence (ECL) kits (Amersham Bioscience).

RNA extraction and quantitative real-time PCR
Total RNAs from harvested hepatocytes were isolated using TRIzol reagent (Invitrogen, Carlsbad, CA). Gene expression was measured by quantitative real-time PCR (qPCR) using the fluorescent TaqMan 5'nuclease assay on an Applied Biosystems 7000 sequence detection system (Foster City, CA, USA). qPCR was performed using cDNA with 2× TaqMan Master Mix and the 20 × premade TaqMan gene expression assays (Applied Biosystems). qPCR conditions were 95 °C for 10 min, followed by 40 cycles of 95 °C for 15 s and 60 °C for 1 min. The PCR primer mix for mouse PPARγ (Mm00440940_m1), FABP4 (Mm00445878_m1), adiponectin (Mm00456425_m1), and fatty acid synthase (Mm00662319_m1) were used. The mRNA of β-actin was quantified as an endogenous control, using primers: 5'-CGATGCTCCC CGGGCTGTAT-3' and 5'-TGGGGTACTTCAGGGTCAGG-3'.

Transfection with siRNAs for gene silencing in cells
siRNA oligonucleotides (20 nM) specific for AMPKα 1/2 were purchased from Santa Cruz Biotechnology. To suppress gene expression, cell transfection was performed with Lipofectamine 2000 (Invitrogen) according to the manufacturer's instructions. In brief, the cells were grown to 60% - 70% confluence, followed by serum starvation for 12 h after 3 T3-L1 cell differentiation. The cells were transfected with validated siRNA or scramble siRNA at a final concentration of 20 nM in the presence of transfection reagent. After transfection, the cells were harvested at 36 h for protein extraction and additional analysis.

Enzyme linked immunosorbent assay (ELISA)

Mouse serum TNFα and MCP-1 were measured with each ELISA kit (R&D Systems, Minneapolis, MN, USA) following the manufacturer's instructions.

Measurement of glucose uptake and acetyl-CoA and ATP content

Glucose uptake levels were measured using Glucose Uptake Assay Kit™ (Abcam, Cambridge, MA, USA). Briefly, proliferating and differentiating 3 T3-L1 cells were seeded at 5×10^5 cells/well in black walled / clear bottom 96-well plates (Corning, Inc., Corning, NY, USA) in DMEM containing 10% FBS. Upon reaching a confluency of 95%, differentiation was induced with differentiating media. After 48 h, media was changed to media containing 10 μg/ml LPS or 0–30 μM BAIBA for 10 days. Following treatment, media was removed from wells and treated with 10 nM insulin and 1 mM 2-Deoxyglucose (2-DG) for 30 min. Afterwards plates were centrifuged for 1 min at 58 g and incubated for 1 h at room temperature. After 2-DG taken up by the cells were extracted by extraction buffer in kit, 2-DG uptake levels were then measured at a wavelength of OD 412 nm on a BioTek Synergy HT plate reader (BioTek Instruments, Inc., Winooski, VT, USA). Intracellular levels of acetyl-CoA were measured using PicoProbe Acetyl CoA Assay Kit™ (Abcam) and intracellular ATP levels were measured using ATP Assay Kit™ (Abcam) in differentiated 3 T3-L1 cells were measured according to the manufacturer's instructions.

Long-chain acyl-CoA dehydrogenase (LCAD) expression in intact cells

LCAD expression was measured with Fatty Acid Oxidation Human In-Cell ELISA kit™ (Abcam) following the manufacturer's directions.

Cell viability assay

Cell viability was determined by 3-(4,5-dimethylthiazol-2-yl)-2,5-diphenyltetrazolium bromide (MTT) assay. In brief, MTT solution (Sigma) was added to experimental cell cultures in 96-well plates and incubated at 37 °C for 1 h. After washing five times with PBS, accumulated red formazan in the experimental cells was dissolved in dimethyl sulfoxide (DMSO) (Sigma). The optical density was used as an indicator of cell viability and was measured at 550 nm.

Statistical analysis

Results are presented as the relative values (means ± SEM). All experiments were performed at least three times. Student's t test or two-way ANOVA were used for statistical analysis. All analyses were performed using the SPSS/PC statistical program (version 12.0 for Windows; SPSS, Chicago, IL, USA).

Results

BAIBA suppresses lipid accumulation during differentiation of 3 T3-L1 cells

BAIBA has been reported to suppress high fat diet-associated hepatic lipogenesis [13]. Therefore, we examined the effect of BAIBA on differentiation in 3 T3-L1 cells. As shown in Fig. 1, treatment of 3 T3-L1 cells with BAIBA significantly suppressed lipid accumulation (Fig. 1a) and lipogenesis-mediated PPARγ, FABP4, adiponectin, and fatty acid synthase mRNA expression (Fig. 1b-e).

BAIBA ameliorates LPS-induced inflammation in differentiated 3 T3-L1 cells via AMPK-mediated pathway

BAIBA prevented LPS-induced inflammatory signaling such as phosphorylation of NFκB and IκB and TNFα and MCP-1 secretion in differentiated 3 T3-L1 cells (Fig. 2). Since AMPK is a key target for the treatment of insulin resistance and type 2 diabetes [17] and AICAR ameliorates inflammatory responses [18], we next evaluated the effect of BAIBA on phosphorylation of AMPK in differentiated 3 T3-L1 cells. We found that BAIBA caused AMPK phosphorylation in a dose-dependent manner (Fig. 2a). Conversely, BAIBA inhibited adiponectin expression in differentiated 3 T3-L1 cells (Fig. 2a) similar with previous reports [19, 20]. These results suggest that BAIBA stimulates AMPK phosphorylation in an adiponectin-independent fashion. We next examined whether BAIBA-induced AMPK phosphorylation contributes to the suppression of LPS-induced inflammation in differentiated 3 T3-L1 cells. The suppressive effects of BAIBA on LPS-induced inflammation were significantly abrogated by siRNA for AMPK (Fig. 2b-d).

BAIBA attenuates LPS-induced impairment of insulin signaling and insulin-stimulated glucose uptake in differentiated 3 T3-L1 cells via AMPK-dependent pathway

LPS treatment suppressed insulin-stimulated phosphorylation of IRS-1 and Akt, and glucose uptake in differentiated 3 T3-L1 cells. However, BAIBA blocked LPS-induced impairment of insulin signaling and insulin-stimulated glucose uptake (Fig. 3a and b). We also examined whether BAIBA-induced AMPK phosphorylation contributes to the suppression of LPS-induced insulin resistance in differentiated 3 T3-L1 cells. In Fig. 3a and b, siRNA for AMPK significantly abrogated the inhibitory effects of BAIBA on LPS-induced insulin resistance.

BAIBA ameliorated LPS-induced impairment of fatty acid oxidation in differentiated 3 T3-L1 cells through AMPK signaling

Koves et al. reported that mitochondrial overload and incomplete fatty acid oxidation cause insulin resistance in skeletal muscle [21]. Enhanced fatty acid oxidation

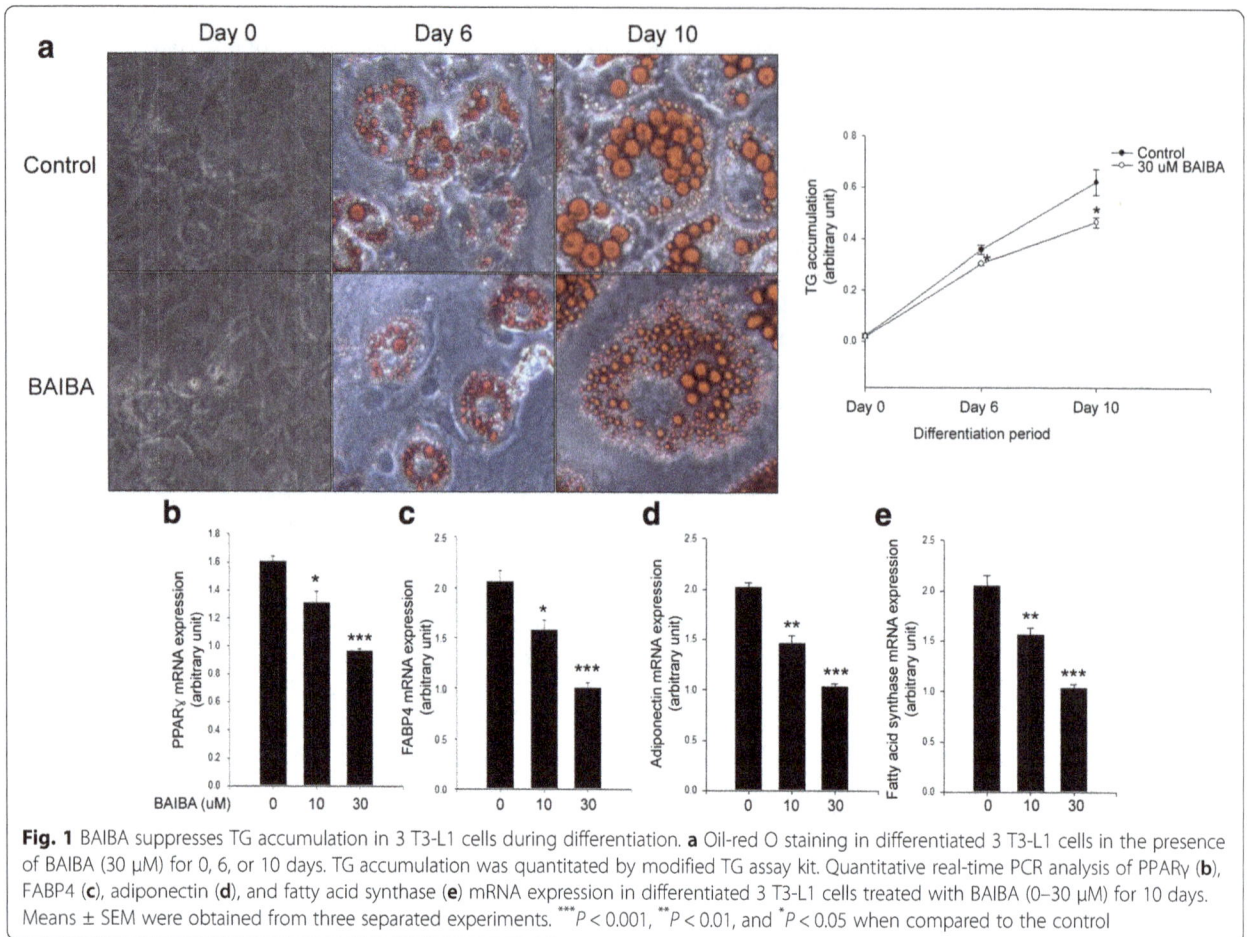

Fig. 1 BAIBA suppresses TG accumulation in 3 T3-L1 cells during differentiation. **a** Oil-red O staining in differentiated 3 T3-L1 cells in the presence of BAIBA (30 μM) for 0, 6, or 10 days. TG accumulation was quantitated by modified TG assay kit. Quantitative real-time PCR analysis of PPARγ (**b**), FABP4 (**c**), adiponectin (**d**), and fatty acid synthase (**e**) mRNA expression in differentiated 3 T3-L1 cells treated with BAIBA (0–30 μM) for 10 days. Means ± SEM were obtained from three separated experiments. $^{***}P < 0.001$, $^{**}P < 0.01$, and $^{*}P < 0.05$ when compared to the control

improves insulin sensitivity in palmitate-treated adipocytes [22]. AMPK have been reported to augment fatty acid oxidation [23]. However, to the best of our knowledge, the effect of BAIBA on fatty acid oxidation in adipocytes has not been elucidated. Therefore, we next evaluated whether BAIBA-induced AMPK could induce fatty acid oxidation. To confirm the stimulation of fatty acid oxidation by BAIBA, we measured levels of acetyl-CoA and ATP, products of fatty acid oxidation, LCAD expression, ACC phosphorylation, and CPT1 expression. As expected, BAIBA treatment significantly elevated intracellular acetyl-CoA, ATP levels, ACC phosphorylation, and CPT1 expression in fully differentiated 3 T3-L1 cells. Furthermore, BAIBA treatment increased LCAD expression in intact human primary adipocytes. However, suppression of AMPK by siRNA or compound C, a specific AMPK inhibitor, restored these changes (Fig. 4).

AMPK plays a critical role in BAIBA-mediated attenuation of inflammation and insulin resistance

To reaffirm importance of AMPK role in the beneficial effects of BAIBA, we examined the effects of glimepiride,

an AMPK-independent drug, and metformin, an AMPK activator on inflammation and insulin resistance during same treatment time with BAIBA. Initially, we selected the treatment concentrations (1 μM glimepiride and 0. 1 mM metformin for 10 days; 1 μM glimepiride and 10 mM metformin for 24 h) which do not affect cell viability and show maximal suppressive effects on inflammation (Additional file 1: Figure S1 and Additional file 2: Figure S2). BAIBA, metformin, and glimepiride ameliorated LPS-induced pro-inflammatory cytokines secretion and glucose uptake impairment. Notably, the effects of BAIBA and metformin on inflammation and insulin resistance are stronger than glimepiride for 10 days. Metformin and glimepiride treatment for 24 h showed similar results to results from 10 days treatment, whereas BAIBA had no effects on inflammation and insulin resistance (Additional file 3: Figure S3), suggesting that 24 h may be insufficient for BAIBA to work.

Discussion

Obesity causes a low-grade chronic inflammatory state within adipose tissue accompanying elevated pro-inflammatory cytokine expression and infiltration of

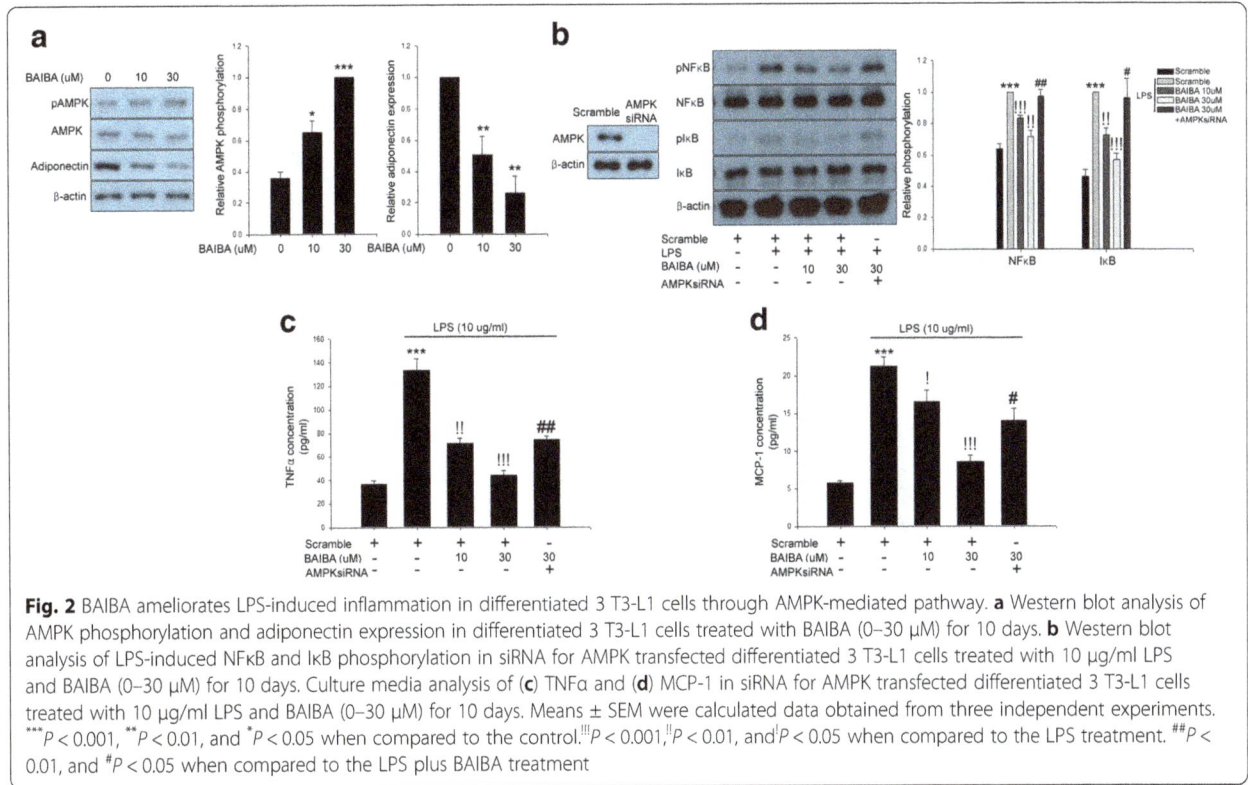

Fig. 2 BAIBA ameliorates LPS-induced inflammation in differentiated 3 T3-L1 cells through AMPK-mediated pathway. **a** Western blot analysis of AMPK phosphorylation and adiponectin expression in differentiated 3 T3-L1 cells treated with BAIBA (0–30 μM) for 10 days. **b** Western blot analysis of LPS-induced NFκB and IκB phosphorylation in siRNA for AMPK transfected differentiated 3 T3-L1 cells treated with 10 μg/ml LPS and BAIBA (0–30 μM) for 10 days. Culture media analysis of (**c**) TNFα and (**d**) MCP-1 in siRNA for AMPK transfected differentiated 3 T3-L1 cells treated with 10 μg/ml LPS and BAIBA (0–30 μM) for 10 days. Means ± SEM were calculated data obtained from three independent experiments. $^{***}P < 0.001$, $^{**}P < 0.01$, and $^{*}P < 0.05$ when compared to the control. $^{!!!}P < 0.001$, $^{!!}P < 0.01$, and $^{!}P < 0.05$ when compared to the LPS treatment. $^{##}P < 0.01$, and $^{#}P < 0.05$ when compared to the LPS plus BAIBA treatment

immune cells such as neutrophils and macrophages, further disseminating the inflammatory response and stimulating systemic inflammation [24, 25]. Adipose tissue and infiltrated macrophages secrete various pro-inflammatory cytokines that contribute to further immune cell infiltration leading to impaired hepatic and skeletal metabolic homeostasis and finally systemic insulin resistance [3, 26, 27].

Furthermore, Adipose tissue dysfunction caused by chronic inflammation leads to improper release and increase serum levels of free fatty acids (FFAs), which are known to contribute to insulin resistance through interfering insulin signaling [28]. The impairment of insulin signaling, leading to insulin resistance is a main characteristic of metabolic disorders and type 2 diabetes.

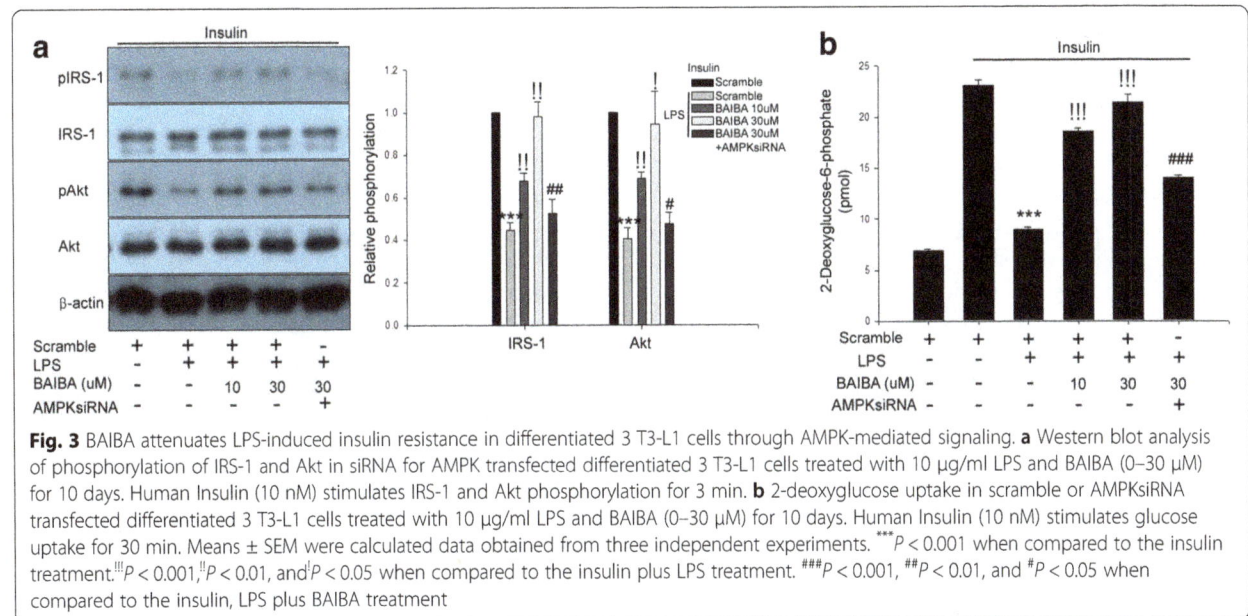

Fig. 3 BAIBA attenuates LPS-induced insulin resistance in differentiated 3 T3-L1 cells through AMPK-mediated signaling. **a** Western blot analysis of phosphorylation of IRS-1 and Akt in siRNA for AMPK transfected differentiated 3 T3-L1 cells treated with 10 μg/ml LPS and BAIBA (0–30 μM) for 10 days. Human Insulin (10 nM) stimulates IRS-1 and Akt phosphorylation for 3 min. **b** 2-deoxyglucose uptake in scramble or AMPKsiRNA transfected differentiated 3 T3-L1 cells treated with 10 μg/ml LPS and BAIBA (0–30 μM) for 10 days. Human Insulin (10 nM) stimulates glucose uptake for 30 min. Means ± SEM were calculated data obtained from three independent experiments. $^{***}P < 0.001$ when compared to the insulin treatment. $^{!!!}P < 0.001$, $^{!!}P < 0.01$, and $^{!}P < 0.05$ when compared to the insulin plus LPS treatment. $^{###}P < 0.001$, $^{##}P < 0.01$, and $^{#}P < 0.05$ when compared to the insulin, LPS plus BAIBA treatment

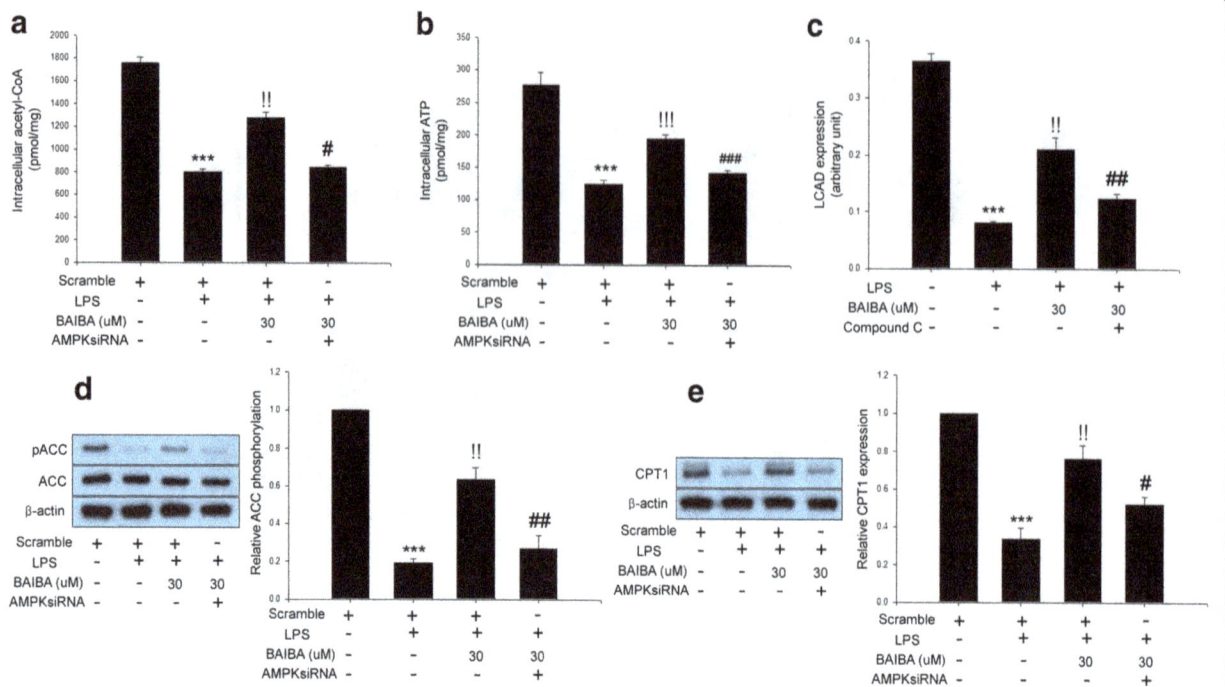

Fig. 4 BAIBA stimulates fatty acid oxidation through AMPK signaling. Intracellular acetyl-CoA (**a**) and ATP levels (**b**) in scramble or AMPKsiRNA transfected differentiated 3 T3-L1 cells treated with 10 μg/ml LPS and BAIBA (0–30 μM) for 10 days. **c** LCAD expression levels in intact human primary adipocytes treated with 10 μg/ml LPS and BAIBA (0–30 μM) for 10 days and compound C (10 μM) for 24 h. Western blot analysis of ACC phosphorylation (**d**) and CPT1 expression (**e**) in differentiated 3 T3-L1 cells treated with 10 μg/ml LPS and BAIBA (0–30 μM) for 10 days. Means ± SEM were obtained from three separated experiments. $^{***}P < 0.001$ when compared to the insulin treatment. $^{!!!}P < 0.001, ^{!!}P < 0.01$, and $^{!}P < 0.05$ when compared to the insulin plus LPS treatment. $^{###}P < 0.001, ^{##}P < 0.01$, and $^{#}P < 0.05$ when compared to the insulin, LPS plus BAIBA treatment

BAIBA has been previously reported to exert potent anti-inflammatory in hepatocytes [5] and skeletal muscle cells [12] and anti-diabetic effects in skeletal muscle cells [12] and hepatocytes [13]. In the current study, we investigated BAIBA effects on LPS-induced inflammation and insulin resistance in mouse adipocytes.

Herein, treatment of differentiated 3 T3-L1 cells with BAIBA led to the prevention of NFκB-mediated pro-inflammatory pathway activation and we also observed a significant decrease in pro-inflammatory cytokines TNFα and MCP-1 after LPS treatment. These results suggest that the anti-inflammatory effects of BAIBA in adipocytes are likely mediated by suppression of NFκB-mediated signaling and its downstream molecules.

The phosphatidylinositol 3-kinase (PI3K)/Akt pathway plays a central role in regulation of various intracellular signaling such as cell survival, proliferation, and differentiation [29]. This Akt activity is suppressed under obese conditions because of the phosphorylation of serine residues in IRS-1, resulting in impairment of the IRS-1-induced PI3K-mediated pathway [30] and inhibition of IRS-1-mediated Akt activation [31, 32]. We previously reported that BAIBA treatment reversed hyperlipidemia-induced inhibition of insulin signaling in both differentiated

C2C12 cells and mouse skeletal muscle [12]. In the current study, we report for the first time that BAIBA treatment significantly increased insulin-stimulated IRS-1 and Akt phosphorylation, and glucose uptake in mouse adipocytes, suggesting that BAIBA has an anti-diabetic effect.

Jung et al. have documented that BAIBA exerts its anti-obesity effect by stimulating fatty acid oxidation in skeletal muscle [12]. In the current study, we found that BAIBA treatment reduced lipogenic-genes (*Fabp4, Ppary, adiponectin, FAS*) mRNA expression accompanying a decrease in lipid accumulation during differentiation of 3 T3-L1 cells. Furthermore, BAIBA stimulated fatty acid oxidation. These results suggest that BAIBA has potential anti-obesity effects in adipocytes. Furthermore, these results support data describing body weight loss by BAIBA administration in a previous study [12]. However, further investigation is required to elucidate detailed mechanisms for suppression of adipocyte differentiation by BAIBA.

Glimepiride, a third-generation diabetes drug sulfonylurea, has demonstrated not to have any effects on AMPK [33]. In this study, we demonstrated that glimepiride attenuated LPS-induced pro-inflammatory cytokines secretion and glucose uptake impairment, but it

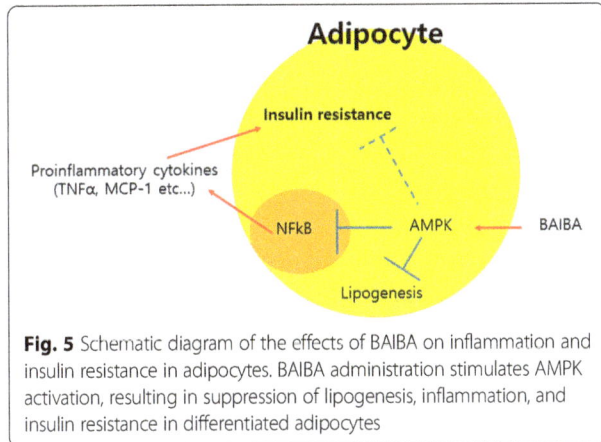

Fig. 5 Schematic diagram of the effects of BAIBA on inflammation and insulin resistance in adipocytes. BAIBA administration stimulates AMPK activation, resulting in suppression of lipogenesis, inflammation, and insulin resistance in differentiated adipocytes

was less effective than BAIBA (Additional file 3: Figure S3). Therefore, AMPK plays a crucial role in the beneficial effects of BAIBA on inflammation and insulin resistance in differentiated adipocytes. We next compared the effects of BAIBA on inflammation and insulin resistance with metformin, an anti-diabetic drug via AMPK activation [34]. Metformin demonstrated the strongest suppressive effects. But, BAIBA is less effective than metformin (Additional file 3: Figure S3). These results demonstrate that metformin is the most effective for suppression of inflammation and insulin resistance. However, side effects such as hypoglycemia (sulfonylurea; [35]), weight gain (sulfonylurea; [35]) or hepatotoxicity (metformin; [36]), may be less, because BAIBA is an endogenous substance. In addition, doses of BAIBA are much less than metformin. Therefore, BAIBA seems to be worth developing as a safer drug for treatment of insulin resistance at least from the perspective of adipocytes.

In summary, we investigated the effects of BAIBA on fully differentiated 3 T3-L1 cells to elucidate whether BAIBA could ameliorate inflammatory responses in adipocytes and subsequently obesity-induced low-grade chronic inflammation in adipose tissue. Our current findings verify that BAIBA alleviates LPS-induced inflammatory responses via AMPK-associated suppression of NFκB-dependent signaling. Not only did BAIBA prevent lipid accumulation during differentiation of 3 T3-L1 cells, but it also ameliorated insulin resistance in differentiated 3 T3-L1 cells.

Conclusion

The present study found that BAIBA ameliorates LPS-induced pro-inflammatory responses and insulin resistance in differentiated adipocytes through AMPK-mediated signaling. Furthermore, BAIBA markedly suppresses lipid accumulation during 3 T3-L1 cell differentiation and stimulates fatty acid oxidation via AMPK pathway (Fig. 5). Attenuation of pro-inflammatory cytokines such as IL-6, TNFα, and IL-1β secreted by immune cells [27, 37] and adipocytes [38, 39] may be a therapeutic approach for treating

systemic low-grade chronic inflammation-associated with metabolic syndrome. Therefore, our report may suggest a novel strategy for obesity-associated metabolic disorders including insulin resistance.

Additional files

Additional file 1: Figure S1. Selection of optimized concentrations of glimepiride and metformin for cell treatment. Cell viability measured by MTT assay in differentiated 3 T3-L1 cells treated with (a) BAIBA (0–30 μM), (b) glimepiride (0–5 μM), or (c) metformin (0–20 mM) for 10 days. Culture media analysis of TNFα and MCP-1 in differentiated 3 T3-L1 cells treated with 10 μg/ml LPS for 24 h and glimepiride (0–5 μM) (d) or metformin (0–200 μM) (e) for 10 days. Means ± SEM were calculated data obtained from three independent experiments. ***$P < 0.001$ and **$P < 0.01$ when compared to the control.$^{III}P < 0.001$,$^{II}P < 0.01$, and$^{I}P < 0.05$ when compared to the LPS treatment (TIFF 4230 kb)

Additional file 2: Figure S2. Selection of optimized concentrations of glimepiride and metformin for cell treatment. Cell viability measured by MTT assay in differentiated 3 T3-L1 cells treated with (a) BAIBA (0–30 μM), (b) glimepiride (0–5 μM), or (c) metformin (0–20 mM) for 24 h. Culture media analysis of TNFα and MCP-1 in differentiated 3 T3-L1 cells treated with 10 μg/ml LPS for 24 h and glimepiride (0–5 μM) (d) or metformin (0–20 mM) (e) for 24 h. Means ± SEM were calculated data obtained from three independent experiments. ***$P < 0.001$ when compared to the control.$^{III}P < 0.001$,$^{II}P < 0.01$, and$^{I}P < 0.05$ when compared to the LPS treatment (TIFF 4230 kb)

Additional file 3: Figure S3. Comparison of BAIBA, metformin, and glimepiride effects on inflammation and insulin resistance. (a) Culture media analysis of TNFα and MCP-1 and (b) 2-deoxyglucose uptake in differentiated 3 T3-L1 cells treated with 10 μg/ml LPS for 24 h and BAIBA (30 μM), metformin (0.1 mM) or glimepiride (5 μM) for 10 days. (c) Culture media analysis of TNFα and MCP-1 and (d) 2-deoxyglucose uptake in differentiated 3 T3-L1 cells treated with 10 μg/ml LPS and BAIBA (30 μM), metformin (10 mM) or glimepiride (5 μM) for 24 h. Human Insulin (10 nM) stimulates glucose uptake for 30 min. Means ± SEM were calculated data obtained from three independent experiments. ***$P < 0.001$ when compared to the control or insulin treatment.$^{III}P < 0.001$,$^{II}P < 0.01$, and$^{I}P < 0.05$ when compared to the LPS treatment or insulin plus LPS treatment. ###$P < 0.001$, ##$P < 0.01$, and #$P < 0.05$ when compared to the LPS plus BAIBA treatment (TIFF 3804 kb)

Abbreviations
AMPK: AMP-activated protein kinase; BAIBA: β-aminoisobutyric acid; LPS: Lipopolysaccharide; NFκB: Nuclear factor kappa beta; siRNA: Small interfering RNA

Acknowledgements
Not applicable.

Funding
This work was supported by a National Research Foundation (NRF) grant funded by the Ministry of Science, ICT, and Future Planning (2016R1C1B2012674), Republic of Korea.

Authors' contributions
TWJ, HSP, GHC, DHK, and TSL: substantial contribution to conception and design; TWJ, HSP, and TSL: acquisition of data, analysis and interpretation of data; TWJ: drafting and revising of the manuscript. All authors approved the final version of the manuscript. TWJ and TSL are responsible for the integrity of the work as a whole.

Competing interests
All authors declare that they have no competing interests.

Author details
[1]Research Administration Team, Seoul National University Bundang Hospital, 166 Gumi-ro, Bundang-gu, Seongnam 463-707, Korea. [2]Department of Surgery, Seoul National University Bundang Hospital, Seoul National University College of Medicine, 166 Gumi-ro, Bundang-gu, Seongnam 463-707, Korea. [3]Department of Surgery, Seoul National University College of Medicine, Seoul, Korea.

References
1. Bluher M. Adipose tissue dysfunction in obesity. Exp Clin Endocrinol Diabetes. 2009;117(6):241–50.

2. Hajer GR, van Haeften TW, Visseren FL. Adipose tissue dysfunction in obesity, diabetes, and vascular diseases. Eur Heart J. 2008;29(24):2959–71.

3. Xu H, Barnes GT, Yang Q, Tan G, Yang D, Chou CJ, Sole J, Nichols A, Ross JS, Tartaglia LA, Chen H. Chronic inflammation in fat plays a crucial role in the development of obesity-related insulin resistance. J Clin Invest. 2003;112(12):1821–30.

4. Okabe TA, Kishimoto C, Murayama T, Yokode M, Kita T. Effects of exercise on the development of atherosclerosis in apolipoprotein E-deficient mice. Exp Clin Cardiol. 2006;11(4):276–9.

5. Begriche K, Massart J, Abbey-Toby A, Igoudjil A, Letteron P, Fromenty B. Beta-aminoisobutyric acid prevents diet-induced obesity in mice with partial leptin deficiency. Obesity. 2008;16(9):2053–67.

6. Roberts LD, Bostrom P, O'Sullivan JF, Schinzel RT, Lewis GD, Dejam A, Lee YK, Palma MJ, Calhoun S, Georgiadi A, Chen MH, Ramachandran VS, Larson MG, Bouchard C, Rankinen T, Souza AL, Clish CB, Wang TJ, Estall JL, Soukas AA, Cowan CA, Spiegelman BM, Gerszten RE. Beta-Aminoisobutyric acid induces browning of white fat and hepatic beta-oxidation and is inversely correlated with cardiometabolic risk factors. Cell Metab. 2014;19(1):96–108.

7. Hardie DG. AMP-activated protein kinase: an energy sensor that regulates all aspects of cell function. Genes Dev. 2011;25(18):1895–908.

8. Salminen A, Hyttinen JM, Kaarniranta K. AMP-activated protein kinase inhibits NF-kappaB signaling and inflammation: impact on healthspan and lifespan. J Mol Med. 2011;89(7):667–76.

9. Kjobsted R, Treebak JT, Fentz J, Lantier L, Viollet B, Birk JB, Schjerling P, Bjornholm M, Zierath JR, Wojtaszewski JF. Prior AICAR stimulation increases insulin sensitivity in mouse skeletal muscle in an AMPK-dependent manner. Diabetes. 2015;64(6):2042–55.

10. Iglesias MA, Ye JM, Frangioudakis G, Saha AK, Tomas E, Ruderman NB, Cooney GJ, Kraegen EW. AICAR administration causes an apparent enhancement of muscle and liver insulin action in insulin-resistant high-fat-fed rats. Diabetes. 2002;51(10):2886–94.

11. Liong S, Lappas M. Activation of AMPK improves inflammation and insulin resistance in adipose tissue and skeletal muscle from pregnant women. J Physiol Biochem. 2015;71(4):703–17.

12. Jung TW, Hwang HJ, Hong HC, Yoo HJ, Baik SH, Choi KM. BAIBA attenuates insulin resistance and inflammation induced by palmitate or a high fat diet via an AMPK-PPARdelta-dependent pathway in mice. Diabetologia. 2015; 58(9):2096–105.

13. Shi CX, Zhao MX, Shu XD, Xiong XQ, Wang JJ, Gao XY, Chen Q, Li YH, Kang YM, Zhu GQ. Beta-aminoisobutyric acid attenuates hepatic endoplasmic reticulum stress and glucose/lipid metabolic disturbance in mice with type 2 diabetes. Sci Rep. 2016;6:21924.

14. Wang H, Qian J, Zhao X, Xing C, Sun B. Beta-Aminoisobutyric acid ameliorates the renal fibrosis in mouse obstructed kidneys via inhibition of renal fibroblast activation and fibrosis. J Pharmacol Sci. 2017;133(4):203–13.

15. Kanda Y, Matsuda M, Tawaramoto K, Kawasaki F, Hashiramoto M, Matsuki M, Kaku K. Effects of sulfonylurea drugs on adiponectin production from 3T3-L1 adipocytes: implication of different mechanism from pioglitazone. Diabetes Res Clin Pract. 2008;81(1):13–8.

16. Caton PW, Kieswich J, Yaqoob MM, Holness MJ, Sugden MC. Metformin opposes impaired AMPK and SIRT1 function and deleterious changes in core clock protein expression in white adipose tissue of genetically-obese db/db mice. Diabetes Obes Metab. 2011;13(12):1097–104.

17. Zhang BB, Zhou G, Li C. AMPK: an emerging drug target for diabetes and the metabolic syndrome. Cell Metab. 2009;9(5):407–16.

18. Yang Z, Wang X, He Y, Qi L, Yu L, Xue B, Shi H. The full capacity of AICAR to reduce obesity-induced inflammation and insulin resistance requires myeloid SIRT1. PLoS One. 2012;7(11):e49935.

19. Li Y, Wang P, Zhuang Y, Lin H, Li Y, Liu L, Meng Q, Cui T, Liu J, Li Z. Activation of AMPK by berberine promotes adiponectin multimerization in 3T3-L1 adipocytes. FEBS Lett. 2011;585(12):1735–40.

20. Prieto-Hontoria PL, Fernandez-Galilea M, Perez-Matute P, Martinez JA, Moreno-Aliaga MJ. Lipoic acid inhibits adiponectin production in 3T3-L1 adipocytes. J Physiol Biochem. 2013;69(3):595–600.

21. Koves TR, Ussher JR, Noland RC, Slentz D, Mosedale M, Ilkayeva O, Bain J, Stevens R, Dyck JR, Newgard CB, Lopaschuk GD, Muoio DM. Mitochondrial overload and incomplete fatty acid oxidation contribute to skeletal muscle insulin resistance. Cell Metab. 2008;7(1):45–56.

22. Malandrino MI, Fucho R, Weber M, Calderon-Dominguez M, Mir JF, Valcarcel L, Escote X, Gomez-Serrano M, Peral B, Salvado L, Fernandez-Veledo S, Casals N, Vazquez-Carrera M, Villarroya F, Vendrell JJ, Serra D, Herrero L. Enhanced fatty acid oxidation in adipocytes and macrophages reduces lipid-induced triglyceride accumulation and inflammation. Am J Physiol Endocrinol Metab. 2015;308(9):E756–69.

23. Osler ME, Zierath JR. Adenosine 5'-monophosphate-activated protein kinase regulation of fatty acid oxidation in skeletal muscle. Endocrinology. 2008; 149(3):935–41.

24. Chawla A, Nguyen KD, Goh YP. Macrophage-mediated inflammation in metabolic disease. Nat Rev Immunol. 2011;11(11):738–49.

25. Huh JY, Park YJ, Ham M, Kim JB. Crosstalk between adipocytes and immune cells in adipose tissue inflammation and metabolic dysregulation in obesity. Mol Cells. 2014;37(5):365–71.

26. Hotamisligil GS, Shargill NS, Spiegelman BM. Adipose expression of tumor necrosis factor-alpha: direct role in obesity-linked insulin resistance. Science. 1993;259(5091):87–91.

27. Weisberg SP, McCann D, Desai M, Rosenbaum M, Leibel RL, Ferrante AW Jr. Obesity is associated with macrophage accumulation in adipose tissue. J Clin Invest. 2003;112(12):1796–808.

28. Boden G. Role of fatty acids in the pathogenesis of insulin resistance and NIDDM. Diabetes. 1997;46(1):3–10.

29. Sinor AD, Lillien L. Akt-1 expression level regulates CNS precursors. J Neurosci. 2004;24(39):8531–41.

30. Gao Z, Hwang D, Bataille F, Lefevre M, York D, Quon MJ, Ye J. Serine phosphorylation of insulin receptor substrate 1 by inhibitor kappa B kinase complex. J Biol Chem. 2002;277(50):48115–21.

31. Guo S. Molecular basis of insulin resistance: the role of IRS and Foxo1 in the control of diabetes mellitus and its complications. Drug Discov Today Dis Mech. 2013;10(1–2):e27–33.

32. Zick Y. Ser/Thr phosphorylation of IRS proteins: a molecular basis for insulin resistance. Scie STKE. 2005;2005(268):pe4.

33. Inukai K, Watanabe M, Nakashima Y, Takata N, Isoyama A, Sawa T, Kurihara S, Awata T, Katayama S. Glimepiride enhances intrinsic peroxisome proliferator-activated receptor-gamma activity in 3T3-L1 adipocytes. Biochem Biophys Res Commun. 2005;328(2):484–90.

34. Wu W, Tang S, Shi J, Yin W, Cao S, Bu R, Zhu D, Bi Y. Metformin attenuates palmitic acid-induced insulin resistance in L6 cells through the AMP-activated protein kinase/sterol regulatory element-binding protein-1c pathway. Int J Mol Med. 2015;35(6):1734–40.

35. Sola D, Rossi L, Schianca GP, Maffioli P, Bigliocca M, Mella R, Corliano F, Fra GP, Bartoli E, Derosa G. Sulfonylureas and their use in clinical practice. Arch Med Sci. 2015;11(4):840–8.

36. Miralles-Linares F, Puerta-Fernandez S, Bernal-Lopez MR, Tinahones FJ, Andrade RJ, Gomez-Huelgas R. Metformin-induced hepatotoxicity. Diabetes Care. 2012;35(3):e21.

37. Lumeng CN, DelProposto JB, Westcott DJ, Saltiel AR. Phenotypic switching of adipose tissue macrophages with obesity is generated by spatiotemporal differences in macrophage subtypes. Diabetes. 2008; 57(12):3239–46.

38. de Luca C, Olefsky JM. Inflammation and insulin resistance. FEBS Lett. 2008; 582(1):97–105.

39. Mohamed-Ali V, Goodrick S, Rawesh A, Katz DR, Miles JM, Yudkin JS, Klein S, Coppack SW. Subcutaneous adipose tissue releases interleukin-6, but not tumor necrosis factor-alpha, in vivo. J Clin Endocrinol Metab. 1997;82(12): 4196–200.

12

Differential genome-wide profiling of alternative polyadenylation sites in nasopharyngeal carcinoma by high-throughput sequencing

Ya-Fei Xu[2†], Ying-Qing Li[1†], Na Liu[1], Qing-Mei He[1], Xin-Ran Tang[1], Xin Wen[1], Xiao-Jing Yang[1], Ying Sun[1], Jun Ma[1*] and Ling-Long Tang[1*]

Abstract

Background: Alternative polyadenylation (APA) is a widespread phenomenon in the posttranscriptional regulation of gene expression that generates mRNAs with alternative 3'-untranslated regions (3'UTRs). APA contributes to the pathogenesis of various diseases, including cancer. However, the potential role of APA in the development of nasopharyngeal carcinoma (NPC) remains largely unknown.

Methods: A strategy of sequencing APA sites (SAPAS) based on second-generation sequencing technology was carried out to explore the global patterns of APA sites and identify genes with tandem 3'UTRs in samples from 6 NPC and 6 normal nasopharyngeal epithelial tissue (NNET). Sequencing results were then validated using quantitative RT-PCR in a larger cohort of 16 NPC and 16 NNET samples.

Results: The sequencing data showed that the use of tandem APA sites was prevalent in NPC, and numerous genes with APA-switching events were discovered. In total, we identified 195 genes with significant differences in the tandem 3'UTR length between NPC and NNET; including 119 genes switching to distal poly (A) sites and 76 genes switching to proximal poly (A) sites. Several gene ontology (GO) terms were enriched in the list of genes with switched APA sites, including regulation of cell migration, macromolecule catabolic process, protein catabolic process, proteolysis, small conjugating protein ligase activity, and ubiquitin-protein ligase activity.

Conclusions: APA site-switching events are prevalent in NPC. APA-mediated regulation of gene expression may play an important role in the development of NPC, and more detailed studies targeting genes with APA-switching events may contribute to the development of novel future therapeutic strategies for NPC.

Keywords: Alternative polyadenylation, Genome-wide profiling, High-throughput sequencing, Nasopharyngeal carcinoma

Background

Nasopharyngeal carcinoma (NPC) is an epithelial malignancy of the head and neck with a highly unbalanced ethnic and geographic distribution. It occurs mainly in Southern China and Southeast Asia, where the incidence can be as high as 20 to 50 cases per 100,000 person-years [1–3]. Although the 5-year overall survival rate is approximately 60% [4] and has increased with the advent of intensity-modulated radiation therapy [5], the prognosis of NPC is still very poor due to recurrence or/and distant metastasis [6]. The etiology of NPC is multi-factorial; including genetic components, Epstein-Barr virus (EBV) infection, environmental factors, and interactions between these factors [7–9]. Among these factors, genetic components play a vital role in the development of NPC and various genes related to NPC have been identified [10–13]. However,

* Correspondence: majun2@mail.sysu.edu.cn; tangll@sysucc.org.cn
†Ya-Fei Xu and Ying-Qing Li contributed equally to this work.
[1]Sun Yat-sen University Cancer Center; State Key Laboratory of Oncology in South China; Collaborative Innovation Center for Cancer Medicine; Guangdong Key Laboratory of Nasopharyngeal Carcinoma Diagnosis and Therapy, Guangzhou 510060, People's Republic of China
Full list of author information is available at the end of the article

genomic abnormalities in NPC tumorigenesis remain largely unidentified. It is particularly important that the genomic foundations of NPC are clearly defined to identify genes contributing to the initiation and progression of NPC, and further guide the development of novel therapeutic strategies for NPC patients.

Posttranscriptional regulation at the mRNA level is generally mediated by miRNAs and RNA-binding proteins which recognize and bind to elements within the 3′-untranslated region (3′UTR). Dysregulation of this can perturb gene expression and contribute to the pathogenesis of various diseases, including several types of cancer [14, 15]. The eukaryotic transcriptome is particularly complicated due to its use of alternative polyadenylation (APA) sites, which can generate diverse mRNA isoforms from a single gene that differ either in their coding sequence, their 3′UTRs, or both [16]. APA is a widespread phenomenon, with more than half of the genes in humans and over 30% in mice having numerous APA sites [17]. Recent studies have shown that APA-switching events may occur in a tissue- or disease-specific manner [18]. The mRNA transcripts in placenta, ovaries and blood are characterized by preferential usage of proximal poly(A) sites (generating isoforms with shorter 3′UTRs), whereas in nervous system and brain, they tend to use distal poly(A) sites (generating isoforms with longer 3′UTRs) [19].

Tandem 3′UTRs can also affect mRNA stability, translation efficiency, and subcellular localization by causing loss of regulatory elements, especially miRNA binding sites in the 3′UTR [20–22]. APA-switching events can influence a number of critical biological processes, including embryonic development and cell differentiation [23–25], cell proliferation [26, 27], immune response [22], neuron activation [28, 29], and tumorigenesis [27, 30–32]. It has been shown that activated T lymphocytes [22] and cancer cells [27] generally use shorter 3′UTRs, and that shortening of tandem 3′UTRs is associated with cell proliferation [22] while the lengthening of tandem 3′UTRs has been observed during cell differentiation [24, 33]. study by Mayr et al. showed that shortening of tandem 3′UTRs was preferentially used by several oncogenes in cancer cell lines [27], suggesting APA-mediated gene expression may play an important role in cancer development. Recent studies also reported that APA-switching events occurred in various types of cancer, including breast cancer [30], colorectal carcinoma [32], glioblastoma [34], and gastric cancer [35]. Nevertheless, whether APA-switching events are integral to the development and progression of NPC remains unknown.

In this study, for the first time, we performed genome-wide profiling of APA sites, with a sequencing APA sites (SAPAS) technology using second-generation sequencing, in NPC and normal nasopharyngeal epithelial tissues (NNET) to identify genes with 3′UTR switching that participate in NPC development. Gene Ontology (GO) and pathway analysis were performed to better understand the function of genes with 3′UTR switching. Subsequently, we validated our sequencing results by quantitative RT-PCR in a larger sample size. Our research provides a novel insight into the tumorigenesis of NPC.

Methods

Clinical specimens

Sixteen NPC fresh tissue samples were collected at the Department of Radiation Oncology of Sun Yat-sen University Cancer Center (Guangzhou, China) between 16 Jan 2010 and 25 Feb 2013. All samples were reassessed by two pathologists and the percentage of tumor cells was 70% or more in all samples. None of the patients had received radiotherapy or chemotherapy before biopsy sampling. 16 NNET tissue samples were collected from outpatients, showed no evidence of cancer, and the tissue samples showed normal histology. This study was approved by the Human Ethics Approval Committee at Sun Yat-sen University Cancer Center. Written informed consent was obtained from each study subject.

RNA extraction

Total RNA was extracted using TRIzol reagent (Life Technologies, Grand Island, NY, USA) according to the manufacturer's instructions. Genomic DNA was removed from total RNA by TURBO DNase (Ambion, Austin, TX, USA). The quantity of RNA was determined using a NanoDrop2000 spectrophotometer (Thermo Scientific, Wilmington, DE, USA) and RNA purity was assessed by the ratio of absorbance at 260 and 280 nm. RNA quality was assessed using electrophoresis in a 1.5% agarose gel stained with ethidium bromide.

Construction of the 3′UTR library

The SAPAS sequencing libraries were constructed as described previously [30, 36]. In brief, total RNA was randomly fragmented by heating. The first strand cDNA was generated by a template-switch reverse transcription (RT) reaction, in which contains an anchored oligo d(T) primer, a 5′ template switching adaptor, and Super-Script II kits (Invitrogen Life Technologies, Karlsruhe, Germany). Then, ds-cDNA was amplified by PCR using known primers tagged with Illumina adaptors. The sequences of all primers were consistent with previous studies [30, 37]. PAGE gel-excision was carried out to select the PCR products with the fragments of 300-500 bp with a QIAquick Gel Extraction Kit (Qiagen, Valencia, CA). The final pooled fragments were sequenced from their 3′end on the Illumina HiSeq 2000 system in dark cycle mode. Finally 58 bp reads were generated.

Illumina reads filtering and mapping

Reads were filtered and trimmed with in-house Perl-scripts, and the trimmed reads were aligned to the human genome (hg19) with Bowtie. Internal priming filtering was performed by analyzing the genomic sequences located 1 to 20 bases downstream of poly(A) cleavage sites, containing the sequence motifs 5'-AAAAAAAA-3', 5'-GAAAA +GAAA+G-3' ("+" means "or more"), or more than 12 "A"s. Sites with only one read were removed.

Poly(A) sites identification and annotation

Cleavage sites were clustered into poly(A) sites as described previously [17, 30]. Briefly, the reads of which 3' ends located within 24 nt from each other and which aligned to the same strand of a chromosome were clustered. Then, cleavage clusters with two or more reads were assigned as poly(A) sites. Next, poly(A) sites were grouped into three types according to the known poly(A) sites in the UCSC transcript ends database [38] and Tian's database [17]: 1) UCSC known genes, where the poly(A) site was located within 24 nt from the 3' transcription end of a UCSC gene; 2) Tian poly(A) DB, where the poly(A) site was located within 24 nt from a poly(A) site in Tian's poly(A) DB; 3) Putative novel poly(A) sites, containing the following six attributes: 3'UTR; located <= 1 kb nt downstream of a UCSC gene; CDS; intron; intergenic; and non-coding gene. Meanwhile, poly(A) sites with reads that overlapped Ensemble-annotated 3'UTR(s) were defined as tandem poly(A) sites. The expression of mRNAs were accumulated by reads of all poly(A) sites, and then the differential expressed genes were identified by edgeR [39]. The raw sequencing data can be accessed from the NCBI Bioproject (http://www.ncbi.nlm.nih.gov/bioproject) under accession no. PRJNA299088.

3'UTR switching analysis between NPC and NNET and functional annotation

3'UTR switching of each gene between 6 NPC and 6 NNET tissues was detected by a pair-wise case-control analysis, which sequentially compared NPC samples to NNET samples to identify genes with 3'UTR switching in each pair. They were then filtered using the Benjamini-Hochberg false discovery rate (FDR), whereby those estimated to be below 0.01 (using R software, version 2.15) were kept. In total, genes with 3'UTR switching that occurrences in more than 10 pairs were defined as genes with tandem 3'UTR between NPC and NNET. Functional annotation analysis of these genes was performed using DAVID Bio-informatics Resources (http://david.abcc.ncifcrf.gov/) [40]. The miRNA targets involved in APA-switching events were identified by TargetScan database [41].

Validation of quantitative RT-PCR analysis

To validate the sequencing data, quantitative RT-PCR was carried out in 16 NPC and 16 NNET tissues for eight genes (JAG1, IRF1, EGLN1, TIMP3, WDR5, SMAD3, FNDC3B, and XRCC5) with extreme 3'UTR length differences between NPC and NNET. Based on SAPAS data, the poly(A) sites of each gene were divided into two supersites: "proximal sites" and "distal sites". Two gene-specific primer sets were specifically designed for "proximal sites" and "distal sites", as described previously [30]. Primer sequences are listed in Additional file 1. The quantitative RT-PCR was performed on the CFX96TouchTM sequence detection system (Bio-Rad, Hercules, CA, USA) using Platinum SYBR Green qPCR SuperMix-UDG reagents (Invitrogen) according to the manufacturer's instructions. GAPDH was used as a control for normalization. For each gene, the relative expression ratio of the proximal site to the distal site was calculated using the $2^{-\Delta\Delta CT}$ method [42].

Statistical analysis

SPSS 16.0 software was used for statistical analysis. All of the data were presented as the mean ± SD. The Student's t-test was used to determine whether significant differences existed in the usage of poly(A) sites of genes between two groups, and two-tailed $P < 0.05$ was considered significant.

Results

Global deep sequencing of 3' ends of mRNA

We used the SAPAS strategy to profile APA sites of 6 NPC and 6 NNET tissues. In total, 20.99 to 26.97 million raw reads with lengths of 58 bp were obtained from Illumina sequencing. A statistical summary of the data is shown in Table 1. Approximately 20.83 to 26.64 million reads harbored the modified anchor oligo d(T), of which 13.02 to 15.71 million reads uniquely mapped to the human nucleus genome (hg19) [43]. Furthermore, 9.83 to 12.68 million reads that could be used directly to infer transcript cleavage sites were obtained after filtering the reads with internal priming. In total, 21,095 UCSC canonical genes were sequenced by at least one read, which accounted for 27.2% of all canonical genes.

A comprehensive inventory of poly(A) sites

As shown in Fig. 1a, the majority of filtered reads (82.17%) were mapped to known poly(A) sites listed in the UCSC transcripts ends database [38] and Tian's database [17]. An additional 5.49% and 1.29% of reads were mapped to the 3'UTR and 1 kb region downstream from the UCSC canonical genes, respectively. The distribution of the number of all reads is shown in Fig. 1b. As a result of the heterogeneity of cleavage sites at poly(A) sites, we took the cleavage clusters with more than one

Table 1 Summary of the SAPAS data from Illumina HiSeq 2000 sequencing

	NPC						NNET					
	NPC1	NPC2	NPC3	NPC4	NPC5	NPC6	NNET1	NNET2	NNET3	NNET4	NNET5	NNET6
Raw reads(M*)	26.08	23.81	24.48	25.29	25.14	20.99	25.94	23.91	25.77	24.87	26.97	24.56
Clean reads(M)	25.90	23.54	24.06	24.94	24.94	20.83	25.77	23.59	25.33	24.70	26.64	24.42
Mapped to genome(M)	21.73	19.75	20.02	21.06	21.39	17.45	21.28	19.49	21.09	19.53	19.46	21.10
Uniquely mapped to genome(M)	17.02	16.42	16.11	16.82	17.29	14.33	17.45	15.87	17.75	16.17	15.72	17.48
Mapped to nuclear genome(M)	13.32	14.63	13.11	13.02	14.69	13.34	15.21	14.45	15.71	14.57	13.92	14.76
Passed Internal Priming filter(M)	11.51	9.83	10.18	10.30	12.68	11.36	12.00	11.47	10.01	12.50	12.06	12.36
Genes sampled by reads(10 K)	1.78	1.89	1.88	1.90	1.80	1.83	1.86	1.88	1.91	1.88	1.73	1.87
Poly(A) sites(10 K)	13.70	29.99	17.36	19.04	13.82	12.50	22.75	18.14	36.03	16.28	12.45	14.90
Known poly(A) sites sampled(10 K)	2.75	2.90	2.89	2.89	2.82	2.87	2.84	2.92	2.86	2.97	2.67	2.90
Putative novel poly(A) sites(10 K)	10.95	27.09	14.47	16.15	11.00	9.63	19.91	15.21	33.17	13.31	9.78	12.01
Genes sampled by poly(A) sites(10 K)	1.62	1.72	1.71	1.73	1.63	1.66	1.73	1.72	1.73	1.72	1.53	1.72

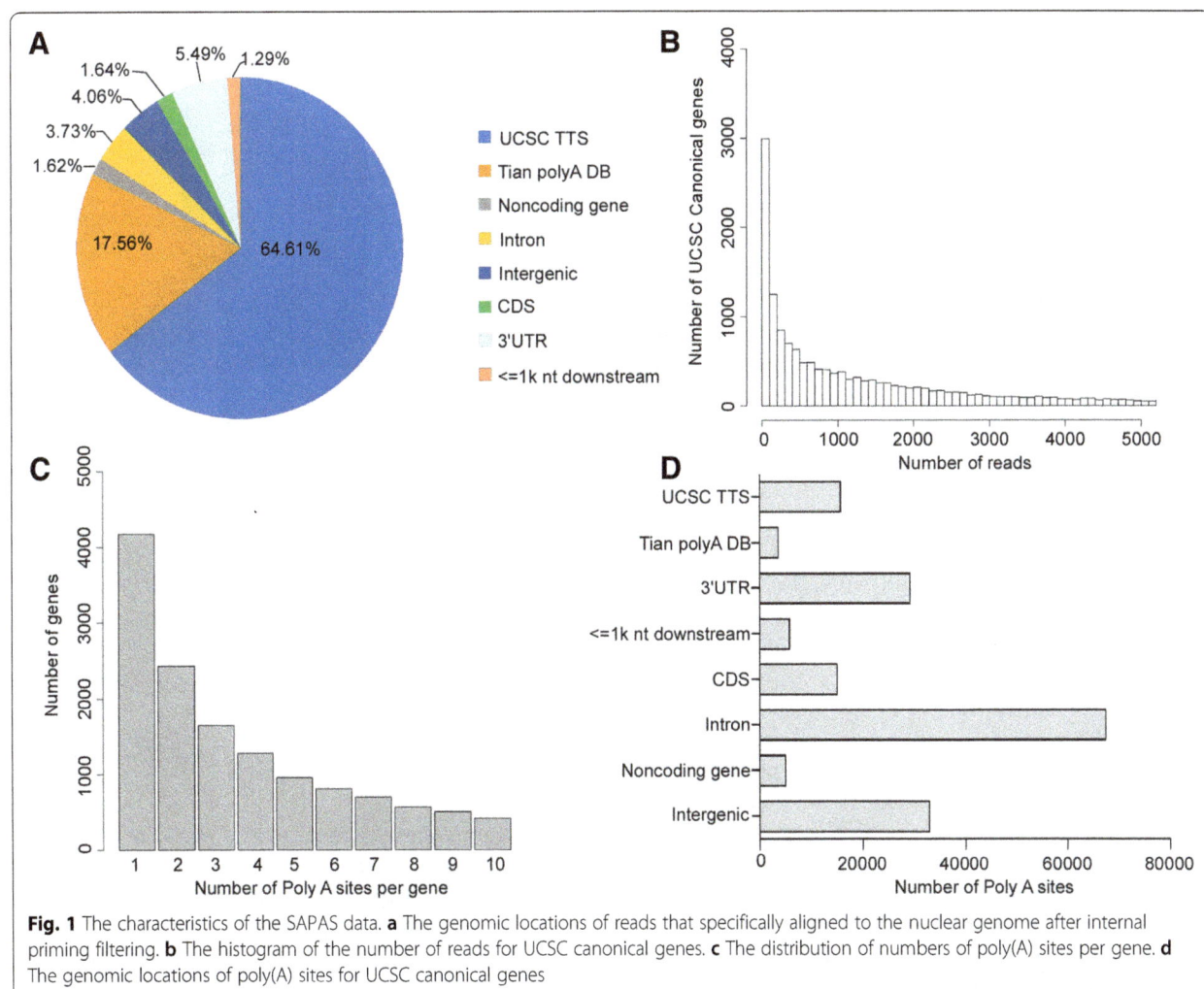

Fig. 1 The characteristics of the SAPAS data. **a** The genomic locations of reads that specifically aligned to the nuclear genome after internal priming filtering. **b** The histogram of the number of reads for UCSC canonical genes. **c** The distribution of numbers of poly(A) sites per gene. **d** The genomic locations of poly(A) sites for UCSC canonical genes

read as poly(A) sites. We observed that 13,181 genes had more than one tandem APA site, among which 10,753 genes harbored more than two tandem APA sites (Fig. 1c). In total, 174,931 poly(A) sites were identified from all twelve samples. Only 11.04% of these sites were found in the UCSC and Tian databases. Another 16.78% of the poly(A) sites were found in the 3'UTRs, 3.31% within 1 kb downstream from the UCSC canonical genes,18.86% in intergenic, 38.57% in intron, 2.87% in noncoding genes, and 8.56% in CDS from the UCSC canonical genes (Fig. 1d).

Differential usage of poly(A) between NPC and NNET

Previous studies have demonstrated that most cancer cells [27] and cancer tissues [31, 32] tend to use shortened 3'UTRs. In contrast to these results for primary cancers, however, one study reported that a greater number of genes with lengthened 3'UTRs existed in a metastasis cell line [30]. In our study, the 3'UTR length of each gene was calculated according to the distance between the poly(A) sites and the stop codon. Subsequently, a pair-wise case-control analysis between NPC and NNET tissues was performed, and a total of 36 pairs were obtained. 3'UTR switching for each gene within each pair was detected using a test of linear trend alternative to independence [44]. A positive Pearson correlation coefficient (r) indicates that NPC tissue contains more lengthened tandem 3'UTRs than NNET, while a negative indicates that NPC tissue harbors more shortened tandem 3'UTRs. The genes with 3'UTR switching between NPC and NNET obtained for each pair are shown in Table 2. We further analyzed the 3'UTR switching frequency for each gene in 36 pairs and found that the frequency of the genes with 3'UTR switching was the highest in at least 10 pairs (Additional file 2). Therefore, we set 10 pairs as the selection criteria for further screening of genes with 3'UTR switching. As a result, we identified 195 genes with significantly different 3'UTR lengths (false discovery rate [FDR] < 0.01, $P <$ 0.01), of which 119 genes switched to longer 3'UTRs and 76 genes switched to shorter 3'UTRs in NPC. Details of the 195 genes with significant differences between NPC and NNET are shown in Additional file 3.

Functional annotation analysis of the genes with switched APA sites

To explore the biological significance of these APA site-switching genes, a functional annotation of the above 195 genes was performed with Database for Annotation, Visualization and Integrated Discovery (DAVID) Bio-informatics Resources, where single-UTR genes were set as the background. The results of Gene Ontology (GO) terms analysis showed that genes with tandem 3'UTRs were mainly enriched in the regulation

Table 2 Genes with APA site switching between NPC and NNET tissues using a pair-wise case-control analysis

Pairs	3'UTR shortened genes	3'UTR lengthened genes	Combined
NPC1 vs. NNET1	104	372	476
NPC1 vs. NNET2	179	192	371
NPC1 vs. NNET3	144	247	391
NPC1 vs. NNET4	58	242	300
NPC1 vs. NNET5	99	446	545
NPC1 vs. NNET6	51	123	174
NPC2 vs. NNET1	55	85	140
NPC2 vs. NNET2	91	13	104
NPC2 vs. NNET3	108	38	146
NPC2 vs. NNET4	100	85	185
NPC2 vs. NNET5	123	234	357
NPC2 vs. NNET6	184	106	290
NPC3 vs. NNET1	63	143	206
NPC3 vs. NNET2	104	23	127
NPC3 vs. NNET3	51	26	77
NPC3 vs. NNET4	79	103	182
NPC3 vs. NNET5	68	178	246
NPC3 vs. NNET6	149	111	260
NPC4 vs. NNET1	62	167	229
NPC4 vs. NNET2	210	104	314
NPC4 vs. NNET3	136	115	251
NPC4 vs. NNET4	158	236	394
NPC4 vs. NNET5	156	355	511
NPC4 vs. NNET6	133	125	258
NPC5 vs. NNET1	158	377	535
NPC5 vs. NNET2	193	116	309
NPC5 vs. NNET3	150	153	303
NPC5 vs. NNET4	55	112	167
NPC5 vs. NNET5	107	286	393
NPC5 vs. NNET6	66	82	148
NPC6 vs. NNET1	102	202	304
NPC6 vs. NNET2	137	24	161
NPC6 vs. NNET3	147	99	246
NPC6 vs. NNET4	53	58	111
NPC6 vs. NNET5	90	172	262
NPC6 vs. NNET6	139	76	215

of cell migration, macromolecule catabolic process, protein catabolic process, proteolysis, small conjugating protein ligase activity, and ubiquitin-protein ligase activity (Table 3). Additionally, genes with tandem 3'UTRs involved in the ubiquitin-mediated proteolysis pathway ($P = 0.022$), lysosomepathway ($P = 0.048$), colorectal

Table 3 Enrichment of genes with tandemed 3'UTR isoforms involved in various GO functional categories

GO category		Count	P-value
GOTERM_BP_FAT	Regulation of cell migration	9	0.0004
GOTERM_BP_FAT	Regulation of locomotion	9	0.001
GOTERM_BP_FAT	Regulation of cell motion	9	0.001
GOTERM_BP_FAT	Macromolecule catabolic process	19	0.0015
GOTERM_BP_FAT	Protein catabolic process	16	0.0024
GOTERM_BP_FAT	Proteolysis	20	0.015
GOTERM_MF_FAT	Small conjugating protein ligase activity	7	0.0052
GOTERM_MF_FAT	Acid-amino acid ligase activity	7	0.013
GOTERM_MF_FAT	Ubiquitin-protein ligase activity	6	0.013
KEGG_PATHWAY	Ubiquitin mediated proteolysis	6	0.022
KEGG_PATHWAY	Lysosome	5	0.048
KEGG_PATHWAY	Colorectal cancer	5	0.017
KEGG_PATHWAY	Renal cell carcinoma	4	0.049

cancer($P = 0.017$) and renal cell carcinoma pathway ($P = 0.049$) were enriched (Table 3). We also performed GO analysis and pathway enrichment analysis by separating the 195 genes into two groups (switching to distal poly(A) and proximal poly(A)), and results were showed in Additional files 4, 5. Since distant metastasis occurs in 20–30% of NPC patients and is the major cause of death in NPC [6], it is noteworthy that we identified 9 genes with enriched tandem 3'UTRs that are involved in the regulation of cell migration; namely *SMAD3*, *JAG1*, *Pikr1*, *Ptp4a1*, *Rac1*, *RRAS2*, *Spag9*, *TRIP6*, and *TRIB1* (Table 4). These results indicate APA site-switching events can influence a number of critical biological processes and may play an important role in the development of NPC.

The effects of APA-site switching events on gene expression and miRNA targeting sites

To further explore the functional effects of APA-site switching events, we firstly analyzed the relationship between the APA switched sites and the mRNA levels of 195 genes. A total of 275 genes with significant differences in the mRNA levels between NPC and NNET were identified, including 198 genes that were up-regulated and 77 genes that were down-regulated in NPC (Additional file 6). Further analyses revealed that among the 119 genes that switched to longer 3'UTRs in NPC, 4 genes were up-regulated and none was down-regulated; and among the 76 genes that switched to shorter 3'UTRs, only one gene was found to be up-regulated or down-regulated in NPC (Additional file 7).

Table 4 Nine genes enriched in GO terms associated with cell migration

UCSC ID	Gene Symbol	Gene Name	r-value
uc002aqj.2	SMAD3[a]	SMAD family member 3	0.086
uc002wnw.2	JAG1[a]	jagged 1 (Alagille syndrome)	−0.351
uc003jva.2	Pikr1	phosphoinositide-3-kinase, regulatory subunit 1 (alpha)	0.0007
uc003pek.2	Ptp4a1	protein tyrosine phosphatase type IVA, member 1	0.929
uc003spw.2	Rac1	ras-related C3 botulinum toxin substrate 1 (rho family, small GTP binding protein Rac1)	0.175
uc009ygq.2	RRAS2	related RAS viral (r-ras) oncogene homolog 2; similar to related RAS viral (r-ras) oncogene homolog 2	−0.564
uc002ita.2	Spag9	sperm associated antigen 9	0.411
uc003uww.2	TRIP6	thyroid hormone receptor interactor 6	0.182
uc003yrx.2	TRIB1	tribbles homolog 1 (Drosophila)	−0.206

[a]genes selected for quantitative RT-PCR validation
r-value: a positive value of r indicates a longer tandem 3'UTR in NPC, and vice versa

These results suggest that the APA-site switching events could not change the mRNA expression levels, and it may affect the translation efficiency and subcellular localization by causing loss of regulatory elements, especially miRNA binding sites in the 3'UTR.

Furthermore, we identified potential miRNA targeting sites between the "proximal polyA sites" and "distal polyA sites" of 195 genes using the publicly available databases TargetScan to explore the effect of APA-switching events on the gain-of or loss-of miRNA targeting sites in their 3'UTR. The results showed that for the 119 genes switched to longer 3'UTRs in NPC, totally 706 miRNA targeting sites were gained and for the 76 genes switched to shorter 3'UTRs in NPC, totally 325 miRNA targeting sites were lost (Additional file 8). These result suggests that APA-switching events can result in the gain or loss of miRNA binding sites in the 3'UTR in the development of NPC.

Real-time RT-PCR validation of selected APA switched sites

To further validate the SAPAS sequencing data, we randomly selected eight genes (*JAG1*, *IRF1*, *EGLN1*, *TIMP3*, *WDR5*, *SMAD3*, *FNDC3B*, and *XRCC5*) with switched APA sites for quantitative RT-PCR validation in 16 NPC and 16 NNET samples. Results of six genes were similar to the sequencing data (Fig. 2). *JAG1*, *IRF1*, *EGLN1*, *WDR5*, and *SMAD3* tended to use lengthened 3'UTR transcripts, whereas *FNDC3B* tended to use shortened 3'UTR transcripts ($P < 0.05$). Consistent with the sequencing data, there appeared to be a higher tendency for lengthened 3'UTR transcripts from the genes *TIMP3* and *XRCC5* to be present in NPC than NNET, however no statistical differences were observed. These tendencies suggest that APA-switching events were more prevalent in NPC tissues.

Discussion

APA allows a single gene to encode multiple mRNA transcripts by changing the mRNA 3'UTR length and plays an important role in various physiological and pathological processes, including tumorigenesis [27, 30, 45, 46]. In this study, we performed genome-wide profiling of tandem APA sites in NPC and NNET tissues using SAPAS based on second-generation sequencing technology. In total, we identified 195 genes whose tandem 3'UTR length differed significantly between NPC and NNET, including 119 genes switching to distal poly(A) sites and 76 genes switching to proximal poly(A) sites. Several gene ontology (GO) terms were enriched in the list of genes with switched APA sites, including regulation of cell migration, macromolecule catabolic process, protein catabolic process, proteolysis, small conjugating protein ligase

activity, and ubiquitin-protein ligase activity. The sequencing results were further validated using quantitative RT-PCR.

APA, which leads to alterations in 3'UTR length and content of genes, shows dynamic characteristics in a variety of tumors. A previous analysis of 27 cancer cell lines derived from sarcomas and breast, lung and colon cancers showed that tumor cells generally use the shorter 3'UTRs [27]. Similarly, Lin et al. found that shorter 3'UTRs isoforms were preferentially upregulated in breast, colon, kidney, liver and lung cancer tissues [31]. Likewise, Morriset al. demonstrated that more genes tended to use shorter 3'UTRs isoforms in colorectal carcinoma compared to colorectal adenoma and normal colon mucosa [32]. However, a recent discovery showed that longer 3'UTRs isoforms were significantly upregulated in MB231, a human breast cancer line that is estrogen independent and highly invasive [30]. Nordlund et al. demonstrated that more genes preferentially used longer 3'UTRs in acute lymphoblastic leukemia [47]. These findings suggest that APA-switching events are more complicated and may occur in a tissue- or disease-specific manner. In this study, we found that 119 genes tended to use longer 3'UTRs and 76 genes tended to use shorter 3'UTRs in NPC, which is the first genome-wide research to investigate APA in NPC.

Furthermore, 3'UTRs harbor several cis-elements, such as U-rich elements (USE), poly A signals (PAS), ARE (AU-rich elements), cytoplasmic polyadenylation elements, miRNA target sites and other unknown elements [46]. Therefore, APA-induced alterations in 3'UTR length and content may result in loss or gain of these regulatory motifs, resulting in series of changes in cell biological function by affecting mRNA stability, transcript export and translation efficiency [48]. Recent studies have revealed that shorter 3'UTRs could lead to greater mRNA stability and increased protein output, and were also associated with elevated cell proliferation rates or transformation [27]. In this study, we identified 195 genes with tandem 3'UTRs isoforms, which were involved in various cellular biological functions, including regulation of cell migration, macromolecule catabolic processes, protein catabolic processes, proteolysis, small conjugating protein ligase activity, and ubiquitin-protein ligase activity. This result is not unexpected because it has been confirmed that metastasis occurs in 20–30% of NPC patients and is the major cause of death in NPC [6]. It is important to note that our study effectively identified genes that were involved in NPC tumorigenesis.

To date, several possible mechanisms have been reported to influence the regulation of APA-switching events. Previous studies have demonstrated that the usage of APA could be influenced by the expression level of genes encoding 3'-end-processing factors and the

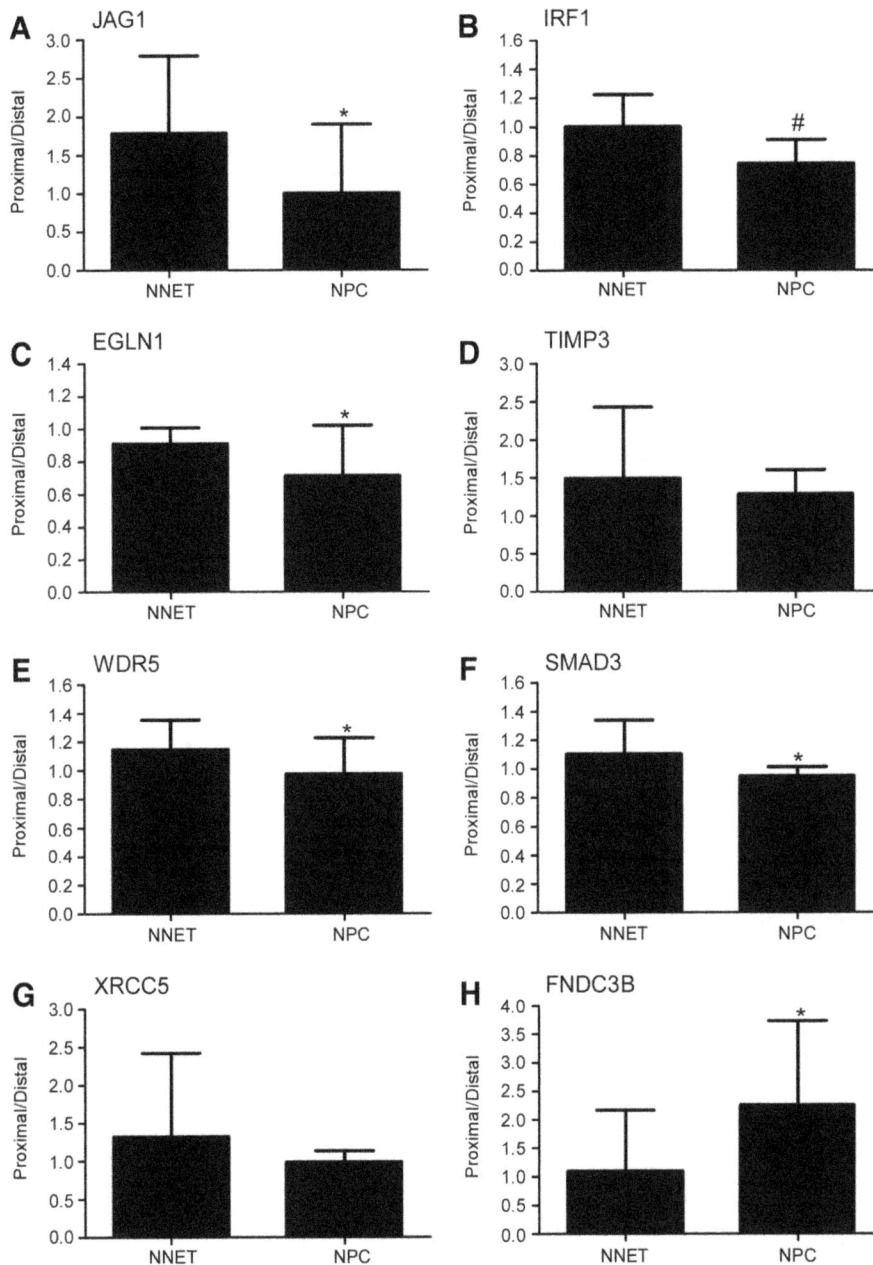

Fig. 2 Validation of 3'UTR switching in 16 NPC and NNET samples with quantitative RT-PCR. **a** *JAG1*; (B) *IRF1*; (**c**) *EGLN1*; (**d**) *TIMP3*; (**e**) *WDR5*; (**f**) *SMAD3*; (**g**) *XRCC5*; (**h**) *FNDC3B*. Proximal/Distal indicates the expression ratio of the shortened 3'UTR to the lengthened 3'UTR

transcription rate of polymerase II [45]. In other studies, differential selection of APA could be ascribed to the strength of different poly(A) signals (weak or strong), and the expression levels of cleavage and polyadenylation specificity factor and cleavage-stimulating factor [49–52]. Furthermore, poly(A)-binding protein nuclear 1, a general factor of polyadenylation, could prevent the usage of proximal poly(A) sites by direct binding to non-canonical poly(A) signals [53–55]. Moreover, the different usage of APA could change the 3'UTR length and content, leading to the loss or gain of regulatory motifs, including miRNA binding sites [20]. In our study, we found that the APA-site switching events could not change the mRNA expression levels, and it could result in the gain or loss of miRNA binding sites in the 3'UTR. For the 119 genes switched to longer 3'UTRs in NPC, totally 706 miRNA targeting sites were gained; and for the 76 genes switched to shorter 3'UTRs, totally 325 miRNA targeting sites were lost. Among them, FNDC3B was identified as the direct and functional target of miR-143 in liver and prostate cancer [56, 57]. In our study, we found that FNDC3B tended to use proximal APA sites and produced mRNAs with shorter 3'UTRs in NPC. Interesting, we noticed that only the longer 3'UTRs harbored the binding sites of miR-143, suggesting that shorter mRNA transcripts can escape from miR-143 regulation. In addition, Zhang et al. reported that *SMAD3* was a direct and functional target of miR-23b [58]. Here, we found that *SMAD3* was prone to using distal APA sites and produced mRNAs with longer 3'UTRs in NPC and using bioinformatics analysis we confirmed that only the longer 3'UTRs harbored the binding sites of miR-23b [59]. These findings provide new insights into how APA mediate the miRNA regulation of gene expression and further affect cell biological function.

Conclusions

In summary, APA site-switching of 3'UTRs are prevalent in NPC, and APA-mediated regulation of gene expression may play important roles in NPC development and progression. Several GO terms and pathways were enriched in genes that undergo APA-switching events, including regulation of cell migration, macromolecule catabolic process, protein catabolic process, proteolysis, small conjugating protein ligase activity, and ubiquitin-protein ligase activity. These findings suggest that more detailed studies targeted genes undergoing APA site-switching events may provide novel insights into clarifying the pathogenesis of NPC and contribute to the development of novel therapeutic strategies for NPC.

Additional files

Additional file 1: PCR primers used in quantitative RT-PCR for APA switching genes (PDF 134 kb)

Additional file 2: The frequency distribution of the genes with lengthened 3'UTR (A) and shortened 3'UTR (B) in different pairs, comparing NPC and NNET. (PDF 123 kb)

Additional file 3: Details of the 195 genes with significant differences in 3'UTR lengths between NPC and NNET. (XLSX 96 kb)

Additional file 4: Enrichment of genes with shortened 3'UTR isoforms involved in various GO functional categories. (PDF 144 kb)

Additional file 5: Enrichment of genes with lengthened 3'UTR isoforms involved in various GO functional categories. (PDF 63 kb)

Additional file 6: Details of the 275 genes with significant differences in the mRNA levels between NPC and NNET. (XLSX 94 kb)

Additional file 7: The effect of APA switching events on gene expression. "Blue" and "red" colors indicate up-regulated or down-regulated genes; "Green" and "yellow" colors indicate genes that switched to longer or shorter 3'UTRs. (PDF 200 kb)

Additional file 8: The gain or loss of miRNA binding sites in the 3'UTR of genes with APA-switching events. (XLSX 26 kb)

Acknowledgements
We greatly appreciated the help of Hailiang Liu (CapitalBio Genomics Co., Ltd) for next generation sequencing data analysis.

Funding
This work was supported by grants from the National Natural Science Foundation of China (81572962, 81802705); the Natural Science Funding of Shenzhen (JCYJ20160422091914681); the Natural Science Foundation of Guang Dong Province (2017A030312003, 2017A030310468); the Health & Medical Collaborative Innovation Project of Guangzhou City, China (201803040003); the Innovation Team Development Plan of the Ministry of Education (IRT_17R110); and the Overseas Expertise Introduction Project for Discipline Innovation (B14035).

Authors' contributions
LLT, JM, and YFX were responsible for study design. YFX, YQL, and LLT carried out the bioinformatic analysis of the sequencing data. YFX performed the quantitative RT-PCR, analyzed the results and drafted the manuscript. NL, XRT, XW, YS, JM participated in the data analysis. QMH and XJY collected tissue samples and performed total RNA extraction. All authors have read and approved the final manuscript.

Competing interests
The authors declare that they have no competing interest.

Author details
[1]Sun Yat-sen University Cancer Center; State Key Laboratory of Oncology in South China; Collaborative Innovation Center for Cancer Medicine; Guangdong Key Laboratory of Nasopharyngeal Carcinoma Diagnosis and Therapy, Guangzhou 510060, People's Republic of China. [2]Department of Cell Biology and Genetics, Shenzhen University Health Science Center, Shenzhen 518060, People's Republic of China.

References
1. Yu MC, Yuan JM. Epidemiology of nasopharyngeal carcinoma. Semin Cancer Biol. 2002;12:421–9.
2. Feng BJ, Huang W, Shugart YY, Lee MK, Zhang F, Xia JC, et al. Genome-wide scan for familial nasopharyngeal carcinoma reveals evidence of linkage to chromosome 4. Nat Genet. 2002;31:395_9.
3. Ou SH, Zell JA, Ziogas A, Anton-Culver H. Epidemiology of nasopharyngeal carcinoma in the United States: improved survival of Chinese patients within the keratinizing squamous cell carcinoma histology. Ann Oncol. 2007;18:29–35.
4. Ma J, Mai HQ, Hong MH, Cui NJ, Lu TX, Lu LX, et al. Is the 1997 AJCC staging system for nasopharyngeal carcinoma prognostically useful for Chinese patient populations? Int J Radiat Oncol Biol Phys. 2001;50:1181–9.
5. Xiao WW, Huang SM, Han F, Wu SX, Lu LX, Lin CG, et al. Local control, survival, and late toxicities of locally advanced nasopharyngeal carcinoma treated by simultaneous modulated accelerated radiotherapy combined with cisplatin concurrent chemotherapy: long-term results of a phase 2 study. Cancer. 2011;117:1874_83.
6. Lai SZ, Li WF, Chen L, Luo W, Chen YY, Liu LZ, et al. How does intensity-modulated radiotherapy versus conventional two-dimensional radiotherapy influence the treatment results in nasopharyngeal carcinoma patients? Int J Radiat Oncol Biol Phys. 2011;80:661–8.

7. Lung ML, Cheung AK, Ko JM, Lung HL, Cheng Y, Dai W. The interplay of host genetic factors and Epstein-Barr virus in the development of nasopharyngeal carcinoma. Chin J Cancer. 2014;33:556–68.

8. Xu FH, Xiong D, Xu YF, Cao SM, Xue WQ, Qin HD, et al. An epidemiological and molecular study of the relationship between smoking, risk of nasopharyngeal carcinoma, and Epstein-Barr virus activation. J Natl Cancer Inst. 2012;104:1396–410.

9. Young LS, Dawson CW. Epstein-Barr virus and nasopharyngeal carcinoma. Chin J Cancer. 2014;33:581–90.

10. Bei JX, Li Y, Jia WH, Feng BJ, Zhou G, Chen LZ, et al. A genome-wide association study of nasopharyngeal carcinoma identifies three new susceptibility loci. Nat Genet. 2010;42:599–603.

11. Jia WH, Pan QH, Qin HD, Xu YF, Shen GP, Chen L, et al. A case-control and a family-based association study revealing an association between CYP2E1 polymorphisms and nasopharyngeal carcinoma risk in Cantonese. Carcinogenesis. 2009;30:2031–6.

12. Jiang RC, Qin HD, Zeng MS, Huang W, Feng BJ, Zhang F, et al. A functional variant in the transcriptional regulatory region of gene LOC344967 cosegregates with disease phenotype in familial nasopharyngeal carcinoma. Cancer Res. 2006;66:693–700.

13. Qin HD, Shugart YY, Bei JX, Pan QH, Chen L, Feng QS, et al. Comprehensive pathway-based association study of DNA repair gene variants and the risk of nasopharyngeal carcinoma. Cancer Res. 2011;71:3000–8.

14. Cooper TA, Wan L, Dreyfuss G. RNA and disease. Cell. 2009;136:777–93.

15. Lee SK, Calin GA. Non-coding RNAs and cancer: new paradigms in oncology. Discov Med. 2011;11:245–54.

16. Nilsen TW, Graveley BR. Expansion of the eukaryotic proteome by alternative splicing. Nature. 2010;463:457–63.

17. Tian B, Hu J, Zhang H, Lutz CS. A large-scale analysis of mRNA polyadenylation of human and mouse genes. Nucleic Acids Res. 2005;33:201–12.

18. Xia Z, Donehower LA, Cooper TA, Neilson JR, Wheeler DA, Wagner EJ, et al. Dynamic analyses of alternative polyadenylation from RNA-seq reveal a 3'-UTR landscape across seven tumour types. Nat Commun. 2014;5:5274.

19. Zhang H, Lee JY, Tian B. Biased alternative polyadenylation in human tissues. Genome Biol. 2005;6:R100.

20. Boutet SC, Cheung TH, Quach NL, Liu L, Prescott SL, Edalati A, et al. Alternative polyadenylation mediates microRNA regulation of muscle stem cell function. Cell Stem Cell. 2012;10:327–36.

21. Ribas J, Ni X, Castanares M, Liu MM, Esopi D, Yegnasubramanian S, et al. A novel source for miR-21 expression through the alternative polyadenylation of VMP1 gene transcripts. Nucleic Acids Res. 2012;40:6821–33.

22. Sandberg R, Neilson JR, Sarma A, Sharp PA, Burge CB. Proliferating cells express mRNAs with shortened 3' untranslated regions and fewer microRNA target sites. Science. 2008;320:1643–7.

23. Hilgers V, Perry MW, Hendrix D, Stark A, Levine M, Haley B. Neural-specific elongation of 3' UTRs during Drosophila development. Proc Natl Acad Sci U S A. 2011;108:15864–9.

24. Ji Z, Tian B. Reprogramming of 3' untranslated regions of mRNAs by alternative polyadenylation in generation of pluripotent stem cells from different cell types. PLoS One. 2009;4:e8419.

25. Ulitsky I, Shkumatava A, Jan CH, Subtelny AO, Koppstein D, Bell GW, et al. Extensive alternative polyadenylation during zebrafish development. Genome Res. 2012;22:2054–66.

26. Elkon R, Drost J, van Haaften G, Jenal M, Schrier M, Oude Vrielink JA, et al. E2F mediates enhanced alternative polyadenylation in proliferation. Genome Biol. 2012;13:R59.

27. Mayr C, Bartel DP. Widespread shortening of 3'UTRs by alternative cleavage and polyadenylation activates oncogenes in cancer cells. Cell. 2009;138:673–84.

28. An JJ, Gharami K, Liao GY, Woo NH, Lau AG, Vanevski F, et al. Distinct role of long 3' UTR BDNF mRNA in spine morphology and synaptic plasticity in hippocampal neurons. Cell. 2008;134:175–87.

29. Lau AG, Irier HA, Gu J, Tian D, Ku L, Liu G, et al. Distinct 3'UTRs differentially regulate activity-dependent translation of brain-derived neurotrophic factor (BDNF). Proc Natl Acad Sci U S A. 2010;107:15945–50.

30. Fu Y, Sun Y, Li Y, Li J, Rao X, Chen C, et al. Differential genome-wide profiling of tandem 3' UTRs among human breast cancer and normal cells by high-throughput sequencing. Genome Res. 2011;21:741–7.

31. Lin Y, Li Z, Ozsolak F, Kim SW, Arango-Argoty G, Liu TT, et al. An in-depth map of polyadenylation sites in cancer. Nucleic Acids Res. 2012;40:8460–71.

32. Morris AR, Bos A, Diosdado B, Rooijers K, Elkon R, Bolijn AS, et al. Alternative cleavage and polyadenylation during colorectal cancer development. Clin Cancer Res. 2012;18:5256–66.

33. Shepard PJ, Choi EA, Lu J, Flanagan LA, Hertel KJ, Shi Y. Complex and dynamic landscape of RNA polyadenylation revealed by PAS-Seq. RNA. 2011;17:761–72.

34. Masamha CP, Xia Z, Yang J, Albrecht TR, Li M, Shyu AB, et al. CFIm25 links alternative polyadenylation to glioblastoma tumour suppression. Nature. 2014;510:412–6.

35. Lai DP, Tan S, Kang YN, Wu J, Ooi HS, Chen J, et al. Genome-wide profiling of polyadenylation sites reveals a link between selective polyadenylation and cancer metastasis. Hum Mol Genet. 2015;24:3410–7.

36. Li Y, Sun Y, Fu Y, Li M, Huang G, Zhang C, et al. Dynamic landscape of tandem 3' UTRs during zebrafish development. Genome Res. 2012;22:1899–906.

37. Tian P, Sun Y, Li Y, Liu X, Wan L, Li J, et al. A global analysis of tandem 3'UTRs in eosinophilic chronic rhinosinusitis with nasal polyps. PLoS One. 2012;7:e48997.

38. Rhead B, Karolchik D, Kuhn RM, Hinrichs AS, Zweig AS, Fujita PA, et al. The UCSC genome browser database: update 2010. Nucleic Acids Res. 2010;38:D613–9.

39. Robinson MD, McCarthy DJ, Smyth GK. edgeR: a Bioconductor package for differential expression analysis of digital gene expression data. Bioinformatics. 2010;26:139–40.

40. Huang da W, Sherman BT, Lempicki RA. Systematic and integrative analysis of large gene lists using DAVID bioinformatics resources. Nat Protoc. 2009;4:44–57.

41. Lewis BP, Burge CB, Bartel DP. Conserved seed pairing, often flanked by adenosines of human genes are microRNA targets. Cell. 2005;120:15–20.

42. Livak KJ, Schmittgen TD. Analysis of relative gene expression data using real-time quantitative PCR and the 2(−Delta Delta C(T)) method. Methods. 2001;25:402–8.

43. Langmead B, Trapnell C, Pop M, Salzberg SL. Ultrafast and memory-efficient alignment of short DNA sequences to the human genome. Genome Biol. 2009;10:R25.

44. Agresti A. Categorical data analysis, Second Edition. Hoboken, New Jersey: John Wiley & Sons, Inc.; 2002.

45. Elkon R, Ugalde AP, Agami R. Alternative cleavage and polyadenylation: extent, regulation and function. Nat Rev Genet. 2013;14:496–506.

46. Sun Y, Fu Y, Li Y, Xu A. Genome-wide alternative polyadenylation in animals: insights from high-throughput technologies. J Mol Cell Biol. 2012;4:352–61.

47. Nordlund J, Kiialainen A, Karlberg O, Berglund EC, Goransson-Kultima H, Sonderkaer M, et al. Digital gene expression profiling of primary acute lymphoblastic leukemia cells. Leukemia. 2012;26:1218–27.

48. Lutz CS. Alternative polyadenylation: a twist on mRNA 3' end formation. ACS Chem Biol. 2008;3:609–17.

49. Proudfoot NJ. Ending the message: poly(A) signals then and now. Genes Dev. 2011;25:1770–82.

50. Yang Q, Coseno M, Gilmartin GM, Doublie S. Crystal structure of a human cleavage factor CFI(m)25/CFI(m)68/RNA complex provides an insight into poly(A) site recognition and RNA looping. Structure. 2011;19:368–77.

51. Shell SA, Hesse C, Morris SM Jr, Milcarek C. Elevated levels of the 64-kDa cleavage stimulatory factor (CstF-64) in lipopolysaccharide-stimulated macrophages influence gene expression and induce alternative poly(A) site selection. J Biol Chem. 2005;280:39950–61.

52. Takagaki Y, Seipelt RL, Peterson ML, Manley JL. The polyadenylation factor CstF-64 regulates alternative processing of IgM heavy chain pre-mRNA during B cell differentiation. Cell. 1996;87:941–52.

53. de Klerk E, Venema A, Anvar SY, Goeman JJ, Hu O, Trollet C, et al. Poly(A) binding protein nuclear 1 levels affect alternative polyadenylation. Nucleic Acids Res. 2012;40:9089–101.

54. Jenal M, Elkon R, Loayza-Puch F, van Haaften G, Kuhn U, Menzies FM, et al. The poly(A)-binding protein nuclear 1 suppresses alternative cleavage and polyadenylation sites. Cell. 2012;149:538–53.

55. Simonelig M. PABPN1 shuts down alternative poly(A) sites. Cell Res. 2012;22:1419–21.

56. Zhang X, Liu S, Hu T, He Y, Sun S. Up-regulated microRNA-143 transcribed by nuclear factor kappa B enhances hepatocarcinoma metastasis by repressing fibronectin expression. Hepatology. 2009;50:490–9.

57. Fan X, Chen X, Deng W, Zhong G, Cai Q, Lin T. Up-regulated microRNA-143 in cancer stem cells differentiation promotes prostate cancer cells metastasis by modulating FNDC3B expression. BMC Cancer. 2013;13:61.

58. Zhang X, Yang J, Zhao J, Zhang P, Huang X. MicroRNA-23b inhibits the proliferation and migration of heat-denatured fibroblasts by targeting Smad3. PLoS One. 2015;10:e0131867.

59. Lewis BP, Burge CB, Bartel DP. Conserved seed pairing, often flanked by adenosines, indicates that thousands of human genes are microRNA targets. Cell. 2005;120:15–20.

13

Dengue virus non-structural protein 1: a pathogenic factor, therapeutic target, and vaccine candidate

Hong-Ru Chen[1†], Yen-Chung Lai[1†] and Trai-Ming Yeh[2*]⬤

Abstract

Dengue virus (DENV) infection is the most common mosquito-transmitted viral infection. DENV infection can cause mild dengue fever or severe dengue hemorrhagic fever (DHF)/dengue shock syndrome (DSS). Hemorrhage and vascular leakage are two characteristic symptoms of DHF/DSS. However, due to the limited understanding of dengue pathogenesis, no satisfactory therapies to treat nor vaccine to prevent dengue infection are available, and the mortality of DHF/DSS is still high. DENV nonstructural protein 1 (NS1), which can be secreted in patients' sera, has been used as an early diagnostic marker for dengue infection for many years. However, the roles of NS1 in dengue-induced vascular leakage were described only recently. In this article, the pathogenic roles of DENV NS1 in hemorrhage and vascular leakage are reviewed, and the possibility of using NS1 as a therapeutic target and vaccine candidate is discussed.

Keywords: Dengue virus (DENV), Nonstructural protein 1 (NS1), Hemorrhage, Coagulopathy, Vascular leakage, Vaccine

Background
General information about dengue

Dengue virus (DENV) is the most common mosquito-borne flavivirus and threatens people in tropic and subtropical areas. The World Health Organization estimates that more than 2.5 billion people representing over 40% of the world's population are at risk of dengue infection [1]. Dengue virus infections are often asymptomatic or cause a flu-like syndrome with fever and rash. However, a small proportion of cases develop into severe illness, which is termed dengue hemorrhagic fever (DHF). DHF is characterized by vascular leakage, thrombocytopenia, and coagulopathy [2]. Vascular leakage results in hemoconcentration and serous effusions, leading to circulatory collapse, which further develops into life-threatening dengue shock syndrome (DSS) [2]. An estimated 390 million infections occur each year globally, and approximately 960,000 people with severe dengue require hospitalization [1]. Children contribute to a large proportion of the severe disease cases. In 1958, DHF was reported to carry a case fatality rate (CFR)

of 13.9% in Bangkok [3]. Even with standardized diagnosis and management, the CFR remained in the range of 0.5–1.7% from 2000–2011 in the Philippines [4]. Despite the high mortality of DHF/DSS, no promising viral-specific drugs or vaccines are available due to the limited understanding of the complicated pathogenic mechanism.

Several hypotheses have been proposed to explain the pathogenesis of DHF/DSS [5]. Among them, antibody-dependent enhancement (ADE) has been proposed to explain why most DHF/DSS cases occur in children who are secondarily infected with a different serotype of DENV from the previous one [6]. Based on ADE, antibodies that are generated by a single DENV infection contribute to lasting homotypic immunity but may permit heterotypic DENV infection. Furthermore, these serotype non-specific antibodies may augment heterotypic virus entry and replication in Fcγ receptor-bearing macrophages, leading to enhanced viremia, antigenemia and cytokine storm [7]. This scenario may also explain why infants who passively acquire maternal anti-dengue antibodies are more likely to develop DHF/DSS following primary infection [8]. However, ADE dose not explain why vascular leakage and hemorrhage occur in DHF/DSS patients. Only when we better understand the molecular mechanisms of DENV pathogenesis can a more effective and specific therapy or vaccine against DHF/DSS be

* Correspondence: today@mail.ncku.edu.tw
†Hong-Ru Chen and Yen-Chung Lai contributed equally to this work.
[2]Department of Medical Laboratory Science and Biotechnology, College of Medicine, National Cheng Kung University, Tainan, Taiwan
Full list of author information is available at the end of the article

developed. In this review, we focus on the pathogenic roles of DENV non-structural protein 1 (NS1) in the pathogenesis of DHF/DSS. The potential of NS1 as a drug target or vaccine candidate to treat or prevent dengue will be discussed.

DENV structure

The DENV particle is approximately 500 Å in diameter and includes a positive-sense RNA genome with ~10,700 nucleotides and 3 structural proteins: capsid (C, 100 amino acids), precursor membrane (prM, 75 amino acids), and envelope (E, 495 amino acids) [9]. The capsid protein and the viral RNA genome form a nucleocapsid that buds at the endoplasmic reticulum (ER) in association with 180 copies of prM and E and carries host-derived lipids to form the immature virion [10]. Initially, the immature virion is covered by 60 spikes, each of which is composed of E trimers with associated prM proteins. The maturation process requires the host protease furin, which cleaves prM into the pr and M proteins in the Golgi after the noninfectious virion passes through the cell's secretory system, which is an acidic environment. This cleavage results in a rearrangement of E to the immature dimer structure, in which E maintains interactions with pr and M [11]. After budding from the cell via exocytosis, the neutral pH of the extracellular environment dissociates E and pr to form mature virions, which are available to infect new cells [11]. In addition to the structural proteins, the RNA genome of dengue virus encodes 7 nonstructural proteins that are essential for viral replication (NS1, NS2A, NS2B, NS3, NS4A, NS4B and NS5).

NS1 structure, expression and secretion

DENV NS1 is a 48-kDa glycoprotein that is highly conserved among all flaviviruses [12]. NS1 is essential for viral replication with an unknown mechanism that possibly involves interactions with NS4A and NS4B [13, 14]. Initially, NS1 is expressed as a monomer in infected cells. After post-translational modification in the ER lumen, it forms homodimers associated with organelle membranes and the cell membrane [12]. Despite the lack of a transmembrane region, NS1 anchors to the cell membrane through several pathways. The mechanisms are unclear, but anchorage of NS1 to glycosyl-phosphatidylinositol and lipid rafts has been shown [15, 16]. In addition, NS1 is the only protein that is continuously secreted by infected host cells. NS1 is secreted in a hexamer form, which is composed of three dimers with a detergent-sensitive hydrophobic central cavity that carries a cargo of ~70 lipid molecules; the composition is similar to a high-density lipoprotein [17, 18]. This lipid-rich structure may help secreted NS1 attach to the cell membrane by associating with glycosaminoglycans (GAGs) [19]. Due to the similarity between NS1 and high-density lipoprotein, NS1 has been proposed to disrupt the coagulation cascade possibly through interfering with the interaction or biogenesis

of endogenous lipoprotein particles [18]. Accumulation of secreted NS1 in DHF/DSS patient sera has been observed during the critical phase [20]. The serum concentration of NS1 in DHF/DSS patients can reach as high as 50 μg/ml, and the concentration is positively correlated with the disease severity [21–23]. During the recovery phase, NS1 is cleared from the circulation by antibody-mediated effects. Because secreted NS1 can interact with complement protein, it was first described as a soluble complement-fixing (SCF) antigen that could promote C4 degradation and in turn possibly protect DENV from complement-dependent lysis [24–26]. Recently, pathogenic roles for secreted NS1 in DHF/DSS have been demonstrated due to its involvement in systemic immunity and endothelial cell activation. In this review, we focus on the molecular mechanisms underlying how NS1 may contribute to vascular leakage, coagulopathy and thrombocytopenia during dengue infection. The possibility of targeting NS1 as a drug and vaccine development target against dengue infection will also be discussed.

The pathogenic roles of NS1 in vascular leakage

Pathogenic factors of vascular leakage in dengue pathogenesis

Based upon in vitro data or mouse models, it was once concluded that endothelial cell apoptosis led to vascular permeability during DENV infections and that this was because direct infection of endothelial cells by DENV or damage by antibodies (Abs) against NS1 which can cross-react with endothelial cells [27–34]. However, plasma leakage improves within 1 to 2 days in DHF/DSS patients who receive appropriate fluid resuscitation, and tissue samples from these patients show little structural damage in their vessels. Therefore, apoptosis of endothelial cells induced by DENV infection or anti-NS1 antibodies is not sufficient to support the clinical outcome. As a result, endothelial dysfunction but not apoptosis induced by a dengue-specific factor is currently considered to play a more important role in causing vascular leakage in DHF/DSS [35–37].

Contribution of the NS1 protein to vascular leakage

DENV NS1-induced vascular leakage has been widely discussed since 2015. A previous study demonstrated that NS1 proteins induced vascular leakage, and applying anti-NS1 antibodies attenuated NS1-induced vascular leakage as well as the mortality rate in mice [38]. However, the mediating receptor of NS1 remains controversial. One study suggested that blocking TLR2 or TLR6 attenuated DENV NS1-induced secretion of TNF-α and IL-6 by peripheral blood mononuclear cells (PBMCs) [39]. TLR6 deficiency also reduced DENV NS1-induced mortality in mice [39]. However, another study demonstrated that NS1-activated TNF-α and IL-1β mRNA expression and IL-6 secretion were attenuated by blocking TLR4 in PBMCs [40]. In contrast, TLR2 inhibition did not alter the effects induced by NS1 in PBMCs [40]. These authors also showed that blocking TLR4 rescued NS1-induced endothelial hyperpermeability, indicating that NS1-induced vascular leakage was mediated by TLR4 [40]. Later, the same group published a short communication to explain that the different results might be caused by contamination of *Escherichia coli*-derived recombinant NS1 with multiple TLR ligands and that TLR4 should be regarded as the real NS1 receptor [41]. However, it has also been shown that DENV NS1 induces similar levels of vascular leakage in TLR4-receptor-deficient mice and wild-type animals, which indicates that NS1-induced vascular leakage can be independent of TLR4 [42]. Taken together, these results suggest that NS1 may contribute to vascular leakage through both TLR4-dependent and independent mechanisms.

In our previous study, we demonstrated that autophagy-mediated junction disruption was involved in DENV NS1-induced vascular leakage, which may explain why vascular leakage in dengue patients is a quick and reversible pathogenic change [43]. NS1-induced macrophage migration inhibitory factor (MIF) secretion is involved in NS1-induced autophagy of endothelial cells [43]. An in vitro study also showed that DENV-infected cells induced MIF secretion, which can cause endothelial hyperpermeability. Furthermore, Mif$^{-/-}$ mice exhibited reduced pathogenesis in a model of severe dengue [44], indicating the importance of MIF in dengue pathogenesis [45]. In fact, several clinical studies have shown that the MIF concentration is elevated in dengue patients [46, 47] and that the MIF concentration is higher in DHF patients who die than in DHF survivors and DF patients [48].

In addition to disrupting endothelial junctions, NS1 also causes vascular leakage by inducing endothelial glycocalyx degradation mediated by heparanase-1 (HPA-1) [42, 49]. The glycocalyx is a thin, negatively charged network consisting of glycoproteins, proteoglycans, and glycosaminoglycans at the luminal side of endothelial cells lining blood vessels throughout the body [50]. To maintain homeostasis, the glycocalyx acts as a barrier that controls numerous physiological processes, such as regulating vascular permeability, preventing the adhesion of leukocytes and blood platelets to the vessel walls [51, 52], mediating shear stress [53, 54], and modulating inflammatory and hemostatic processes. Damage of the endothelial glycocalyx correlates to several vascular pathologies, including ischemia/reperfusion, hypoxia, sepsis, volume overload, diabetes and atherosclerosis [50, 55].

Shedding of the endothelial glycocalyx is related to activation of the heparan sulfate-specific glucuronidase HPA-1 [52, 56]. HPA-1 is synthesized as a 65-kDa non-active precursor that subsequently undergoes proteolytic cleavage to yield 8-kDa and 50-kDa subunits that heterodimerize to form an active enzyme. Activated HPA-1 enhances shedding of the transmembrane heparan sulfate proteoglycan

syndecan-1 (CD138) and elevates the CD138 level in the bloodstream [57, 58]. In addition to HPA-1, metalloproteinase (MMP) family proteins are also important proteases that are capable of digesting the endothelial glycocalyx [59, 60] and increased MMP levels correlate with vascular leakage in DHF/DSS [61–64]. In 2017, Glasner suggested that DENV NS1-induced vascular leakage was independent of inflammatory cytokines, including TNF-α, IL-6 and IL-8, but was dependent on endothelial glycocalyx components, including cathepsin L and HPA-1 [42]. Recently, we further demonstrated that MIF is involved in DENV NS1-induced HPA-1 and MMP-9 secretion and degradation of the endothelial glycocalyx [65]. Taken together, the mechanisms of the vascular leakage that occurs during DENV infection may be very complex and may involve both the virus and the host immune response. The possible mechanisms by which DENV NS1 contributes to vascular leakage are shown in Fig. 1.

The pathogenic roles of NS1 in coagulopathy and thrombocytopenia

In addition to vascular leakage, DENV NS1 may also contribute to severe dengue by disrupting coagulation. The NS1/thrombin complex was found in the sera of dengue patients, and binding of NS1 to prothrombin inhibited its activation, leading to a prolonged activated partial thromboplastin time [66]. However, whether NS1 is involved in thrombocytopenia is still unclear. It is known that LPS can induce platelet activation and potentiate platelet aggregation via TLR4/MyD88 signal transduction [67]. Since both NS1 and LPS can activate immune cells through TLR4, NS1 may induce platelet activation and enhance aggregation, possibly leading to over-destruction of platelets during dengue infection. Collectively, increasing evidence suggest that NS1 plays a crucial role in dengue pathogenesis by contributing to both vascular leakage and hemorrhage in dengue disease.

DENV NS1 as a therapeutic target
Current status of DENV treatment

Although many dengue patients only experience asymptomatic or mild signs of a flu-like illness followed by self-recovery within one week, some patients develop worse dengue symptoms that become life-threatening. To date, the treatment of dengue disease has been mostly supportive, and no licensed therapeutic drug is available. An effective drug against DENV infection is in great demand until a satisfactory vaccine becomes available. Because earlier observational studies stated that disease severity positively correlated with the viremia level and febrile phase during infections [68, 69], dengue researchers have put great effort into anti-viral approaches targeting different structural or nonstructural proteins. The inhibitory mechanisms of viral entry [70],

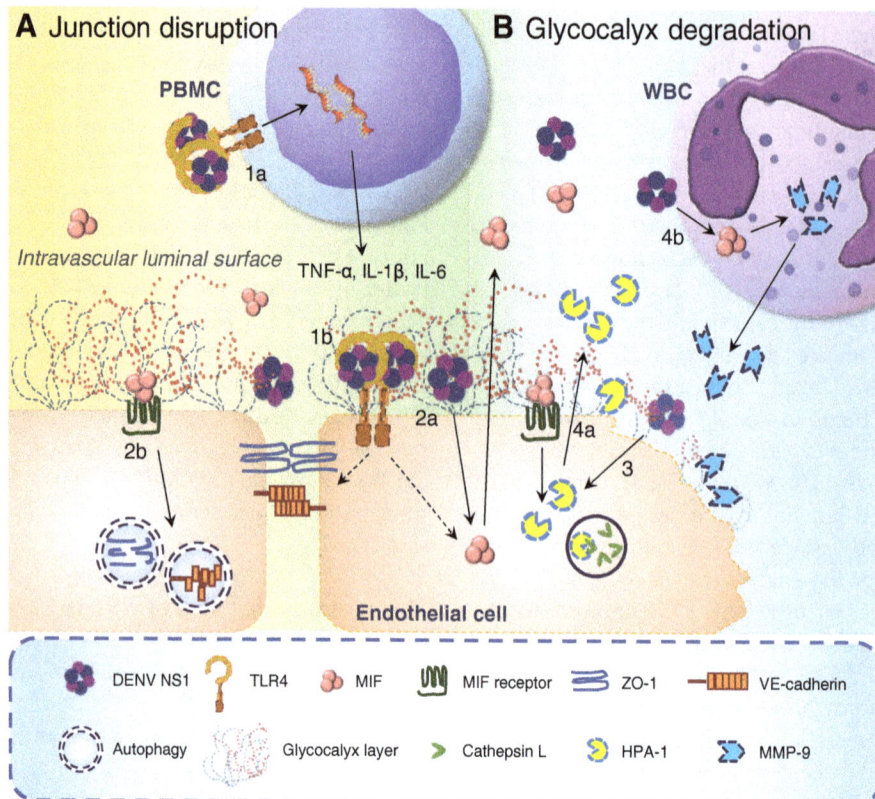

Fig. 1 The possible mechanisms by which DENV NS1 causes vascular leakage. (1a) NS1 binding to TLR4 of PBMCs induces the expression and secretion of TNF-α, IL-1β and IL-6 cytokines, which may disrupt the tight junction, leading to vascular leakage [40]. (1b) NS1 binding to TLR4 or (2a) other molecules on endothelial cells induces the secretion of MIF [43]. (2b) MIF binding to its receptor on endothelial cells induces junction disruption through autophagic degradation of junction proteins such as ZO-1 and VE-cadherin [43]. (3) Binding of NS1 to endothelial cells also induces HPA-1 activation through cathepsin L, leading to endothelial glycocalyx degradation and vascular leakage [42, 49]. (4a) Additionally, NS1-induced MIF secretion is also involved in HPA-1 secretion of endothelial cells, and (4b) MMP-9 secretion of WBCs which can also contribute to endothelial glycocalyx degradation [65]

pH-dependent viral fusion [71, 72], enzymes required for transcription/replication [73–77], and viral protein modifications [78] have been widely investigated. From this perspective, some off-patent drugs and antibiotics have also been tested for repurposing [79, 80], which is beneficial for shortening development time and costs. Although some drugs lead to significant viral reduction and provide effective anti-viral activity both in vitro and in animal models, in real world situations, these types of antiviral drugs face other limitations and challenges, probably due to untimely treatment in the clinic. People often enroll in clinical studies until their viremia declines during the later phase of illness. As a result, most cases, unfortunately, fail to meet the therapeutic endpoint measurements in clinical trials [71].

From another perspective, other studies have provided different insights into host modulation and immune regulation as therapeutic targets, which include targeting host dependency factors, host restriction factors, and host-mediated pathogenesis pathways [81]. In contrast to viral targets, host-targeting antiviral approaches are believed to avoid the rapid drug resistance or mutations that arise during viral evolution. Strategies targeting host factors have been widely reviewed using advanced mass screening approaches [82–84]. For instance, turn-on targets of antiviral responses are often reported to act as defensive therapies [85, 86]. Interferons exert diverse antiviral functions against viral replication, which can activate interferon-stimulated genes and related mechanisms. In addition, regulation of host metabolic pathways required for viral replication, such as glycolysis and autophagy, has been studied recently [87, 88]. However, these approaches can nonspecifically regulate the functions of different cells, and most of these approaches fail in clinical trials [89]. Recently, we found that minocycline, a semi-synthetic tetracycline-derivative antibiotic, attenuates DENV replication through inhibition of MIF secretion and autophagy formation both in vitro and in vivo [90]. In addition, minocycline treatment can prolong the survival of ICR suckling mice after DENV infection. Therefore, minocycline may modulate both virus replication and the host immune response. Further clinical trials of minocycline in dengue patients may help to verify its therapeutic protection against DHF/DSS.

Antibody against NS1 as a therapeutic drug for dengue disease

In addition to small molecule drugs, antibody therapies are appreciated for their specificity against diseases. To date, many murine- or human-derived monoclonal antibodies have been developed to test their therapeutic effects against DENV infection in different studies. Antibodies targeting structural proteins, such as envelope and prM/M, have been characterized; these antibodies are termed "neutralizing antibodies" due to their blockage of viral entry and inhibition of viral attachment to host cells. However, safety issues and insufficient efficacy against all four DENV serotypes are often challenged due to the risk of ADE. The enhancement of viral infection by antibodies against DENV has been not only evaluated both in vitro and in vivo but also emphasized in a clinical cohort study [91]. Nevertheless, many researchers have identified mAbs that can neutralize DENV infection without ADE as a side effect. One study indicated that single-dose administration of human Ab513, which recognizes a linear epitope of envelope domain III, prevented DENV-induced thrombocytopenia in humanized mice with ADE [92]. Another study suggested that antibodies that recognized the envelope dimer epitope (EDE) were highly potent and broadly neutralizing

antibodies [93, 94]. In addition, the human-derived mAb SIgN-3C with a LALA mutant abrogated the ADE effect and protected mice from lethal DENV-2 infection [95].

In contrast to Abs against structural proteins on the virion, such as E and PrM/M, which are effective only in the viremic phase, anti-NS1 Abs can provide different therapeutic mechanisms, by not only reducing viral propagation from infected cells in the early viremic phase but also attenuating NS1-induced disease development during the critical phase. In addition, because NS1 is not a viral structural protein, anti-NS1 Abs will not induce ADE. Indeed, anti-NS1 Abs can reduce viral replication by complement-dependent cytotoxicity (CDC) of infected cells and have been demonstrated in several flaviviruses, including DENV, in vitro and in vivo [96–99]. In addition, anti-NS1 Abs can block NS1-elicited pathogenic effects both in vitro and in vivo [38] and reduce DENV-induced mortality and morbidity in different mouse models (Table 1).

However, as previously described, many anti-NS1 Abs can cross-react with host proteins; thus, antibodies generated from NS1 immune sera may contain cross-reactive Abs with undesired side effects [32, 100]. Therefore, we need to identify a subclass of protective anti-NS1 Abs that can block the activity of all four different dengue NS1 serotypes without cross-reactivity to host proteins. In our previous study, we analyzed a mAb against NS1 and identified Abs against a region of the NS1 wing domain that

Table 1 Administration of Abs against DENV NS1 in different mouse models

Approach	Antibody administration	Challenge/routes	Mice	Outcomes	Reference
NS1 polyclonal antisera	500 l (i.p.) 24 h prior to challenge	100 LD50 of DENV2 (NGC) /i.c.	BALB/c	100% survival	[113]
Monoclonal ascitic fluid	1-10 mg/mouse (i.p.) 24 h prior to challenge	100 LD50 of DENV2 (NGC) /i.c.	BALB/c	50-93% survival	[113]
NS1 polyclonal antisera	300 µl (i.p.) cotreatment	NS1 (10 mg/kg) + 1×106 PFU of DENV2 (adapted strain D220)/ i.v.	Ifnar−/−C57BL/6	100% survival	[38]
Anti-NS1 mAb (1H7.4)	200 µg (i.p.) cotreatment	NS1 (10 mg/kg) +1×106 PFU of DENV2 (adapted strain D220)/ i.v.	Ifnar−/−C57BL/6	100% survival	[38]
Anti-DJ NS1 and anti-ΔC[a] NS1 polyclonal Abs	50-150 µg/mouse (i.p.) 24 h after challenge	9×107 PFU of DENV2 (16681)/ i.d.; 1×107 PFU of DENV2 (454009A)/i.v.	C3H/HeN	Reduce hemorrhage; rescue partial bleeding prolonged	[96, 114]
Anti-NS1 mAb (33D2)	100 µg/mouse (i.p.) 24 h after challenge	2×108 PFU of DENV1-4/i.d.; 4×107 PFU of DENV2 (454009A)/i.v.	C3H/HeN; STAT1-/-C57BL/6	80% survival; reduce viremia and NS1 antigenemia; reduce hemorrhage; rescue partial bleeding prolong	[97]
Anti-DJ[b] NS1 polyclonal Abs	Two doses of 150 µg/mouse (i.p.) 24 and 48 h after challenge	1×107 PFU/mouse DENV2 (16681)/i.d.	STAT1-/- C57BL/6	Reduce mast cell degranulation, macrophage infiltration and chemokine production	[115]
Anti-NS1 mAb (2E8)	One dose of 50-150 µg/mouse (i.p.) either 1, 3, or 4 days after challenge	1×107 PFU/mouse	STAT1-/-C57BL/6	Reduce viremia and NS1 antigenemia; rescue partial bleeding prolong	[114]

[a]ΔC NS1: full-length DENV NS1 lacking the C-terminal amino acids (a.a.) 271-352
[b]Chimeric DJ NS1: consisting of N-terminal DENV NS1 (a.a. 1-270) and C-terminal Japanese encephalitis virus NS1 (a.a. 271-352)

were protective against DENV infection in mice. Further-more, the amount of these anti-NS1 Abs was inversely correlated with the severity of disease in dengue patients, indicating that the Abs were protective in patients [97]. Therefore, a mAb against this region of NS1 may repre-sent an alternative choice for a therapeutic drug that is specific against DENV infection while avoiding the risk of ADE (Fig. 2).

DENV NS1 as a vaccine candidate
Current status of DENV vaccine development
The only licensed dengue vaccine currently available was developed by Sanofi Pasteur and has been approved in many countries. This live-attenuated tetravalent dengue vaccine (CYD-TDV; Dengvaxia) contains DENV E and prM proteins from the four serotypes in the yellow fever 17D backbone and has been used to induce preventive humoral and cell-mediated immune responses [101, 102]. Although CYD-TDV induced neutralizing Abs against all four DENV serotypes, this vaccine rendered only partial protection against serotype 2 DENV infection. In addition

to the unequal efficacy of CYD-TDV against all four DENV serotypes, vaccination of this vaccine may induce non-protective Abs that enhance disease severity in persons who had not been exposed to dengue before. Indeed, it is reported that among children younger than nine years of age, the vaccine is associated with an increased incidence of hospitalization for severe dengue disease [103]. Therefore, the vaccination of seronegative individuals with Dengvaxia may enhance dengue disease severity but not protection due to ADE [104]. Conversely, some studies have suggested that the dengue vaccine fails to provide full protection, pos-sibly due to the lack of T cell immunity elicited against non-structural proteins or an NS1-induced protective immune response [105]. Collectively, these concerns make nonstruc-tural proteins, including NS1, alternative options for den-gue vaccine development.

NS1 as a vaccine candidate against DENV infection
Both humoral and T cell-mediated cellular immune re-sponses are critical for protection against DENV infection. Viral structural proteins have been regarded as potent

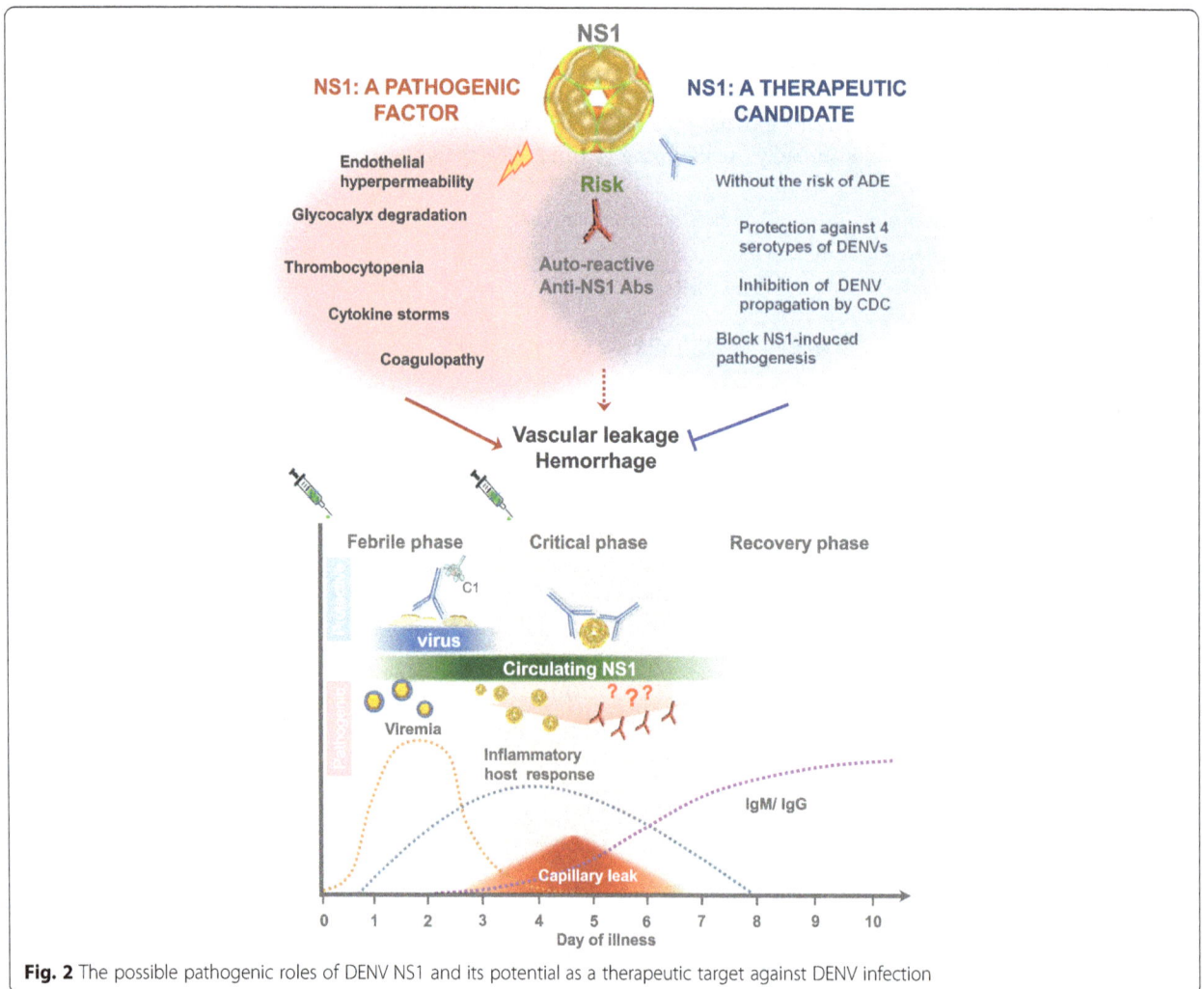

Fig. 2 The possible pathogenic roles of DENV NS1 and its potential as a therapeutic target against DENV infection

targets to induce neutralizing Abs but are associated with the intractable issue of ADE. As a nonstructural protein, NS1 does not induce Abs against the virion. NS1 is the only nonstructural protein of DENV that can be both anchored on the surface of infected cells as a membrane-associated homodimer and released from infected cells into circulation as a hexamer. These properties of NS1 make it able to trigger both cellular and humoral immunity. Because NS1 is exposed on infected cells, the complement cascade can be triggered by NS1-bound anti-NS1 Abs [106]. Complement activation can lyse infected cells via CDC and eventually reduce viral titers through suppression of viral propagation. Studies have shown that immunization with DENV NS1 via different approaches can induce protective immune responses against DENV infection in mice, as shown in Table 2.

However, immunization of mice with full length of DENV NS1 can induce Abs cross-react with host proteins have also been demonstrated by different groups and these cross-reactive Abs can cause pathological effects both in vitro and in mice [107–109]. Although the contributions of these cross-reactive Abs in dengue pathogenesis are still under debate, the potential side effects induced by vaccination with full-length NS1 should be avoided in dengue vaccine design. Since most of these cross-reactive Abs recognize the C-terminal region of NS1. [110], different approaches have been applied to prevent the induction of cross-reactive Abs by NS1 immunization. For instance, NS1 lacking its C-terminus (ΔC NS1) was used to immunize mice; the results showed that ΔC NS1-elicited Abs provided better protection against DENV infection than immunization with full-length NS1 [96]. However, in addition to the C-terminus, other regions of NS1 also show molecular mimicry to host proteins and can elicit auto-reactive Abs against endothelial cells and coagulation factors [111, 112]. To avoid the risk of the induction of cross-reactive antibodies by NS1 immunization, a short modified NS1 peptide containing an 11-a.a. conserved wing domain region of NS1 was designed; this peptide modified the critical pathogenic amino acids to reduce cross-reactivity but maintain immunogenicity. Importantly, both active immunization with the modified NS1 peptide and passive transfer of polyclonal Abs against the modified NS1 peptide provided protection against DENV in a hemorrhagic mouse model and a lethal infection mouse model [97].

Table 2 Different NS1-based vaccine strategies in mouse models

Vaccine type	Approaches	Challenge/routes	Mouse	Outcome	Reference
Protein	Full length NS1 + CFA adjuvant	Lethal amount of DENV2 (NGC) from suckling mouse brain/i.c.	CD1	88% survival; 35% reduction in morbidity	[98]
	Recombinant vaccinia virusexpressed NS1	100 IC50 of DENV4 (H241) or DENV2 (NGC)/i.c.	BALB/c	63-100% survival	[116]
	rEC204-NS1N65 – protein A	100 LD50 of DENV2 (NGC)/i.c.	BALB/c	100% survival	[117]
	rNS1+ LTG33D adjuvant	4.32 log10 PFU of DENV2 (NGC)/i.c.	BALB/c	50% survival; 10% reduction in morbidity	[118]
	ΔC NS1# + CFA adjuvant	9×107 PFU of DENV2 (16681)/ i.d.	C3H/HeN	66% reduction in hemorrhage; rescue partial bleeding prolong	[96]
	Chimeric DJ NS1## + CFA adjuvant	9×107 PFU of DENV2 (16681)/ i.d.	C3H/HeN	66% reduction in hemorrhage; rescue partial bleeding prolong	[96]
	Full DENV 1-4 NS1 + MPLA/AddaVax adjuvant	1×107 of DENV2 (adapted strain D220)/i.v.	Ifnar −/−C57BL/6	60-100% survival; reduce viremia and NS1 antigenemia	[38]
Subunit peptide	Modified NS1-WD[a]+ CFA adjuvant	2×108 PFU of DENV1-4/i.d.; 4×107 PFU of DENV2 (454009A)/i.v.	C3H/HeN; STAT1-/-C57BL/6	100% survival; reduce viremia and NS1 antigenemia; 70-90% reduction in hemorrhage; rescue partial bleeding prolong	[97]
	pD2NS1/pD2NS1+ pIL-2	5×106 -107 PFU of DENV2 (PL046)/i.v.	C3H	50-80% survival; 70-80% reduction in morbidity	[119]
DNA vaccine	pcTPANS1[b]	4.32 log10 PFU of DENV2 (NGC)/i.c.	BALB/C	100% survival	[120, 121]
	pcENS1[c]	4.32 log10 PFU of DENV2 (NGC)/i.c.	BALB/C	86.7% survival; 60% reduction in morbidity	[122]

[a]NS1-WD: wing domain region of NS1
[b]TPA: human tissue plasminogen activator; a secretory signal sequence.
[c]pcENS1: encoding the C-terminal E protein plus the full NS1 region

Conclusions

Collectively, this review discusses the critical pathogenic roles of NS1 in dengue pathogenesis. NS1 is considered a unique "viral toxin" in dengue disease. Therapeutic approaches and vaccine development targeting NS1 may provide different opportunities to combat dengue disease.

Abbreviations

CFR: Case-fatality rate; CXCR: CXC chemokine receptors; DENV: Dengue virus; DF: Dengue fever; DHF: Dengue hemorrhagic fever; DSS: Dengue shock syndrome; E: Envelope protein; ER: Endoplasmic reticulum; GAG: Glycosaminoglycan; IL: Interleukin; iNOS: Inducible NO synthase; MIF: Macrophage migration inhibitory factor; MMP: Matrix metalloproteinase; NO: nitric oxide; NS1: Nonstructural protein 1; PBMCs: Peripheral blood mononuclear cells; prM: Pre-membrane protein; TLR: Toll-like receptor; TNF: Tumor necrosis factor

Acknowledgements

We thank the members of the Center of Infectious Disease and Signaling Research of NCKU for their invaluable inputs and insights throughout the course of this study.

Funding

This study was supported by grants from the Ministry of Science and Technology of Taiwan (102-2320-B-006-025-MY3) (105-2321-B-006-023) and (106-2321-B-006 -011).

Authors' contributions

T-M.Y. provided the main ideas and organized and directed this article. H-R.C. contributed to "The role of NS1 in the pathogenesis of dengue" section and Y-C.L. wrote the "NS1 as a target protein for treatment and vaccination" section. All authors read and approved the final manuscript.

Competing interests

The authors declare that they have no competing interests.

Author details

[1]The Institute of Basic Medical Sciences, College of Medicine, National Cheng Kung University, Tainan, Taiwan. [2]Department of Medical Laboratory Science and Biotechnology, College of Medicine, National Cheng Kung University, Tainan, Taiwan.

References

1. Bhatt S, Gething PW, Brady OJ, Messina JP, Farlow AW, Moyes CL, Drake JM, Brownstein JS, Hoen AG, Sankoh O, et al. The global distribution and burden of dengue. Nature. 2013;496(7446):504–7.
2. Dengue haemorrhagic fever. diagnosis, treatment, prevention and control. 2nd ed. Geneva: World Health Organization; 1997.
3. Kalayanarooj S. Standardized Clinical Management: Evidence of Reduction of Dengue Haemorrhagic Fever Case-Fatality Rate in Thailand. Dengue Bulletin. 1999;23:10–7.
4. Bravo L, Roque VG, Brett J, Dizon R, L'Azou M. Epidemiology of dengue disease in the Philippines (2000-2011): a systematic literature review. PLoS Negl Trop Dis. 2014;8(11):e3027.
5. Lei HY, Yeh TM, Liu HS, Lin YS, Chen SH, Liu CC. Immunopathogenesis of dengue virus infection. J Biomed Sci. 2001;8(5):377–88.
6. Kliks SC, Nisalak A, Brandt WE, Wahl L, Burke DS. Antibody-dependent enhancement of dengue virus growth in human monocytes as a risk factor for dengue hemorrhagic fever. Am J Trop Med Hyg. 1989;40(41):444–51.
7. Halstead SB, Venkateshan CN, Gentry MK, Larsen LK. Heterogeneity of infection enhancement of dengue 2 strains by monoclonal antibodies. J Immunol. 1984;132(31):1529–32.
8. Kliks SC, Nimmanitya S, Nisalak A, Burke DS. Evidence that maternal dengue antibodies are important in the development of dengue hemorrhagic fever in infants. Am J Trop Med Hyg. 1988;38(21):411–9.
9. Kuhn RJ, Zhang W, Rossmann MG, Pletnev SV, Corver J, Lenches E, Jones CT, Mukhopadhyay S, Chipman PR, Strauss EG, et al. Structure of dengue virus: implications for flavivirus organization, maturation, and fusion. Cell. 2002; 108(5):717–25.
10. Byk LA, Gamarnik AV. Properties and Functions of the Dengue Virus Capsid Protein. Annu Rev Virol. 2016;3(1):263–81.
11. Christian EA, Kahle KM, Mattia K, Puffer BA, Pfaff JM, Miller A, Paes C, Davidson E, Doranz BJ. Atomic-level functional model of dengue virus Envelope protein infectivity. Proc Natl Acad Sci USA. 2013;110(46):18662–7.
12. Muller DA, Young PR. The flavivirus NS1 protein: Molecular and structural biology, immunology, role in pathogenesis and application as a diagnostic biomarker. Antiviral Res. 2013;98(2):192–208.
13. Youn S, Li T, McCune BT, Edeling MA, Fremont DH, Cristea IM, Diamond MS. Evidence for a genetic and physical interaction between nonstructural proteins NS1 and NS4B that modulates replication of West Nile virus. J Virol. 2012;86(13):7360–71.
14. Lindenbach BD, Rice CM. Genetic interaction of flavivirus nonstructural proteins NS1 and NS4A as a determinant of replicase function. J Virol. 1999; 73(6):4611–21.
15. Jacobs MG, Robinson PJ, Bletchly C, Mackenzie JM, Young PR. Dengue virus nonstructural protein 1 is expressed in a glycosyl-phosphatidylinositol-linked form that is capable of signal transduction. FASEB J. 2000;14(11):1603–10.
16. Noisakran S, Dechtawewat T, Avirutnan P, Kinoshita T, Siripanyaphinyo U, Puttikhunt C, Kasinrerk W, Malasit P, Sittisombut N. Association of dengue virus NS1 protein with lipid rafts. J Gen Virol. 2008;89(Pt 10):2492–500.
17. Edeling MA, Diamond MS, Fremont DH. Structural basis of Flavivirus NS1 assembly and antibody recognition. Proc Natl Acad Sci U S A. 2014;111(11):4285–90.
18. Gutsche I, Coulibaly F, Voss JE, Salmon J, d'Alayer J, Ermonval M, Larquet E, Charneau P, Krey T, Megret F, et al. Secreted dengue virus nonstructural protein NS1 is an atypical barrel-shaped high-density lipoprotein. Proc Natl Acad Sci U S A. 2011;108(19):8003–8.
19. Avirutnan P, Zhang L, Punyadee N, Manuyakorn A, Puttikhunt C, Kasinrerk W, Malasit P, Atkinson JP, Diamond MS. Secreted NS1 of dengue virus attaches to the surface of cells via interactions with heparan sulfate and chondroitin sulfate E. PLoS Pathog. 2007;3(11):e183.
20. Chuang YC, Wang SY, Lin YS, Chen HR, Yeh TM. Re-evaluation of the pathogenic roles of nonstructural protein 1 and its antibodies during dengue virus infection. J Biomed Sci. 2013;20:42.
21. Alcon S, Talarmin A, Debruyne M, Falconar A, Deubel V, Flamand M. Enzyme-linked immunosorbent assay specific to Dengue virus type 1 nonstructural protein NS1 reveals circulation of the antigen in the blood during the acute phase of disease in patients experiencing primary or secondary infections. J Clin Microbiol. 2002;40(2):376–81.
22. Libraty DH, Young PR, Pickering D, Endy TP, Kalayanarooj S, Green S, Vaughn DW, Nisalak A, Ennis FA, Rothman AL. High circulating levels of the dengue virus nonstructural protein NS1 early in dengue illness correlate with the development of dengue hemorrhagic fever. J Infect Dis. 2002;186(8):1165–8.
23. Young PR, Hilditch PA, Bletchly C, Halloran W. An antigen capture enzyme-linked immunosorbent assay reveals high levels of the dengue virus protein NS1 in the sera of infected patients. J Clin Microbiol. 2000;38(3):1053–7.
24. Avirutnan P, Fuchs A, Hauhart RE, Somnuke P, Youn S, Diamond MS, Atkinson JP. Antagonism of the complement component C4 by flavivirus nonstructural protein NS1. J Exp Med. 2010;207(4):793–806.
25. Avirutnan P, Hauhart RE, Somnuke P, Blom AM, Diamond MS, Atkinson JP. Binding of flavivirus nonstructural protein NS1 to C4b binding protein modulates complement activation. J Immunol. 2011;187(1):424–33.
26. Smith TJ, Brandt WE, Swanson JL, McCown JM, Buescher EL. Physical and biological properties of dengue-2 virus and associated antigens. J Virol. 1970;5(41):524–32.
27. Liao H, Xu J, Huang J. FasL/Fas pathway is involved in dengue virus induced apoptosis of the vascular endothelial cells. J Med Virol. 2010;82(8):1392–9.

28. Long X, Li Y, Qi Y, Xu J, Wang Z, Zhang X, Zhang D, Zhang L, Huang J. XAF1 contributes to dengue virus-induced apoptosis in vascular endothelial cells. FASEB J. 2013;27(3):1062–73.

29. Chen HC, Hofman FM, Kung JT, Lin YD, Wu-Hsieh BA. Both virus and tumor necrosis factor alpha are critical for endothelium damage in a mouse model of dengue virus-induced hemorrhage. J Virol. 2007;81(11):5518–26.

30. Cheng HJ, Luo YH, Wan SW, Lin CF, Wang ST, Hung NT, Liu CC, Ho TS, Liu HS, Yeh TM, et al. Correlation between serum levels of anti-endothelial cell autoantigen and anti-dengue virus nonstructural protein 1 antibodies in dengue patients. Am J Trop Med Hyg. 2015;92(5):989–95.

31. Lin CF, Lei HY, Shiau AL, Liu HS, Yeh TM, Chen SH, Liu CC, Chiu SC, Lin YS. Endothelial cell apoptosis induced by antibodies against dengue virus nonstructural protein 1 via production of nitric oxide. J Immunol. 2002;169(2):657–64.

32. Chen CL, Lin CF, Wan SW, Wei LS, Chen MC, Yeh TM, Liu HS, Anderson R, Lin YS. Anti-dengue virus nonstructural protein 1 antibodies cause NO-mediated endothelial cell apoptosis via ceramide-regulated glycogen synthase kinase-3beta and NF-kappaB activation. J Immunol. 2013;191(4):1744–52.

33. Lin CF, Chiu SC, Hsiao YL, Wan SW, Lei HY, Shiau AL, Liu HS, Yeh TM, Chen SH, Liu CC, et al. Expression of cytokine, chemokine, and adhesion molecules during endothelial cell activation induced by antibodies against dengue virus nonstructural protein 1. J Immunol. 2005;174(1):395–403.

34. Cheng HJ, Lin CF, Lei HY, Liu HS, Yeh TM, Luo YH, Lin YS. Proteomic analysis of endothelial cell autoantigens recognized by anti-dengue virus nonstructural protein 1 antibodies. Exp Biol Med (Maywood). 2009;234(1):63–73.

35. Avirutnan P, Punyadee N, Noisakran S, Komoltri C, Thiemmeca S, Auethavornanan K, Jairungsri A, Kanlaya R, Tangthawornchaikul N, Puttikhunt C, et al. Vascular leakage in severe dengue virus infections: a potential role for the nonstructural viral protein NS1 and complement. J Infect Dis. 2006;193(8):1078–88.

36. Thomas SJ. NS1: A corner piece in the dengue pathogenesis puzzle? Sci Transl Med. 2015;7(304):304fs337.

37. Halstead SB. Pathogenesis of Dengue: Dawn of a New Era. F1000Res. 2015;4:1353–60.

38. Beatty PR, Puerta-Guardo H, Killingbeck SS, Glasner DR, Hopkins K, Harris E. Dengue virus NS1 triggers endothelial permeability and vascular leak that is prevented by NS1 vaccination. Sci Transl Med. 2015;7(304):304ra141.

39. Chen J, Ng MM, Chu JJ. Activation of TLR2 and TLR6 by Dengue NS1 Protein and Its Implications in the Immunopathogenesis of Dengue Virus Infection. PLoS Pathog. 2015;11(7):e1005053.

40. Modhiran N, Watterson D, Muller DA, Panetta AK, Sester DP, Liu L, Hume DA, Stacey KJ, Young PR. Dengue virus NS1 protein activates cells via Toll-like receptor 4 and disrupts endothelial cell monolayer integrity. Sci Transl Med. 2015;7(304):304ra142.

41. Modhiran N, Watterson D, Blumenthal A, Baxter AG, Young PR, Stacey KJ. Dengue virus NS1 protein activates immune cells via TLR4 but not TLR2 or TLR6. Immunol Cell Biol. 2017;95(5):491–5.

42. Glasner DR, Ratnasiri K, Puerta-Guardo H, Espinosa DA, Beatty PR, Harris E. Dengue virus NS1 cytokine-independent vascular leak is dependent on endothelial glycocalyx components. PLoS Pathog. 2017;13(11):e1006673.

43. Chen HR, Chuang YC, Lin YS, Liu HS, Liu CC, Perng GC, Yeh TM. Dengue Virus Nonstructural Protein 1 Induces Vascular Leakage through Macrophage Migration Inhibitory Factor and Autophagy. PLoS Negl Trop Dis. 2016;10(7):e0004828.

44. Assuncao-Miranda I, Amaral FA, Bozza FA, Fagundes CT, Sousa LP, Souza DG, Pacheco P, Barbosa-Lima G, Gomes RN, Bozza PT, et al. Contribution of macrophage migration inhibitory factor to the pathogenesis of dengue virus infection. FASEB J. 2010;24(1):218–28.

45. Chuang YC, Lei HY, Liu HS, Lin YS, Fu TF, Yeh TM. Macrophage migration inhibitory factor induced by dengue virus infection increases vascular permeability. Cytokine. 2011;54(2):222–31.

46. Ferreira RA, de Oliveira SA, Gandini M, Ferreira Lda C, Correa G, Abiraude FM, Reid MM, Cruz OG, Kubelka CF. Circulating cytokines and chemokines associated with plasma leakage and hepatic dysfunction in Brazilian children with dengue fever. Acta Trop. 2015;149:138–47.

47. Yong YK, Tan HY, Jen SH, Shankar EM, Natkunam SK, Sathar J, Manikam R, Sekaran SD. Aberrant monocyte responses predict and characterize dengue virus infection in individuals with severe disease. J Transl Med. 2017;15(1):121.

48. Chen LC, Lei HY, Liu CC, Shiesh SC, Chen SH, Liu HS, Lin YS, Wang ST, Shyu HW, Yeh TM. Correlation of serum levels of macrophage migration inhibitory factor with disease severity and clinical outcome in dengue patients. Am J Trop Med Hyg. 2006;74(1):142–7.

49. Puerta-Guardo H, Glasner DR, Harris E. Dengue Virus NS1 Disrupts the Endothelial Glycocalyx, Leading to Hyperpermeability. PLoS Pathog. 2016;12(7):e1005738.

50. Reitsma S, Slaaf DW, Vink H, van Zandvoort MA, oude Egbrink MG. The endothelial glycocalyx: composition, functions, and visualization. Pflugers Arch. 2007;454(3):345–59.

51. Lipowsky HH. The endothelial glycocalyx as a barrier to leukocyte adhesion and its mediation by extracellular proteases. Ann Biomed Eng. 2012;40(4):840–8.

52. Schmidt EP, Yang Y, Janssen WJ, Gandjeva A, Perez MJ, Barthel L, Zemans RL, Bowman JC, Koyanagi DE, Yunt ZX, et al. The pulmonary endothelial glycocalyx regulates neutrophil adhesion and lung injury during experimental sepsis. Nat Med. 2012;18(8):1217–23.

53. Bai K, Wang W. Spatio-temporal development of the endothelial glycocalyx layer and its mechanical property in vitro. J R Soc Interface. 2012;9(74):2290–8.

54. Dull RO, Cluff M, Kingston J, Hill D, Chen H, Hoehne S, Malleske DT, Kaur R. Lung heparan sulfates modulate K(fc) during increased vascular pressure: evidence for glycocalyx-mediated mechanotransduction. Am J Physiol Lung Cell Mol Physiol. 2012;302(9):L816–28.

55. Becker BF, Chappell D, Jacob M. Endothelial glycocalyx and coronary vascular permeability: the fringe benefit. Basic Res Cardiol. 2010;105(6):687–701.

56. Chappell D, Jacob M, Rehm M, Stoeckelhuber M, Welsch U, Conzen P, Becker BF. Heparinase selectively sheds heparan sulphate from the endothelial glycocalyx. Biol Chem. 2008;389(1):79–82.

57. Yang Y, Macleod V, Miao HQ, Theus A, Zhan F, Shaughnessy JD Jr, Sawyer J, Li JP, Zcharia E, Vlodavsky I, et al. Heparanase enhances syndecan-1 shedding: a novel mechanism for stimulation of tumor growth and metastasis. J Biol Chem. 2007;282(18):13326–33.

58. Purushothaman A, Uyama T, Kobayashi F, Yamada S, Sugahara K, Rapraeger AC, Sanderson RD. Heparanase-enhanced shedding of syndecan-1 by myeloma cells promotes endothelial invasion and angiogenesis. Blood. 2010;115(12):2449–57.

59. Mulivor AW, Lipowsky HH. Inhibition of glycan shedding and leukocyte-endothelial adhesion in postcapillary venules by suppression of matrixmetalloprotease activity with doxycycline. Microcirculation (New York, NY : 1994). 2009;16(8):657–66.

60. Lipowsky HH. Protease Activity and the Role of the Endothelial Glycocalyx in Inflammation. Drug Discov Today Dis Models. 2011;8(1):57–62.

61. Voraphani N, Khongphatthanayothin A, Srikaew K, Tontulawat P, Poovorawan Y. Matrix metalloproteinase-9 (mmp-9) in children with dengue virus infection. Jpn J Infect Dis. 2010;63(5):346–8.

62. Her Z, Kam YW, Gan VC, Lee B, Thein TL, Tan JJ, Lee LK, Fink K, Lye DC, Renia L, et al. Severity of Plasma Leakage Is Associated With High Levels of Interferon gamma-Inducible Protein 10, Hepatocyte Growth Factor, Matrix Metalloproteinase 2 (MMP-2), and MMP-9 During Dengue Virus Infection. J Infect Dis. 2017;215(1):42–51.

63. Luplertlop N, Misse D. MMP cellular responses to dengue virus infection-induced vascular leakage. Jpn J Infect Dis. 2008;61(4):298–301.

64. Suwarto S, Sasmono RT, Sinto R, Ibrahim E, Suryamin M. Association of Endothelial Glycocalyx and Tight and Adherens Junctions With Severity of Plasma Leakage in Dengue Infection. J Infect Dis. 2017;215(6):992–9.

65. Chen HR, Chao CH, Liu CC, Ho TS, Tsai HP, Perng GC, Lin YS, Wang JR, Yeh TM. Macrophage migration inhibitory factor is critical for dengue NS1-induced endothelial glycocalyx degradation and hyperpermeability. PLoS Pathog. 2018;14(4):e1007033.

66. Lin SW, Chuang YC, Lin YS, Lei HY, Liu HS, Yeh TM. Dengue virus nonstructural protein NS1 binds to prothrombin/thrombin and inhibits prothrombin activation. J Infect. 2012;64(3):325–34.

67. Zhang G, Han J, Welch EJ, Ye RD, Voyno-Yasenetskaya TA, Malik AB, Du X, Li Z. Lipopolysaccharide stimulates platelet secretion and potentiates platelet aggregation via TLR4/MyD88 and the cGMP-dependent protein kinase pathway. J Immunol. 2009;182(12):7997–8004.

68. Vaughn DW, Green S, Kalayanarooj S, Innis BL, Nimmannitya S, Suntayakorn S, Endy TP, Raengsakulrach B, Rothman AL, Ennis FA, et al. Dengue viremia titer, antibody response pattern, and virus serotype correlate with disease severity. J Infect Dis. 2000;181(1):2–9.

69. Wang WK, Chao DY, Kao CL, Wu HC, Liu YC, Li CM, Lin SC, Ho ST, Huang JH, King CC. High levels of plasma dengue viral load during defervescence in patients with dengue hemorrhagic fever: implications for pathogenesis. Virology. 2003;305(2):330–8.

70. Altmeyer R. Virus attachment and entry offer numerous targets for antiviral therapy. Curr Pharm Des. 2004;10(30):3701–12.

71. Tricou V, Minh NN, Van TP, Lee SJ, Farrar J, Wills B, Tran HT, Simmons CP. A randomized controlled trial of chloroquine for the treatment of dengue in Vietnamese adults. PLoS Negl Trop Dis. 2010;4(8):e785.

72. De La Guardia C, Lleonart R. Progress in the identification of dengue virus entry/fusion inhibitors. Biomed Res Int. 2014;2014:825039.

73. Nguyen NM, Tran CN, Phung LK, Duong KT, Huynh Hle A, Farrar J, Nguyen QT, Tran HT, Nguyen CV, Merson L, et al. A randomized, double-blind placebo controlled trial of balapiravir, a polymerase inhibitor, in adult dengue patients. J Infect Dis. 2013;207(9):1442–50.

74. Rothan HA, Han HC, Ramasamy TS, Othman S, Rahman NA, Yusof R. Inhibition of dengue NS2B-NS3 protease and viral replication in Vero cells by recombinant retrocyclin-1. BMC Infect Dis. 2012;12:314.

75. van Cleef KWR, Overheul GJ, Thomassen MC, Kaptein SJF, Davidson AD, Jacobs M, Neyts J, van Kuppeveld FJM, van Rij RP. Identification of a new dengue virus inhibitor that targets the viral NS4B protein and restricts genomic RNA replication. Antivir Res. 2013;99(2):165–71.

76. Wang QY, Kondreddi RR, Xie XP, Rao R, Nilar S, Xu HY, Qing M, Chang D, Dong HP, Yokokawa F, et al. A Translation Inhibitor That Suppresses Dengue Virus In Vitro and In Vivo. Antimicrob Agents Ch. 2011;55(9):4072–80.

77. Mastrangelo E, Pezzullo M, De Burghgraeve T, Kaptein S, Pastorino B, Dallmeier K, de Lamballerie X, Neyts J, Hanson AM, Frick DN, et al. Ivermectin is a potent inhibitor of flaviviruses replication specifically targeting NS3 helicase activity: new prospects for an old drug. J Antimicrob Chemoth. 2012;67(8):1884–94.

78. Rathore APS, Paradkar PN, Watanabe S, Tan KH, Sung C, Connolly JE, Low J, Ooi EE, Vasudevan SG. Celgosivir treatment misfolds dengue virus NS1 protein, induces cellular pro-survival genes and protects against lethal challenge mouse model. Antivir Res. 2011;92(3):453–60.

79. Simanjuntak Y, Liang JJ, Lee YL, Lin YL. Repurposing of prochlorperazine for use against dengue virus infection. J Infect Dis. 2015;211(3):394–404.

80. Leela SL, Srisawat C, Sreekanth GP, Noisakran S, Yenchitsomanus PT, Limjindaporn T. Drug repurposing of minocycline against dengue virus infection. Biochem Bioph Res Co. 2016;478(1):410–6.

81. Krishnan MN, Garcia-Blanco MA. Targeting host factors to treat West Nile and dengue viral infections. Viruses. 2014;6(2):683–708.

82. de Chassey B, Meyniel-Schicklin L, Vonderscher J, Andre P, Lotteau V. Virus-host interactomics: new insights and opportunities for antiviral drug discovery. Genome Med. 2014;6(11):115.

83. Savidis G, McDougall WM, Meraner P, Perreira JM, Portmann JM, Trincucci G, John SP, Aker AM, Renzette N, Robbins DR, et al. Identification of zika virus and dengue virus dependency factors using functional genomics. Cell Rep. 2016;16(1):232–46.

84. Wang Y, Zhang P. Recent advances in the identification of the host factors involved in dengue virus replication. Virol Sin. 2017;32(1):23–31.

85. Yu JS, Wu YH, Tseng CK, Lin CK, Hsu YC, Chen YH, Lee JC. Schisandrin A inhibits dengue viral replication via upregulating antiviral interferon responses through STAT signaling pathway. Sci Rep. 2017;7:45171.

86. Zainal N, Chang CP, Cheng YL, Wu YW, Anderson R, Wan SW, Chen CL, Ho TS, AbuBakar S, Lin YS. Resveratrol treatment reveals a novel role for HMGB1 in regulation of the type 1 interferon response in dengue virus infection. Sci Rep. 2017;7:42998.

87. Datan E, Roy SG, Germain G, Zali N, McLean JE, Golshan G, Harbajan S, Lockshin RA, Zakeri Z. Dengue-induced autophagy, virus replication and protection from cell death require ER stress (PERK) pathway activation. Cell Death Dis. 2016;7:e2127.

88. Fontaine KA, Sanchez EL, Camarda R, Lagunoff M. Dengue virus induces and requires glycolysis for optimal replication. J Virol. 2015;89(4):2358–66.

89. Low JG, Ooi EE, Vasudevan SG. Current status of dengue therapeutics research and development. J Infect Dis. 2017;215(suppl_2):S96–S102.

90. Lai YC, Chuang YC, Chang CP, Lin YS, Perng GC, Wu HC, Hsieh SL, Yeh TM. Minocycline suppresses dengue virus replication by down-regulation of macrophage migration inhibitory factor-induced autophagy. Antiviral Res. 2018;155:28–38.

91. Katzelnick LC, Gresh L, Halloran ME, Mercado JC, Kuan G, Gordon A, Balmaseda A, Harris E. Antibody-dependent enhancement of severe dengue disease in humans. Science. 2017;358(6365):929–32.

92. Robinson LN, Tharakaraman K, Rowley KJ, Costa VV, Chan KR, Wong YH, Ong LC, Tan HC, Koch T, Cain D, et al. Structure-guided design of an anti-dengue antibody directed to a non-immunodominant epitope. Cell. 2015; 162(3):493–504.

93. Rouvinski A, Guardado-Calvo P, Barba-Spaeth G, Duquerroy S, Vaney MC, Kikuti CM, Navarro Sanchez ME, Dejnirattisai W, Wongwiwat W, Haouz A,

et al. Recognition determinants of broadly neutralizing human antibodies against dengue viruses. Nature. 2015;520(7545):109–13.

94. Dejnirattisai W, Wongwiwat W, Supasa S, Zhang X, Dai X, Rouvinski A, Jumnainsong A, Edwards C, Quyen NTH, Duangchinda T, et al. A new class of highly potent, broadly neutralizing antibodies isolated from viremic patients infected with dengue virus. Nat Immunol. 2015;16(2):170–7.

95. Xu M, Zuest R, Velumani S, Tukijan F, Toh YX, Appanna R, Tan EY, Cerny D, MacAry P, Wang CI, et al. A potent neutralizing antibody with therapeutic potential against all four serotypes of dengue virus. NPJ Vaccines. 2017;2:2.

96. Wan SW, Lu YT, Huang CH, Lin CF, Anderson R, Liu HS, Yeh TM, Yen YT, Wu-Hsieh BA, Lin YS. Protection against dengue virus infection in mice by administration of antibodies against modified nonstructural protein 1. PLoS One. 2014;9(3):e92495.

97. Lai YC, Chuang YC, Liu CC, Ho TS, Lin YS, Anderson R, Yeh TM. Antibodies against modified NS1 wing domain peptide protect against dengue virus infection. Sci Rep. 2017;7(1):6975.

98. Schlesinger JJ, Brandriss MW, Walsh EE. Protection of mice against dengue 2 virus encephalitis by immunization with the dengue 2 virus non-structural glycoprotein NS1. J Gen Virol. 1987;68(Pt 3):853–7.

99. Krishna VD, Rangappa M, Satchidanandam V. Virus-specific cytolytic antibodies to nonstructural protein 1 of Japanese encephalitis virus effect reduction of virus output from infected cells. J Virol. 2009;83(10):4766–77.

100. Lin CF, Wan SW, Chen MC, Lin SC, Cheng CC, Chiu SC, Hsiao YL, Lei HY, Liu HS, Yeh TM, et al. Liver injury caused by antibodies against dengue virus nonstructural protein 1 in a murine model. Lab Invest. 2008;88(10):1079–89.

101. Vigne C, Dupuy M, Richetin A, Guy B, Jackson N, Bonaparte M, Hu B, Saville M, Chansinghakul D, Noriega F, et al. Integrated immunogenicity analysis of a tetravalent dengue vaccine up to 4 y after vaccination. Hum Vaccin Immunother. 2017;13(9):2004–16.

102. Guy B, Jackson N. Dengue vaccine: hypotheses to understand CYD-TDV-induced protection. Nat Rev Microbiol. 2016;14(1):45–54.

103. Hadinegoro SR, Arredondo-Garcia JL, Capeding MR, Deseda C, Chotpitayasunondh T, Dietze R, Muhammad Ismail HI, Reynales H, Limkittikul K, Rivera-Medina DM, et al. Efficacy and Long-Term Safety of a Dengue Vaccine in Regions of Endemic Disease. N Engl J Med. 2015;373(13):1195–206.

104. Halstead SB. Dengvaxia sensitizes seronegatives to vaccine enhanced disease regardless of age. Vaccine. 2017;35(47):6355–8.

105. Halstead SB. Licensed dengue vaccine: Public health conundrum and scientific challenge. Am J Trop Med Hyg. 2016;95(4):741–5.

106. Avirutnan P, Hauhart RE, Marovich MA, Garred P, Atkinson JP, Diamond MS. Complement-mediated neutralization of dengue virus requires mannose-binding lectin. MBio. 2011;2(6):e00276–11.

107. Lin YS, Yeh TM, Lin CF, Wan SW, Chuang YC, Hsu TK, Liu HS, Liu CC, Anderson R, Lei HY. Molecular mimicry between virus and host and its implications for dengue disease pathogenesis. Exp Biol Med. 2011;236(5):515–23.

108. Lin CF, Wan SW, Cheng HJ, Lei HY, Lin YS. Autoimmune pathogenesis in dengue virus infection. Viral Immunology. 2006;19(2):127–32.

109. Sun DS, King CC, Huang HS, Shih YL, Lee CC, Tsai WJ, Yu CC, Chang HH. Antiplatelet autoantibodies elicited by dengue virus non-structural protein 1 cause thrombocytopenia and mortality in mice. J Thromb Haemost. 2007; 5(11):2291–9.

110. Chen MC, Lin CF, Lei HY, Lin SC, Liu HS, Yeh TM, Anderson R, Lin YS. Deletion of the C-terminal region of dengue virus nonstructural protein 1 (NS1) abolishes anti-NS1-mediated platelet dysfunction and bleeding tendency. J Immunol. 2009;183(3):1797–803.

111. Liu IJ, Chiu CY, Chen YC, Wu HC. Molecular mimicry of human endothelial cell antigen by autoantibodies to nonstructural protein 1 of dengue virus. J Biol Chem. 2011;286(11):9726–36.

112. Chuang YC, Lin YS, Liu HS, Yeh TM. Molecular mimicry between dengue virus and coagulation factors induces antibodies to inhibit thrombin activity and enhance fibrinolysis. J Virol. 2014;88(23):13759–68.

113. Henchal EA, Henchal LS, Schlesinger JJ. Synergistic interactions of anti-NS1 monoclonal antibodies protect passively immunized mice from lethal challenge with dengue 2 virus. J Gen Virol. 1988;69(Pt 8):2101–7.

114. Wan SW, Chen PW, Chen CY, Lai YC, Chu YT, Hung CY, Lee H, Wu HF, Chuang YC, Lin J, et al. Therapeutic effects of monoclonal antibody against dengue virus NS1 in a STAT1 knockout mouse model of dengue infection. J Immunol. 2017;199(8):2834–44.

115. Chu YT, Wan SW, Chang YC, Lee CK, Wu-Hsieh BA, Anderson R, Lin YS. Antibodies against nonstructural protein 1 protect mice from dengue virus-induced mast cell activation. Lab Invest. 2017;97(5):602.

116. Falgout B, Bray M, Schlesinger JJ, Lai CJ. Immunization of mice with recombinant vaccinia virus expressing authentic dengue virus nonstructural protein NS1 protects against lethal dengue virus encephalitis. J Virol. 1990; 64(9):4356–63.

117. Srivastava AK, Putnak JR, Warren RL, Hoke CH. Mice immunized with a dengue type-2 virus-E and NS1 fusion protein made in Escherichia-Coli are protected against lethal dengue virus-infection. Vaccine. 1995;13(13):1251–8.

118. Amorim JH, Diniz MO, Cariri FAMO, Rodrigues JF, Bizerra RSP, Goncalves AJS, Alves AMD, Ferreira LCD. Protective immunity to DENV2 after immunization with a recombinant NS1 protein using a genetically detoxified heat-labile toxin as an adjuvant. Vaccine. 2012;30(5):837–45.

119. Wu SF, Liao CL, Lin YL, Yeh CT, Chen LK, Huang YF, Chou HY, Huang JL, Shaio MF, Sytwu HK. Evaluation of protective efficacy and immune mechanisms of using a non-structural protein NS1 in DNA vaccine against dengue 2 virus in mice. Vaccine. 2003;21(25-26):3919–29.

120. Costa SM, Freire MS, Alves AMB. DNA vaccine against the non-structural 1 protein (NS1) of dengue 2 virus. Vaccine. 2006;24(21):4562–4.

121. Goncalves AJ, Oliveira ER, Costa SM, Paes MV, Silva JF, Azevedo AS, Mantuano-Barradas M, Nogueira AC, Almeida CJ, Alves AM. Cooperation between CD4+ T Cells and humoral immunity is critical for protection against dengue using a DNA vaccine based on the NS1 antigen. PLoS Negl Trop Dis. 2015;9(12):e0004277.

122. Costa SM, Azevedo AS, Paes MV, Sarges FS, Freire MS, Alves AMB. DNA vaccines against dengue virus based on the ns1 gene: The influence of different signal sequences on the protein expression and its correlation to the immune response elicited in mice. Virology. 2007;358(2):413–23.

14

Nucleocapsid protein-dependent assembly of the RNA packaging signal of Middle East respiratory syndrome coronavirus

Wei-Chen Hsin[1], Chan-Hua Chang[1], Chi-You Chang[1], Wei-Hao Peng[2], Chung-Liang Chien[2], Ming-Fu Chang[3*] and Shin C. Chang[1*] (iD)

Abstract

Background: Middle East respiratory syndrome coronavirus (MERS-CoV) consists of a positive-sense, single-stranded RNA genome and four structural proteins: the spike, envelope, membrane, and nucleocapsid protein. The assembly of the viral genome into virus particles involves viral structural proteins and is believed to be mediated through recognition of specific sequences and RNA structures of the viral genome.

Methods and Results: A culture system for the production of MERS coronavirus-like particles (MERS VLPs) was determined and established by electron microscopy and the detection of coexpressed viral structural proteins. Using the VLP system, a 258-nucleotide RNA fragment, which spans nucleotides 19,712 to 19,969 of the MERS-CoV genome (designated PS258(19712–19969)$_{ME}$), was identified to function as a packaging signal. Assembly of the RNA packaging signal into MERS VLPs is dependent on the viral nucleocapsid protein. In addition, a 45-nucleotide stable stem-loop substructure of the PS258(19712–19969)$_{ME}$ interacted with both the N-terminal domain and the C-terminal domain of the viral nucleocapsid protein. Furthermore, a functional SARS-CoV RNA packaging signal failed to assemble into the MERS VLPs, which indicated virus-specific assembly of the RNA genome.

Conclusions: A MERS-oV RNA packaging signal was identified by the detection of GFP expression following an incubation of MERS VLPs carrying the heterologous mRNA GFP-PS258(19712–19969)$_{ME}$ with virus permissive Huh7 cells. The MERS VLP system could help us in understanding virus infection and morphogenesis.

Keywords: MERS-CoV, RNA packaging signal, Nucleocapsid protein

Background

Middle East respiratory syndrome coronavirus (MERS-CoV) is a novel coronavirus that causes acute respiratory syndrome with a high mortality rate in human [1]. The first case of MERS-CoV was identified in September 2012 in Saudi Arabia. From the initial outbreak to April 2018, MERS-CoV spread through 27 countries and caused approximately 2144 cases and 750 deaths (http://www.who.int/emergencies/mers-cov/en/). Dipeptidyl peptidase 4, which is also known as CD26, was identified as a functional receptor for MERS-CoV [2, 3]. Coronaviruses are enveloped, positive-sense, single-stranded RNA viruses with approximately 26–32 kb genomic RNA [4–6]. The 5′ two-thirds of the viral genome consists of open reading frames (ORF) 1a and 1b that encode the viral nonstructural proteins (nsps), whereas the 3′ one-third consists of ORFs that encode the viral structural proteins, including the spike (S), membrane (M), envelope (E) and nucleocapsid (N), and accessory proteins. The S, M and E proteins form the viral envelope [7–9], whereas the N protein is considered the most important protein that interacts with the viral genomic RNA and packages the RNA into virus particles by recognizing a specific sequence, which is termed the packaging signal [10–12].

Studies on mouse hepatitis virus (MHV), which is a lineage A betacoronavirus, localized the packaging signal

* Correspondence: mfchang@ntu.edu.tw; scchang093@ntu.edu.tw
[3]Institute of Biochemistry and Molecular Biology, College of Medicine, National Taiwan University, No. 1, Jen-Ai Road, First Section, Taipei 100, Taiwan
[1]Institute of Microbiology, College of Medicine, National Taiwan University, No. 1, Jen-Ai Road, First Section, Taipei 100, Taiwan
Full list of author information is available at the end of the article

to the 3'-end of ORF 1b of the viral genome in the gene that encodes the nsp15 endoribonuclease [13–15]. A stable stem-loop of 69-nucleotides (nt) was identified as sufficient for RNA packaging. Computer analysis further revealed conservation of the packaging signal in both the sequence and RNA secondary structure between MHV and bovine coronavirus (BCoV) and among other lineage A betacoronaviruses [16–18]. Our previous studies on severe acute respiratory syndrome coronavirus (SARS-CoV), which is a lineage B betacoronavirus, identified a 580-nt RNA fragment with a stable stem-loop structure as a functional signal to drive packaging of coexpressed RNA of a green fluorescent protein (GFP) into virus-like particles (VLPs) [19]. This SARS-CoV packaging signal spanned the viral genome from nt 19,715 to 20,294 and was localized to a subdomain of the nsp15 gene different from the packaging signal of lineage A betacoronaviruses. However, studies on alphacoronavirus transmissible gastroenteritis virus (TGEV) localized the RNA packaging signal to the 5'-end of the viral genome [20, 21], and sequences in the 5'-UTR and/or 3'-UTR may be required for the RNA packaging of gammacoronavirus infectious bronchitis virus (IBV) [22, 23].

In addition to the packaging signal, the viral structural proteins may also play roles in the assembly of the viral genome. Studies on MHV indicated that M and E proteins are sufficient for the assembly of VLPs [9]. Through a specific interaction between the viral M protein and the packaging signal, a coexpressed RNA fragment carrying the viral packaging signal can be packaged into VLPs in the absence of N protein [24, 25]. Nevertheless, studies argue for the involvement of the N protein in RNA genome packaging. The carboxy-terminal domain (CTD) of the N protein was demonstrated to be the major determinant of MHV packaging signal recognition [11]; and the further downstream carboxy-terminal tail coordinates the selectivity of genome packaging and couples genome encapsidation to the virion assembly [26]. In addition, our earlier study on SARS-CoV indicated N protein-dependent assembly of the viral RNA packaging signal [19]. To date, the RNA packaging signal of MERS-CoV has not been determined, and it is unclear whether the N protein is essential for the MERS-CoV RNA package.

In this study, a putative RNA packaging signal of the MERS-CoV genome was predicted by bioinformatics analysis. MERS VLPs carrying RNA sequences of GFP fused to a 258-nt RNA fragment consisting of the putative RNA packaging signal and its flanking sequences were generated and incubated with MERS-CoV-permissive Huh7 cells for functional analysis. The results indicate that the RNA fragment spanning nt 19,712 to 19,969 of the viral genome is sufficient to function as a packaging signal and assemble into the MERS VLPs. In addition, packaging of the MERS-CoV RNA depends on the viral N protein.

Methods

Cell lines and culture condition

Human embryonic kidney cells 293 T and hepatocellular carcinoma Huh7 cells were maintained in Dulbecco's modified Eagle medium (GIBCO) supplemented with 10% heat-inactivated fetal bovine serum, 1% 100X non-essential amino acids plus 100 U of penicillin and 100 μg of streptomycin per ml in a humidified 5% CO_2 atmosphere at 37 °C.

Plasmids

(i) Plasmids pcDNA-ctrl-V5HisTopo, pcDNA-MERS-E, pcDNA-MERS-M, and pcDNA-MERS-N. Plasmid pcDNA-ctrl-V5HisTopo was generated by inserting a DNA fragment containing multiple cloning sites derived from annealing of two oligonucleotides, CACCATGGA ATTCATCGATCTAGATCCGCGGCCGCACTCGAGT and its complementary sequences, into pcDNA3.1D/ V5-His-TOPO (Invitrogen). Plasmids pcDNA-MERS-E, pcDNA-MERS-M, and pcDNA-MERS-N encode the V5- and His-tagged E, M, and N protein, respectively, of MERS-CoV and were generated by inserting their corresponding cDNA fragments into pcDNA-ctrl-V5HisTopo. The MERS-CoV cDNA fragments were chemically synthesized (Invitrogen) according to GenBank (HCoV-EMC strain; accession number NC_019843.3) and used as templates for PCR amplification with the following primer sets: CS-ME-E1 (GGAATTCATGTTACCCTTTG) and CS-ME-E2 (ATCAACCCACTCGTCAGG) for the E gene, CS-ME-M1 (GGAATTCATGTCTAATATGACGC) and CS-ME-M2 (ATCAGCTCGAAGCAATGCAAG) for the M gene, and CS-ME-N-f(RI) (GGAATTCATGGCAT CCCCT) and CS-ME-N-r(RI) (GGAATTCATCAGTG TTAACATC) for the N gene. The PCR products of E and M gene were treated with EcoRI and EcoRV restriction endonucleases, and inserted into the EcoRI and EcoRV sites of pcDNA-ctrl-V5HisTopo to generate plasmids pcDNA-MERS-E and pcDNA-MERS-M, respectively. The PCR product of N gene was treated with EcoRI restriction endonuclease, and inserted into the EcoRI site of pcDNA-ctrl-V5HisTopo to generate plasmid pcDNA-MERS-N.

(ii) Plasmid pcDNA-MERS-S. For construction of plasmid pcDNA-MERS-S, pcDNA-MERS-S1 was first generated following a treatment of plasmid pCR4-MERS-S1-Topo (kindly provided by Haagmans BL and Osterhaus AD, Department of Viroscience, Erasmus Medical Center, Rotterdam, Netherlands) with EcoRI restriction endonuclease and insertion of the resultant DNA fragment containing the MERS-CoV S protein coding sequences from nt 1 to 2238 into the EcoRI site of pcDNA-ctrl-V5HisTopo. A DNA fragment representing the MERS-CoV S protein coding sequences from nt 2230 to 4062 with ScaI site at the 5' end and EcoRV at the 3' end was then generated by PCR amplification from a chemically synthesized template (Invitrogen) and inserted into the ScaI site of the plasmid pcDNA-MERS-S1 located at nt 2229 of the MERS-CoV S coding sequences to generate plasmid pcDNA-MERS-S.

(iii) Plasmids pET-MERS-N, pET-MERS-N(1–156), and pET-MERS-N(1–263). Plasmids pET-MERS-N, pET-MERS-N(1–156), and pET-MERS-N(1–263) encode the His-tagged full-length MERS-CoV N protein, the N-terminal domain from amino acid residues 1 to 156, and 1 to 263, respectively. For construction of pET-MERS-N, plasmid pcDNA-MERS-N was treated with EcoRI restriction endonuclease and the resultant DNA fragment of the N gene was inserted into the EcoRI site of pET-28a (Novagen). Plasmid pET-MERS-N(1–156) was derived from pET-MERS-N following a digestion with HindIII restriction endonuclease and self-ligation of the resultant 5.8-kb DNA fragment. For construction of plasmid pET-MERS-N(1–263), a 321-bp HindIII fragment was obtained from pET-MERS-N and inserted into the HindIII site of pET-MERS-N(1–156).

(iv) Plasmids pET-MERS-N(239–413) and pET-MERS-N(264–413). Plasmids pET-MERS-N(239–413) and pET-MERS-N(264–413) encode the His-tagged MERS-CoV N protein from amino acid residues 239 to 413 and 264 to 413, respectively. For generation of plasmid pET-MERS-N(239–413), pET-MERS-N was used as the template for PCR amplification with the primer set CS-ME-N715(NheI)-f (GGGGCTAGCACTAAGAAAG ATGCTGC) and CS-ME-N-r(RI) (GGAATTCATCAGTG TTAACATC). The resultant PCR product representing the DNA fragment of N(239–413) was treated with NheI and EcoRI restriction endonucleases and then inserted into the NheI and EcoRI sites of pET-28a. For generation of plasmid pET-MERS-N(264–413), a 468-bp DNA fragment obtained from the treatment of pET-MERS-N with HindIII restriction endonuclease was inserted into the HindIII site of pET-28a.

(v) Plasmids pEGFP-PS258(19712–19969)ME and pEGFP-N1-PS580. Plasmid pEGFP-PS258(19712–19969)ME represents the cDNA of the putative packaging signal of MERS-CoV genomic RNA inserted into the 3′ noncoding region of the GFP gene. For construction of the plasmid pEGFP-PS258(19712–19969)ME, a DNA fragment representing MERS-CoV genomic RNA from nt 19,712 to 19,969 with NotI site on both ends was first obtained following PCR amplification from a chemically synthesized template (Invitrogen) and a treatment of the PCR product with NotI restriction endonuclease. The DNA fragment was then inserted into the NotI site of pEGFP-N1 to generate plasmid pEGFP-PS258(19712–19969)ME. Plasmid pEGFP-N1-PS580 has been previously described [19]. It represents the cDNA of the packaging signal of SARS-CoV genomic RNA from nt 19,715 to

20,294 inserted into the 3′ noncoding region of the GFP gene.

Transient transfection and harvest of cell lysates

Transient transfection was performed with T-Pro Non-liposome transfection Reagent II (Genestar Biotech) according to the manufacturer's protocol. Briefly, the expression plasmid was diluted into Opti-MEM (GIBCO) and mixed with T-Pro Non-liposome transfection Reagent II at the ratio of 1 μg DNA to 2 μl transfection Reagent. Two days posttransfection, cells were lysed using a RIPA buffer consisting of 50 mM Tris-HCl, pH 7.5, 150 mM NaCl, 0.5% sodium deoxycholate, 1% NP-40, 0.1% SDS, and 1% complete EDTA-free protease inhibitor (Roche).

Production and harvest of virus like particles (VLPs)

For production of MERS VLPs, cotransfection was performed with plasmids encoding the MERS-CoV structural proteins E, M, and S, in the presence or absence of the N-expressing plasmid and the MERS-CoV packaging signal plasmid pEGFP-PS258(19712–19969)ME, the SARS-CoV packaging signal plasmid pEGFP-N1-PS580, or the vector control pEGFP-N1. Production of MERS VLPs in the transfected cells was examined by electron microscopy three days posttransfection. For the collection of supernatant VLPs, culture medium was clarified by centrifugation at 1000 rpm in an RS-240 rotor (Kubota 2010) for 5 min, passed through a 0.45 μm filter, and subjected to ultracentrifugation at 36000 rpm in an SW41 rotor (Beckman) for 3 h at 4 °C. The VLP pellet was resuspended in PBS and stored at − 80 °C. For collecting cellular VLPs, the transfected cells were resuspended in PBS containing 1% complete EDTA-free protease inhibitor and subjected to three cycles of freeze (− 80 °C) and thaw (37 °C) prior to the centrifugation at 1000 rpm. In addition, for separation of supernatant VLPs with different structure compositions, the VLP suspension was further loaded on a discontinuous sucrose gradient consisting of 20, 30, 50, and 60% sucrose in 20 mM HEPES (pH 7.4) and 0.1% BSA and centrifuged at 36000 rpm for 15 h at 4 °C. The density of VLPs was determined by a refractometer (ATAGO). Expression of MERS-CoV structural proteins in the VLPs were examined by Western blot analysis.

Electron microscopic analysis of MERS VLPs

Three days following cotransfection of the plasmids encoding the MERS-CoV structural proteins, cells were fixed with 4% glutaraldehyde in 0.1 M phosphate buffer for 24 h at 4 °C and post-fixed 1% aqueous osmium tetroxide diluted in the same phosphate buffer at room temperature for 1 h. After washing, the fixed cells were dehydrated in a graded ethanol series and embedded in a Polybed 812-Araldite mixture (EMS, Hatfield, PA).

Semi-thin sections of 1 μm were obtained using an ultramicrotome (Ultracut E, Leica-Reichert Jung, Wetzlar, Germany) and stained with toluidine blue for correlative light microscopy. Ultrathin sections were cut at 70 nm, collected on copper grids (200 meshes) and stained with uranyl acetate and lead citrate. Images were examined in a Hitachi H-7100 electron microscope equipped with a Gatan 832 digital camera (Gatan, Inc.).

Western blot analysis

Protein lysates were resolved by polyacrylamide gel electrophoresis (PAGE) and electrotransferred onto an Immobilon-P membrane (Millipore) as described previously [27]. Mouse monoclonal antibody against V5 epitope (Invitrogen) was used as the primary antibody to detect expression of the V5-tagged recombinant proteins. Following incubation with horseradish peroxidase-conjugated secondary antibodies, specific interactions between antigens and antibodies were detected by the enhanced chemiluminescence system (Advansta).

Immunofluorescence assay

Cells cultured on glass coverslips were fixed with 4% paraformaldehyde for 30 min at room temperature. The fixed cells were permeabilized with 0.5% Triton X-100 and washed with PBS. Following a blocking with 3% BSA for 1 h at room temperature, the cells were incubated with rabbit polyclonal antibodies against GFP for 1 h at room temperature, washed with PBS, and then incubated with secondary antibodies conjugated with Alexa Fluor® 488 (Invitrogen) for 1 h at room temperature. Cell nuclei were stained with Hoechst. The coverslips were mounted on glass slides. Zeiss Axioskop 40 microscope was used to capture the images.

Expression and purification of MERS-CoV N protein and its subdomains

For expression of recombinant MERS-CoV N protein and its subdomains, plasmids pET-MERS-N and its derivatives were individually transformed into *E. coli* BL21(DE3) cells. Protein expression was induced with 0.1 mM isopropyl-β-D-thiogalactopyranoside for 18 h at 16 °C, and purified as previously described [19] with modifications. In brief, cell pellets were subjected to sonication and centrifugation at 6000 rpm in an RA-200 J rotor (Kubota) for 10 min at 4 °C. The supernatants were collected and loaded onto a nickel affinity column. The His-tagged MERS-CoV N proteins were eluted with elution buffers consisting of 50 mM sodium phosphate, pH 8.0, 300 mM NaCl, 6 M urea and a stepwise gradient of imidazole at 10, 50 and 200 mM. The fractions that contain proteins of interest, identified by Coomassie blue staining and Western blot analysis following SDS-PAGE, were pooled together and dialyzed against a dialysis

buffer containing 50 mM sodium phosphate, pH 7.4, 150 mM NaCl, 1 mM EDTA, and 0.01% NaN₃. The purified proteins were concentrated with Amicon Ultra-15 concentrator (Millipore) and kept in 50% glycerol at − 80 °C for filter binding assay.

Filter binding assay

Filter binding assay was carried out as previously described [19] with modifications. In brief, biotinylated RNA fragments were biochemically synthesized (Thermo Fisher; Integrated DNA Technologies) and used as the probes. The probes were heated at 80 °C for 10 min and then incubated at 37 °C for 15 min. Purified proteins pre-incubated independently at 37 °C for 15 min were then mixed with the RNA probe in a filter binding buffer consisting of 20 mM HEPES, pH 7.3, 40 mM KCl, 2 mM MgCl₂, and 2 mM DTT. After an additional incubation for 10 min, the reaction mixture was passed through Immobilon-P membrane that had been activated with methanol and soaked in the filter binding buffer. The membrane was washed three times with the binding buffer. Specific interactions between biotin-labeled RNA probes and purified proteins were detected by the enhanced chemiluminescence system following pre-incubation with streptavidin horseradish peroxidase conjugate. In addition, a biotin-labeled RNA fragment 5′–UCCUGCUUCAACAG UGCUUGGACGGAAC–3′ (Thermo Fisher) was used as the negative control.

Results

Bioinformatics analysis of the MERS-CoV RNA genome

Bioinformatics and functional analysis have previously identified the minimum size packaging signal (approximately 60 to 95 nt) for various coronaviruses. However, the packaging signal of lineage C betacoronavirus MERS-CoV has not been determined. Based on the observations that a stable stem–loop structure is often a prerequisite for an RNA fragment to be a packaging signal and that unique sequences may determine the packaging specificity of different coronavirus lineages, we proposed the analysis of the genome sequence and the structure of different lineage betacoronaviruses for the prediction of the potential packaging signal of MERS-CoV. The whole genome sequence of MERS-CoV was first compared with lineage B betacoronavirus SARS-CoV by alignment with NCBI blastn. This revealed a highly variable region from nt 19,757 to 20,434 of the MERS-CoV genome located at the 3′ end of ORF 1b and between two regions that have the highest conservation (the alignment score was higher than 200; Fig. 1a, top). Interestingly, this variable region overlaps the PS580 RNA fragment spanning nt 19,715 to 20,294 of the SARS-CoV genome, which has been identified as a functional packaging signal [19]. In addition, when the MERS-CoV RNA sequence was compared with that of the lineage A betacoronavirus MHV, the divergent

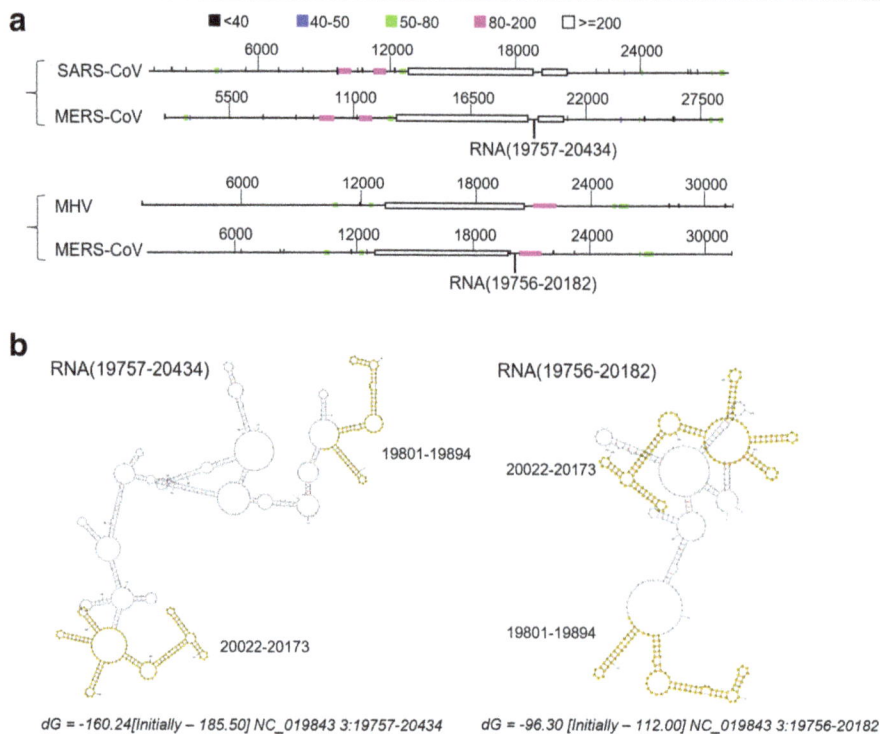

Fig. 1 Sequence similarity among the coronavirus genomic RNAs and secondary structure prediction. **a** Alignment of the whole genome sequence of MERS-CoV (accession number NC_019843.3) with that of SARS-CoV (accession number AY291451.1) and MHV (accession number NC_001846.1) by NCBI blastn. Regions with the highest conservation (alignment score ≧ 200) are indicated by open boxes followed by alignment scores 80–200, 50–80, 40–50, and < 40 as indicated. MERS-CoV RNA fragments spanning nt 19,757 to 20,434 [RNA(19757–20434)] and nt 19,756 to 20,182 [RNA(19756–20182)] with sequence diversity were subjected to secondary structure prediction. **b** Secondary structure prediction. Secondary structure of MERS-CoV RNA(19757–20434) and RNA(19756–20182) were analyzed by Mfold. Two subdomains of 94-nt (nt 19,801 to 19,894) and 152-nt (nt 20,022 to 20,173) that form stable substructures in both RNA fragments were colored yellow

sequence was localized to a similar but shorter fragment spanning nt 19,756 to 20,182 of the MERS-CoV genome (Fig. 1a, bottom). These results located a highly variable region of the genome sequences among the different lineage betacoronaviruses. Secondary structures of the MERS-CoV RNA(19757–20434) and RNA(19756–20182) were then analyzed (Fig. 1b). Two RNA subdomains of 94-nt (nt 19,801 to 19,894) and 152-nt (nt 20,022 to 20,173) that form stable structures in both RNA fragments were identified as potential packaging signals of MERS-CoV.

Identification of PS258(19712–19969)$_{ME}$ as a putative N protein-dependent RNA packaging signal of MERS-CoV

For examination of the RNA packaging of MERS-CoV, a culture system that expresses viral structural proteins and produces MERS VLPs was established. As shown in Fig. 2a, expression of MERS-CoV structural proteins was detected following cotransfection of plasmids encoding the viral proteins M, E, S, and N as indicated. Successful production of MERS VLPs in transfected cells in the absence (VLPdN) or presence of N protein (VLP) was confirmed by electron microscopy (Fig. 2b). In addition,

VLPs that were released into the culture medium (supernatant VLPs) were subjected to a discontinuous sucrose gradient centrifugation. Western blot analysis demonstrated that fractions 6 and 7 likely represent VLPs that contain four structural proteins with densities of 1.151 and 1.207, respectively (Fig. 2c).

A 258-nt RNA fragment, named PS258(19712–19969)$_{ME}$ (Fig. 3a) and that contains the earlier-identified 94-nt stable stem-loop structure (highlighted) as a center domain and extends on both ends, was chosen to begin functional analysis for identification of the putative RNA packaging signal. To examine the packaging activity of the PS258(19712–19969)$_{ME}$ RNA fragment, the plasmid pEGFP-PS258(19712–19969)ME that expresses heterologous mRNA GFP-PS258(19712–19969)$_{ME}$ was generated. Cotransfection was performed with the plasmids encoding MERS-CoV structural proteins and plasmid pEGFP-PS258(19712–19969)ME. In addition, plasmid pEGFP-N-PS580 that encodes the GFP-PS580 RNA fragment containing the SARS-CoV RNA packaging signal was applied to examine the specificity of the viral RNA packaging. As shown in Fig. 3, the expression of the viral structural proteins was detected in cell lysates (panel a)

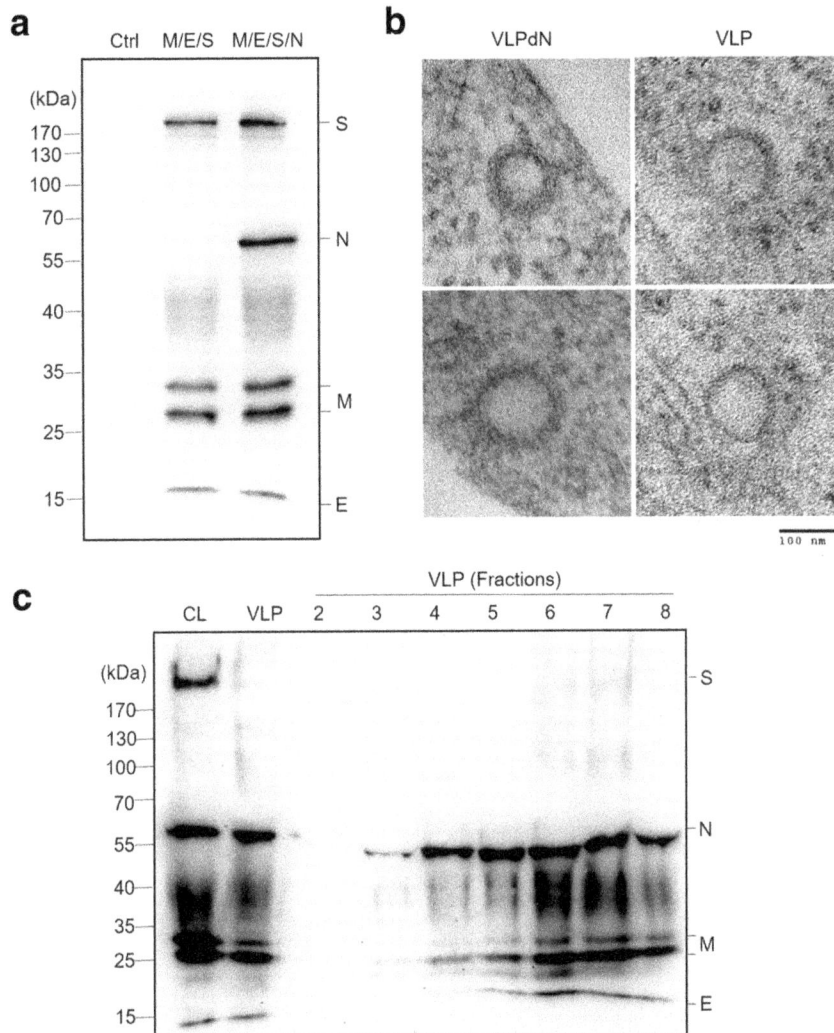

Fig. 2 Production of MERS VLPs in cultured cells. **a** Expression of MERS-CoV structural proteins. Plasmids encoding MERS-CoV structural proteins M, E, S, and N as indicated were cotransfected into 293 T cells and the cell lysates were prepared for Western blot analysis two days posttransfection. Protein lysate prepared from cells transfected with control plasmid was applied as a negative control (lane Ctrl). **b** Electron microscopic analysis of MERS VLPs. The cells were fixed and embedded three days following cotransfection of the plasmids encoding the MERS-CoV structural proteins M, E, and S (VLPdN) or M, E, S, and N (VLP). Images of the sections were examined for the presence of MERS VLPs in a Hitachi H-7100 electron microscope equipped with a Gatan 832 digital camera. **c** Separation of MERS VLPs. MERS VLPs collected from culture medium were subjected to a discontinuous sucrose gradient centrifugation as described in Methods. The fractions were collected for Western blot analysis. Lane CL represents the protein lysates of transfected cells and lane VLP represents the total VLPs prior to the gradient centrifugation

and in both the cellular and supernatant VLPs (panel b; VLP, VLP/PS$_{ME}$, and VLP/PS$_{SA}$). Assembly of the GFP-PS258(19712–19969)$_{ME}$ into MERS VLPs (VLP/PS$_{ME}$) was examined by incubating the VLPs with the virus-permissible Huh7 cells that endogenously express the viral receptor hDPP4 [2]. As shown in Fig. 3c, GFP-PS258(19712–19969)$_{ME}$ RNA that assembled into the VLP/PS$_{ME}$ was evident by the detection of GFP expression upon entering the cells. The expression of GFP was not detected in Huh7 cells coincubating with VLPs collected from the culture medium of cells cotransfected

with plasmids encoding the MERS-CoV structural proteins and the control vector pEGFP-N1 (Fig. 3c; VLP). These results demonstrated that the PS258(19712–19969)$_{ME}$ RNA fragment bears a functional packaging signal that is critical for the assembly of the viral RNA into the MERS VLPs. In the absence of the MERS-CoV RNA sequences, GFP RNA alone was not assembled or expressed in the VLPs. In addition, no GFP expression was detected when the Huh7 cells were incubated with VLPs collected from the culture medium of cells cotransfected with plasmids encoding MERS-CoV structural

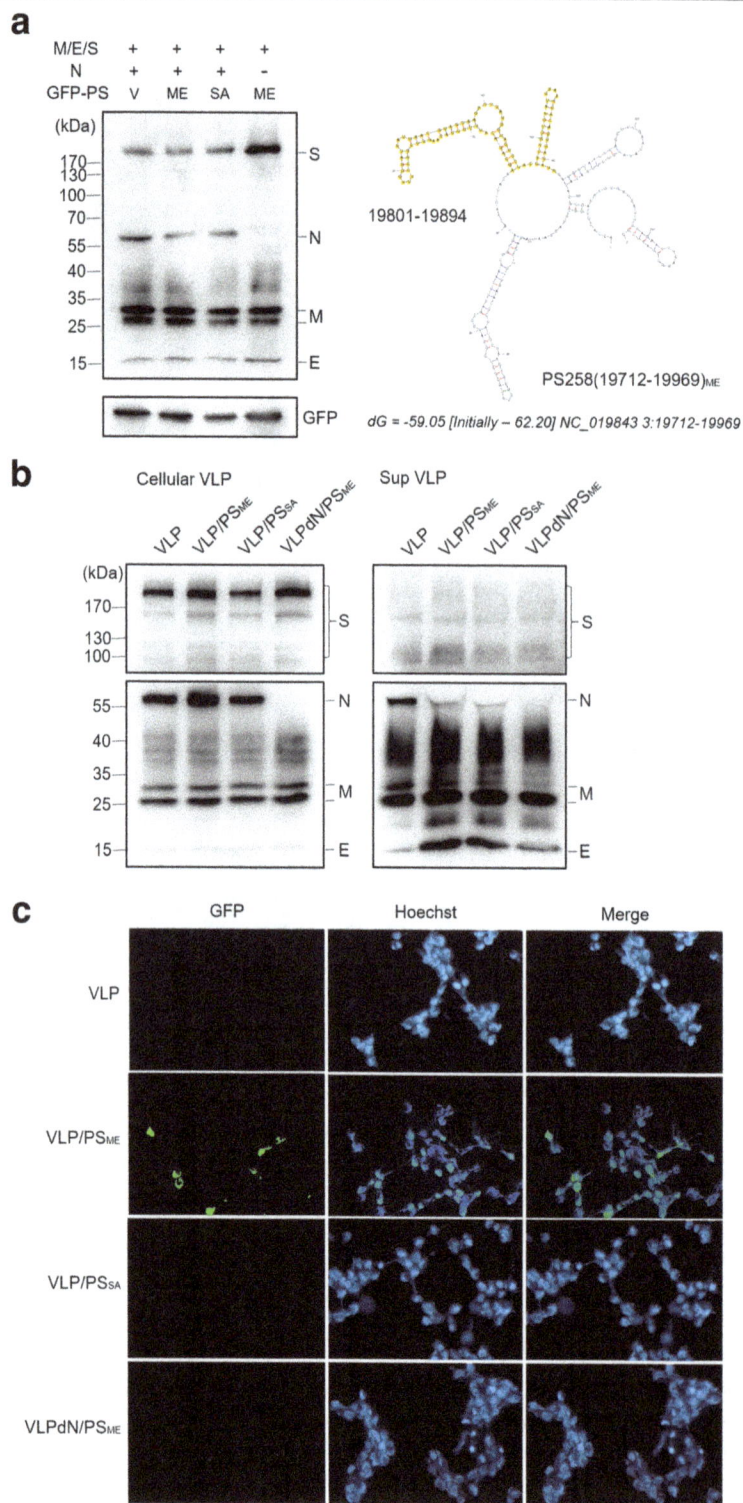

Fig. 3 (See legend on next page.)

(See figure on previous page.)
Fig. 3 Functional analysis of the putative MERS-CoV RNA packaging signal. **a-b** Expression of MERS-CoV structural proteins in transfected cells and VLPs. Western blot analysis was performed with the cell lysates (panel **a**) and both the cellular and supernatant VLPs (panel b) following cotransfection of the plasmids encoding the viral structural proteins and a heterologous GFP-PS mRNA as indicated. The secondary structure of the PS258(19712–19969)$_{ME}$ RNA fragment is shown with the 94-nt stable substructure highlighted as marked in Fig. 1b. **c** Functional analysis of RNA packaging signal. MERS VLPs were collected from the medium of the cultured cells following cotransfection of the plasmids encoding the viral structural proteins S, E, M, and N, and the GFP vector control plasmid pEGFP-N1 (indicated by VLP), the putative MERS-CoV packaging signal plasmid pEGFP-PS258(19712–19969)ME (indicated by VLP/PS$_{ME}$), and the SARS-CoV packaging signal plasmid pEGFP-N1-PS580 (indicated by VLP/PS$_{SA}$). VLPdN/PS$_{ME}$ represents MERSVLPs produced by cotransfection of the plasmids encoding MERS-CoV M, E, and S proteins and plasmid pEGFP-PS258(19712–19969)ME. These MERS VLPs harvested from different cell sources were incubated with naïve Huh7 cells for 48 h. The treated Huh7 cells were then fixed for immunofluorescence staining with GFP antibody and Hoechst

proteins and the plasmid that encodes the heterologous mRNA GFP-PS580 containing the SARS-CoV RNA packaging signal (Fig. 3c; VLP/PS$_{SA}$), which indicated that the SARS-CoV RNA packaging signal could not be assembled into MERS VLPs. This suggests a viral RNA-specific package.

In addition to the packaging signal, viral structural proteins may also play roles in the assembly of the viral genome [9, 11, 19, 24–26]. To elucidate the MERS-CoV RNA packaging, MERS VLPs produced in the absence of the N protein (named VLPdN/PS$_{ME}$) were incubated with Huh7 cells. In contrast to the expression of GFP in cells incubated with MERS VLP/PS$_{ME}$, the GFP signal was not detected in Huh7 cells incubated with VLPdN/PS$_{ME}$ (Fig. 3c). This result indicates that the MERS-CoV RNA packaging is dependent on the viral N protein.

MERS-CoV N protein interacts with a stable stem-loop structure in the viral RNA packaging signal

To investigate the RNA-binding activity of the MERS-CoV N protein, the His-tagged N protein was expressed in *E. coli* BL21(DE3) and purified through a nickel affinity column. As shown in Fig. 4, the His-tagged full-length N protein of approximately 55 kDa was purified by an elution buffer containing 200 mM imidazole (panel a). Fractions 2 and 3, which showed the peak level of the N protein, were pooled together for the filter binding assay. In addition, a 45-nt RNA fragment spanning nt 19,805 to 19,849 (tentatively named SL19805$_{ME}$) of the

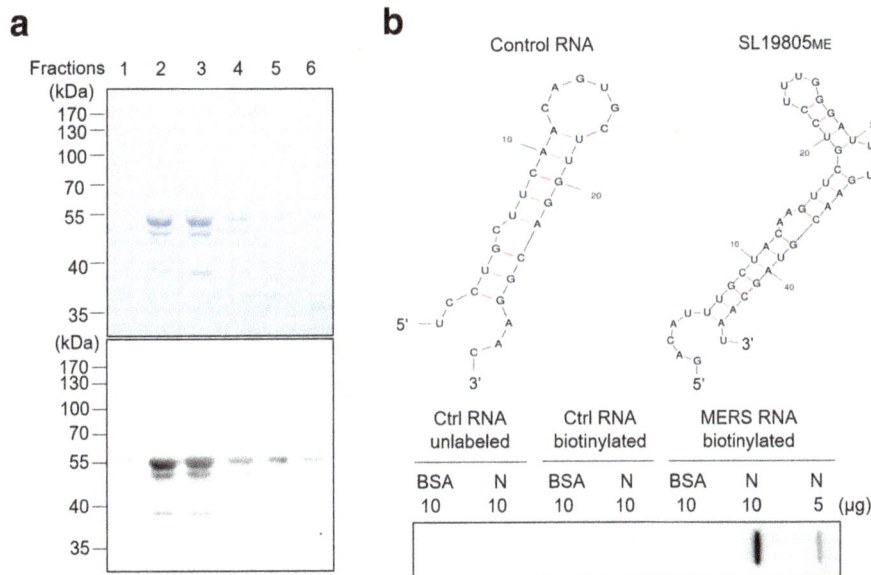

Fig. 4 The RNA binding activity of MERS-CoV N protein. **a** Purification of the His-tagged MERS-CoV full-length N protein. Following expression of the His-tagged MERS-CoV N protein in *E. coli* BL21(DE3), the cells were lysed and cell supernatant collected was subjected to protein purification on a nickel-bead affinity column. The His-tagged MERS-CoV N protein eluted by a buffer containing 200 mM imidazole was detected by Coomassie blue staining (top) and Western blot analysis using antibody against the His-tag (bottom). Fractions 2 and 3 were pooled together for the filter binding assay. **b** Filter binding assay. The interactions between the MERS-CoV N protein and the biotin-SL19805$_{ME}$ probe were analyzed by the filter binding assay. Unlabeled and 3' biotin-labeled RNA fragments with sequences 5'–UCCUGCUUCAACAGUGCUUGGACGGAAC-3' and the predicted structure (as shown) were used as controls for RNA specificity. BSA was used as a protein control

viral genome that constitutes a stable stem-loop substructure of the PS258(19712–19969)$_{ME}$ was used in the RNA binding assay. As shown in Fig. 4b, an interaction between the biotinylated SL19805$_{ME}$ and the MERS-CoV N protein was detected. However, no signals were observed with the protein control BSA and in the control groups of unlabeled and biotin-labeled RNA. These results localized a predicted substructure of the PS258(19712–19969)$_{ME}$ RNA packaging signal to interact with the viral N protein.

Although the structure of the full-length MERS-CoV N protein has not been determined, a recent study revealed structural features of the N-terminal region of MERS-CoV in common with SARS-CoV and other coronaviruses [28–30]. The N protein of coronavirus is structurally organized into two domains, the N-terminal domain (NTD) and C-terminal domain (CTD), which are separated by a flexible linker (Fig. 5). The NTD structure is organized as an antiparallel β-sheet core domain with disordered loops, whereas the CTD is composed of mainly α-helices. Previous studies demonstrated that the CTD of the SARS-CoV N protein is involved in oligomerization to form a capsid structure, whereas both domains may be involved in RNA binding [19, 30–34]. In addition, the linker is able to modulate the RNA binding activity of the NTD and CTD [35]. In this study, the RNA-binding characteristics of the MERS-CoV N protein were examined by analyzing the interactions between the SL19805$_{ME}$ RNA and various fragments of the N protein. Following expression and purification of the His-tagged N proteins (Fig. 5a), a filter binding assay was performed. The results demonstrated the RNA binding activities of the full-length N protein and both the N(1–263) and N(239–413) fragments that represent the NTD plus the flexible linker and the CTD, respectively (Fig. 5b). Nevertheless, when deleting a part of the β-sheet structure of the NTD, the N(1–156) fragment had a lower RNA-binding activity compared to that of the N(1–263) fragment, which indicated that the structural integrity of the NTD could be important for RNA binding. However, a 25-amino-acid N-terminal deletion from the N(239–413) fragment, which generated the N(264–413) fragment, had little effect on the RNA-binding

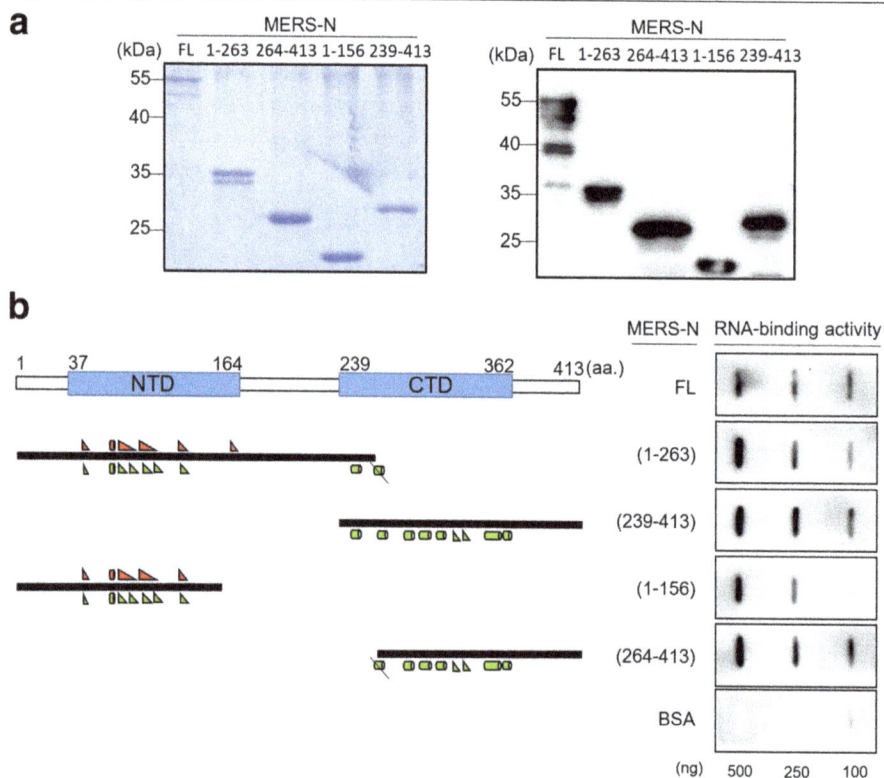

Fig. 5 The RNA binding activity of MERS-CoV N fragments. a Purification of various N fragments. Purification of the full-length (FL) N protein and its subdomains N(1–263), N(264–413), N(1–156), and N(239–413) followed the procedures as described in the legend of Fig. 4. Coomassie blue staining and Western blot analysis are shown. b Schematic representation of the N subdomains and the filter binding assay. The N protein of coronavirus is organized into two structural domains (NTD and CTD) separated by a flexible linker. The NTD structure mainly has an antiparallel β-sheet core domain, whereas the CTD is composed of mainly α-helices [29, 30, 33]. The secondary structural elements are indicated by triangles for β-sheets and cylinders for α-helices, and those shown above the N protein fragments (closed boxes) correspond to the structure of the MERS-CoV N protein, whereas those shown under the boxes correspond to the SARS-CoV N protein. The filter binding assay was conducted with the biotin-SL19805$_{ME}$ and increasing amounts of the N proteins and BSA control as indicated

activity. These results indicate that both the NTD and CTD of the MERS-CoV N protein could interact with SL19805$_{ME}$, which is a 45-nt stable stem-loop structure in the viral RNA packaging signal.

Furthermore, although the heterologous mRNA GFP-PS580 containing the SARS-CoV RNA packaging signal could not be assembled into MERS VLPs (Fig. 3c; VLP/PS$_{SA}$), the SL19893$_{SA}$ that represents a 50-nt conserved stem-loop structure within the PS580 showed its ability to interact with the MERS-CoV N protein (Fig. 6). Nevertheless, the binding activity was much lower than that of the SL19805$_{ME}$. This result suggests that interaction of the viral RNA with the N protein may be a prerequisite but not sufficient for RNA packaging into VLPs. Virus-specific RNA sequences and structures may determine the binding activity of the N protein. In addition, subsequent interactions between the N protein and other viral structural proteins may facilitate assembly of the viral RNA into VLPs.

Discussion

Our previous study on SARS-CoV indicated an N protein-dependent package of the viral RNA. The RNA packaging signal was biologically identified and located within the viral genome spanning nt 19,715 to 20,294 [19]. In this study, the prediction from the sequence and

structure analysis localized the putative MERS-CoV packaging signal to the 3' end of the ORF 1b of the viral genome (Fig. 1). Further studies demonstrated that the 258-nt PS258(19712–19969)$_{ME}$ RNA fragment could function as a packaging signal and drive the packaging of the heterologous GFP gene into the MERS VLPs (Fig. 3c). Minimum sequences and structures required for RNA packaging need to be further elucidated. Nevertheless, the in vitro RNA binding assay demonstrated an interaction between the viral N protein and a 45-nt stable stem-loop structure within the functionally identified packaging signal of the MERS-CoV RNA (Figs. 4 and 5).

Previously, studies on MHV mapped a 69-nt stem-loop RNA structure as the core packaging signal of MHV, and a 190-nt RNA fragment containing the core packaging signal has a much higher packaging activity [13, 25]. In addition, the packaging signal selectively interacts with the viral M protein, which drives the packaging of the viral RNA into the virus particles [25]. Studies on various coronaviruses indicate that coronaviruses could package the RNA fragments containing their own packaging signals [15, 16, 19]. In this study, we further demonstrated that MERS VLPs could package the PS258(19712–19969)$_{ME}$ RNA fragment of MERS-CoV, but not the SARS-CoV packaging signal PS580 (Fig. 3c). This suggests a specificity of the

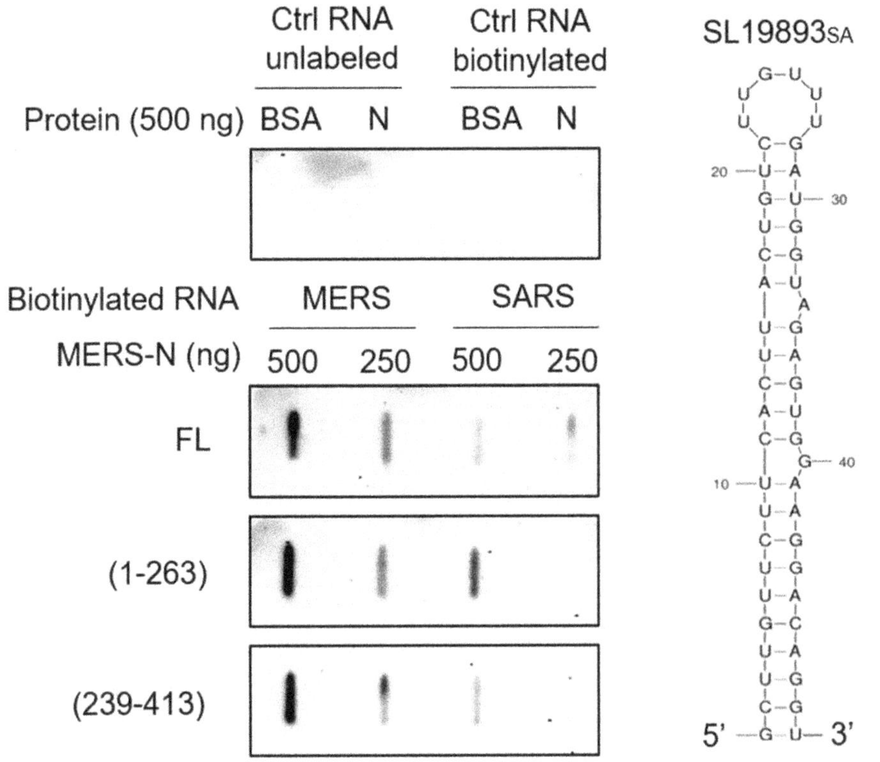

Fig. 6 The RNA binding activity of the MERS-CoV N protein on SL19805$_{ME}$ and SL19893$_{SA}$. A filter binding assay was performed with MERS-CoV N proteins and the 50-nt biotin-labeled SARS-CoV RNA (SL19893$_{SA}$). The control RNAs and proteins are described in the legend of Fig. 4

MERS-CoV RNA packaging. In addition, the involvement of the N protein in genome packaging may vary among the different coronaviruses. Previous studies demonstrate an N-dependent packaging of the SARS-CoV RNA packaging signal [19], but an N-independent packaging of the MHV RNA fragment was also suggested [24, 25]. In this study, an N-dependent packaging of MERS-CoV RNA was demonstrated (Fig. 3c).

The N protein of coronaviruses can be divided into two structural domains (NTD and CTD) and three intrinsically disordered regions (the N-arm, central linker region and C-tail) [10, 36]. Previous studies demonstrated the involvement of both the structural domains in binding the RNA of SARS-CoV and MHV (either independently or cooperatively as a bipartite) and showed the involvement of the C-terminal domain in oligomerization of the N protein [19, 30–34, 36–38]. In this study, the RNA-binding activity was demonstrated for the full-length N protein and both the N(1–263) and N(239–413) fragments that represent the NTD plus the flexible central linker region and the CTD, respectively (Fig. 5). The reduced RNA-binding activity of the N(1–156) fragment may indicate a critical role of the structural integrity of NTD. Alternatively, the central linker region may play a role in RNA binding. However, the N(264–413) fragment that lacks the N-terminal 25 amino acids of the N(239–413) fragment has an RNA-binding activity comparable to the N(239–413). This is different from the observation that the absence of the N-terminal 22 amino acids of SARS CoV N protein CTD significantly diminished its interaction with RNA [31]. Critical structures and sequences of the MERS-CoV N protein involved in RNA binding could be further studied. The MERS VLP system, which was established here for studying virus assembly and infection, could be used as a model system for evaluation of the efficacy of antiviral drugs.

Conclusions

In this study, a MERS-CoV RNA packaging signal was identified by the detection of GFP expression following incubation of the MERS VLPs carrying the heterologous mRNA GFP-PS258(19712–19969)$_{ME}$ with the virus permissive Huh 7 cells. Both the NTD and CTD of the MERS-CoV N protein showed binding activity to the 45-nt SL19805$_{ME}$ RNA fragment that forms a stable stem-loop substructure of the viral RNA packaging signal PS258(19712–19969)$_{ME}$. The MERS VLP system could help us understand virus infection and morphogenesis.

Acknowledgements
We gratefully acknowledge Haagmans BL and Osterhaus AD for providing plasmid pCR4-MERS-S1-Topo.

Funding
This work was supported by Research Grants 102–2321-B-002-028 and 107–2321-B-002-023 from the Ministry of Science and Technology, Republic of China.

Authors' contributions
WCH and CHC conceived the study, carried out most of the experiments and analyzed data. WCH drafted the manuscript. WCH, CHC, and CYC all participated in plasmid construction. CYC, WHP, and CLC provided technical assistance on the electron microscopic analysis of MERS VLPs. MFC and SCC conceived the study, participated in its design and coordination, provided technical assistance and revised the manuscript. All authors read and approved the final version of the manuscript.

Competing interests
The authors declare that they have no competing interests.

Author details
[1]Institute of Microbiology, College of Medicine, National Taiwan University, No. 1, Jen-Ai Road, First Section, Taipei 100, Taiwan. [2]Institute of Anatomy and Cell Biology, College of Medicine, National Taiwan University, No. 1, Jen-Ai Road, First Section, Taipei 100, Taiwan. [3]Institute of Biochemistry and Molecular Biology, College of Medicine, National Taiwan University, No. 1, Jen-Ai Road, First Section, Taipei 100, Taiwan.

References
1. Zaki AM, van Boheemen S, Bestebroer TM, Osterhaus AD, Fouchier RA. Isolation of a novel coronavirus from a man with pneumonia in Saudi Arabia. N Engl J Med. 2012;367:1814–20.
2. Raj VS, Mou H, Smits SL, Dekkers DH, Muller MA, Dijkman R, Muth D, Demmers JA, Zaki A, Fouchier RA, Thiel V, Drosten C, Rottier PJ, Osterhaus AD, Bosch BJ, Haagmans BL. Dipeptidyl peptidase 4 is a functional receptor for the emerging human coronavirus-EMC. Nature. 2013;495:251–4.
3. Lu G, Hu Y, Wang Q, Qi J, Gao F, Li Y, Zhang Y, Zhang W, Yuan Y, Bao J, Zhang B, Shi Y, Yan J, Gao GF. Molecular basis of binding between novel human coronavirus MERS-CoV and its receptor CD26. Nature. 2013;500:227–31.
4. Pasternak AO, Spaan WJ, Snijder EJ. Nidovirus transcription: how to make sense...? J Gen Virol. 2006;87:1403–21.
5. Stadler K, Masignani V, Eickmann M, Becker S, Abrignani S, Klenk HD, Rappuoli R. SARS–beginning to understand a new virus. Nat Rev Microbiol. 2003;1:209–18.
6. Dires B, Dawo F. Review on Middle East respiratory syndrome. Open Acc Lib J. 2015;2:e1749.
7. Boscarino J, Logan H, Lacny J, Gallagher T. Envelope protein palmitoylations are crucial for murine coronavirus assembly. J Virol. 2008;82:2989–99.
8. de Haan CA, Vennema H, Rottier PJ. Assembly of the coronavirus envelope: homotypic interactions between the M proteins. J Virol. 2000;74:4967–78.
9. Vennema H, Godeke GJ, Rossen JW, Voorhout WF, Horzinek MC, Opstelten DJ, Rottier PJ. Nucleocapsid-independent assembly of coronavirus-like particles by co-expression of viral envelope protein genes. EMBO J. 1996;15:2020–8.
10. Chang CK, Lo SC, Wang YS, Hou MH. Recent insights into the development of therapeutics against coronavirus diseases by targeting N protein. Drug Discov Today. 2016;21:562–72.
11. Kuo L, Koetzner CA, Hurst KR, Masters PS. Recognition of the murine coronavirus genomic RNA packaging signal depends on the second RNA-binding domain of the nucleocapsid protein. J Virol. 2014;88:4451–65.
12. Molenkamp R, Spaan WJM. Identification of a specific interaction between the coronavirus mouse hepatitis virus A59 nucleocapsid protein and packaging signal. Virology. 1997;239:78–86.
13. Fosmire JA, Hwang K, Makino S. Identification and characterization of a coronavirus packaging signal. J Virol. 1992;66:3522–30.
14. Kuo L, Masters PS. Functional analysis of the murine coronavirus genomic RNA packaging signal. J Virol. 2013;87:5182–92.

15. Woo K, Joo M, Narayanan K, Kim KH, Makino S. Murine coronavirus packaging signal confers packaging to nonviral RNA. J Virol. 1997;71:824–7.

16. Cologna R, Hogue BG. Identification of a bovine coronavirus packaging signal. J Virol. 2000;74:580–3.

17. Chen SC, van den Born E, van den Worm SH, Pleij CW, Snijder EJ, Olsthoorn RC. New structure model for the packaging signal in the genome of group IIa coronaviruses. J Virol. 2007;81:6771–4.

18. Chen SC, Olsthoorn RC. Group-specific structural features of the 5′-proximal sequences of coronavirus genomic RNAs. Virology. 2010;401:29–41.

19. Hsieh PK, Chang SC, Huang CC, Lee TT, Hsiao CW, Kou YH, Chen IY, Chang CK, Huang TH, Chang MF. Assembly of severe acute respiratory syndrome coronavirus RNA packaging signal into virus-like particles is nucleocapsid dependent. J Virol. 2005;79:13848–55.

20. Escors D, Izeta A, Capiscol C, Enjuanes L. Transmissible gastroenteritis coronavirus packaging signal is located at the 5′ end of the virus genome. J Virol. 2003;77:7890–902.

21. Morales L, Mateos-Gomez PA, Capiscol C, del Palacio L, Enjuanes L, Sola I. Transmissible gastroenteritis coronavirus genome packaging signal is located at the 5′ end of the genome and promotes viral RNA incorporation into virions in a replication-independent process. J Virol. 2013;87:11579–90.

22. Penzes Z, Tibbles K, Shaw K, Britton P, Brown TD, Cavanagh D. Characterization of a replicating and packaged defective RNA of avian coronavirus infectious bronchitis virus. Virology. 1994;203:286–93.

23. Dalton K, Casais R, Shaw K, Stirrups K, Evans S, Britton P, Brown TD, Cavanagh D. Cis-acting sequences required for coronavirus infectious bronchitis virus defective-RNA replication and packaging. J Virol. 2001;75: 125–33.

24. Narayanan K, Chen CJ, Maeda J, Makino S. Nucleocapsid-independent specific viral RNA packaging via viral envelope protein and viral RNA signal. J Virol. 2003;77:2922–7.

25. Narayanan K, Makino S. Cooperation of an RNA packaging signal and a viral envelope protein in coronavirus RNA packaging. J Virol. 2001;75:9059–67.

26. Kuo L, Koetzner C, Masters PS. A key role for the carboxy-terminal tail of the murine coronavirus nucleocapsid protein in coordination of genome packaging. Virology. 2016;494:100–7.

27. Chang MF, Sun CY, Chen CJ, Chang SC. Functional motifs of delta antigen essential for RNA binding and replication of hepatitis delta virus. J Virol. 1993;67:2529–36.

28. Chang CK, Hou MH, Chang CF, Hsiao CD, Huang TH. The SARS coronavirus nucleocapsid protein–forms and functions. Antivir Res. 2014;103:39–50.

29. Papageorgiou N, Lichière J, Baklouti A, Ferron F, Sévajol M, Canard B, Coutard B. Structural characterization of the N-terminal part of the MERS-CoV nucleocapsid by X-ray diffraction and small-angle X-ray scattering. Acta Crystallogr D Struct Biol. 2016;72:192–202.

30. Saikatendu KS, Joseph JS, Subramanian V, Neuman BW, Buchmeier MJ, Stevens RC, Kuhn P. Ribonucleocapsid formation of severe acute respiratory syndrome coronavirus through molecular action of the N-terminal domain of N protein. J Virol. 2007;81:3913–21.

31. Chen CY, Chang CK, Chang YW, Sue SC, Bai HI, Riang L, Hsiao CD, Huang TH. Structure of the SARS coronavirus nucleocapsid protein RNA-binding dimerization domain suggests a mechanism for helical packaging of viral RNA. J Mol Biol. 2007;368:1075–86.

32. Luo H, Chen J, Chen K, Shen X, Jiang H. Carboxyl terminus of severe acute respiratory syndrome coronavirus nucleocapsid protein: self-association analysis and nucleic acid binding characterization. Biochemistry. 2006;45: 11827–35.

33. Takeda M, Chang CK, Ikeya T, Güntert P, Chang YH, Hsu YL, Huang TH, Kainosho M. Solution structure of the C-terminal dimerization domain of SARS coronavirus nucleocapsid protein solved by the SAIL-NMR method. J Mol Biol. 2008;380:608–22.

34. Yu IM, Gustafson CL, Diao J, Burgner JW II, Li Z, Zhang J, Chen J. Recombinant severe acute respiratory syndrome (SARS) coronavirus nucleocapsid protein forms a dimer through its C-terminal domain. J Biol Chem. 2005;280:23280–6.

35. Chang CK, Hsu YL, Chang YH, Chao FA, Wu MC, Huang YS, Hu CK, Huang TH. Multiple nucleic acid binding sites and intrinsic disorder of severe acute respiratory syndrome coronavirus nucleocapsid protein: implications for ribonucleocapsid protein packaging. J Virol. 2009;83:2255–64.

36. Chang CK, Sue SC, Yu TH, Hsieh CM, Tsai CK, Chiang YC, Lee SJ, Hsiao HH, Wu WJ, Chang WL, Lin CH, Huang TH. Modular organization of SARS coronavirus nucleocapsid protein. J Biomed Sci. 2006;13:59–72.

37. Hurst K, Koetzner C, Masters P. Identification of in vivo interacting domains of the murine coronavirus nucleocapsid protein. J Virol. 2009; 83:7221–34.

38. Ma Y, Tong X, Xu X, Li X, Lou Z, Rao Z. Structures of the N- and C-terminal domains of MHV-A59 nucleocapsid protein corroborate a conserved RNA-protein binding mechanism in coronavirus. Protein Cell. 2010;1:688–97.

15

H. pylori infection and extra-gastroduodenal diseases

Feng-Woei Tsay[1,2] and Ping-I Hsu [1*]

Abstract

Helicobacter pylori infection is the principal cause of peptic ulcer disease, gastric adenocarcinoma and gastric mucosa-associated lymphoid tissue lymphoma. Recent studies have shown that it may interfere with many biological processes and determine or influence the occurrence of many diseases outside the stomach. Currently, the role of *H. pylori* in idiopathic thrombocytopenic purpura and iron deficiency anemia is well documented. Emerging evidence suggests that it may also contribute to vitamin B12 deficiency, insulin resistance, metabolic syndrome, diabetes mellitus and non-alcoholic liver disease. Additionally, it may increase the risk of acute coronary syndrome, cerebrovascular disease, neurodegenerative disease and other miscellaneous disorders. Different pathogenic mechanisms have been hypothesized, including the occurrence of molecular mimicry and the induction of a low-grade inflammation. This review summarizes the results of the most relevant studies on the extra-gastroduodenal manifestations of *H. pylori* infection.

Keywords: *Helicobacter pylori*, Iron deficiency anemia, Idiopathic thrombocytopenic purpura and vitamin B12 deficiency

Background

Helicobacter pylori infection is the principal cause of chronic gastritis, gastric ulcer, duodenal ulcer, gastric adenocarcinoma and gastric mucosa-associated lymphoid tissue lymphoma [1, 2]. In recent decades, many articles have published on the fascinating topic of extragastroduodenal manifestations of *H. pylori* infection, including hematological, metabolic, cardiovascular, neurodegenerative and allergic disorders [3–13]. Different pathogenic mechanisms have been hypothesized, including the occurrence of molecular mimicry and the induction of a low-grade inflammation. Indeed, *H. pylori* infection is a very good model for studying host-bacterial interactions and very attractive for those interested in the role of gut microbiota in health and diseases. Here, we summarize the results of the most relevant studies on the extragastroduodenal manifestations of *H. pylori* infection.

* Correspondence: williamhsup@yahoo.com.tw
[1]Division of Gastroenterology and Hepatology, Department of Internal Medicine, Kaohsiung Veterans General Hospital and National Yang-Ming University, 386 Ta Chung 1st Road, Kaohsiung 813, Taiwan, Republic of China
Full list of author information is available at the end of the article

Iron deficiency anemia

The link between Iron deficiency anemia (IDA) and *H. pylori* infection was reported firstly in 1991 by Blecker et al., who cured IDA of a 15 year-old female presenting with anemia-related syncope and *H. pylori*-induced chronic active hemorrhagic gastritis by eradication therapy without iron supplements [14]. The association of *H. pylori* infection with unexplained IDA has been proven in adult and pediatric populations [15, 16] though a few investigations didn't show this link [17, 18]. Recently, Qu et al. conducted a meta-analysis of 15 case-control studies to investigate the relation between *H. pylori* infection and IDA [19]. *H. pylori* infection was diagnosed by endoscopy and histological examination in five studies, in which patients with peptic ulcer disease and gastric cancer were not included. The other 10 studies confirmed *H. pylori* infection by serology or urea breath test. The data showed an increased risk of IDA in patients with *H. pylori* infection with an odds ratio (OR) of 2.2 (95% confidence interval [CI]:1.5–3.2) [19]. Several works also demonstrated recovery from IDA by successful eradication of *H. pylori* without iron supplements [20]. Yuan et al. performed a meta-analysis of 16 randomized controlled trials involving 956 patients to assess the impact of *H. pylori* eradication therapy on IDA [21]. In this work, the diagnosis of *H. pylori* infection was based on rapid urease test or histology in eight studies, in which patients with peptic ulcer disease were excluded. The other eight studies confirmed *H. pylori* infection by urea breath test. The follow-up time in these studies ranged from 1 to 3 months. The difference from baseline to endpoint of hemoglobin, serum iron, and serum ferritin in the meta-analysis was statistically significantly different between anti-*H. pylori* treatment plus oral iron and oral iron alone (differences: Hb, 1.48 g/dL; serum iron: 1.15 mol/L; serum ferritin, 1.84 ng/mL) [21].

H. pylori causes IDA by several mechanisms. First, increased iron loss can be due to hemorrhagic gastritis, peptic ulcer disease and gastric adenocarcinoma [22]. Second, CagA protein of *H. pylori* has been shown to participate in iron acquisition from interstitial holotransferrin [23]. Iron uptake by *H. pylori* is enhanced during the growth of the bacteria [24]. Third, *H. pylori*-related corporal gastritis may decrease acid secretion due to gland atrophy and results in the reduction of iron absorption from diet [25].

In summary, the association of *H. pylori* and IDA has been conclusively proven in numerous studies. Current international and national guidelines recommend eradication of *H. pylori* infection in patients with unexplained IDA [26, 27].

Immune thrombocytopenic purpura

Gasbarrini et al. reported the first case of *H. pylori* infection associated with immune thrombocytopenic purpura (ITP) in 1998 [28]. An observation study from Japan also found a good platelet response in ITP patients treated by *H. pylori* eradication [29]. A randomized controlled trial by Brito et al. revealed that *H. pylori* eradication resulted in a significant platelet response in children and adolescents affected by ITP [30]. The role of *H. pylori* infection in ITP has also been confirmed by several other studies [31, 32]. Nonetheless, some studies from countries with low prevalence of infection, like France and the United States, did not find the link between *H. pylori* infection and ITP [33, 34]. Recently, Stasi et al. conducted a meta-analysis of 25 studies to investigate the impact of anti-*H. pylori* therapy on ITP [34]. The assessing time for platelet response ranged from one to six months. The data showed that the rates of complete response (platelet count $\geq 100 \times 10^9$/L) and overall response (platelet count $\geq 30 \times 10^9$/L and at least doubling of the basal count) after successful eradication of *H. pylori* were 42.7 and 50.3%, respectively [35]. The predictors of a good response to eradication therapy were countries with higher prevalence of *H. pylori* infection (such as Japan and Italy) and patients with milder degree of thrombocytopenia [35]. In the majority of ITP

patients responding to anti-*H. pylori* therapy, the durability of platelet response is more than 7 years, indicating the disease is cured [36]. Another meta-analysis by Arnold et al. performed a meta-analysis to determine the effect of *H. pylori* eradication therapy in patients with ITP by comparing the platelet response in ITP patients with and without *H. pylori* infection [37]. The odds of achieving a platelet count response following eradication therapy were 14.5 higher (95% CI: 4.2 to 83.0) in patients with *H. pylori* infection than in those without infection (response rate: 51.2% vs. 8.8%). These findings strengthen the causal association between *H. pylori* infection and ITP. Several mechanisms regarding *H. pylori*-associated ITP have been proposed [38]. One intriguing hypothesis concerning molecular mimicry is that cross-reactive antibodies are produced that react both *H. pylori* components and platelet surface antigens. Takahashi et al. showed that platelet elutes from *H. pylori*-infected ITP patients recognized CagA protein in immunoblots, but those from *H. pylori*-infected non-ITP patients did not [39]. Bai et al. also reported that monoclonal antibodies generated against *H. pylori* urease B react with GP IIb/IIIa expressed on the platelet surface [40]. While these findings suggest molecular mimicry between *H. pylori* components and platelet surface antigens, the exact pathogenic roles of these cross-reactive antibodies remain obscure. In another potential mechanism, *H. pylori* infection may alter Fcγ receptor balance of moncytes/macrophages and induce autoantibody formation. A recent study showed that the FcγR II B expression on circulating monocytes was down-regulated in *H. pylori*-infected ITP patients [41]. Therefore, *H. pylori* may alter Fcγ receptor balance of moncytes/macrophages through downregulation of the inhibitory receptor FcγR II B.

In conclusion, many studies support the association between *H. pylori* infection and ITP. Current international and national guidelines recommend that *H. pylori* infection should be sought and treated in patients with ITP [27].

Vitamin B12 deficiency

The link between vitamin B12 deficiency and *H. pylori* infection was reported firstly in 1984 by O'Connor et al. who showed Campylobacter-like organisms in patients with type A gastritis and pernicious anemia [42]. Studies have demonstrated a link between chronic *H. pylori* infection and malabsorption of vitamin B12 [43]. Sarari et al. showed that vitamin B12 deficiency was present in 67.4% (29/43) of the patients with *H. pylori* infection [44]. Shuval-Sudai et al. found a higher prevalence of *H. pylori* infection in patients at the lower end of the normal range of serum vitamin B12 levels [45]. However, most studies regarding the association between vitamin B12 and *H. pylori* infection focus on testing *H. pylori* status and measuring serum levels of vitamin B12. No adequate interventional studies proving the effect of anti-*H. pylori* therapy on vitamin B12 deficiency exist.

Metabolic syndrome and diabetes mellitus (DM)

Many epidemiological studies have supported a link between insulin resistance, metabolic syndrome and *H. pylori* infection [46, 47]. Chen et al. demonstrated that *H. pylori*-infected subjects had a higher prevalence of metabolic syndrome than those without *H. pylori* infection [48]. Additionally, Yang et al. showed a significant association between *H. pylori* infection and DM [49]. Similar results were also observed by other investigators [50]. Furthermore, Horikawa et al. revealed that *H. pylori* infection worsened glycemia control in diabetic patients [51]. Polyzos et al. conducted a systemic review including nine studies and showed a trend toward a positive association between *H. pylori* infection and insulin resistance [47]. In contrast, several studies did not find the link between *H. pylori* infection and insulin resistance or metabolic syndrome [52]. Naja et al. showed no association between *H. pylori* infection and metabolic syndrome in a Lebanese population [53]. A meta-analysis of 18 studies found no strong correlation between *H. pylori* infection and serum concentrations of total cholesterol and triglyceride [54]. Wada et al. also found that successful eradication of *H. pylori* could not improve glucose control of DM in Japanese patients [55]. Furthermore, a recent randomized controlled trial involving 49 *H. pylori*-infected subjects in a prediabetes stage showed that *H. pylori* eradication resulted in an increased Homeostatic model assessment of insulin resistance (HOMA-IR) [56].

Several studies reported a reverse link between *H. pylori* infection and obesity [57–60]. A case-control study from Taiwan demonstrated an inverse relationship between morbid obesity and *H. pylori* seropositivity [57]. An ecological study also showed an inverse correlation between *H. pylori* prevalence and rate of overweight/obesity in countries of the developed world [58]. However, a large case-control study including 8820 participants from China showed body mass index was significantly and positively associated with *H. pylori* infection [59]. An intervention trial demonstrated serum ghrelin concentrations were inversely related to the severity of *H. pylori*-associated gastritis in prepubertal children [60]. Eradication of *H. pylori* infection resulted in a significant increase in body mass index along with a significant decrease in circulating ghrelin levels and an increase in leptin levels [60].

In summary, the issue of the association between *H. pylori* infection and metabolic syndrome or DM remains contradictory.

Nonalcoholic fatty liver disease (NAFLD)

A cohort study by Kim et al. demonstrated that the subjects with *H. pylori* infection had a higher incidence of NAFLD than those without infection (hazard ratio: 1.21 [95% CI: 1.1–1.3]) [61]. Polyzos et al. also revealed that patients with NAFLD had higher anti-*H. pylori* IgG titers, together with lower circulating adiponectin and higher tumor necrosis factor-α levels, compared to non-NAFLD subjects [62]. However, opposite results from Korea and Japan showed no association between *H. pylori* infection and NAFLD [63, 64]. Recently, a meta-analysis demonstrated a significantly increased risk of NAFLD in patients with *H. pylori* infection [65]. Nonetheless, the mechanism underlying the association between *H. pylori* infection and NAFLD remains unclear, and interventional studies proving the effect of anti-*H. pylori* therapy on NAFLD are fairly limited.

In summary, the association between *H. pylori* infection and NAFLD remains contradictory.

Coronary artery disease (CAD)

Mendall et al. first showed a link between *H. pylori* and CAD in 1994 [66]. Several studies reported that CagA-postive strains of *H. pylori* were associated with atherosclerosis [67–69]. Al-Ghamdi et al found that *H. pylori* plays an important role in the development of CAD by altering the lipid profile and enhancement of chronic inflammation [70]. Figura et al. also revealed that CagA-postive strains of *H. pylori* were associated with high serum levels of interleukin-6 and B-type natriuretic peptide in patients with CAD [71]. A nationwide retrospective cohort study demonstrated that *H. pylori* infection increased the risk of acute coronary syndrome [72]. In addition, a meta-analysis of 26 studies involving more than 20,000 patients also showed a significant association between *H. pylori* infection and the risk of myocardial infarction (OR: 2.10; 95% CI: 1.8–2.5) [73]. However some studies from Indian and German did not find the association between *H. pylori* and CAD [74, 75]. Additionally, there are still no interventional studies proving the beneficial effect of *H. pylori* eradication in decreasing the incidence of CAD.

There are several proposed mechanisms underlying the association between *H. pylori* infection and CAD. *H. pylori* has been detected in human carotid atherosclerotic plaques [76]. Oshima et al. demonstrated the association of *H. pylori* infection with systemic inflammation and endothelial dysfunction in healthy male subjects [77]. They proposed that *H. pylori* infection may cause atherogenesis through persistent low-grade inflammation. Recently, molecular mimicry between CagA antigen of *H. pylori* and atherosclerotic plaque peptides has also been proposed as a possible mechanism [78].

In conclusion, there is controversial evidence linking *H. pylori* infection and CAD. No adequate interventional trials demonstrating a lower incidence of CAD as a result of anti-*H. pylori* therapy exit.

Cerebrovascular disease

Wincup et al. first reported a link between *H. pylori* infection and stroke in 1996 (OR = 1.57, 95% CI 0.95 to 2.60) [79]. A Mexican study found that levels of antibodies to *H. pylori* predict incident stroke in fully adjusted models (OR: 1.58; 95% CI: 1.1 to 2.3) [80]. Recently, Wang et al. performed a meta-analysis of 4041 Chinese patients, and found an association between *H. pylori* infection and non-cardioembolic stroke [81]. However, a cohort study of 9895 cases from the United States found a reverse link between *H. pylori* infection and stroke mortality, and this reverse association was stronger for *H. pylori* cagA positivity [82]. In summary, there is controversial evidence linking *H. pylori* infection and cerebrovascular disease.

Other miscellaneous disorders

Some studies also disclosed the relationship of *H. pylori* with dementia and Alzheimer's disease (AD) [83, 84]. A study in Greece by Kountouras et al. found higher prevalence of *H. pylori* infection in patients with AD than in the control group [85]. Hung et al. designed a study for the relationship between *H. pylori* infection and non-Alzheimer's dementia (non-AD) using a nation-wide population-based dataset in Taiwan, and found that patients with *H. pylori* infection were 1.6-fold more likely to develop non-AD than those without infection [83]. A retrospective cohort study using nationwide database in Taiwan showed that eradication of *H. pylori* was associated with a decreased progression of dementia as compared to no eradication of *H. pylori* in AD patients with peptic ulcers [86]. However, further prospective randomized control trials are needed to clarify these findings.

The inverse relationship between *H. pylori* infection and allergic asthma has been reported. A meta-analysis by Zhou et al... in 2013 found lower prevalence rate of *H. pylori* infection in patients with allergic asthma [87]. Higher prevalence rate of *H. pylori* infection has been found in cirrhotic patients with hepatoencephalopathy than in those without hepatoencephalopathy [88]. Jaing et al also showed the association of *H. pylori* infection with elevated blood ammonia levels in cirrhotic patients

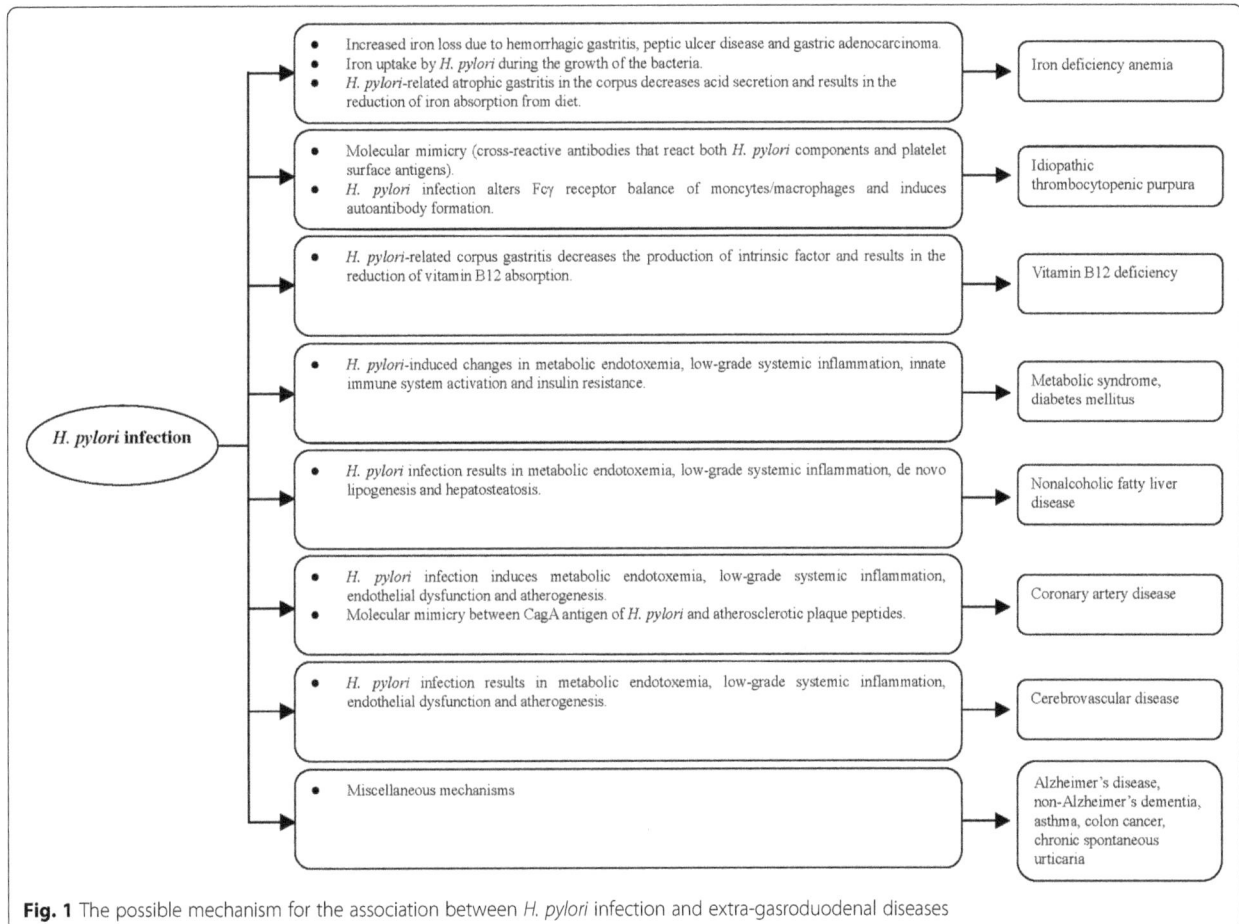

Fig. 1 The possible mechanism for the association between *H. pylori* infection and extra-gasroduodenal diseases

Table 1 The relevant studies on the associations between *H. pylori* infection and extra-gastroduodenal diseases

	Extra-gastroduodenal disease	Key evidences	Conclusion
1	Iron deficiency anemia (IDA)	Pros: 1. Qu et al. [19]: an increased risk of IDA in patients with *H. pylori* infection (meta-analysis of case-control studies). 2. Yuan et al. [21]: Eradication of *H. pylori* could improve the levels of hemoglobin and serum ferritin in patients with IDA (meta-analysis of intervention trials). Cons: 1. Sandstrom et al. [18]: no association between *H. pylori* infection and IDA in female adolescents (case-control study).	Eradication of *H. pylori* infection is recommended for patients with unexplained IDA.
2	Immune thrombocytopenic purpura (ITP)	Pros: 1. Stasi et al. [35]: The overall response rate of increased platelet count was 50.3% after successful eradication of *H. pylori* in ITP patients (meta-analysis of intervention trials). 2. Arnold et al. [37]: The odds of achieving a platelet count response following eradication therapy were 14.5 higher in ITP patients with *H. pylori* infection than in those without infection (response rate: 51.2% vs. 8.8%) (meta-analysis of intervention trials). Cons: 1. Michel et al. [34]: Seroprevalence of *H. pylori* in patients with ITP was not significantly different from that in control subjects (case-control study).	*H. pylori* infection should be sought and treated in patients with ITP.
3	Vitamin B12 deficiency	Pros: 1. Sarari et al. [44]: There was significant association between the presence of *H. pylori* infection and vitamin B12 deficiency (case-control study). 2. Shuval-Sudai et al. [45]: Prevalence of *H. pylori* seropositivity was significantly higher among subjects with borderline (> 145–180 pg/mL) or low normal (> 180–250 pg/mL) vitamin B12 levels than among those with vitamin B12 > 250 pg/mL (case-control study).	*H. pylori* infection is associated with vitamin B12 deficiency.
4	Metabolic syndrome and diabetes mellitus (DM)	Pros: 1. Chen et al. [48]: *H. pylori*-infected subjects had a higher prevalence of metabolic syndrome than those without *H. pylori* infection (case-control study). 2. Yang et al. [49]: *H. pylori* infection was associated with risk of DM (case-control study). Cons: 1. Naja et al. [53]: no association between *H. pylori* infection and metabolic syndrome (case-control study). 2. Wada et al. [55]: The eradication of Helicobacter pylori does not affect glycemic control in Japanese subjects with type 2 diabetes (intervention trial).	The association between *H. pylori* infection and metabolic syndrome or DM is contradictory.
5	Nonalcoholic fatty liver disease (NAFLD)	Pros: 1. Kim et al. [61]: The subjects with *H. pylori* infection had a higher incidence of NAFLD than those without infection (cohort study). 2. Wijarnpreecha et al. [65]: a significantly increased risk of NAFLD in patients with *H. pylori* infection (meta-analysis of case-control studies). Cons: 1. Okushin et al. [63]: no association between *H. pylori* infection and NAFLD (case-control study).	The association between *H. pylori* infection and NAFLD remains contradictory.
6	Coronary artery disease (CAD)	Pros: 1. Yu et al. [73]: significant association between *H. pylori* infection and the risk of myocardial infarction (meta-analysis of case-control studies). Cons: 1. Schottker et al. [75]: no association between *H. pylori* infection and the risk of CAD (cohort study).	The association between *H. pylori* infection and CAD is contradictory.

Table 1 The relevant studies on the associations between *H. pylori* infection and extra-gastroduodenal diseases *(Continued)*

	Extra-gastroduodenal disease	Key evidences	Conclusion
7	Cerebrovascular disease	Pros: 1. Wang et al. [81]: significant association between *H. pylori* infection and non-cardioembolic stroke (meta-analysis of case-control studies). Cons: 1. Chen et al. [82]: a reverse link between *H. pylori* infection and stroke mortality (cohort study).	There is controversial evidence linking *H. pylori* infection and cerebrovascular disease.

[89]. Several studies have also reported that *H. pylori* infection increases the risk of colon adenocarcinoma and adenoma [90–92]. Recently, an association between *H. pylori* infection and chronic spontaneous urticaria has been reported but remains controversial. Fukuda et al. demonstrated a significant improvement of chronic spontaneous urticaria by anti-*H. pylori* therapy in Japanese patients [93]. This work was consistent with a systemic review of 10 studies by Federman et al. [94]. However, Moreira et al. did not find the association between *H. pylori* infection and chronic spontaneous urticaria [95].

In summary, there are still controversial evidences linking *H. pylori* infection and aforementioned miscellaneous disorders. Adequate interventional trials are needed to clarify these associations.

Conclusions

Recent studies have shown that *H. pylori* may interfere with many biological processes and determine or influence the occurrence of many diseases outside the stomach (Table 1 and Fig. 1). Currently, its role in ITP and IDA is well documented. Emerging evidence suggests that it may also contribute to vitamin B12 deficiency, insulin resistance, metabolic syndrome, diabetes mellitus and non-alcoholic liver disease. Additionally, it may also increase the risk of acute coronary syndrome, cerebrovascular disease, and neurodegenerative disease, *H. pylori* infection is a perfect model for the study of interplay between human beings and bacteria. Further studies are mandatory to clarify the pathogenesis of extragastroduodenal diseases induced by *H. pylori* infection.

Abbreviations
AD: Alzheimer's disease; CI: Confidence interval; DM: Diabetes mellitus; IDA: Iron deficiency anemia; ITP: Immune thrombocytopenic purpura; NAFLD: Nonalcoholic fatty liver disease; OR: Odds ratio

Authors' contributions
Drs. PIH and FWT reviewed the articles and wrote the manuscript. Both authors read and approved the final manuscript.

Competing interests
The authors declare that they have no competing interests.

Author details
[1]Division of Gastroenterology and Hepatology, Department of Internal Medicine, Kaohsiung Veterans General Hospital and National Yang-Ming University, 386 Ta Chung 1st Road, Kaohsiung 813, Taiwan, Republic of China. [2]Cheng Shiu University, Kaohsiung, Taiwan, Republic of China.

References
1. Suerbaum S, Michetti P. Helicobacter pylori infection. N Engl J Med. 2002;347(15):1175–86.
2. Graham DY. Helicobacter pylori update: gastric cancer, reliable therapy, and possible benefits. Gastroenterology. 2015;148(4):719–31.
3. Realdi G, Dore MP, Fastame L. Extradigestive manifestations of helicobacter pylori infection: fact and fiction. Dig Dis Sci. 1999;44(2):229–36.
4. Suzuki H, Franceschi F, Nishizawa T, et al. Extragastric manifestations of helicobacter pylori infection. Helicobacter. 2011;16(Suppl 1):65–9.
5. Banic M, Franceschi F, Babic Z, et al. Extragastric manifestations of helicobacter pylori infection. Helicobacter. 2012;17(Suppl 1):49–55.
6. Deng B, Li Y, Zhang Y, et al. Helicobacter pylori infection and lung cancer: a review of an emerging hypothesis. Carcinogenesis. 2013;34(6):1189–95.
7. Papagiannakis P, Michalopoulos C, Papalexi F, et al. The role of helicobacter pylori infection in hematological disorders. Eur J Intern Med. 2013;24(8):685–90.
8. Buzas GM. Metabolic consequences of helicobacter pylori infection and eradication. World J Gastroenterol. 2014;20(18):5226–34.
9. Campuzano-Maya G. Hematologic manifestations of helicobacter pylori infection. World J Gastroenterol. 2014;20(36):12818–38.
10. Franceschi F, Tortora A, Gasbarrini G, et al. Helicobacter pylori and extragastric diseases. Helicobacter. 2014;19(Suppl 1):52–8.
11. Franceschi F, Zuccala G, Roccarina D, et al. Clinical effects of helicobacter pylori outside the stomach. Nat Rev Gastroenterol Hepatol. 2014;11(4):234–42.
12. Wong F, Rayner-Hartley E, Byrne MF. Extraintestinal manifestations of helicobacter pylori: a concise review. World J Gastroenterol. 2014;20(34):11950–61.
13. Chmiela M, Gajewski A, Rudnicka K. Helicobacter pylori vs coronary heart disease - searching for connections. World J Cardiol. 2015;7(4):187–203.
14. Blecker U, Renders F, Lanciers S, et al. Syncopes leading to the diagnosis of a helicobacter pylori positive chronic active haemorrhagic gastritis. Eur J Pediatr. 1991;150(8):560–1.
15. Ortiz M, Rosado-Carrion B, Bredy R. Role of helicobacter pylori infection in Hispanic patients with anemia. Bol Asso Med P R. 2014;106:13–8.
16. Sato Y, Yoneyama O, Azumaya M, et al. The relationship between iron deficiency in patients with helicobacter pylori-infected nodular gastritis and the serum prohepcidin level. Helicobacter. 2015;20:11–8.
17. Bazmamoun H, Razavi Z, Esfahani H, et al. Evaluation of iron deficiency anemia and BMI in children suffering from helicobacter pylori infection. Iran J Ped Hematol Oncol. 2014;4:167–71.
18. Sandstrom G, Rodjer S, Kaijser B, et al. Helicobacter pylori antibodies and iron deficiency in female adolescents. PLoS One. 2014;9:e113059.

19. Qu XH, Huang XL, Xiong P, et al. Does helicobacter pylori infection play a role in iron deficiency anemia? A meta-analysis World J Gastroenterol. 2010;16(7):886–96.

20. Annibale B, Marginani M, Monarca B, et al. Reversal of iron deficiency anemia after helicobacter pylori eradication in patients with asymptomatic gastritis. Ann Intern Med. 1999;131:668–72.

21. Yuan W, Li Y, Yang K, et al. Iron deficiency anemia in helicobacter pylori infection: meta-analysis of randomized controlled trials. Scand J Gastroenterol. 2010;45(6):665–76.

22. Tan HJ, Goh KL. Extragastrointestinal manifestations of Helicobacter pylori infection: facts or myth? A critical review. J Dig Dis. 2012;13:342–9.

23. Boyanova L. Role of helicobacter pylori virulence factors for iron acquisition from gastric epithelial cells of the host and impact on bacterial colonization. Future Microbiol. 2011;6(8):843–6.

24. Muhsen K, Cohen D. Helicobacter pylori infection and iron stores: a systemic review and meta-analysis. Helicobacter. 2008;13:323–40.

25. Capurso G, Lahner E, Marcheggiano A, et al. Involvement of the corporal mucosa and related changes in gastric acid secretion characterize patients with iron deficiency anaemia associated with helicobacter pylori infection. Aliment Pharmacol Ther. 2001;15:1753–61.

26. Goddard AF, James MW, McIntyre AS, et al. Guidelines for the management of iron deficiency anemia. Gut. 2011;60:1309–16.

27. Malfertheiner P, Megraud F, O'Morain CA, et al. Management of Helicobacter pylori infection--the Maastricht IV/ Florence consensus report. Gut. 2012;61(5):646–64.

28. Gasbarrini A, Franceschi F, Tartaglione R, et al. Regression of autoimmune thrombocytopenia after eradication of helicobacter pylori. Lancet. 1998;352(9131):878.

29. Kikuchi T, Kobayashi T, Yamashita T, et al. Eight-year follow-up of patients with immune thrombocytopenic purpura related toH. Pyloriinfection. Platelets. 2011;22(1):61–4.

30. Brito HS, Braga JA, Loggetto SR, et al. Helicobacter pylori infection and immune thrombocytopenia purpura in children and adolescents: a randomized controlled trial. Platelet. 2014;15:1–6.

31. Kim H, Lee WS, Lee KH, et al. Efficacy of helicobacter pylori eradication for the 1st-line treatment of immune thrombocytopenia patients with moderate thrombocytopenia. AnnHematol. 2015;94:939–46.

32. Noonavath RN, Lakshmi CP, Dutta TK, et al. Helicobacter pylori eradication in patients with chronic immune thrombocytopenic purpura. World J Gastroenterol. 2014;20:6918–23.

33. Michel M, Cooper N, Jean C, et al. Does helicobacter pylori initiate or perpetuate immune thrombocytopenic purpura? Blood. 2004;103(3):890–6.

34. Michel M, Khellaf M, Desforges L, et al. Autoimmune thrombocytopenic purpura and helicobacter pylori infection. Arch Intern Med. 2002;162(9):1033–6.

35. Stasi R, Sarpatwari A, Segal JB, et al. Effects of eradication of helicobacter pylori infection in patients with immune thrombocytopenic purpura: a systematic review. Blood. 2009;113(6):1231–40.

36. Tsumoto C, Tominaga K, Okazaki H, et al. Long-term efficacy of helicobacter pylori eradication in patients with idiopathic thrombocytopenia purpura: 7-year follow-up prospective study. Ann Hematol. 2009;88:789–93.

37. Arnold DM, Bernotas A, Nazi I, et al. Platelet count response to H. Pylori treatment in patients with immune thrombocytopenic purpura with and without H. Pylori infection: a systematic review. Haematologica. 2009;94(6):850–6.

38. Kuwana M. Helicobacter pylori-associated immune thrombocytopenia: clinical features and pathogenic mechanisms. World J Gastroenterol. 2014;20:714–23.

39. Takahashi T, Yujiri T, Shinohara K, et al. Molecular mimicry by helicobacter pylori CagA protein may be involved in the pathogenesis of H. Pylori-associated chronic idiopathic thrombocytopenic purpura. Br J Haematol. 2004;124:91–6.

40. Bai Y, Wang Z, Bai X, et al. Cross reaction of antibody against helicobacter pylori urease B with platelet glycoprotein IIIa and its significance in the pathogenesis of immune thrombocytopenic purpura. Int J Hematol. 2009;89:142–9.

41. Wu Z, Zhou J, Prsoon P, et al. Low expression of FCCRIIB in macrophages of immune thrombocytopenia-affected individuals. Int J Hematol. 2012;96:588–93.

42. O'Connor HJ, Axon AT, Dixon MF. Campylobacter-like organisms unusual in type a (pernicious anaemia) gastritis. Lancet. 1984;2(8411):1091.

43. Stabler SP. Vitamin B12 deficiency. N Engl J Med. 2013;368:2041–2.

44. Sarari AS, Farraj MA, Hamoudi W, et al. Helicobacter pylori, a causative agent of vitamin B12 deficiency. J Infect Dev Ctries. 2008;2(5):346–9.

45. Shuval-Sudai O, Granot E. An association between helicobacter pylori infection and serum vitamin B12 levels in healthy adults. J Clin Gastroenterol. 2003;36(2):130–3.

46. Eshraghian A, Hashemi SA, Hamidian Jahromi A, et al. Helicobacter pylori infection as a risk factor for insulin resistance. Dig Dis Sci. 2009;54(9):1966–70.

47. Polyzos SA, Kountouras J, Zavos C, et al. The association between helicobacter pylori infection and insulin resistance: a systematic review. Helicobacter. 2011;16(2):79–88.

48. Chen TP, Hung HF, Chen MK, et al. Helicobacter pylori infection is positively associated with metabolic syndrome in Taiwanese adults: a cross-sectional study. Helicobacter. 2015;20:184–91.

49. Yang GH, Wu JS, Yang YC, et al. Gastric helicobacter pylori infection associated with risk of diabetes mellitus, but not prediabetes. J Gastroenterol Hepatol. 2014;29:1794–9.

50. Bajai S, Rekwal L, Misra SP, et al. Association of Helicobacter pylori infection in patients with type 2 diabetes. Indian J Endocrinol Metab. 2014;18:694–9.

51. Horikawa C, Kodama S, Fujihara K, et al. High risk of failing eradication of helicobacter pylori in patients with diabetes: a meta-analysis. Diabetes Res Clin Pract. 2014;106:81–7.

52. Gillum RF. Infection with helicobacter pylori, coronary heart disease, cardiovascular risk factors, and systemic inflammation: the third National Health and nutrition examination survey. J Natl Med Assoc. 2004;96:1470–6.

53. Naja F, Nasreddine L, Hwalla N, et al. Association of H. Pylori infection with insulin resistance and metabolic syndrome among Lebanese adults. Helicobacter. 2012;17(6):444–51.

54. Danesh J, Peto R. Risk factors for coronary heart disease and infection with helicobacter pylori: meta-analysis of 18 studies. BMJ. 1998;316:1130–2.

55. Wada Y, Hamamoto Y, Kawasaki Y, et al. The eradication of helicobacter pylori does not affect glycemic control in Japanese subjects with type 2 diabetes. Jpn Clin Med. 2013;4:41–3.

56. Kachuei A, Amini M, Sebghatollahi V, et al. Effect of helicobacter pylori eradication on insulin resistance among prediabetic patients: a pilot study and single-blind randomized controlled clinical trial. J Res Med Sci. 2016;21:8.

57. Wu MS, Lee WJ, Wang HH, et al. A case-control study of association of helicobacter pylori infection with morbid obesity in Taiwan. Arch Intern Med. 2005;165:1552–5.

58. Lender N, Talley NJ, Enck P, et al. Associations between helicobacter pylori and obesity--an ecological study. Aliment Pharmacol Ther. 2014;40:24–31.

59. Xu C, Yan M, Sun Y, et al. Prevalence of helicobacter pylori infection and its relation with body mass index in a Chinese population. Helicobacter. 2014;19:437–42.

60. Pacifico L, Anania C, Osborn JF, et al. Long-term effects of helicobacter pylori eradication on circulating ghrelin and leptin concentrations and body composition in prepubertal children. Eur J Endocrinol. 2008;158:323–32.

61. Kim TJ, Sinn DH, Min YW, et al. A cohort study on helicobacter pylori infection associated with non-alcoholic fatty liver disease. J Gastroenterol. 2017;52(11):1201–10.

62. Polyzos SA, Kountouras J, Papatheodorou A, et al. Helicobacter pylori infection in patients with nonalcoholic fatty liver disease. Metabolism. 2013;62:121–6.

63. Okushin K, Takahashi Y, Yamamichi N, et al. Helicobacter pylori infection is not associated with fatty liver disease including non-alcoholic fatty liver disease: a large-scale cross-sectional study in Japan. BMC Gastroenterol. 2015;15:25.

64. Tang DM, Kumar S. The association between helicobacter pylori infection and nonalcoholic fatty liver disease. Curr Gastroenterol Rep. 2017;19:5.

65. Wijarnpreecha K, Thongprayoon C, Panjawatanan P, et al. Helicobacter pylori and risk of nonalcoholic fatty liver disease: a systemic review and meta-analysis. J Gastroenerol. 2017; Jan 17; https://doi.org/10.1097/MCG. 0000000000000784.

66. Mendall MA, Goggin PM, Molineaux N, et al. Relation of helicobacter pylori infection and coronary heart disease. Br Heart J. 1994;71(5):437–9.

67. Mayr M, Kiechl S, Mendall MA, Willeit J, Wick G, Xu QB. Increased risk of atherosclerosis is confined to CagA-positive Helicobacter pylori strains prospective results from the Bruneck study. Stroke. 2003;34:610–5.

68. Park MJ, Choi SH, Kim D, et al. Association between helicobacter pylori Seropositivity and the coronary artery calcium score in a screening population. Gut Liver. 2011;5(3):321–7.

69. Huang B, Chen Y, Xie Q, et al. CagA-positive helicobacter pylori strains enhanced coronary atherosclerosis by increasing serum OxLDL and HsCRP in patients with coronary heart disease. Dig Dis Sci. 2011;56(1):109–14.

70. Al-Ghamdi A, Jiman-Fatani AA, El-Banna H. Role of chlamydia pneumoniae, helicobacter pylori and cytomegalovirus in coronary artery disease. Pak J Pharm Sci. 2011;24(2):95–101.

71. Figura N, Palazzuoli A, Vaira D, et al. Cross-sectional study: CagA-positive helicobacter pylori infection, acute coronary artery disease and systemic levels of B-type natriuretic peptide. J Clin Pathol. 2014;67(3):251–7.

72. Lai CY, Yang TY, Lin CL, et al. Helicobacter pylori infection and the risk of acute coronary syndrome: a nationwide retrospective cohort study. Eur J Clin Microbiol Infect Dis. 2015;34:69–74.

73. Yu XJ, Yang X, Feng L, et al. Association between helicobacter pylori infection and angiographically demonstrated coronary artery disease: a meta-analysis. Exp Ther Med. 2017;13:787–93.

74. Padmavati S, Gupta U, Agarwal HK. Chronic infections & coronary artery disease with special reference to Chalmydia pneumoniae. Indian J Med Res. 2012;135(2):228–32.

75. Schottker B, Adamu MA, Weck MN, et al. Helicobacter pylori infection, chronic atrophic gastritis and major cardiovascular events: a population-based cohort study. Atherosclerosis. 2012;220(2):569–74.

76. Ameriso SF, Fridman EA, Leiguarda RC, et al. Detection of helicobacter pylori in human carotid atherosclerotic plaques. Stroke. 2001;32:385–91.

77. Oshima T, Ozono R, Yano Y, et al. Association of Helicobacter pylori infection with systemic inflammation and endothelial dysfunction in healthy male subjects. J Am Coll Cardiol. 2005;45:1219–22.

78. Kucukazman M, Yavuz B, Sacikara M, et al. The relationship between updated Sydney system score and LDL cholesterol levels in patients infected with helicobacter pylori. Dig Dis Sci. 2009;54:604–7.

79. Whincup PH, Mendall MA, Perry IJ, et al. Prospective relations between helicobacter pylori infection, coronary heart disease, and stroke in middle aged men. Heart. 1996;75(6):568–72.

80. Sealy-Jefferson S, Gillespie BW, Aiello AE, et al. Antibody levels to persistent pathogens and incident stroke in Mexican Americans. PLoS One. 2013;8(6):e65959.

81. Wang ZW, Li Y, Huang LY, et al. Helicobacter pylori infection contributes to high risk of ischemic stroke: evidence from a meta-analysis. J Neurol. 2012;259(12):2527–37.

82. Chen Y, Segers S, Blaser MJ. Association between helicobacter pylori and mortality in the NHANES III study. Gut. 2013;62(9):1262–9.

83. Huang WS, Yang TY, Shen WC, et al. Association between helicobacter pylori infection and dementia. J Clin Neurosci. 2014;21(8):1355–8.

84. Honjo K, van Reekum R, Verhoeff NP. Alzheimer's disease and infection: do infectious agents contribute to progression of Alzheimer's disease? Alzheimers Dement. 2009;5(4):348–60.

85. Kountouras J, Tsolaki M, Gavalas E, et al. Relationship between helicobacter pylori infection and Alzheimer disease. Neurology. 2006;66(6):938–40.

86. Chang YP, Chiu GF, Kuo FC, et al. Eradication of helicobacter pylori is associated with the progression of dementia: a population-based study. Gastroenterol Res Pract. 2013;2013:175729.

87. Zhou X, Wu J, Zhang G. Association between helicobacter pylori and asthma: a meta-analysis. Eur J Gastroenterol Hepatol. 2013;25(4):460–8.

88. Hu BL, Wang HY, Yang GY. Association of Helicobacter pylori infection with hepatic encephalopathy risk: a systematic review. Clin Res Hepatol Gastroenterol. 2013;37(6):619–25.

89. Jiang HX, Qin SY, Min ZG, et al. Association of Helicobacter pylori with elevated blood ammonia levels in cirrhotic patients: a meta-analysis. Yonsei Med J. 2013;54(4):832–8.

90. Zhang Y, Hoffmeister M, Weck MN, et al. Helicobacter pylori infection and colorectal cancer risk: evidence from a large population-based case-control study in Germany. Am J Epidemiol. 2012;175(5):441–50.

91. Wu Q, Yang ZP, Xu P, et al. Association between helicobacter pylori infection and the risk of colorectal neoplasia: a systematic review and meta-analysis. Color Dis. 2013;15(7):e352–64.

92. Chen YS, Xu SX, Ding YB, et al. Helicobacter pylori infection and the risk of colorectal adenoma and adenocarcinoma: an updated meta-analysis of different testing methods. Asian Pac J Cancer Prev. 2013;14(12):7613–9.

93. Fukuda S, Shimoyama T, Umegaki T, et al. Effect of helicobacter pylori eradication in the treatment of Japanese patients with chronic idiopathic urticaria. J Gastroenterol. 2004;39(9):827–30.

94. Federman DG, Kirsner RS, Moriarty JP, et al. The effect of antibiotic therapy for patients infected with helicobacter pylori who have chronic urticaria. J Am Acad Dermatol. 2003;49(5):861–4.

95. Moreira A, Rodrigues J, Delgado L, et al. Is helicobacter pylori infection associated with chronic idiopathic urticaria? Allergol Immunopathol (Madr). 2003;31(4):209–14.

16

The functional interplay of low molecular weight thiols in *Mycobacterium tuberculosis*

C. Sao Emani*⃝, M. J. Williams, I. J. Wiid and B. Baker*

Abstract

Background: Three low molecular weight thiols are synthesized by *Mycobacterium tuberculosis (M.tb)*, namely ergothioneine (ERG), mycothiol (MSH) and gamma-glutamylcysteine (GGC). They are able to counteract reactive oxygen species (ROS) and/or reactive nitrogen species (RNS). In addition, the production of ERG is elevated in the MSH-deficient *M.tb* mutant, while the production of MSH is elevated in the ERG-deficient mutants. Furthermore, the production of GGC is elevated in the MSH-deficient mutant and the ERG-deficient mutants. The propensity of one thiol to be elevated in the absence of the other prompted further investigations into their interplay in *M.tb*.

Methods: To achieve that, we generated two *M.tb* mutants that are unable to produce ERG nor MSH but are able to produce a moderate (ΔegtD-mshA) or significantly high (ΔegtB-mshA) amount of GGC relative to the wild-type strain. In addition, we generated an *M.tb* mutant that is unable to produce GGC nor MSH but is able to produce a significantly low level of ERG (ΔegtA-mshA) relative to the wild-type strain. The susceptibilities of these mutants to various in vitro and ex vivo stress conditions were investigated and compared.

Results: The ΔegtA-mshA mutant was the most susceptible to cellular stress relative to its parent single mutant strains (ΔegtA and ΔmshA) and the other double mutants. In addition, it displayed a growth-defect in vitro, in mouse and human macrophages suggesting; that the complete inhibition of ERG, MSH and GGC biosynthesis is deleterious for the growth of *M.tb*.

Conclusions: This study indicates that ERG, MSH and GGC are able to compensate for each other to maximize the protection and ensure the fitness of *M.tb*. This study therefore suggests that the most effective strategy to target thiol biosynthesis for anti-tuberculosis drug development would be the simultaneous inhibition of the biosynthesis of ERG, MSH and GGC.

Keywords: Thiols, Compensation, Tuberculosis, Therapeutic targets, ROS, RNS

Background

Upon host invasion, *Mycobacterium tuberculosis (M.tb)* encounters various cellular stresses generated by macrophages such as acidic, oxidative and nitrosative stress. However, *M.tb* is able to escape this, multiply, causing active tuberculosis (TB) or become dormant within necrotic macrophages (granuloma) [1, 2]. The host susceptibility to TB depends largely on its ability to fight invading mycobacteria by generating reactive oxygen species (ROS) and reactive nitrogen species (RNS) [3].

This became evident when the NADPH oxidase deficient (NOX2) mice and iNOS (inducible nitric oxide synthase) deficient mice were found to be more susceptible to TB infection than the wild-type mice [4, 5]. In addition, children with chronic granulomatous disease (a disorder characterized by phagocytic oxidative bursts resulting in recurrent pyogenic infections) were found to be highly susceptible to TB and to present complications during BCG vaccination [6]. Previous studies suggest a role of the phagocyte NADPH oxidase in the release of cytokines, implicating an interplay between the production of cytokines and the production of ROS, though the mechanism remains ambiguous. In addition, this interplay may also be implicated in the structural organization and formation of granuloma [7].

* Correspondence: karallia@sun.ac.za; brubaker@sun.ac.za
DST-NRF Centre of Excellence for Biomedical Tuberculosis Research; SAMRC Centre for Tuberculosis Research; Division of Molecular Biology and Human Genetics; Department of Biomedical Sciences, Faculty of Medicine and Health Sciences; Stellenbosch University, PO Box 241, Francie van Zijl Drive, Tygerberg 8000, Cape Town, South Africa

Several enzymes have been implicated in the detoxification of *M.tb* [8–10], however these enzymes required redox buffers during enzymatic reactions. Low molecular weight thiols such as MSH and ERG are efficient redox buffers [8, 11, 12]. Though it was shown that MSH and ERG are required for the survival of mycobacteria during adverse conditions [11, 13–15], the ability to generate mycobacteria mutants deficient in either MSH or ERG or both [11, 13, 16–18], suggests that they are compensated for by another thiol. Recently, another thiol, gamma-glutamylcysteine (GGC), was shown to provide mycobacteria protection against nitrosative and oxidative stress [18]. In addition, the production of ERG is elevated in the absence of MSH and vice versa [11, 15–19], while the production of GGC was found to be elevated in a MSH-deficient mutant and ERG-deficient mutants [18]. Elevation of one thiol following the loss of another as a compensation mechanism to maximize the protection of *M.tb* was therefore investigated in this study. Double mutants lacking MSH and ERG but producing a moderate amount of GGC (Δ*egtD-mshA*), another lacking both MSH and ERG but producing a high level of GGC (Δ*egtB-mshA*) and a last one lacking both MSH and GGC but producing a low level of ERG (Δ*egtA-mshA*) were generated. These were further characterized in vitro and ex vivo. This study demonstrates for the first time the significance of the compensatory roles of ERG, MSH and GGC in *M.tb*.

Methods

Generation and genotyping of *M.tb* double mutants

The gene *mshA* was deleted in the previously generated single *M.tb* CDC1551 mutants (*egtA*, *egtB* and *egtD*) as previously described [18, 20, 21]. To maximize the chances of obtaining the double mutants, plates were supplemented with OADC and ERG during the double cross over step. The deletion of *mshA* was investigated by PCR as previously described [18] and confirmed by southern blotting as follows. The genomic DNA was extracted from each strain as previously described [22]. Following extraction, it was digested (4–6 μg) with ClaI restriction enzyme overnight. Confirmation of complete digestion was performed by running a little amount of the digested DNA on an agarose gel (test gel). The digested genomic DNA along with the digoxigenin (DIG)-labelled molecular weight ladder (Roche) were separated on a 1% agarose gel and depurinated by incubating the gel in 250 mM HCl for 10 min (mins) at room temperature (RT). The gel was later rinsed with distilled H_2O.

Southern transfer of DNA onto the membrane

This was performed as previously described [23] with few modifications. After depurination, the DNA was denatured by incubating the gel at room temperature (RT) for 30 mins in the denaturing buffer (0.5 M NaOH, 1.5 mM NaCl). It was subsequently neutralised in the neutralization buffer (0.5 M Tris/HCl pH 7.5, 1.5 M NaCl) for another 30 mins. Southern transfer was performed using the positively charged nylon membrane (Roche Diagnostic GmbH Mannheim, Germany) overnight in 20X SSC (3 M NaCl, 300 mM sodium citrate, pH 7). The membrane was washed in 2X SSC the following day and baked for 2 h (hrs) at 80 °C between 2 Wattman papers.

The DIG High Prime DNA labelling and detection kit II and the DIG wash and block Buffer set (Roche) were used at this stage. The principle is described briefly as follows. DIG binds to the T and A bases of the single stranded (denatured) probe, which would hybridize to the single stranded fragments from the genomic DNA digestion. Subsequently, an anti-DIG antibody (conjugated to alkaline phosphatase) would be added. The conjugated alkaline phosphatase would be able to dephosphorylate CSPD (Disodium3-(4-methoxyspiro{l,2-dioxetane-3,2'-(5'-chloro)tricyclo[3.3.1.13,7]decan}-4-yl) phenyl phosphate) leading to photons emission at 477 nm.

Probe labelling

An amount of 150–200 ng of the probe DNA was denatured at 100 °C for 10 mins, snapped cooled on ice for 5 mins, added in 1 X DIG High prime and incubated for 24–48 h at 37 °C for the labelling reaction to occur. The reaction was stopped by incubating the mixture at 65 °C for 10 mins.

Prehybridization and hybridization of the membrane

The membrane from the southern transfer, was pre-hybridized at 65 °C for 30–60 min in the pre-hybridization buffer using a shaking water bath (optimal hybridization temperature is equal to the melting temperature of the probes minus forty two). The denatured probe was added in the hybridization buffer and the pre-hybridization buffer was replaced with the hybridization buffer containing the probe. Using a heat sealer, the membrane was sealed without air bubbles in a plastic bag and incubated at 65 °C overnight. The following day, the membrane was washed twice for 5 mins at RT in a high stringency preheated (65 °C) buffer (2X SSC/0.1% SDS (sodium dodecyl sulphate)). It was subsequently washed twice in a preheated (65 °C) low stringency buffer (0.5X SSC/0.1% SDS) for 15 mins. After these washes, the membrane was incubated with shaking at RT for 2 mins in 1X maleate buffer. After discarding the maleate buffer, the membrane was incubated further in the blocking solution for 30 mins to 3 hrs. The blocking solution was discarded and replaced with another blocking solution containing the specific antibody and the membrane was incubated further for another 30 mins. The membrane was subsequently washed twice in 1X washing buffer at RT for 15 mins and equilibrated with the detection buffer for 3 mins.

Detection

The equilibrated membrane was placed in a hybridization bag and 1-3 ml CSPD (chemiluminescent substrate for alkaline phosphatase) was applied to it. After removal of air bubbles, the membrane was heat-sealed. Following, incubation at RT for 5 mins, excess fluid was removed, and the membrane was sealed again and incubated further at 37 °C for 10 mins. Bands detection and image acquisition were performed by the ChemiDoc™ MP System (BioRad; 2000 Alfred Nobel Drive, Hercules, California 94,547, USA).

Quantification of thiols

After culturing mycobacteria for ~ 2 weeks in 7H9 liquid media, 100 μl of each culture was serially diluted and plated for colony forming unit (CFU) counts. Five millilitres of each culture was pelleted by centrifugation. One millilitre of the supernatant was filtered twice (using a syringe filter) and lyophilized overnight. The pellets were washed twice in double distilled water and stored at – 80 °C. Lyophilized supernatants (extracellular fractions) and frozen pellets (intracellular fractions) from all biological replicates were re-suspended in the lysis buffer (50% warm acetonitrile + 20 mM hepes pH 8 + 2 mM monobromobimanne), sonicated in a water bath sonicator for ~ 30 mins at 60 °C and acidified with a final concentration of 1 mM acetic acid. Following centrifugation, they were filtered twice and stored for liquid chromatography tandem mass spectrometry (LC-MS) analyses [24].

Growth curve analysis of the mutants

This was performed as previously described [25]. The growth rate was evaluated by subtracting the OD_{600} at day 4 from the OD_{600} at day 10, which represents the linear exponential phase of growth [26].

Susceptibility testing of the mutants

Mycobacteria from frozen stocks were cultured on plates, 7H11 solid cultures supplemented with 1X OADC (oleic acid, albumin, dextrose and catalase). The lawn of mycobacteria formed on the plates were scrapped off, re-suspended in 7H9 supplemented with 1X ADS (albumin, dextrose, sodium chloride). After disrupting cell aggregates by trituration, cells suspensions were re-suspended to an OD_{600} of ~ 0.02. Then they were exposed in a 96-well plate to either 0.2 mM diamide (DIM), or 5 mM vitamin C (VC) for ~ 72 h, or ~ 4 mM diethylaminetriamine nitric oxide adduct (DETA-NO) for 14 days. Their susceptibilities to diamide (DIM) and vitamin C (VC) were estimated from the CFU counts of the treated cells relatively to the untreated cells. Their susceptibilities to DETA-NO were estimated from the fluorescence intensity of resazurin of the treated cells relative to the untreated cells. Similarly, their susceptibilities to antibiotics were investigated as follows. Logarithmic phase liquid cultures (in ADS) were diluted to an OD_{600} of ~ 0.007 and added to an equal volume of serially diluted drugs in black 96-well plates (optical bottom) and incubated for ~ 7 days at 37 °C. After adding resazurin and incubating the plates for 24–48 h at 37 °C, susceptibilities were estimated from the measured fluorescence intensity of resazurin (excitation at 544 nm and emission at 590 nm) of the treated cells relative to the untreated cells.

Infection of macrophages

Double mutants were inoculated 3–7 days before other strains, to ensure that they are at the same growth stage on the day of infection. On the day of infection, logarithmic phase mycobacteria were washed in phosphate buffer saline (PBS) or in the defined cell media supplemented with 10% fetal bovine serum (RPMI 1640 (Roswell Park Memorial Institute medium) for human primary macrophages or DMEM (Dulbecco's modified Eagle's medium) for RAW 264.7 murine cell lines). Re-suspensions were triturated by mixing with a syringe (25GA × 5/8in (0.5 x16mm)) (≥10X). The OD_{600} was adjusted to 0.1 with the cell culture media and the re-suspension was triturated. Previous optimizations revealed that the concentration of the double mutants, ΔegtA-mshA and ΔegtD-mshA was ~ 10^7/ml, of the ΔegtB and ΔegtB-mshA mutants was ~ 4 X 10^7 and of the other mutants and the wild-type was ~ 3.5 X 10^7/ml at OD_{600} of ~ 0.1. This enabled to calculate the volume required for each strain to obtain the targeted multiplicity of infection (MOI). One ml of each adjusted suspension was added in triplicate and accordingly to each well of a 24-well plate containing seeded macrophages (~ 5 X 10^5 per well). Few microliters of the mycobacterial suspensions added to the macrophages were serially diluted and plated for CFU counts to estimate the number of mycobacteria at time zero (before infection). Macrophages were gently washed (two-four times) after three hours of infection. Following the wash step, they were either lysed with 0.05% SDS in order to estimate the intracellular mycobacteria load at time ~ 4 h or incubated further for later time points. For prolong exposure, additional washes were performed on the third day. M0 macrophages differentiated from peripheral blood mononuclear cells (PBMC) isolated over the Histopaque (Sigma Aldrich) gradient method from the blood of a healthy donor were infected as described above with the only difference in the number of macrophages seeded per plate (~ 3 X 10^5 instead of ~ 5 X 10^5).

Statistical analyses

Statistical analyses were performed with Prism using a multiple t-test approach, assuming a uniform distribution with alpha set to 0.05 *($P < 0.05$), **($P < 0.01$), ***($P < 0.001$), ****($P < 0.0001$).

Results

The *M.tb* mutants deficient in more than one thiol have a growth defect in vitro

The gene *mshA* was deleted in the previously generated Δ*egtA*, Δ*egtB*, Δ*egtD* single thiol-deficient mutants as previously described [18] (Fig. 1). This resulted in the loss of MSH production in the generated double mutants (Table 1). The Δ*egtA-mshA* mutant could not produce GGC, neither MSH, but did produce a low level of ERG, the Δ*egtB-mshA* could not produce ERG neither MSH but produced a significantly high level of GGC, and the Δ*egtD-mshA* mutant was also unable to produce ERG, neither MSH but produced a high level of GGC (Table 1).

Complementation of the Δ*egtA-mshA* by inserting a copy of *egtA* at the attP site of the genome as previously described [18], restored the production of ERG and GGC in this strain (Δ*egtAc-mshA* in Table 1).

The growth profiles of the generated double mutants were evaluated in liquid cultures supplemented with either ADS or OADC. Growth fitness of the strains were evaluated by investigating their growth rate as previously described [26]. All double mutant had a growth defect in media supplemented with ADS or OADC relative to the wild-type strain (Fig. 2a and b). The growth defect of the Δ*egtA-mshA* mutant relative to its parent strains is more pronounced in the media supplemented with ADS (Fig. 2c) relative to media supplemented with OADC (Fig. 2d). This was not the case with the Δ*egtB-mshA* mutant (Fig. 2e and f), but was with the Δ*egtD-mshA* mutant (Fig.2g and h). The production of GGC and ERG is restored (Table 1) in the complemented strain of the Δ*egtA-mshA* mutant and analysis of the growth rate of this complemented strain relative to

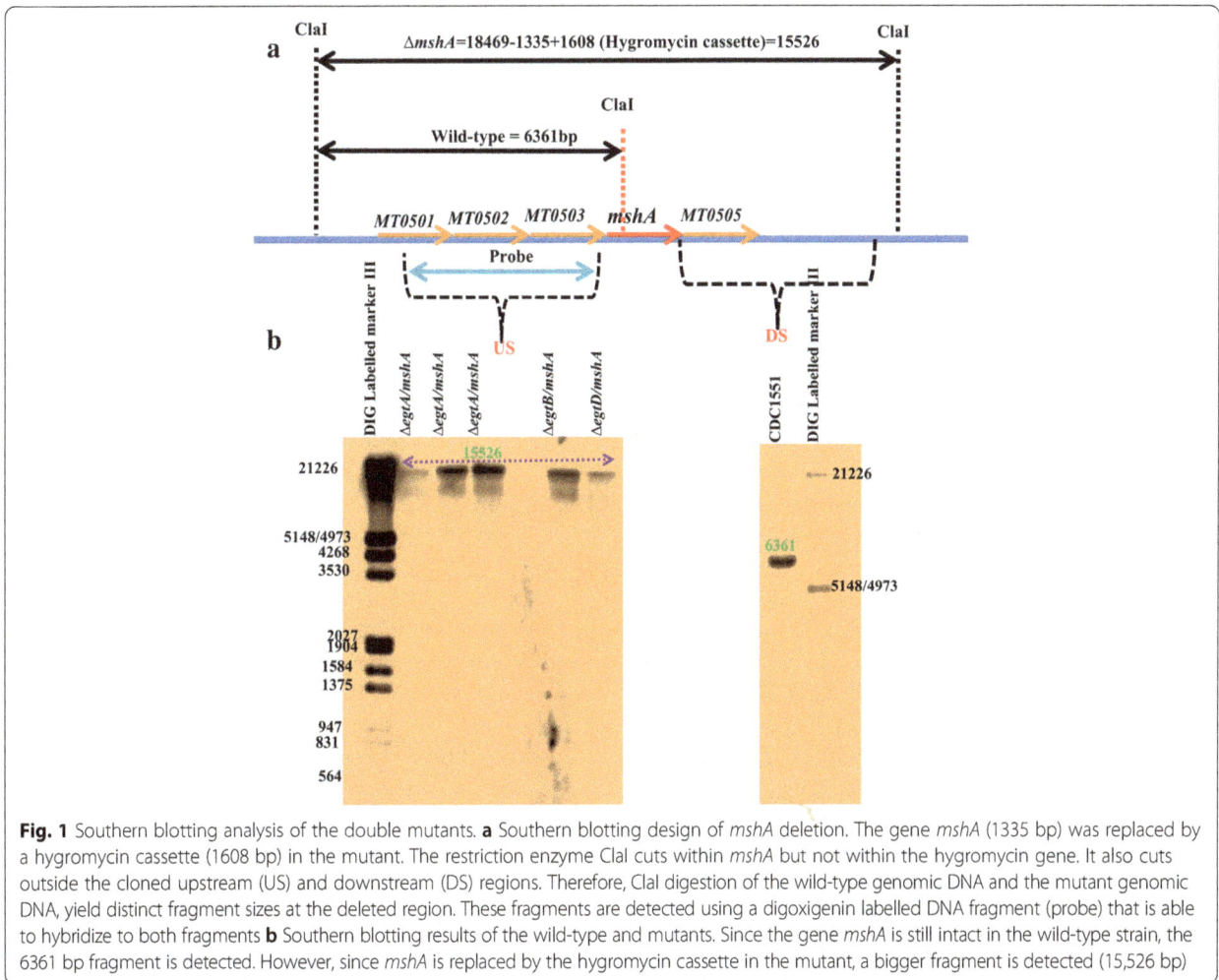

Fig. 1 Southern blotting analysis of the double mutants. **a** Southern blotting design of *mshA* deletion. The gene *mshA* (1335 bp) was replaced by a hygromycin cassette (1608 bp) in the mutant. The restriction enzyme ClaI cuts within *mshA* but not within the hygromycin gene. It also cuts outside the cloned upstream (US) and downstream (DS) regions. Therefore, ClaI digestion of the wild-type genomic DNA and the mutant genomic DNA, yield distinct fragment sizes at the deleted region. These fragments are detected using a digoxigenin labelled DNA fragment (probe) that is able to hybridize to both fragments **b** Southern blotting results of the wild-type and mutants. Since the gene *mshA* is still intact in the wild-type strain, the 6361 bp fragment is detected. However, since *mshA* is replaced by the hygromycin cassette in the mutant, a bigger fragment is detected (15,526 bp)

Table 1 Level of thiols in the generated double mutants pg/10^5CFUs

	Wild-type	$\Delta egtA$-$mshA$	$\Delta egtB$-$mshA$	$\Delta egtD$-$mshA$	$\Delta egtAc$-$mshA$
IE_1	111	10	< 5	< 5	486
EE_1	33	15	< 5	< 5	303
IE_2	296	48	< 5	< 5	184
EE_2	93	44	< 5	< 5	118
IM_1	41	< 5	< 5	< 5	< 5
IM_2	12	< 5	< 5	< 5	< 5
IG_1	1.7	< 5	112	24	25
IG_2	0.6	< 5	91	23	21

IE intracellular ERG, *EE* extracellular ERG, *IM* intracellular MSH, *IG* intracellular gamma-glutamylcysteine

the wild-type reveals that it is not significantly ($P > 0.05$) different (Fig. 2i and j).

The *M.tb* mutant, deficient in all three thiols, is the most sensitive to oxidative and nitrosative stress

Ferric ions (Fe^{3+}) can be reduced by VC to ferrous ions (Fe^{2+}) ($Fe^{3+} + VC = Fe^{2+}$), which in turn can react with oxygen to yield superoxide ($Fe^{2+} + O_2 = O_2^{\circ-} + Fe^{3+}$). The generated superoxide can be converted to hydrogen peroxide by dismutation ($O_2^{\circ-} + 2H^+ = H_2O_2 + O_2$). Hydrogen peroxide can also react with ferrous ions to yield hydroxyl radicals ($H_2O_2 + Fe^{2+} = Fe^{3+} + OH^\circ + OH^-$) [27, 28]. As such, VC is able to generate oxidative stress. Previous studies indicated that the MSH-deficient $\Delta mshA$ mutant is sensitive to VC [29]. Therefore, in order to determine if the loss of more than one thiol would aggravate the sensitivity of *M.tb*, the double mutants with their respective parent single mutants were exposed to VC. While the $\Delta egtA$-$mshA$ mutant was the most sensitive strain (Fig. 3a), all three double mutants were more sensitive than their respective parent strains (Fig. 3a). Compounds such as DIM generate oxidative stress by oxidizing thiols [30, 31]. The mutant $\Delta egtA$-$mshA$ was the most sensitive double mutant to DIM (Fig. 3b). The susceptibility of this mutant to antibiotics known to generate oxidative stress such as rifampicin [32] (RIF) and sulfaguanidine [25] (Su) was investigated. Preliminary investigations at lethal concentrations revealed no significant difference between $\Delta egtA$-$mshA$ and its parent single mutant strains ($\Delta egtA$ and $\Delta mshA$) since they were already highly sensitive to these antibiotics as previously shown [11, 25]. However, sub-lethal concentrations of these drugs significantly inhibited the growth of the $\Delta egtA$-$mshA$ mutant (Fig. 3c). This was not observed with other tested antibiotics namely, streptomycin (Strp) and ethambutol (EmB) (Fig. 3c). It was previously indicated that the high level of MSH in the $\Delta egtA$ mutant was able to protect it against a short exposure to a low concentration of nitric oxide. In addition, the

high level of GGC in the $\Delta mshA$ mutant was able to protect it against an extended exposure to a high concentration of nitric oxide [18]. In this study, the $\Delta egtA$-$mshA$ mutant (deficient in both MSH and GGC, Table 1) was more sensitive to nitric oxide stress generated by DETA-NO than the wild-type, the GGC-deficient $\Delta egtA$ and MSH-deficient $\Delta mshA$ single mutants (Fig. 3d).

The *M.tb* mutant, deficient in all three thiols, has the most severe growth defect in macrophages

During TB infection, human macrophages are able to generate oxidative and nitrosative stress to destroy invading mycobacteria. *M. tuberculosis* is able to escape this defence mechanism to some extent [1]. It was previously shown that the thiol-deficient single mutants survived within the first few days and became sensitive after three days of infection in mouse macrophages at multiplicity of infection (MOI) $\geq$ 5:1 (mycobacteria: macrophages) [11, 33]. The ability of the double thiol-deficient mutants to survive within the first few days of infection of mouse macrophages was therefore investigated. The $\Delta egtA$-$mshA$ mutant was the most sensitive double mutant at MOI 1:1 (Fig. 4a). Investigation at a higher multiplicity of infection MOI 10:1 further confirms that the $\Delta egtA$-$mshA$ mutant was more sensitive than its parent single mutant strains during the first few days of infection (Fig. 4b). However, to ensure that these results could be related to humans treated with potential compounds inhibiting the biosynthesis of all three thiols, human blood monocyte-derived macrophages (HBMM) isolated from a healthy donor were infected with these mutants. As opposed to the observation in mouse macrophages (Fig. 4a and b), the $\Delta egtA$-$mshA$ mutant became more sensitive than its parent strains only after 3 days of infection at MOI 2.5:1 (Fig. 4c), a trend that was observed as well at a higher MOI (MOI 5:1, data not shown).

Discussion

The ability of thiols to protect mycobacteria against oxidative and nitrosative stress is well documented [11, 17, 18, 33–35]. However, it was unclear if the fitness of *M.tb* would be more affected in case all thiols were depleted simultaneously. In this study, by generating a series of double mutants, it was shown that the loss of more than one thiol affects the growth rate of *M.tb*. In addition, the growth defect of the double mutants was more severe relative to their parent strains in the absence of catalase (media supplemented with ADS) (Fig. 2a, b, c, d, g, h). This suggests that catalase may facilitate the growth of these mutants by reducing hydrogen peroxide or peroxynitrite [36]. The growth defect phenotype was partially reversed in the complemented strain of the $\Delta egtA$-$mshA$ mutant ($\Delta egtAc$-$mshA$,

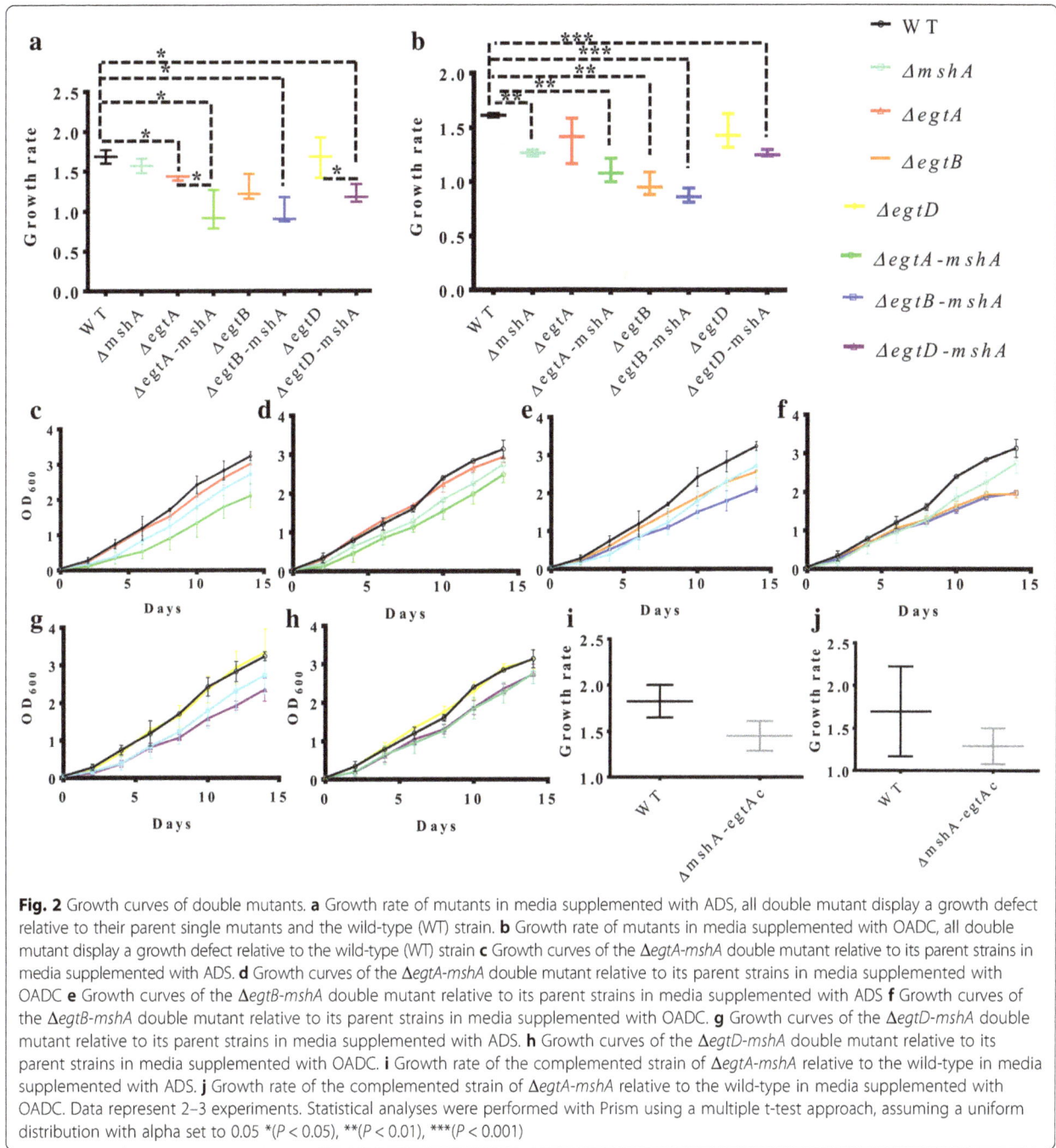

Fig. 2 Growth curves of double mutants. **a** Growth rate of mutants in media supplemented with ADS, all double mutant display a growth defect relative to their parent single mutants and the wild-type (WT) strain. **b** Growth rate of mutants in media supplemented with OADC, all double mutant display a growth defect relative to the wild-type (WT) strain **c** Growth curves of the ΔegtA-mshA double mutant relative to its parent strains in media supplemented with ADS. **d** Growth curves of the ΔegtA-mshA double mutant relative to its parent strains in media supplemented with OADC **e** Growth curves of the ΔegtB-mshA double mutant relative to its parent strains in media supplemented with ADS **f** Growth curves of the ΔegtB-mshA double mutant relative to its parent strains in media supplemented with OADC. **g** Growth curves of the ΔegtD-mshA double mutant relative to its parent strains in media supplemented with ADS. **h** Growth curves of the ΔegtD-mshA double mutant relative to its parent strains in media supplemented with OADC. **i** Growth rate of the complemented strain of ΔegtA-mshA relative to the wild-type in media supplemented with ADS. **j** Growth rate of the complemented strain of ΔegtA-mshA relative to the wild-type in media supplemented with OADC. Data represent 2–3 experiments. Statistical analyses were performed with Prism using a multiple t-test approach, assuming a uniform distribution with alpha set to 0.05 *($P < 0.05$), **($P < 0.01$), ***($P < 0.001$)

Fig. 2i and j). Since the production of ERG and GGC is restored in the complemented strain (Table 1), this suggests that all three thiols are required to ensure the optimal growth of *M.tb*.

On the other hand, though the ΔegtB-mshA and ΔegtD-mshA mutants were more sensitive than their parent single mutant strains to oxidative stress (Fig. 3a), the ΔegtA-mshA mutant was the most sensitive strain to oxidative and nitrosative stress (Fig. 3). In addition, it was sensitive to sub-lethal concentrations of RIF and Su,

but not Strp neither EmB. Since the mode of action of Strp and EmB is not directly associated with the generation of oxidative stress [37], as is of the case for Su [25] and RIF [32], these results suggest that compounds targeting the biosynthesis of all three thiols would reduce the therapeutic dose of drugs that generate oxidative stress such as RIF and Su.

Though it was indicated that ERG is able to scavenge peroxyntrite [38], and decompose S-nitrosoglutathione [39], it is unclear if it is able to protect eukaryotic or prokaryotic

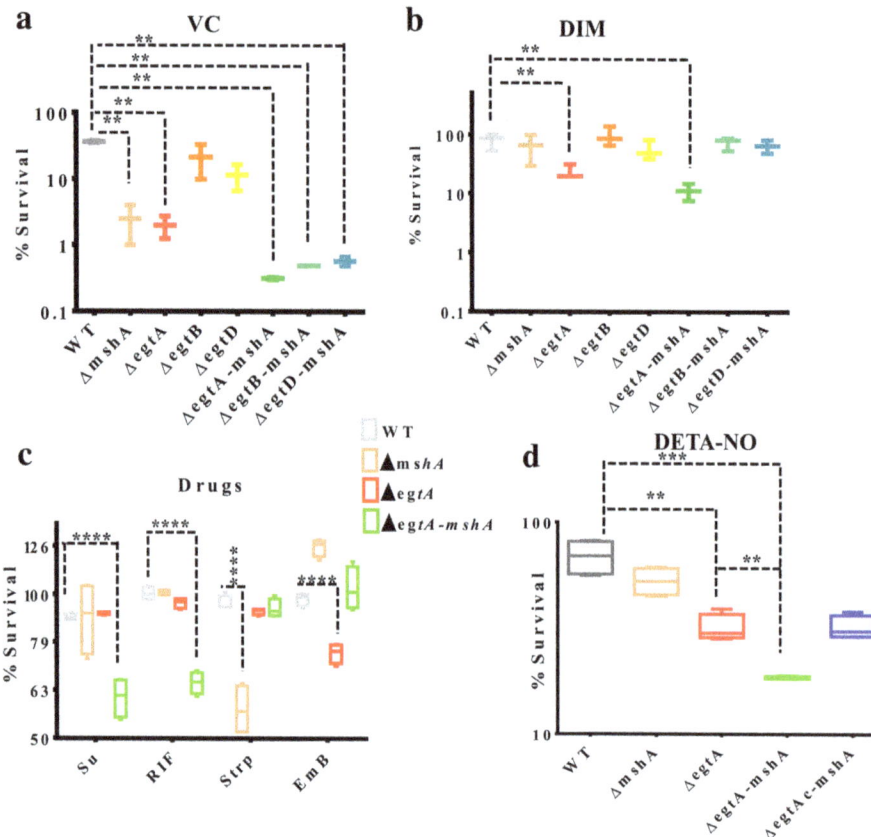

Fig. 3 Susceptibility of the double mutants to oxidative and nitrosative stress. **a** Susceptibility of the mutants to vitamin C (VC) (5 mM for ~ 72 h). Every double mutant was more sensitive than its parent single mutant strains; however, ΔegtA-mshA appeared to be the most sensitive. Data are representative of two experiments. **b** Susceptibility of the mutants to diamide (DIM) (0.2 mM for ~ 72 h), ΔegtA-mshA is the most sensitive mutant. Data are representative of three independent experiments **c** Susceptibility of the mutants to sulfaguanidine (Su, 3.8 μg/ml), rifampicin (RIF, 0.0007 μg/ml), streptomycin (Strp, 0.16 μg/ml) and ethambutol (Emb, 0.6 μg/ml). ΔegtA-mshA is more sensitive than its parent strains to RIF and Su, while ΔmshA is sensitive to Strep and ΔegtA is sensitive to EmB. Data are representative of two experiments and two technical replicates for each experiment. **d** Susceptibility of the mutants to nitric oxide generated by diethylaminetriamine nitric oxide adduct (DETA-NO) (4 mM for 14 days). Even though, the single mutants display a sensitivity trend, ΔegtA-mshA is more sensitive than its parent strains. Data are representative of two experiments and two technical replicates for each experiment. Statistical analyses were performed with Prism using a multiple t-test approach, assuming a uniform distribution with alpha set to 0.05 *(P < 0.05), **(P < 0.01), ***(P < 0.001), ****(P < 0.0001)

cells against nitrosative stress. Preliminary investigations of the susceptibility of all three double mutants to nitrosative stress generated by DETA-NO revealed that the ΔegtA-mshA mutant, which still produced low levels of ERG (Table 1), was more sensitive than the ΔegtB-mshA and ΔegtD-mshA mutants which can't produce ERG (Table 1) (data not shown). In addition, it was shown that chemical complementation of the sensitivity phenotype of the ΔegtA mutant to nitrosative stress generated by DETA-NO could be achieved with GGC but not ERG [18]. Therefore, it is less likely that the high sensitivity of the ΔegtA-mshA mutant to nitrosative stress relative to its parent strains (Fig. 3d) is associated with the depletion of ERG in this strain (Table 1). Nevertheless, according to results in Table 1, dealing with the anti-nitrosative roles of MSH [40] and GGC [18, 41], the sensitivity of the double mutant lacking both thiols (ΔegtA-mshA) is more likely

associated with the loss of both thiols (Table 1) in this strain.

Further investigations of the survival of these mutants revealed that the ΔegtA-mshA mutant had the most severe growth defect within macrophages (Fig. 4), indicating that the elevated GGC in the other double mutants (Table 1) may have protected them during the first three days of infection. The growth defect of the ΔegtA-mshA mutant within the mouse macrophages was observed during early infections (~ 3 days, Fig. 4a and b). On the other hand, the ERG-deficient single mutant strains were shown to display a growth defect within mouse macrophages after 4 days of infection [11, 33]. This suggests that the elevated levels of MSH and GGC in the ERG-deficient single mutants [18, 25] are not enough to protect them during a prolong exposure to ROS and RNS generated by macrophages (after 4 days) but are enough to protect them

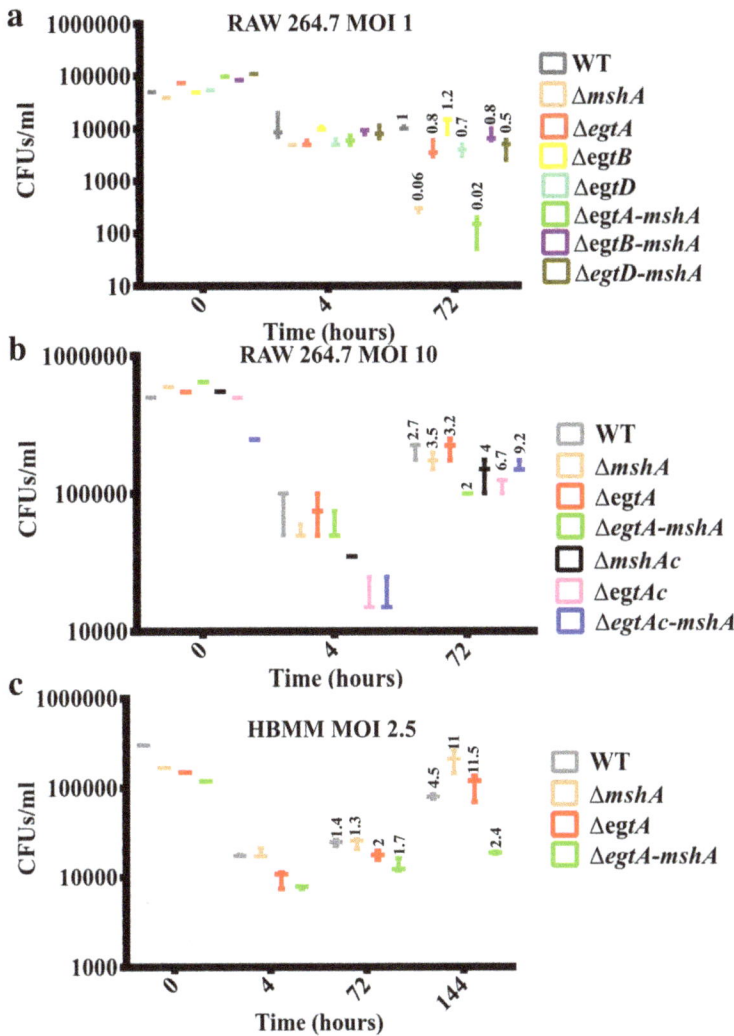

Fig. 4 Survival of thiols-deficient mutants in macrophages. **a** Investigation of the survival of all double mutant relative to their parent strains in murine cell lines RAW264.7 at an MOI of~ 1:1. The *ΔegtA-mshA* double mutant was the most sensitive. **b** Further, investigation of its survival relative to its parent and complemented strains at an MOI of~ 10:1. The *ΔegtA-mshA* mutant was still the most sensitive. **c** This was also observed when human blood monocyte-derived macrophages (HBMM) were infected at an MOI of ~ 2.5:1 and 5:1 (data not shown), however at a later time point. The 0-h time-point represents the amount of mycobacteria added to the macrophages and the 4-h time point represents the amount of mycobacteria taken up by macrophages. For accuracy, the growth index (GI) was determined based on the amount of each ingested mycobacterial strain (4-h time point). The average GI indicated at the top of each whisker, was determined by dividing the CFUs obtained at the defined time point by the CFUs obtained at the 4-h time point (that indicates the uptake amount of each stain). Data are representative of three replicates

during the first few days of infection. Further explaining why, the *ΔegtA-mshA* mutant, deficient in all thiols was the most sensitive during the first few days of infection (Fig. 4a and b). However, this was not the case with human blood monocyte-derived macrophages (HBMM), as the *ΔegtA-mshA* mutant displayed the most severe sensitivity only after 3 days (Fig. 4c). This suggests agreement with previous studies that showed that mycobacteria are better adapted to survive and grow exponentially in the human primary macrophages than in mouse macrophages [42]. Probably, because mouse macrophages display increased iNOS (inducible nitric oxide synthase) activity and consequently increased production of RNS during early infections [43].

The sensitivity phenotype of the *ΔegtA-mshA* double mutant observed during the early time point in mouse macrophages (Fig. 4a and b) may therefore be due to this initial burst, which is not the case in HBMM where the growth defect was only observed at a later time point (6-day) (Fig. 4c). Therefore, thiols interplay to ensure an optimal protection of *M.tb* against nitrosative and oxidative stress. It is also worth noting that the *ΔegtA-mshA* mutant still produced a low level of ERG (Table 1), yet, it displayed the most severe sensitivity (Figs. 3 and 4) suggesting that the absolute simultaneous inhibition of all three thiols could be lethal to *M.tb*. However, this requires further investigations.

Conclusions

In conclusion, thiols are able to protect *M.tb* against various cellular stresses and ensuring their fitness in vitro and within macrophages. However, to ensure the potential complete eradication of invading *M.tb* during infection, this study suggests that targeting the production of all three thiols simultaneously would be more efficient.

Abbreviations

ADS: Albumin, dextrose, sodium chloride; CFU: Colony forming unit; CSPD: Disodium3-(4-methoxyspiro{1,2-dioxetane-3,2′-(5′-chloro)tricyclo[3.3.1.13,7]decan}-4-yl) phenyl phosphate; DETA-NO: Diethylaminetriamine nitric oxide adduct; DIG: digoxigenin; DIM: Diamide; DMEM: Dulbecco's modified Eagle's medium; EmB: Ethambutol; ERG: Ergothioneine; GGC: Gamma-glutamylcysteine; HBMM: Human blood monocyte-derived macrophages; Hr: hour; iNOS: Inducible nitric oxide synthase; *M.tb: Mycobacterium tuberculosis*; Min: minute; MOI: Multiplicity of infection; MSH: Mycothiol; OADC: Oleic acid, albumin, dextrose and catalase; PBMC: Peripheral blood mononuclear cells; PBS: Phosphate buffer saline; RIF: Rifampicin; RNS: Reactive nitrogen species.; ROS: Reactive oxygen species; RPMI 1640: Roswell Park Memorial Institute medium; RT: Room temperature; SDS: Sodium dodecyl sulphate; Strp: Streptomycin; Su: Sulfaguanidine.; TB: Tuberculosis; VC: Vitamin C

Acknowledgements

Authors would also like to thank Abhilasha Madhvi Mishra for collecting and isolating the PBMC, Jomien Mouton and Danicke Willemse for kindly donating the RAW 264.7 cells lines, Andile Ngwane for his intellectual input during the design of the drug testing experiments, Malcolm Taylor and the mass spectrometry unit of the Central Analytical Facilities of Stellenbosch University for performing the LC-MS.

Funding

Research reported in this publication was supported by the South African Medical Research Council (SAMRC) and the DST-NRF Centre of Excellence for Biomedical Tuberculosis Research.

Authors' contributions

CSE, MJW, IJW and BB conceived the experiments, read and revised the manuscript. CSE wrote the manuscript, designed and performed the experiments. All authors read and approved the final manuscript.

Competing interests

The authors declare that they have no competing interests.

References

1. Stallings CL, Glickman MS. Is Mycobacterium tuberculosis stressed out? A critical assessment of the genetic evidence. Microbes Infect [Internet]. NIH Public Access; 2010 [cited 2018 Feb 27];12:1091–101. Available from: https://www.ncbi.nlm.nih.gov/pubmed/20691805.
2. Xu G, Wang J, Gao GF, Liu CH. Insights into battles between Mycobacterium tuberculosis and macrophages. Protein Cell [Internet]. Springer; 2014 [cited 2018 Feb 27];5:728–36. Available from: http://www.ncbi.nlm.nih.gov/pubmed/24938416.
3. Via LE, Lin PL, Ray SM, Carrillo J, Allen SS, Eum SY, et al. Tuberculous granulomas are hypoxic in guinea pigs, rabbits, and nonhuman primates. Infect Immun [Internet]. 2008;76:2333–40. Available from: http://view.ncbi.nlm.nih.gov/pubmed/18347040.
4. MacMicking JD, North RJ, LaCourse R, Mudgett JS, Shah SK, Nathan CF. Identification of nitric oxide synthase as a protective locus against tuberculosis. Proc Natl Acad Sci U S A [Internet]. 1997;94:5243–8. Available from: http://view.ncbi.nlm.nih.gov/pubmed/9144222.
5. Adams LB, Dinauer MC, Morgenstern DE, Krahenbuhl JL. Comparison of the roles of reactive oxygen and nitrogen intermediates in the host response to Mycobacterium tuberculosis using transgenic mice. Tuber Lung Dis Off J Int Union Against Tuberc Lung Dis. 1997;78:237–46.
6. Lee PPW, Chan K-W, Jiang L, Chen T, Li C, Lee T-L, et al. Susceptibility to mycobacterial infections in children with X-linked chronic granulomatous disease: a review of 17 patients living in a region endemic for tuberculosis. Pediatr Infect Dis J. 2008;27:224–30.
7. Deffert C, Cachat J, Krause K-H. Phagocyte NADPH oxidase, chronic granulomatous disease and mycobacterial infections. Cell Microbiol [Internet]. 2014 [cited 2018 Jun 6];16:1168–78. Available from: http://www.ncbi.nlm.nih.gov/pubmed/24916152.
8. Nambi S, Long JE, Mishra BB, Baker R, Murphy KC, Olive AJ, et al. The oxidative stress network of Mycobacterium tuberculosis reveals coordination between radical detoxification systems. Cell Host Microbe. 2015;17:829–37.
9. Bryk R, Lima CD, Erdjument-Bromage H, Tempst P, Nathan C. Metabolic enzymes of mycobacteria linked to antioxidant defense by a thioredoxin-like protein. Sci (80-) [Internet]. 2002;295:1073–7. Available from: http://view.ncbi.nlm.nih.gov/pubmed/11799204.
10. Lee SP, Hwang YS, Kim YJ, Kwon KS, Kim HJ, Kim K, et al. Cyclophilin A Binds to Peroxiredoxins and Activates Its Peroxidase Activity. J Biol Chem. 2001;276:29826–32.
11. Saini V, Cumming BM, Guidry L, Lamprecht DA, Adamson JH, Reddy VP, et al. Ergothioneine Maintains Redox and Bioenergetic Homeostasis Essential for Drug Susceptibility and Virulence of Mycobacterium tuberculosis. Cell Rep. 2016;14(3):572–85.
12. Ordóñez E, Van Belle K, Roos G, De Galan S, Letek M, Gil JA, et al. Arsenate Reductase, Mycothiol, and Mycoredoxin Concert Thiol/Disulfide Exchange. J Biol Chem [Internet]. 2009 [cited 2018 Feb 27];284:15107–15116. Available from: http://www.ncbi.nlm.nih.gov/pubmed/19286650
13. Xu X, Vilchèze C, Av-Gay Y, Gómez-Velasco A, Jacobs WRJ. Precise null deletion mutations of the mycothiol synthesis genes reveal their role in isoniazid and ethionamide resistance in Mycobacterium smegmatis. Antimicrob Agents Chemother [Internet]. 2011;55:3133–9. Available from: http://view.ncbi.nlm.nih.gov/pubmed/21502624
14. Ung KSE, Av-Gay Y. Mycothiol-dependent mycobacterial response to oxidative stress. FEBS Lett. 2006;580:2712–6.
15. Ta P, Buchmeier N, Newton GL, Rawat M, Fahey RC. Organic Hydroperoxide resistance protein and Ergothioneine compensate for loss of Mycothiol in Mycobacterium smegmatis mutants. J Bacteriol [Internet]. 2011;193:1981–90. Available from: http://view.ncbi.nlm.nih.gov/pubmed/21335456
16. Vilchèze C, Av-Gay Y, Attarian R, Liu Z, Hazbón MH, Colangeli R, et al. Mycothiol biosynthesis is essential for ethionamide susceptibility in Mycobacterium tuberculosis. Mol Microbiol [Internet]. 2008;69:1316–1329. Available from: http://view.ncbi.nlm.nih.gov/pubmed/18651841.
17. Sao Emani C, Williams MJ, Wiid IJ, Hiten NF, Viljoen AJ, Pietersen R-DD, et al. Ergothioneine is a secreted antioxidant in Mycobacterium smegmatis. Antimicrob Agents Chemother [Internet]. 2013;57:3202–7. Available from: http://view.ncbi.nlm.nih.gov/pubmed/23629716.
18. Sao Emani C, Williams MJ, Van Helden PD, Taylor MJC, Wiid IJ, Baker B. Gamma-glutamylcysteine protects ergothioneine-deficient Mycobacterium tuberculosis mutants against oxidative and nitrosative stress. Biochem Biophys Res Commun. 2018;495(1):174–8.
19. Shea RJ, Mulks MH. ohr, Encoding an organic hydroperoxide reductase, is an in vivo-induced gene in Actinobacillus pleuropneumoniae. Infect Immun [Internet]. 2002;70:794–802. Available from: http://view.ncbi.nlm.nih.gov/pubmed/11796613.
20. Parish T, Stoker NG. Use of a flexible cassette method to generate a double unmarked Mycobacterium tuberculosis tlyA plcABC mutant by gene replacement. Microbiology [Internet]. 2000 [cited 2018 May 9];146(Pt 8):1969–75. Available from: http://view.ncbi.nlm.nih.gov/pubmed/10931901.

21. Muttucumaru DGN, Parish T. The molecular biology of recombination in mycobacteria: what do we know and how can we use it? Curr Issues Mol Biol [Internet]. 2004;6:145–57. Available from: http://view.ncbi.nlm.nih.gov/pubmed/15119825.

22. Warren R, de Kock M, Engelke E, Myburgh R, Gey van Pittius N, Victor T, et al. Safe Mycobacterium tuberculosis DNA extraction method that does not compromise integrity. J Clin Microbiol [Internet] American Society for Microbiology (ASM); 2006 [cited 2018 Jun 8];44:254–6. Available from: http://www.ncbi.nlm.nih.gov/pubmed/16390984.

23. Warren R, Richardson M, Sampson S, Hauman JH, Beyers N, Donald PR, et al. Genotyping of Mycobacterium tuberculosis with additional markers enhances accuracy in epidemiological studies J Clin Microbiol [Internet]. American Society for Microbiology (ASM); 1996 [cited 2018 Jun 8];34:2219–24. Available from: http://www.ncbi.nlm.nih.gov/pubmed/8862588.

24. Capone DL, Ristic R, Pardon KH, Jeffery DW. Simple Quantitative Determination of Potent Thiols at Ultratrace Levels in Wine by Derivatization and High-Performance Liquid Chromatography–Tandem Mass Spectrometry (HPLC-MS/MS) Analysis. Anal Chem [Internet]. 2015 [cited 2018 Jun 8];87:1226–31. Available from: http://www.ncbi.nlm.nih.gov/pubmed/25562625.

25. Sao Emani C, Williams MJ, Wiid I, Baker B, Carolis C. Compounds with potential activity against Mycobacterium tuberculosis. Antimicrob Agents Chemother [Internet]. American Society for Microbiology; 2018 [cited 2018 Feb 15];AAC.02236-17. Available from: http://www.ncbi.nlm.nih.gov/pubmed/29437626.

26. Sandegren L, Lindqvist A, Kahlmeter G, Andersson DI. Nitrofurantoin resistance mechanism and fitness cost in Escherichia coli. J Antimicrob Chemother [internet]. Oxford University Press; 2008 [cited 2018 Mar 9];62:495–503. Available from: https://academic.oup.com/jac/article-lookup/doi/10.1093/jac/dkn222

27. Haber F, Weiss J. The Catalytic Decomposition of Hydrogen Peroxide by Iron Salts. Proc R Soc A Math Phys Eng Sci [Internet]. The Royal Society; 1934 [cited 2018 Jun 7];147:332–51. Available from: http://rspa.royalsocietypublishing.org/cgi/doi/10.1098/rspa.1934.0221.

28. Burkitt MJ, Gilbert BC. Model studies of the iron-catalysed Haber-Weiss cycle and the ascorbate-driven Fenton reaction. Free Radic Res Commun [Internet]. 1990 [cited 2018 Jun 7];10:265–80. Available from: http://www.ncbi.nlm.nih.gov/pubmed/1963164.

29. Vilchèze C, Hartman T, Weinrick B, Jacobs WRJ. Mycobacterium tuberculosis is extraordinarily sensitive to killing by a vitamin C-induced Fenton reaction. Nat Commun [Internet]. 2013;4:1881. Available from: http://view.ncbi.nlm.nih.gov/pubmed/23695675.

30. Kosower NS, Kosower EM. Diamide: an oxidant probe for thiols. Methods Enzymol [Internet]. 1995 [cited 2018 Jun 6];251:123–33. Available from: http://www.ncbi.nlm.nih.gov/pubmed/7651192.

31. Rudyk O, Eaton P. Biochemical methods for monitoring protein thiol redox states in biological systems. Redox Biol [Internet]. Elsevier; 2014 [cited 2018 Feb 27];2:803–813. Available from: http://www.ncbi.nlm.nih.gov/pubmed/25009782.

32. Piccaro G, Pietraforte D, Giannoni F, Mustazzolu A, Fattorini L. Rifampin Induces Hydroxyl Radical Formation in Mycobacterium tuberculosis. Antimicrob Agents Chemother [Internet]. 2014 [cited 2018 Feb 27];58:7527–33. Available from: http://www.ncbi.nlm.nih.gov/pubmed/25288092.

33. Richard-Greenblatt M, Bach H, Adamson J, Pena-Diaz S, Wu L, Steyn AJC, et al. Regulation of Ergothioneine Biosynthesis and its effect on Mycobacterium tuberculosis Growth and Infectivity. J Biol Chem [Internet]. 2015; Available from: http://view.ncbi.nlm.nih.gov/pubmed/26229105.

34. Newton GL, Buchmeier N, Fahey RC. Biosynthesis and functions of mycothiol, the unique protective thiol of Actinobacteria. Microbiol Mol Biol Rev [Internet]. 2008;72:471–94. Available from: http://view.ncbi.nlm.nih.gov/pubmed/18772286.

35. Saikolappan S, Das K, Dhandayuthapani S. Inactivation of the organic hydroperoxide stress resistance regulator OhrR enhances resistance to oxidative stress and isoniazid in Mycobacterium smegmatis. J Bacteriol [Internet]. 2015;197:51–62. Available from: http://view.ncbi.nlm.nih.gov/pubmed/25313389.

36. Glorieux C, Calderon PB. Catalase, a remarkable enzyme: targeting the oldest antioxidant enzyme to find a new cancer treatment approach. Biol Chem [Internet]. 2017 [cited 2018 Mar 23];398:1095–108. Available from: http://www.ncbi.nlm.nih.gov/pubmed/28384098.

37. Almeida Da Silva PE, Palomino JC. Molecular basis and mechanisms of drug resistance in Mycobacterium tuberculosis: classical and new drugs. J Antimicrob Chemother [Internet]. 2011 [cited 2018 Feb 27];66:1417–30. Available from: http://www.ncbi.nlm.nih.gov/pubmed/21558086.

38. Aruoma OI, Whiteman M, England TG, Halliwell B. Antioxidant Action of Ergothioneine: Assessment of Its Ability to Scavenge Peroxynitrite. Biochem Biophys Res Commun [Internet]. Academic Press; 1997 [cited 2018 Mar 6];231:389–91. Available from: https://www.sciencedirect.com/science/article/pii/S0006291X9796109X.

39. Misiti F, Castagnola M, Zuppi C, Giardina B, Messana I. Role of ergothioneine on S-nitrosoglutathione catabolism. Biochem J [Internet]. Portland Press Limited; 2001 [cited 2018 Mar 6];356:799–804. Available from: http://www.ncbi.nlm.nih.gov/pubmed/11389687.

40. Miller CC, Rawat M, Johnson T, Av-Gay Y. Innate protection of Mycobacterium smegmatis against the antimicrobial activity of nitric oxide is provided by mycothiol. Antimicrob Agents Chemother [Internet]. 2007;51:3364–3366. Available from: http://view.ncbi.nlm.nih.gov/pubmed/17638697.

41. Alqahtani S, Mahmoud AM. Gamma-Glutamylcysteine ethyl Ester protects against cyclophosphamide-induced liver injury and hematologic alterations via upregulation of PPARγ and attenuation of oxidative stress, inflammation, and apoptosis. Oxidative Med Cell Longev. 2016;2016:4016209.

42. Jordao L, Bleck CKE, Mayorga L, Griffiths G, Anes E. On the killing of mycobacteria by macrophages. Cell Microbiol [Internet]. Wiley/Blackwell (10.1111); 2008 [cited 2018 Jun 7];10:529–548. Available from: http://doi.wiley.com/10.1111/j.1462-5822.2007.01067.x.

43. Jordao L, Bleck CKE, Mayorga L, Griffiths G, Anes E. On the killing of mycobacteria by macrophages. Cell Microbiol [Internet]. 2007 [cited 2018 Mar 8];0:071106215315001–???. Available from: http://www.ncbi.nlm.nih.gov/pubmed/17986264.

17

Metformin causes cancer cell death through downregulation of p53-dependent differentiated embryo chondrocyte 1

Shu-Man Hsieh Li[1], Shu-Ting Liu[1], Yung-Lung Chang[1], Ching-Liang Ho[2*] and Shih-Ming Huang[1*] ⓘ

Abstract

Background: Metformin is the most commonly used first-line medicine for type II diabetes mellitus. Acting via AMP-activated protein kinase, it has been used for more than 60 years and has an outstanding safety record. Metformin also offers protection against cancer, but its precise mechanisms remain unclear.

Methods: We first examined the cytotoxic effects of metformin in the HeLa human cervical carcinoma and ZR-75-1 breast cancer cell lines using assays of cell viability, cleaved poly-ADP-ribose polymerase, and Annexin V-fluorescein isothiocyanate apoptosis, as well as flow cytometric analyses of the cell cycle profile and reactive oxygen species (ROS). We later clarified the effect of metformin on p53 protein stability using transient transfection and cycloheximide chase analyses.

Results: We observed that metformin represses cell cycle progression, thereby inducing subG1 populations, and had induced apoptosis through downregulation of p53 protein and a target gene, differentiated embryo chondrocyte 1 (DEC1). In addition, metformin increased intracellular ROS levels, but N-acetyl cysteine, a ROS scavenger, failed to suppress metformin-induced apoptosis. Further results showed that metformin disrupted the electron transport chain and collapsed the mitochondrial membrane potential, which may be the cause of the elevated ROS levels. Examination of the mechanisms underlying metformin-induced HeLa cell death revealed that reduced stability of p53 in metformin-treated cells leads to decreases in DEC1 and induction of apoptosis.

Conclusion: The involvement of DEC1 provides new insight into the positive or negative functional roles of p53 in the metformin-induced cytotoxicity in tumor cells.

Keywords: Metformin, p53, Apoptosis, Reactive oxygen species, DEC1

Background

The biguanide metformin is a first-line oral anti-hyperglycemic agent prescribed to nearly all newly diagnosed type II diabetes mellitus patients. Metformin also appears to have clinical benefits in other diseases, including diabetic nephropathy, stage III chronic kidney disease, and the cardiovascular complications associated with diabetes, such as cardiac hypertrophy and myocardial infarction [1, 2]. Although metformin has been used in Europe since 1957, the precise molecular mechanisms by which it mitigates diabetes are sill not fully understood. Results from an increasing number of studies suggest metformin works in the liver. Metformin enters liver cells primarily via organic cation transporter-1 and then suppresses mitochondrial complex I, which leads to a decrease in ATP levels and a rise in AMP levels [3]. The resultant change in the AMP/ATP ratio leads to activation of AMP-activated protein kinase (AMPK), which suppresses fatty acid synthesis and gluconeogenesis, and exerts insulin sensitizing effects [4].

Several studies indicate that metformin also exerts protective effects against inflammation, age-related pathologies, and cancer [2, 5–8]. Retrospective and prospective evidence suggests taking metformin is related to a decline in the incidences of various cancers, including

* Correspondence: 02241@ndmctsgh.edu.tw; shihming@ndmctsgh.edu.tw
[2]Division of Hematology/Oncology, Department of Medicine, Tri-Service General Hospital, National Defense Medical Center, Taipei City 114, Taiwan, Republic of China
[1]Department of Biochemistry, National Defense Medical Center, Taipei City 114, Taiwan, Republic of China

hepatocellular carcinoma, pancreatic cancer, and colon cancer in diabetic patients [2, 7–10]. At present, there are at least 3860 articles listed in PubMed that are related to the study of metformin in cancer. Consequently, there are large amounts of both in vitro and in vivo data on the antitumor effects of metformin. Metformin is able to not only reduce insulin but also inhibit the mammalian target of rapamycin (mTOR) signaling pathway, which makes it an especially appealing target for evaluating metabolism unique to tumor cells, such as the Warburg effect [2, 9]. It has been proposed that the cancer preventive actions of metformin involve four components: 1) cancer stems cells, 2) microRNAs (miRs), 3) epithelial-to-mesenchymal transition (EMT), and 4) cellular senescence [9, 11, 12]. But as with diabetes, details of the mechanisms by which metformin acts against cancer remain unclear.

p53 is a well-known tumor suppressor gene that plays a vital role in about 50% of human cancers [13, 14]. At the premalignant tumor stage, senescence can be triggered normally by stressors such as DNA damage, oncogenes, and oxidative damage. In response to such stresses, p53 is activated and induces transcription of a variety of target genes to cause cells change their phenotypes from DNA repair to apoptosis and senescence [14, 15]. It appears, for example, that p53 transcriptional regulation of components of both the extrinsic (via a caspase cascade) and intrinsic (via the mitochondria) pathways serves as an apoptosis inducer [16, 17]. Moreover, p53 is also able to promote apoptosis through transcriptional induction of redox-related genes to generate reactive oxygen species (ROS), which in turn cause oxidative degradation of mitochondrial components and cell death [16, 18, 19]. Notably, metformin reduces the abundance of p53 in cases of hepatosteatosis, but enhances p53 stability via USP7 in esophageal cancer [20, 21]. Consequently, there is a need to confirm the availability and function of p53 in cancers treated with metformin in our working system. In the present study, therefore, we examined the cytotoxic effects of metformin in two cancer cell lines, clarifying its effects on apoptosis, ROS generation, mitochondrial function, differentiated embryo chondrocyte 1 (DEC1) expression, and p53 protein stability. Our findings provide new information for the potential reposition of metformin in the treatment of cancer.

Methods
Cell culture and reagents
HeLa cells were cultivated in Dulbecco's modified Eagle's medium (DMEM) supplemented with 10% fetal bovine serum (FBS) and 1% penicillin-streptomycin (Invitrogen, MA, USA). ZR-75-1 breast cancer cells were cultivated in Roswell Park Memorial Institute (RPMI) 1640 medium supplemented with 10% FBS and 1% penicillin-streptomycin

(Invitrogen). Actinomycin D (Act D), cycloheximide (CHX), 2′,7-dichlorofluorescein diacetate (DCFH-DA), hydrogen peroxide (H_2O_2), metformin, MG132, N-acetyl cysteine (NAC), propidium iodide (PI), and thiazolyl blue tetrazlium bromide (MTT) were obtained from Sigma Aldrich (MO, USA). Pifithrin-α and Z-VAD-FMK was from Enzo (CA, USA).

Cell survival analysis
Cells were seeded into 24-well culture plates and incubated for 1 day, after which they were exposed to different concentrations of metformin in fresh DMEM or RPMI 1640 for the indicated periods of time. After adding MTT solution (0.5 mg/ml in phosphate buffered saline, PBS) to each well, the cells were incubated for 1 h at 37 °C. Dimethylsulfoxide (DMSO; 200 μl) was then added, and the absorbance at 570 nm and 620 nm each was measured using an ELISA plate reader (Multiskan EX, Thermo, MA, USA). The control group containing cells cultured in medium only was defined as 100% cell survival.

Western blotting
Cells were lysed at 4 °C in lysis buffer (100 mM Tris-HCl of pH 8.0, 150 mM NaCl, 0.1% SDS, and 1% Triton X-100). Proteins in the lysate were separated by SDS-PAGE, transferred onto polyvinylidene difluoride membranes (Millipore, MA, USA), and probed using antibodies against α-actinin (ACTN), cyclin D1, HSP90 α/β, p53(Santa Cruz Biotechnology, CA, USA), caspase 3, cyclin B1, EGFR, p-Histone H3 (phosphorylation at Ser 10, H3P), cleaved poly-ADP-ribose polymerase (cPARP) (Cell Signaling, MA, USA), and DEC1 (Bethyl Laboratory, TX, USA).

Fluorescence-activated cell sorting (FACS), cell cycle profiles, apoptosis, and ROS analysis
Cells were fixed in 70% ice-cold ethanol and stored at −30 °C overnight, after which they were washed with ice-cold PBS supplemented with 1% FBS twice and stained with PI solution (5 μg/ml PI in PBS, 0.5% Triton X-100, and 0.5 μg/ml RNase A) for 30 min at 37 °C in the dark. The cell cycle distribution was then evaluated based on cellular DNA content using FACS.

The incidence of apoptosis (early and late stages) and necrosis was assessed using a fluorescein isothiocyanate (FITC)-Annexin V Apoptosis Detection Kit (BD Biosciences, CA, USA) according to the manufacturer's protocol.

The fluorescent marker DCFH-DA was used to determine intracellular ROS levels. Cells were incubated for 20 h with the indicated concentrations of metformin or with H_2O_2 as a positive control. Living cells were then stained with DCFH-DA (20 μM) for 40 min at 37 °C and harvested. After washed once with PBS, the cells were evaluated using a FACSCalibur flow cytometer and Cell Quest Pro software (BD Biosciences).

Oxygen consumption rate (OCR)

The cellular OCR was detected using an XF24 bioenergetic assay according to the manufacturer's protocol (Seahorse Bioscience, Billerica, MA, USA). In brief, HeLa cells were seeded onto an XF24 microplate in DMEM supplemented with 5% FBS. They were then incubated for 2 days, after which the medium was replaced with sodium bicarbonate-free DMEM supplemented with 1% FBS. The OCR was measured at a steady state, after which the machine sequentially added the standard samples (0.5 μM and 1 μM), oligomycin (1 μM), carbonyl cyanide 4-[trifluoromethoxy] phenylhydrazone (FCCP; 1 μM) and a mixture of rotenone (1 μM) and myxothiazol (1 μM) into the wells to obtain the maximal and non-mitochondrial respiration rates.

Mitochondrial membrane potential analysis

Mitochondrial potential was measured using a BD™ MitoScreen Flow Cytometry Mitochondrial Membrane Potential Detection Kit (BD Biosciences) according to the manufacturer's protocol. Briefly, HeLa cells were incubated for 18 h in a 6-cm culture plate and treated with metformin. The cells were then trypsinized and pelleted by centrifugation at 1000 rpm, after which the cells were resuspended in PBS and counted, which confirmed there were fewer than 1×10^6 cells per ml. The cells were then stained with JC-1 dye (5,5′,6,6′-tetrachloro-1,1′,3,3′-tetraethylbenzimi-dazolylcarbocyanine iodide) for 10–15 min at 37 °C in a CO_2 incubator. The fluorescence intensity of the JC-1 was evaluated flow cytometrically. The excitation wavelength was 488 nm, while emission wavelengths of 530 nm (FL1-H channel) and 580 nm (FL2-H channel) were used to detect the JC-1 monomer and aggregates, respectively.

Plasmids and transfection

DEC1 construct was produced by inserting the full-length polymerase chain reaction (PCR) product into pEGFP vector using the SacI-EcoRI restriction sites. The pSG5.HA.p53 expression vector was constructed as described previously [22]. jetPEI (PolyPlus-transfection, France) reagent was used according to the manufacturer's instructions to deliver the plasmids into cells cultivated in 6-well plates. The total amount of DNA in each well was adjusted to the same level by adding empty vector.

Subcellular cytoplasmic, membrane, and nuclear extract preparations

HeLa cells were cultivated in 100-mm culture dishes and incubated under the indicated conditions. Cytoplasmic, membrane and nuclear extracts were separated using a Subcellular Protein Fractionation Kit for Cultured Cells according to the manufacturer's protocol (Thermo Fisher Scientific, MA, USA). For the cytoplasmic fraction, cells were lysed in Cytoplasmic Extraction buffer (CEB) at 4 °C, after which the cytoplasmic extract (supernatant) was acquired by centrifugation ($14,000 \times g$, 15 min, 4 °C). For the membrane fraction, CEB-treated pellets were lysed in Membrane Extraction buffer (MEB) at 4 °C, and the membrane extract (supernatant) was acquired by centrifugation ($14,000 \times g$, 15 min, 4 °C). For the nuclear fraction, MEB-treated pellets were lysed in Nuclear Extraction buffer at 4 °C, and nuclear extract (supernatant) was acquired by centrifugation ($14,000 \times g$, 15 min, 4 °C).

Fluorescence microscopy

HeLa cells in 6-well culture plates were cultivated in DMEM supplemented with 10% FBS and 1% penicillin-streptomycin. After transfection with pEGFP.-DEC1 for 5 h, a fluorescence microscope (Model DMURE2, Leica, Wetzlar, Germany) was used to observe cells expressing the encoded proteins, and Image-Pro®Plus software (Media-cybernetics, MD, USA) was utilized to process the images, as previously described [23].

Reverse transcription-polymerase chain reaction (RT-PCR)

Total RNA was obtained using the TRIzol (Thermo Fisher Scientific) reagent according to the manufacturer's protocol, after which 1 μg of the total RNA was reverse transcribed using MMLV reverse transcriptase (Epicentre Biotechnologies, WI, USA) for 60 min at 37 °C. A Veriti Thermal Cycler (Applied Biosystems, CA, USA) was utilized to run the PCR reactions. The PCR primers used were as follows: for GAPDH, 5′-CTTC ATTGACCTCAACTAC-3′ (forward) and 5′-GCCA TCCACAGTCTTCTG-3′ (reverse); for p53, 5′ -GATG AAGCTCCCAGAATGCCAGAG-3′ (reverse) and 5′ -GAGTTCCAAGGCCTCATTCAGCTC-3′ (reverse).

DEC-1 mRNA interference

DEC-1- and LUC-shRNA-containing lentiviral vectors were purchased from the National RNAi Core Facility (Academia Sinica, Taiwan, ROC). HeLa cells were infected with the indicated retroviruses or lentiviruses in selection medium containing 2 mg/ml polybrene. Forty-eight hours after infection, cells were treated with 8 mg/ml puromycin to select for a pool of puromycin-resistant clones. The silencing efficacy was verified by Western blot assay.

Statistical analysis

Student's t-test was used to compare the difference of apoptotic stages and cell viability by indicted agents. Values of $P < 0.05$ were considered significant.

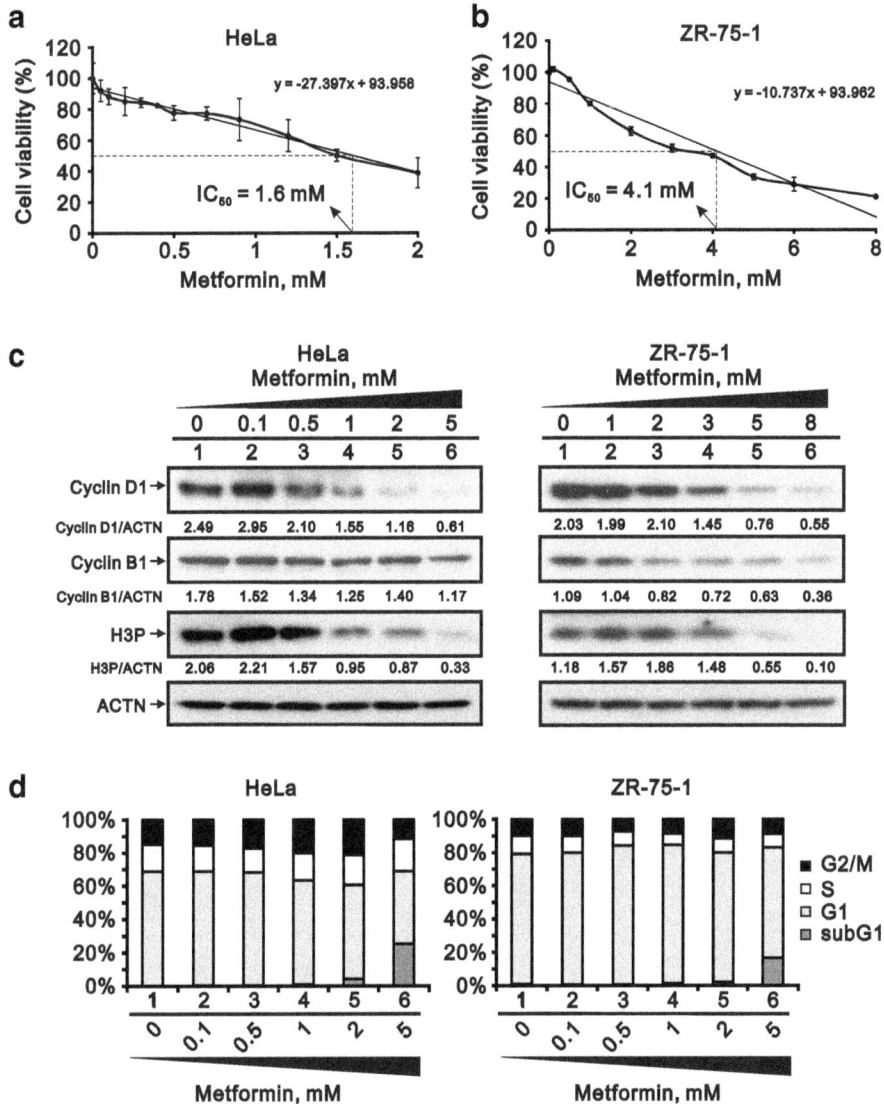

Fig. 1 Cytotoxicity of metformin in HeLa and ZR-75-1 cells. **a** and **b** HeLa cells (**a**) and ZR-75-1 (**b**) cells were treated with the indicated concentration of metformin for 35 h and 70 h, respectively. Cell viability was measured using the MTT method. **c** HeLa and ZR-75-1 cells were incubated with indicated concentration of metformin for 20 h and 25 h, respectively. Cell lysates were subjected to western blot analysis using antibodies against cyclin D1, cyclin B1 and H3P. ACTN was the protein loading control. The protein levels of cyclin D1, cyclin B1 and H3P after normalization with the loading control protein ACTN are presented as fold change. **d** HeLa and ZR-75-1 cells were incubated with the indicated concentration of metformin for 30 h and 57 h, respectively. The cells were then subjected to flow cytometric cell cycle profile analysis. The results are representative of three independent experiments

Results

Metformin reduces cancer cell viability

We found that metformin reduced cell viability in the HeLa cervical carcinoma and ZR-75-1 breast cancer cell lines, exhibiting IC50s of 1.6 mM and 4.1 mM, respectively (Fig. 1a and b). We also observed that three proteins associated with cell cycle progression, cyclin D1 (G1 phase), cyclin B1 (G2 phase) and H3P (M phase), were dose-dependently suppressed by metformin (Fig. 1c). The cell cycle profiles in both cell lines showed that the subG1 population was dose-dependently increased by metformin while the G1 population was reduced (Fig. 1d). Thus cell cycle progression appears to be suppressed by metformin.

Metformin induces apoptosis in HeLa cells

Using FITC labeled Annexin V with PI in HeLa cells, we verified that metformin increases the incidence of apoptosis at both the early and late stages and necrosis (Fig. 2a and b). NAC failed to rescue the late apoptosis and necrosis, whereas it increased the percentage of early apoptosis.

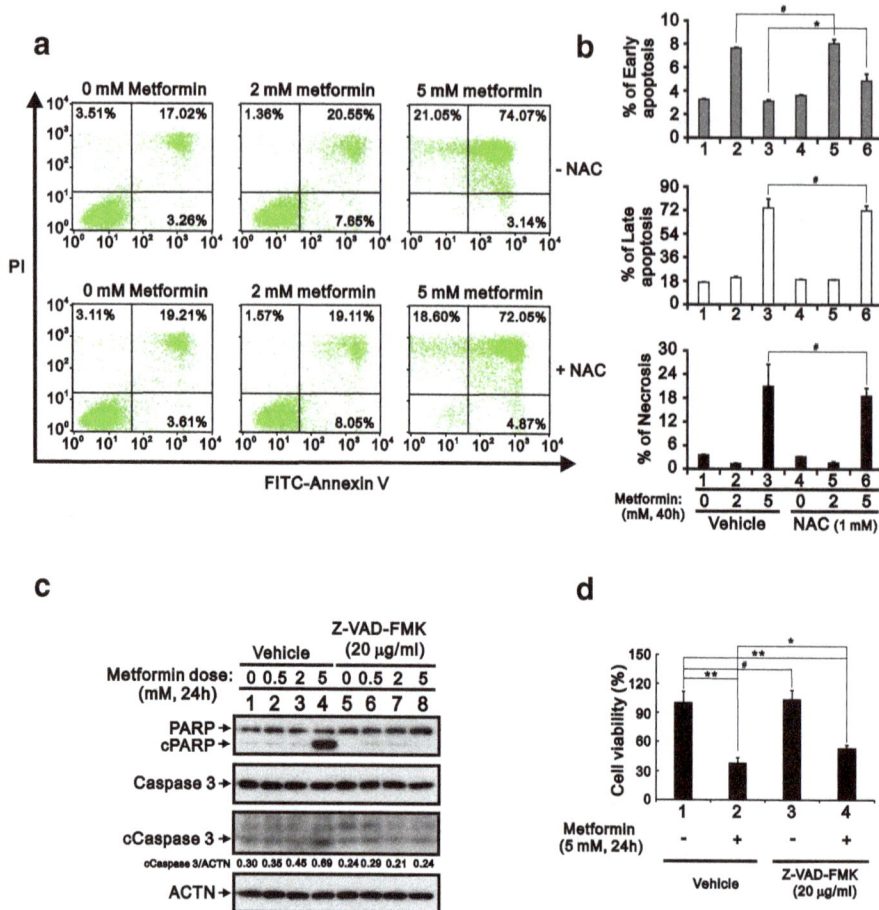

Fig. 2 Metformin-induced apoptosis in HeLa cells. **a** HeLa cells (8×10^4 cells) were incubated with the indicated concentration of metformin for 40 h, after which cell death, apoptosis or necrosis were quantified using FITC-Annexin V and PI and flow cytometry. **b** Quantitative analysis of percentage of indicated stages is presented as the mean ± S.D. of at least three independent experiments; # $p > 0.05$ and * $p < 0.05$ (Student's t-test). **c** HeLa cells were incubated with the indicated concentration of metformin and 20 µg/ml Z-VAD-FMK for 24 h. Cell lysates were then subjected to western blotting with antibodies against PARP and caspase 3. ACTN was the loading control. The protein levels of cleaved Caspase 3 (cCaspase 3) after normalization with the loading control protein ACTN are presented as fold change. **d** HeLa cells (5×10^4 cells) were treated with vehicle (DMSO), 5 mM metformin, 20 µg/ml Z-VAD-FMK, or 5 mM metformin plus 20 µg/ml Z-VAD-FMK for 24 h. Quantitative analysis of cell viability is presented as the mean ± S.D. of at least three independent experiments; # $p > 0.05$, * $p < 0.05$, and ** $p < 0.01$ (Student's t-test)

Consistent with that finding, western blot analysis of lysates from metformin-treated HeLa cell lysates revealed that levels of cPARP were increased in the metformin-treated cells (Fig. 2c). In addition, using the general caspase inhibitor Z-VAD-FMK, we found that metformin induced cleavage of PARP and caspase 3 and that approximately 40% of metformin-induced cell death was significantly rescued by Z-VAD-FMK (Fig. 2c and d). Taken together, these results suggest apoptosis may be a main cause of the cell death induced by metformin.

Metformin promotes cytotoxic ROS generation unrelated to apoptosis

We also used flow cytometry with DCFH-DA to examine the effect of metformin on intracellular ROS levels in HeLa cells. The results summarized in Fig. 3a show that with increases in the metformin concentration, ROS levels were obviously elevated relative the increases elicited by H_2O_2, which served as a positive control. Although ROS reportedly promote apoptosis [24], we discovered that the antioxidant NAC failed to prevent cPARP cleavage (Fig. 3b), but nevertheless partially suppressed metformin-induced cell death (Fig. 3c). Figs. 2 and 3 suggests ROS may contribute to metformin-induced cytotoxicity, though not via an apoptosis pathway.

Alternatively, cellular ROS production could lead to disruption of mitochondrial respiration and/or collapse of the mitochondrial membrane potential [25, 26]. Metformin not only lowers blood glucose but also suppresses complex-I in the electric transport

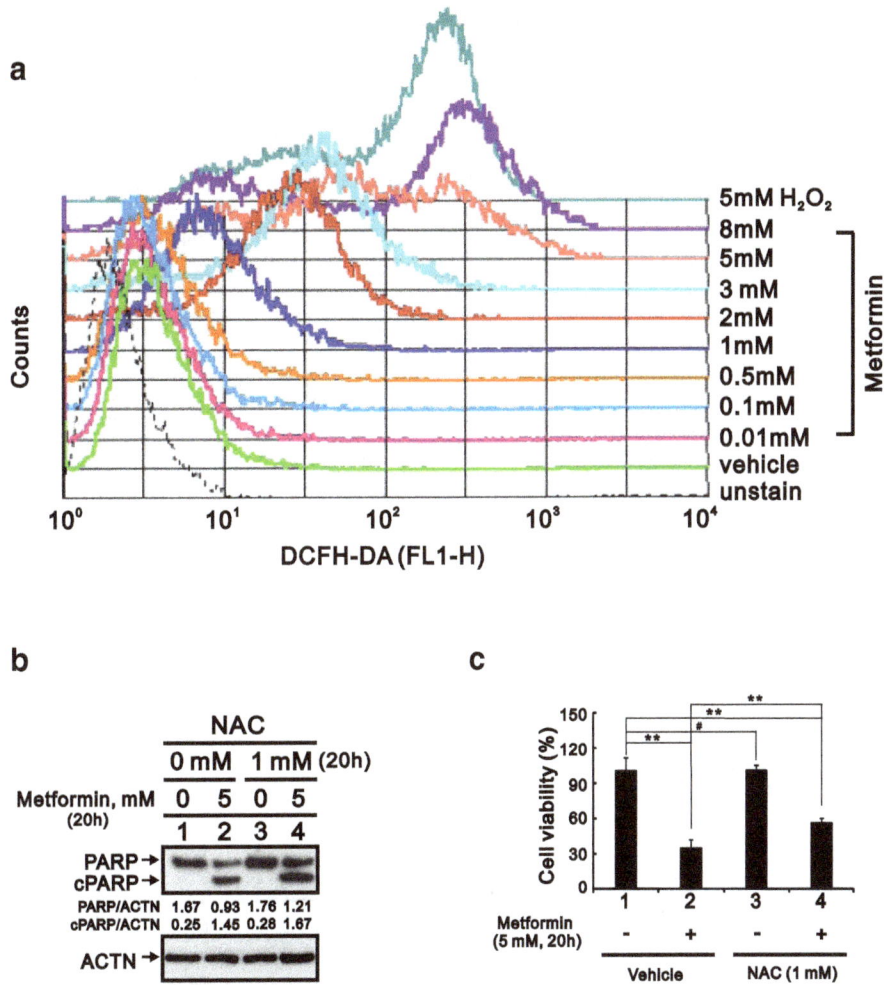

Fig. 3 Induction of ROS generation by metformin in HeLa cells. **a** HeLa cells were incubated for 20 h with various concentrations of metformin, after which the live cells was stained with 10 μM DCFH-DA for 40 min at 37 °C and assayed using a flow cytometer. **b** HeLa cells were incubated for 20 h with 5 mM metformin and/or 1 mM NAC. The cell lysates were then subjected to western blotting with an antibody against PARP. ACTN was the loading control. The protein levels of PARP and cleaved PARP (cPARP) after normalization with the loading control protein ACTN are presented as fold change. **c** HeLa cells (5×10^4 cells) were incubated for 20 h with vehicle (DMSO), 5 mM metformin, 1 mM NAC, or 5 mM metformin plus 1 mM NAC. Quantitative analysis of cell viability is presented as the mean ± S.D. of at least three independent experiments; # $p > 0.05$, * $p < 0.05$, and ** $p < 0.01$ (Student's t-test)

chain [27, 28]. For that reason, we measured the OCR and found that metformin decreased basal respiration, maximal respiratory capacity, and ATP-linked respiration in HeLa cells (Fig. 4a). To further examine the effect of metformin on mitochondrial membrane integrity, we used JC-1 staining to monitor the mitochondrial membrane potential. The results showed the metformin elicited increases in FL1-H (JC-1 monomers) and decreases in FL2-H (JC-1 aggregates) (Fig. 4b and c), which is indicative of depolarization of the mitochondrial membrane. This suggests metformin-induced ROS production in HeLa cells may reflect disruption of mitochondrial function.

The functional role of DEC1 in metformin-induced apoptosis

There is a link between the transcription factor DEC1 and apoptosis [29]. We observed that metformin reduced DEC1 levels and increased expression of cPARP proteins (Figs. 5a and 2b), which prompted us to evaluate DEC1's involvement in metformin-induced apoptosis. We initially determined the localization of DEC1 by separately examining the cytoplasmic, membrane, and nuclear fractions of HeLa cells. HSP90α/β, EGFR and PARP served as markers of cytoplasm, cell membrane and nuclei, respectively. We found that DEC1 was present mainly in the nucleus, and that MG132, a proteasome inhibitor, had little or no effect of DEC1 levels.

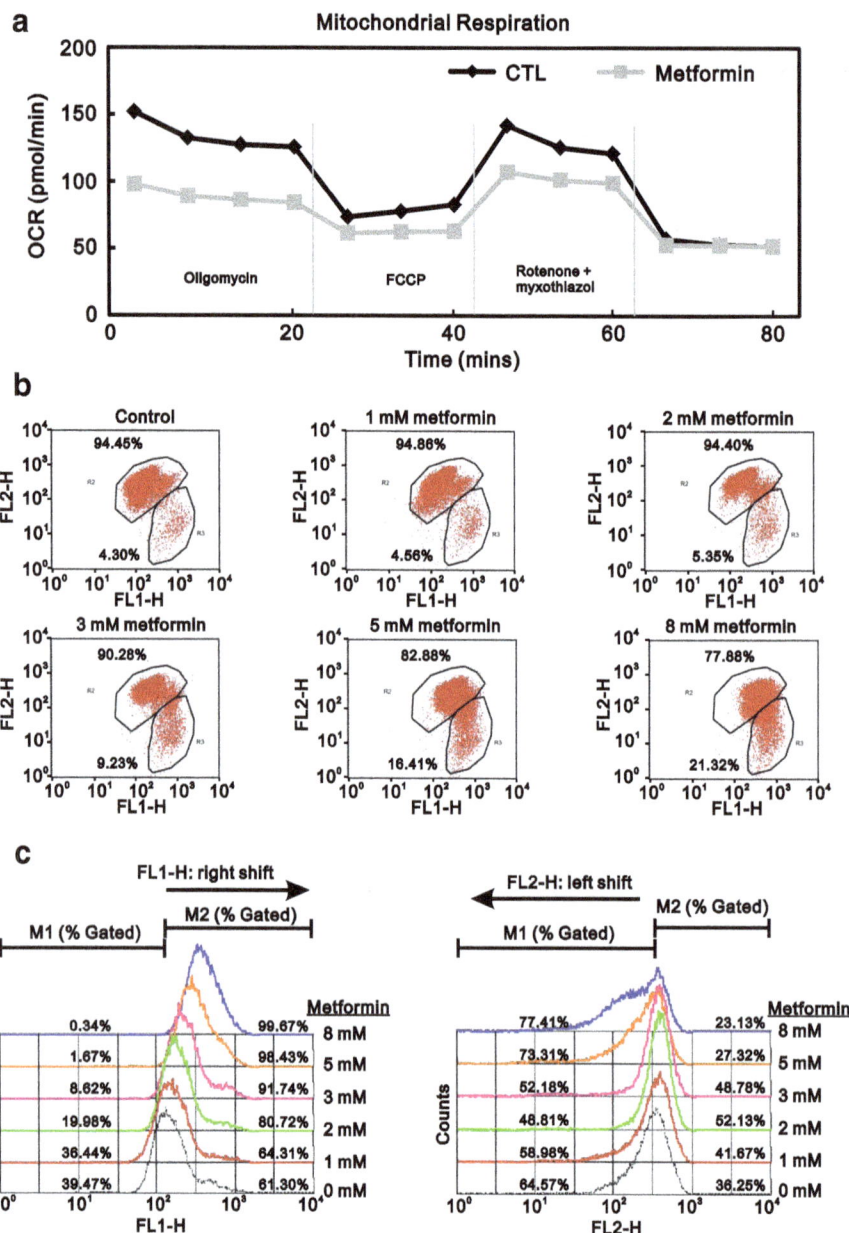

Fig. 4 Effect of metformin on mitochondrial function in HeLa cells. **a** HeLa cells were incubated for 20 h with 5 mM metformin, after which the cellular OCR was measured in XF24 bioenergetic assays. **b** HeLa cells were incubated for 16 h with the indicated concentrations of metformin, after which JC-1 staining was analyzed using flow cytometry. **c** Changes in FL1-H and FL2-H were further evaluated using a FACS Calibur flow cytometer. The results are representative of two independent experiments

By contrast, metformin induced DEC1 degradation in all three fractions (Fig. 5b). Ectopic overexpression of pEGFP-DEC1 in HeLa cells confirmed that DEC1 localized primarily in the nucleus (Fig. 5c). To determine the relationship between DEC1 and apoptosis, HeLa cells were treated with metformin alone or in combination with ectopic DEC1 expression. Subsequent western blot analysis showed that ectopic DEC1 expression partially suppressed metformin-induced apoptosis (Fig. 5d), suggesting metformin may

trigger apoptosis through downregulation of DEC1 expression.

Involvement of p53 in metformin-induced apoptosis

Early studies indicate *DEC1* gene is a target gene of p53 [30]. We found that metformin dose-dependently decreased levels of both p53 and DEC1 while making cells apoptotic. Overexpression of p53 partially rescued DEC1 levels and decreased the extent of apoptosis (Fig. 6a). These results suggest metformin may induce apoptosis

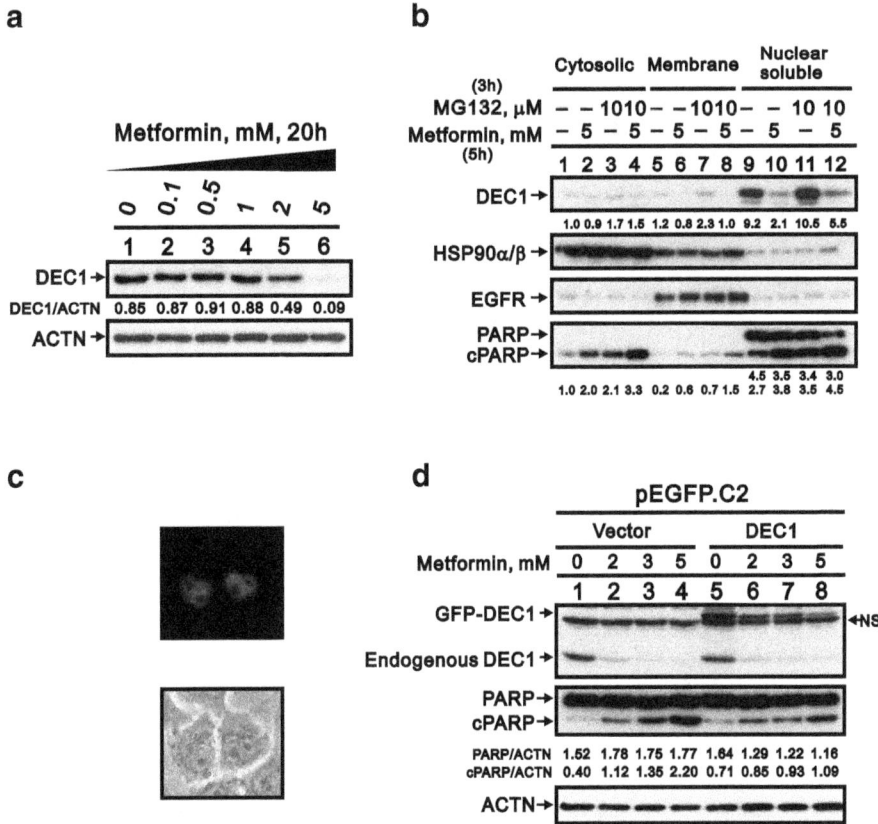

Fig. 5 Function of DEC1 in metformin-induced apoptosis in HeLa cells. **a** HeLa cells were incubated for 20 h with the indicated concentrations of metformin, after which the cell lysates were subjected to western blotting with an antibody against DEC1. ACTN was the loading control. The protein levels of DEC1 after normalization with the loading control protein ACTN are presented as fold change. **b** HeLa cells were incubated with 5 mM metformin with and without 10 μM MG132 for the indicated times. They were then lysed; divided into cytoplasmic, membrane, and nuclear fractions; and subjected to western blotting with antibodies against DEC1, HSP90α/β (cytoplasmic fraction), EGFR (membrane fraction) and PARP (intact: nuclear fraction; cleaved: nuclear and cytoplasmic fractions). The protein levels of cleaved DEC1, PARP, and cPARP are presented as fold change. **c** HeLa cells were transiently transfected with 2 μg pEGFP.DEC1 for 5 h and then were observed with fluorescence-microscopy. **d** HeLa cells were transiently transfected with 2 μg of pEGFP vector and pEGFP.DEC1 and incubated for 13 h with 5 mM metformin. The cell lysates were subjected to western blotting with antibodies against DEC1 and PARP. ACTN was the loading control. The protein levels of PARP and cleaved PARP (cPARP) after normalization with the loading control protein ACTN are presented as fold change. The results are representative of three independent experiments

in HeLa cells by acting on p53 upstream of DEC1. To better understand the mechanism underlying the downregulation of p53 by metformin, we first used MG132 to determine whether metformin induces degradation of p53 via a proteasome-dependent pathway. We observed that p53 degradation was mediated through the proteasomes, but MG132 failed to fully suppress p53 degradation elicited by metformin (Fig. 6b). Subsequent application of RNA and protein synthesis inhibitors (actinomycin D and cycloheximide, respectively) revealed no effect of metformin on p53 expression (Fig. 6c, compare lanes 1–4). Moreover, actinomycin D appeared to increased p53 levels and to exert a protective effect against metformin-induced p53 degradation (Fig. 6d, compare lanes 5–8).

Treatment with cycloheximide for 12 h elicited no further effect on p53 levels, most likely because p53 has a short half-life in HeLa cells (Fig. 6d, compare lanes 9–12) [31]. To overcome the time-window limitation for cycloheximide treatment, we re-examined the timing of metformin treatment and the stability of endogenous p53. Metformin-induced p53 degradation was first detected after around 2 h of treatment (Fig. 6e), but it was difficult to detect p53 in HeLa cells after only 10 min of cycloheximide treatment (50 μg/ml) (Fig. 6f), which is consistent with our earlier study [31]. We therefore decreased the cycloheximide concentration from 50 μg/ml to 50 ng/ml and increased the concentration of metformin from 5 to 10 mM. Under those conditions, metformin accelerated the degradation of p53 in the presence of cycloheximide. It thus appears that metformin reduces p53 levels in HeLa cells by reducing the protein's stability (Fig. 6g).

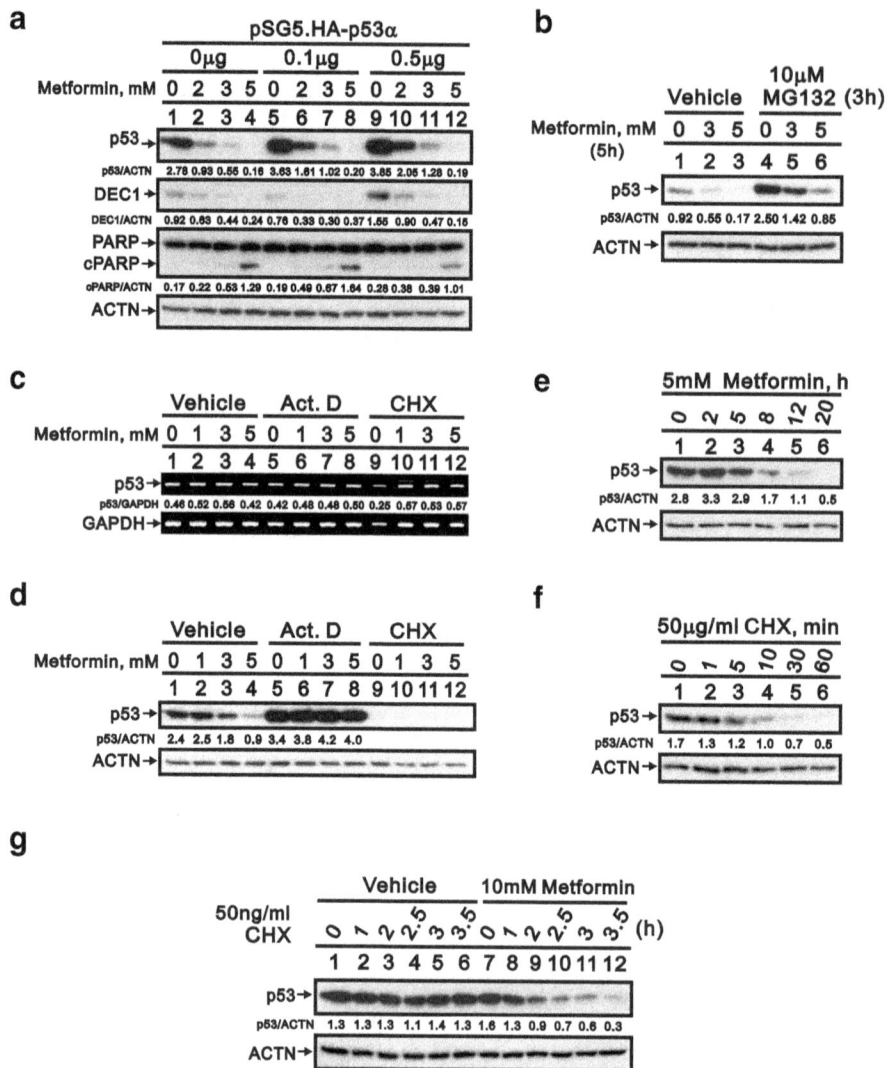

Fig. 6 Transcriptional and translational regulation of p53 in HeLa cells. **a** HeLa cells were transiently transfected with 0.5 µg of pSG5.HA vector or the indicated amount of pSG5.HA.p53 and incubated for 12 h with 5 mM metformin. The cell lysates were subjected to western blotting with antibodies against p53, DEC1, and PARP. ACTN was the loading control. The protein levels of p53, DEC1, and cPARP after normalization with the loading control protein ACTN are presented as fold change. **b** HeLa cells were incubated for 5 h with the indicated concentrations of metformin with or without 10 µM MG132, after which the cell lysates were subjected to western blotting with an antibody against p53. ACTN was the loading control. The protein levels of p53 after normalization with the loading control protein ACTN are presented as fold change. **c** and **d** HeLa cells were incubated for 12 h with the indicated concentrations of metformin with and without 0.1 µM actinomycin D (Act D) or 50 µg/ml cycloheximide (CHX). Levels of p53 mRNA and protein were then assayed in the cell lysates using RT-PCR (**c**) and western blotting (**d**), respectively. GAPDH mRNA was the mRNA loading control; ACTN was the protein loading control. **e** and **f** HeLa cells were incubated with 5 mM metformin (**e**) or 50 µg/ml CHX (**f**) for the indicated times, after which cell lysates were subjected to western blotting with an antibody against p53. **g** HeLa cells were incubated for the indicated times with 10 mM metformin with and without 50 ng/ml CHX. The cell lysates were then subjected to western blotting with an antibody against p53. **d-g** The protein levels of p53 after normalization with the loading control protein ACTN are presented as fold change. The results are representative of three independent experiments

Loss-of-function of p53 and DEC1 for metformin-induced apoptosis

To further verify the contribution of p53 and DEC1 to metformin-induced apoptosis, we applied a small-molecule inhibitor of p53, pifithrin-α, which reportedly inhibits several p53-dependent processes in vitro, including UV-induced expression of cyclin G, p21, and MDM-2 [32]. We also assessed the effect of DEC1 knockdown using a short-hairpin silencing system (Fig. 7). Our results showed that, by itself, pifithrin-α had no apparent effect on PARP cleavage. When combined 10 mM metformin, however, it dramatically increased levels of cPARP and caspase 3 (Fig. 7a). Knocking down DEC1 also increased levels of cPARP (Fig. 7b, compare lanes 9 with 7). In

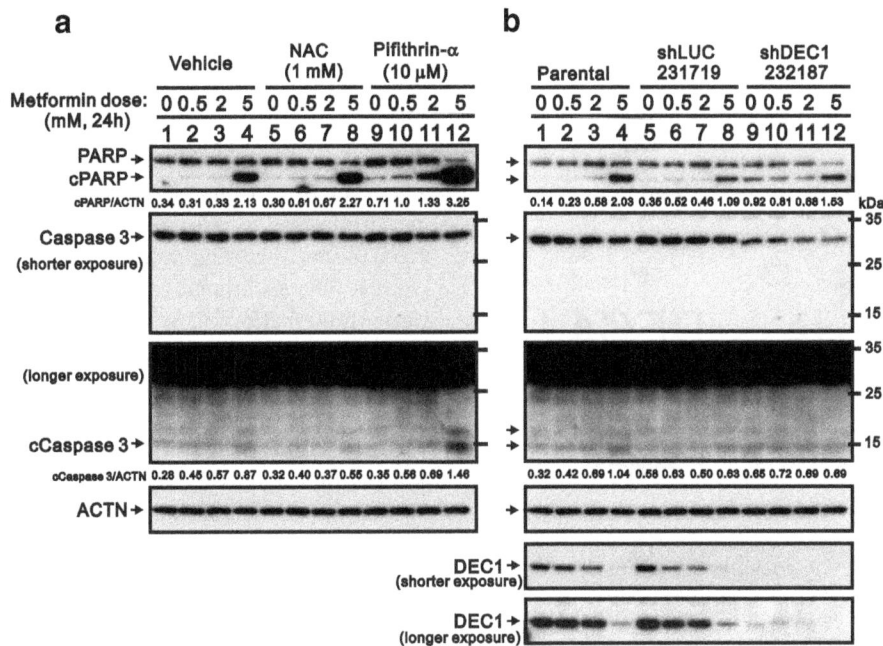

Fig. 7 Verification of p53 and DEC1 into the metformin-induced apoptosis in HeLa cells. **a** HeLa cells were incubated for 24 h with the indicated concentrations of metformin, 1 mM NAC, and 10 µM pifithrin-α. The cell lysates were then subjected to western blotting with antibodies against PARP and caspase 3. ACTN was the loading control. **b** Following DEC1 knockdown in HeLa cells, the cells were incubated for 24 h with the indicated concentration of metformin. The cell lysates were then subjected to western blotting with antibodies against PARP and Caspase 3. ACTN was the loading control and DEC1 was the silencing efficiency of shDEC1. The protein levels of cPARP and cCaspase 3 after normalization with the loading control protein ACTN are presented as fold change. The results are representative of three independent experiments

contrast to previously reported effects [33, 34], we observed that pifithrin-α induced apoptosis in HeLa cells, which is consistent with its promotion of p53-mediated apoptosis in JB6 cells [35].

Discussion

Among the three biguanides (buformin, metformin. and phenformin) developed for the treatment of diabetes, increased cardiac mortality and risk of lactic acidosis led to withdrawal of buformin and phenformin in the early 1970s [2]. On the other hand, the lower risk and beneficial characteristics of metformin has enabled it to become one of the most popular medications in the world. Moreover, higher doses of biguanides may have direct antitumor effects [36]. Our findings suggest the antitumor effects of high-dose metformin are mediated through multiple pathways involving apoptosis, ROS generation, and downregulation of p53-related proteins. We propose that metformin may directly decrease p53 abundance in sensitive cells, which in turn leads to downregulation of p53 target genes (e.g., *DEC1*) and to induction of apoptosis. Metformin also induces ROS generation by suppressing the mitochondrial respiration rate and membrane potential. All of the abovementioned effects contribute to metformin-induced cell death (Fig. 8), and several clinical trials have shown promising results

with metformin against various cancers, including breast cancer, gastric cancer, and pancreatic ductal adenocarcinoma, among others [37–39]. It is therefore crucial to further realize the molecular mechanisms of biguanides, which have the potential to contribute to the development in therapies for not only diabetes but also cancer.

Autophagy and apoptosis are two major cell death pathways [40]. One study showed that suppressing autophagy using chloroquine enhanced palmitic acid-induced apoptosis while increasing ROS generation [41]. However, our findings showed that NAC, a well-known ROS scavenger failed to inhibit the metformin-induced apoptosis and the cleavage of PARP. These results suggest that in our study apoptosis may be induced through suppression of autophagy, not through ROS generation. The precise relationship between autophagy and apoptosis remains to be further elucidated in HeLa cells. Several studies have demonstrated that metformin decreases ROS production through reduction of NAD (P) H oxidase activity [42, 43]. In addition to the inhibition of NAD (P) H oxidase activity, metformin may increase the ROS generation through other mechanisms in various cell types [44–46]. One study showed that there is complex interplay among processes regulating ROS, autophagy and apoptosis in response to expression of p53-inducible glycolysis and apoptosis regulator (TIGAR), which functions as a fructose

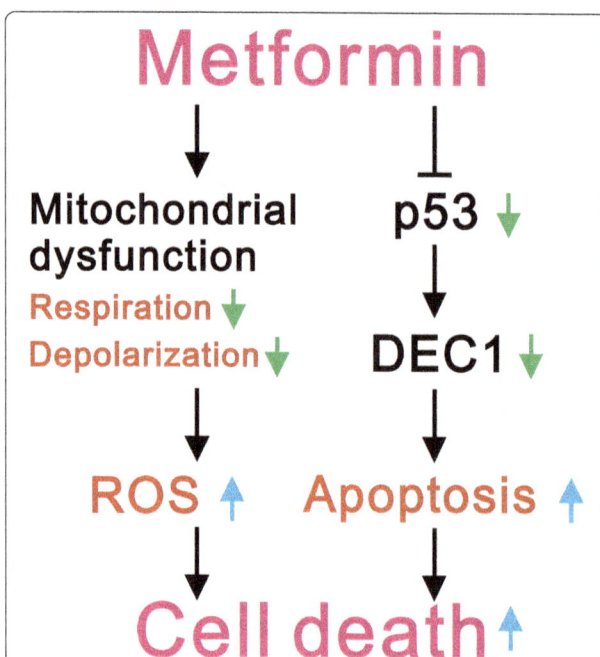

Fig. 8 Proposed working mechanisms of metformin in cancer cells. Metformin may directly decrease p53 in sensitive cells, which would in turn downregulate expression of its target gene, *DEC1*, leading to apoptosis. Metformin not only induces cellular apoptosis but also induces ROS generation through repression of mitochondrial respiration and membrane potential to kill cancer cells. Thus, apoptosis, mitochondrial dysfunction, and ROS generation all contribute to the induction of HeLa cell death by metformin

2,6-bisphosphatase [15]. TIGAR promotes activity in the pentose phosphate pathway and helps lower intracellular ROS. In the present study, metformin-mediated reduction in endogenous p53 may have led to ROS generation via downregulation of TIGAR expression.

The transcription factor p53 is a known tumor suppressor and is stabilized and activated for cellular responses to a variety of stresses, including hypoxia, DNA damage, and oncogene expression. These cellular responses include cell cycle arrest, apoptosis, senescence, and so on [13, 14]. It is commonplace for p53 activity and the activities of other tumor suppressors to be inhibited within tumors so as to inactivate cell-death pathways. Because HeLa cells are infected by human papillomavirus (HPV), they are able to express oncoprotein E6 to maintain endogenous wild-type p53 at low levels for human cervical tumorigenesis [22, 47]. Our findings in the present study suggest that as described in our earlier DXR work [48], metformin modulates levels of endogenous p53 to trigger various cellular activities altering expression of p53 target genes, including p21 (cell cycle inhibitor) [49], Bax (apoptosis inducer) [50], DNA damage regulated autophagy modulator 1 (autophagy inducer) [51], DEC1 (senescence inducer) [30], and survivin (apoptosis inhibitor) [52]. Given that p53 is an

apoptosis inducer, the loss of survivin's anti-apoptosis effect may explain why metformin, alone or in combination with pifithrin-α, induces apoptosis despite the reduction in p53 [52, 53]. However, further experiments will be needed to determine the contributions made by p53 and its target genes to the various dose-dependent effects of metformin. Several studies have shown that metformin may increase or decrease endogenous p53 via mechanisms involving miR-34a, USP7, and mitophagy [20, 21, 54]. Additional experiments will be required to clarify how metformin selectively mediates increases or decreases in the levels of p53.

It was recently reported that metformin reduces the risk of cervical cancer [55]. Although the mechanisms underlying the reduced risk remain to be explored, the authors of that study suggest the reduction in risk reflects metformin's ability to reduce inflammation via inhibition of nuclear factor κB and STAT3 pathways. Taken together, that work and our present findings suggest metformin has the potential to suppress the proliferation and growth of cervical cancer cells and may be a useful addition to the currently used methods for the prevention and treatment of cervical cancer.

Conclusions

In the present study, we demonstrated that metformin has several actions that suppress cell survival, including induction of apoptosis and ROS generation. The regulatory mechanisms of metformin may reflect its ability to reduce the stability, and thus the abundance, of endogenous wild-type p53. This would be expected to alter expression of many p53-dependent target genes responsible for various cell death pathways. Our work fully supports the reposition of metformin for cancer treatment or combination therapy with currently used cancer therapeutic agents.

Abbreviations
Act D: Actinomycin D; ACTN: α-actinin; AMPK: AMP-activated protein kinase; CEB: cytoplasmic extraction buffer; CHX: cycloheximide; cPARP: cleaved poly-ADP-ribose polymerase; DCFH-DA: 2′,7-dichlorofluorescein diacetate; DEC1: Differentiated Embryo Chondrocyte 1; DMEM: Dulbecco's modified Eagle's medium; EMT: epithelial-to-mesenchymal transition; FACS: fluorescence- activated cell sorting; FBS: fetal bovine serum; FCCP: carbonyl cyanide 4-[trifluoromethoxy] phenylhydrazone; FITC: fluorescein isothiocyanate; H₂O₂: hydrogen peroxide; H3P: phosphorylation at Ser 10 Histone H3; JC-1: 5,5′,6,6′-tetrachloro-1,1′,3,3′-tetraethylbenzimidazolylcarbocyanine iodide; MEB: membrane extraction buffer; miRs: microRNAs; MTT: thiazolyl blue tetrazlium bromide; NAC: N-acetyl cysteine; NEB: nuclear extraction buffer; OCR: oxygen consumption rate; OCT1: organic cation transporter-1; HPV: human papillomavirus; PBS: phosphate buffered saline; PI: propidium iodide; ROS: reactive oxygen species; RPMI: Roswell Park Memorial Institute; RT-PCR: reverse transcription-polymerase chain reaction; TIGAR: TP53-inducible glycolysis and apoptosis regulator

Acknowledgements
We gratefully acknowledge all of the funding sources.

Funding
This work was supported by grants from the Ministry of National Defense-Medical Affairs Bureau [MAB–106–20 to S-M HUANG], the Ministry of Science

and Technology [MOST 105–2314–B–016–047 to C-L HO], and Teh-Tzer Study Group for Human Medical Research Foundation [A106–1017 to C-L HO], Taiwan, ROC.

Authors' contributions
SMHL conceived and, analyzed data and wrote the paper. STL and YLC carried out experiments and analyzed data. CLH and SMH conceived of the study, and participated in its design and coordination and helped to draft the manuscript. All authors read and approved the final manuscript.

Competing interests
The authors declare that they have no competing interests.

References
1. American Diabetes Association. Standards of medical care in diabetes--2014. Diabetes Care. 2014;37(Suppl 1):S14–80.
2. Foretz M, Guigas B, Bertrand L, Pollak M, Viollet B. Metformin: from mechanisms of action to therapies. Cell Metab. 2014;20:953–66.
3. Gong L, Goswami S, Giacomini KM, Altman RB, Klein TE. Metformin pathways: pharmacokinetics and pharmacodynamics. Pharmacogenet Genomics. 2012;22:820–7.
4. Viollet B, Guigas B, Sanz Garcia N, Leclerc J, Foretz M, Andreelli F. Cellular and molecular mechanisms of metformin: an overview. Clin Sci (Lond). 2012;122:253–70.
5. Novelle MG, Ali A, Dieguez C, Bernier M, de Cabo R. Metformin. A Hopeful Promise in Aging Research. CSH Perspect Med. 2016;6:a025932.
6. Scheen AJ, Esser N, Paquot N. Antidiabetic agents. Potential anti-inflammatory activity beyond glucose control. Diabetes Metab. 2015;41:183–94.
7. Kasznicki J, Sliwinska A, Drzewoski J. Metformin in cancer prevention and therapy. Ann Transl Med. 2014;2:57.
8. Rizos CV, Elisaf MS. Metformin and cancer. Eur J Pharmacol. 2013;705:96–108.
9. Del Barco S, Vazquez-Martin A, Cufi S, Oliveras-Ferraros C, Bosch-Barrera J, Joven J, Martin-Castillo B, Menendez JA. Metformin: multi-faceted protection against cancer. Oncotarget. 2011;2:896–917.
10. Jalving M, Gietema JA, Lefrandt JD, de Jong S, Reyners AK, Gans RO, de Vries EG. Metformin: taking away the candy for cancer? Eur J Cancer. 2010;46:2369–80.
11. Bao B, Azmi AS, Ali S, Zaiem F, Sarkar FH. Metformin may function as anti-cancer agent via targeting cancer stem cells: the potential biological significance of tumor-associated miRNAs in breast and pancreatic cancers. Ann Transl Med. 2014;2:59.
12. Barriere G, Tartary M, Rigaud M. Metformin: a rising star to fight the epithelial mesenchymal transition in oncology. Anti Cancer Agents Med Chem. 2013;13:333–40.
13. Bieging KT, Mello SS, Attardi LD. Unravelling mechanisms of p53-mediated tumour suppression. Nat Rev Cancer. 2014;14:359–70.
14. Oren M. Decision making by p53: life, death and cancer. Cell Death Differ. 2003;10:431–42.
15. Bensaad K, Tsuruta A, Selak MA, Vidal MN, Nakano K, Bartrons R, Gottlieb E, Vousden KH. TIGAR, a p53-inducible regulator of glycolysis and apoptosis. Cell. 2006;126:107–20.
16. Haupt S, Berger M, Goldberg Z, Haupt Y. Apoptosis - the p53 network. J Cell Sci. 2003;116:4077–85.
17. Schuler M, Green DR. Mechanisms of p53-dependent apoptosis. Biochem Soc Trans. 2001;29:684–8.
18. Polyak K, Xia Y, Zweier JL, Kinzler KW, Vogelstein B. A model for p53-induced apoptosis. Nature. 1997;389:300–5.
19. Speidel D. Transcription-independent p53 apoptosis: an alternative route to death. Trends Cell Biol. 2010;20:14–24.
20. Song YM, Lee WK, Lee YH, Kang ES, Cha BS, Lee BW. Metformin restores Parkin-mediated Mitophagy, suppressed by cytosolic p53. Int J Mol Sci. 2016;17:122.
21. Xu Y, Lu S. Metformin inhibits esophagus cancer proliferation through upregulation of USP7. Cell Physiol Biochem. 2013;32:1178–86.
22. Huang SM, Schonthal AH, Stallcup MR. Enhancement of p53-dependent gene activation by the transcriptional coactivator Zac1. Oncogene. 2001;20:2134–43.
23. Huang SM, Huang SP, Wang SL, Liu PY. Importin alpha1 is involved in the nuclear localization of Zac1 and the induction of p21WAF1/CIP1 by Zac1. Biochem J. 2007;402:359–66.
24. Mukhopadhyay S, Das DN, Panda PK, Sinha N, Naik PP, Bissoyi A, Pramanik K, Bhutia SK. Autophagy protein Ulk1 promotes mitochondrial apoptosis through reactive oxygen species. Free Radic Biol Med. 2015;89:311–21.
25. Starkov AA. The role of mitochondria in reactive oxygen species metabolism and signaling. Ann N Y Acad Sci. 2008;1147:37–52.
26. Venditti P, Di Stefano L, Di Meo S. Mitochondrial metabolism of reactive oxygen species. Mitochondrion. 2013;13:71–82.
27. Owen MR, Doran E, Halestrap AP. Evidence that metformin exerts its anti-diabetic effects through inhibition of complex 1 of the mitochondrial respiratory chain. Biochem J. 2000;348:607–14.
28. Birsoy K, Possemato R, Lorbeer FK, Bayraktar EC, Thiru P, Yucel B, Wang T, Chen WW, Clish CB, Sabatini DM. Metabolic determinants of cancer cell sensitivity to glucose limitation and biguanides. Nature. 2014;508:108–12.
29. Li Y, Xie M, Yang J, Yang D, Deng R, Wan Y, Yan B. The expression of antiapoptotic protein survivin is transcriptionally upregulated by DEC1 primarily through multiple sp1 binding sites in the proximal promoter. Oncogene. 2006;25:3296–306.
30. Qian Y, Zhang J, Yan B, Chen X. DEC1, a basic helix-loop-helix transcription factor and a novel target gene of the p53 family, mediates p53-dependent premature senescence. J Biol Chem. 2008;283:2896–905.
31. Lu GY, Huang SM, Liu ST, Liu PY, Chou WY, Lin WS. Caffeine induces tumor cytotoxicity via the regulation of alternative splicing in subsets of cancer-associated genes. Int J Biochem Cell Biol. 2014;47:83–92.
32. Komarov PG, Komarova EA, Kondratov RV, Christov-Tselkov K, Coon JS, Chernov MV, Gudkov AV. A chemical inhibitor of p53 that protects mice from the side effects of cancer therapy. Science. 1999;285:1733–7.
33. Zhu X, Yu QS, Cutler RG, Culmsee CW, Holloway HW, Lahiri DK, Mattson MP, Greig NH. Novel p53 inactivators with neuroprotective action: syntheses and pharmacological evaluation of 2-imino-2,3,4,5,6,7-hexahydrobenzothiazole and 2-imino-2,3,4,5,6,7-hexahydrobenzoxazole derivatives. J Med Chem. 2002;45:5090–7.
34. Culmsee C, Zhu X, Yu QS, Chan SL, Camandola S, Guo Z, Greig NH, Mattson MP. A synthetic inhibitor of p53 protects neurons against death induced by ischemic and excitotoxic insults, and amyloid beta-peptide. J Neurochem. 2001;77:220–8.
35. Kaji A, Zhang Y, Nomura M, Bode AM, Ma WY, She QB, Dong Z. Pifithrin-alpha promotes p53-mediated apoptosis in JB6 cells. Mol Carcinog. 2003;37:138–48.
36. Menendez JA, Quirantes-Pine R, Rodriguez-Gallego E, Cufi S, Corominas-Faja B, Cuyas E, Bosch-Barrera J, Martin-Castillo B, Segura-Carretero A, Joven J. Oncobiguanides: Paracelsus' law and nonconventional routes for administering diabetobiguanides for cancer treatment. Oncotarget. 2014;5:2344–8.
37. Sonnenblick A, Agbor-Tarh D, Bradbury I, Di Cosimo S, Azim HA Jr, Fumagalli D, Sarp S, Wolff AC, Andersson M, Kroep J, et al. Impact of diabetes, insulin, and metformin use on the outcome of patients with human epidermal growth factor receptor 2-positive primary breast Cancer: analysis from the ALTTO phase III randomized trial. J Clin Oncol. 2017;35:1421–9.
38. Lee CK, Jung M, Jung I, Heo SJ, Jeong YH, An JY, Kim HI, Cheong JH, Hyung WJ, Noh SH, et al. Cumulative metformin use and its impact on survival in gastric Cancer patients after gastrectomy. Ann Surg. 2016;263:96–102.
39. Amin S, Mhango G, Lin J, Aronson A, Wisnivesky J, Boffetta P, Lucas AL. Metformin improves survival in patients with pancreatic ductal adenocarcinoma and pre-existing diabetes: a propensity score analysis. Am J Gastroenterol. 2016;111:1350–7.
40. Yonekawa T, Thorburn A. Autophagy and cell death. Essays Biochem. 2013;55:105–17.
41. Jiang XS, Chen XM, Wan JM, Gui HB, Ruan XZ, Du XG. Autophagy protects against palmitic acid-induced apoptosis in podocytes in vitro. Sci Rep. 2017;7:42764.
42. Kelly B, Tannahill GM, Murphy MP, O'Neill LA. Metformin inhibits the production of reactive oxygen species from NADH:ubiquinone oxidoreductase to limit induction of interleukin-1beta (IL-1beta) and boosts Interleukin-10 (IL-10) in lipopolysaccharide (LPS)-activated macrophages. J Biol Chem. 2015;290:20348–59.
43. Ouslimani N, Peynet J, Bonnefont-Rousselot D, Therond P, Legrand A, Beaudeux JL. Metformin decreases intracellular production of reactive

oxygen species in aortic endothelial cells. Metabolism. 2005;54:829–34.

44. Wang X, Li R, Zhao X, Yu X, Sun Q. Metformin promotes HaCaT cell apoptosis through generation of reactive oxygen species via Raf-1-ERK1/2-Nrf2 inactivation. Inflammation. 2018;41:948–58.

45. Mogavero A, Maiorana MV, Zanutto S, Varinelli L, Bozzi F, Belfiore A, Volpi CC, Gloghini A, Pierotti MA, Gariboldi M. Metformin transiently inhibits colorectal cancer cell proliferation as a result of either AMPK activation or increased ROS production. Sci Rep. 2017;7:15992.

46. Veleba J, Kopecky J Jr, Janovska P, Kuda O, Horakova O, Malinska H, Kazdova L, Oliyarnyk O, Skop V, Trnovska J, et al. Combined intervention with pioglitazone and n-3 fatty acids in metformin-treated type 2 diabetic patients: improvement of lipid metabolism. Nutr Metab (Lond). 2015;12:52.

47. May P, May E. Twenty years of p53 research: structural and functional aspects of the p53 protein. Oncogene. 1999;18:7621–36.

48. Chang YL, Lee HJ, Liu ST, Lin YS, Chen TC, Hsieh TY, Huang HS, Huang SM. Different roles of p53 in the regulation of DNA damage caused by 1,2-heteroannelated anthraquinones and doxorubicin. Int J Biochem Cell Biol. 2011;43:1720–8.

49. El-Deiry WS, Tokino T, Velculescu VE, Levy DB, Parsons R, Trent JM, Lin D, Mercer WE, Kinzler KW, Vogelstein B. WAF1, a potential mediator of p53 tumor suppression. Cell. 1993;75:817–25.

50. Chipuk JE, Kuwana T, Bouchier-Hayes L, Droin NM, Newmeyer DD, Schuler M, Green DR. Direct activation of Bax by p53 mediates mitochondrial membrane permeabilization and apoptosis. Science. 2004;303:1010–4.

51. Crighton D, Wilkinson S, O'Prey J, Syed N, Smith P, Harrison PR, Gasco M, Garrone O, Crook T, Ryan KM. DRAM, a p53-induced modulator of autophagy, is critical for apoptosis. Cell. 2006;126:121–34.

52. Mirza A, McGuirk M, Hockenberry TN, Wu Q, Ashar H, Black S, Wen SF, Wang L, Kirschmeier P, Bishop WR, et al. Human survivin is negatively regulated by wild-type p53 and participates in p53-dependent apoptotic pathway. Oncogene. 2002;21:2613–22.

53. Altieri DC. Survivin, versatile modulation of cell division and apoptosis in cancer. Oncogene. 2003;22:8581–9.

54. Do MT, Kim HG, Choi JH, Jeong HG. Metformin induces microRNA-34a to downregulate the Sirt1/Pgc-1alpha/Nrf2 pathway, leading to increased susceptibility of wild-type p53 cancer cells to oxidative stress and therapeutic agents. Free Radic Biol Med. 2014;74:21–34.

55. Tseng CH. Metformin use and cervical cancer risk in female patients with type 2 diabetes. Oncotarget. 2016;7:59548–55.

18

Personalized risk assessment for dynamic transition of gastric neoplasms

Jean Ching-Yuan Fann[1], Tsung-Hsien Chiang[2,3,4], Amy Ming-Fang Yen[5*], Yi-Chia Lee[2,6,7*] (iD), Ming-Shiang Wu[2] and Hsiu-Hsi Chen[6,7]

Abstract

Background: To develop an individually-tailored dynamic risk assessment model following a multistep, multifactorial process of the Correa's gastric cancer model.

Methods: First, we estimated the state-to-state transition rates following Correa's five-step carcinogenic model and assessed the effect of risk factors, including *Helicobacter pylori* infection, history of upper gastrointestinal disease, lifestyle, and dietary habits, on the step-by-step transition rates using data from a high-risk population in Matsu Islands, Taiwan. Second, we incorporated information on the gastric cancer carcinogenesis affected by genomic risk factors (including inherited susceptibility and irreversible genomic changes) based on literature to generate a genetic and epigenetic risk assessment model by using a simulated cohort identical to the Matsu population. The combination of conventional and genomic risk factors enables us to develop the personalized transition risk scores and composite scores.

Results: The state-by-state transition rates per year were 0.0053, 0.7523, 0.1750, and 0.0121 per year from normal mucosa to chronic active gastritis, chronic active gastritis to atrophic gastritis, atrophic gastritis to intestinal metaplasia, and intestinal metaplasia to gastric cancer, respectively. Compared with the median risk group, the most risky decile had a 5.22-fold risk of developing gastric cancer, and the least risky decile around one-twelfth of the risk. The median 10-year risk for gastric cancer incidence was 0.77%. The median lifetime risk for gastric cancer incidence was 5.43%. By decile, the 10-year risk ranged from 0.06 to 4.04% and the lifetime risk ranged from 0.42 to 21.04%.

Conclusions: We demonstrate how to develop a personalized dynamic risk assessment model with the underpinning of Correa's cascade to stratify the population according to their risk for progression to gastric cancer. Such a risk assessment model not only facilitates the development of an individually-tailored preventive strategy with treatment for *H. pylori* infection and endoscopic screening but also provides short-term and long-term indicators to evaluate the program effectiveness.

Keywords: Gastric cancer, Prevention, *Helicobacter pylori*, Endoscopy

Background

Gastric cancer poses a great threat to global health that takes more than 720,000 tolls per year worldwide [1]. The current approach to gastric cancer management largely relies on endoscopic detection followed by muco-sectomy, gastrectomy and/or chemotherapy; however, in the absence of early detection, gastric cancer is associated with a high fatality rate, and the 5-year survival rate for patients with locally advanced disease is only about 40% despite aggressive treatment [2].

Early detection and treatment of gastric cancer and its precancerous lesion is very feasible as carcinogenesis of gastric cancer often follows a multistage process (i.e., the Correa's model) that develops from chronic active gastritis (CAG) to atrophic gastritis (AG), intestinal metaplasia (IM), dysplasia, and finally to carcinoma [3]. *Helicobacter pylori* is now recognized as the main risk factor that initiates this process. An estimated 89% of infection-related cancers can be prevented if *H. pylori* can be eradicated from the population of interest [4]; hence, *H. pylori* eradication is now considered the most effective way to

* Correspondence: amyyen@tmu.edu.tw; yichialee@ntu.edu.tw
[5]School of Oral Hygiene, College of Oral Medicine, Taipei Medical University, No. 250, Wu-Hsing Street, Xinyi District, Taipei 110, Taiwan
[2]Department of Internal Medicine, College of Medicine, National Taiwan University Hospital, No. 7, Chung-Shan South Road, Taipei 10002, Taiwan
Full list of author information is available at the end of the article

ameliorate the burden of gastric cancer [5–7]. The age-adjusted incidence of gastric cancer has shown a steady decline, which is not only attributed to improvements in sanitation and hygiene but also to the eradication of *H. pylori* that has become a routine clinical practice in the treatment of peptic ulcers. Nevertheless, the annual number of new cases of gastric cancer in the globe is expected to still remain stable until 2030 [1]. This projection suggests universal approach to the prevention of gastric cancer may not be sufficient as the risk of developing gastric cancer varies from individual to individual and also does the acceptance of screening, compliance with the referral, and clinical workup for confirmatory diagnosis.

In the setting of mass screening, irreversible damage may already have occurred after patients have harbored *H. pylori* infection for decades before they undergo screening and treatment for *H. pylori*. This observation is supported by a recent meta-analysis, based on 8 randomized controlled trials and 16 cohort studies, of the benefit of eradication therapy; on average, gastric cancer risk was reduced only about 50% in adult patients [8]. Therefore, to efficiently eliminate the threat of gastric cancer, a population-based program should focus on both early treatment and early detection. The advent of genomics and the urgent need to prevent gastric cancer in areas with high prevalence of *H. pylori* infection and high incidence of gastric cancer have increasingly gained attention to the potential benefits of developing individually-tailored preventive strategies [9–11]. However, there is lacking of the personalized risk assessment, namely, quantitative risk-score-based stratification of the underlying population, for the development of an effective strategy that consists of *H. pylori* eradication and endoscopic screening for each individual.

Since gastric cancer is a multistep and multifactorial progressive disease, findings from basic researches should help inform the development of preventive measures [12]. Various factors may influence the transitions between stages in the development of gastric cancer, including *H. pylori* infection, genetic polymorphisms and epigenetic changes, consumption of tobacco and alcohol, and dietary habits [12, 13]. In the current study, we aimed to develop a multistep and multifactorial dynamic risk assessment model by taking into account the current evidence on environmental, genetic, and epigenetic risk factors responsible for gastric carcinogenesis. We also provided short-term (such as premalignant gastric lesions) and long-term (such as incidence and mortality of gastric cancer) indicators to support the effectiveness when such a personalized prevention program was implemented on a high-risk population.

Methods

Evolution of community-based prevention campaign on Matsu Islands

There are three phases of community-based prevention program gradually offered for residents on the Matsu Islands, an island archipelago located in the Taiwan Strait (also an offshore island between Taiwan and China). The residents had a high gastric cancer burden, with an incidence rate 3–5 folds higher than that of the main island of Taiwan and the highest mortality rate from gastric cancer among all Taiwanese populations. Therefore, a two-stage screening program targeting the premalignant gastric lesions and early-stage gastric cancer was conducted in 1996–1998 using the serum anti-*H. pylori* immunoglobin G antibody test and serum pepsinogen measurement as the first stage and those who tested positive were referred to the second-stage endoscopy for confirmatory diagnosis and histological assessment; the results have been described in full elsewhere [10]. The second phase was to launch a community-based integrated screening since 2002 onwards with five common cancers in combination with other examinations for chronic diseases [14]. The program invited residents aged 30 and above on the Matsu Islands to participate annually with various inter-screening intervals for different items. The third phase was to introduce a chemopreventive program for gastric cancer by using the mass eradication of *H. pylori* infection since 2004 [9, 11]. The effects of *H. pylori* infection and conventional risk factors were estimated from the empirical data collected from three phases of the community-based screening programs.

Gastric cancer prevention programs

As the current paper places emphasis on the prevention of gastric cancer, here we detail the evolution of prevention programs for gastric cancer. In 1996–1998, a screening program mainly based on the serological biomarkers was conducted. The first stage included the serum anti-*H. pylori* immunoglobin G antibody test and serum pepsinogen measurement. Those with positive results in the first stage were referred to confirmatory endoscopy and histological assessment. Among 3541 residents aged 30 years or older registered in population list, a total of 2184 residents participated in the first stage of the screening project. Among 946 who had first-stage positive results, 523 complied with second-stage endoscopic examination, 325 underwent endoscopic biopsy for histological evaluation, and 2 gastric cancers were detected endoscopically.

The second gastric cancer prevention program was launched in 2004, which included the first stage with C^{13}-urea breath test and the second stage with endoscopic examination and histological evaluation. In 2004, a total of 4121 participants participated and 2598 (63%) tested positive for *H. pylori* infection. Endoscopy was done for 1762 *H. pylori* carriers for histological assessment and 4 gastric cancers were found. Histology was classified using the updated Sydney system [15]. The overall eradication rate was 97.7% following 2 courses of antibiotic treatments.

The study flow chart for collecting information on this cohort is depicted in Fig. 1. Because these two programs were in conjunction with a community-based integrated screening program, in addition to the transition between states (normal → CAG, CAG → AG, AG → IM, and IM → gastric cancer), information on the state-specific risk factors, such as the demographic data, lifestyle factors, diet habits, and family and medical histories, were available. Further searching for the information of genetic susceptibility and genetic/epigenetic alternations from literature, we can build up the following personalized multistate risk assessment model.

Personalized multistate risk assessment model

We constructed a multistep and multifactorial disease natural history in the light of the Correa's model that can be delineated as follows: normal → CAG → AG → IM → gastric cancer [3], superimposed with state-specific factors in each state transition. The relative risk of *H. pylori* infection, history of upper gastrointestinal disease, exercise habit, fruit intake, chicken intake, dry fish intake, and salt fish intake on different transitions were estimated on the basis of the empirical data from the Matsu Islands [10, 11, 13, 14]. The relative risks associated with genetic and epigenetic

factors were extracted from the literature and were fitted with empirical data [16–21].

Figure 2 shows the five-state Markov model for gastric cancer. In the light of recognized risk factors, we calculated the incidences of the transition from normal to CAG (λ_{12}), the transition from CAG to AG (λ_{23}), from AG to IM (λ_{34}), and from IM to gastric cancer (λ_{45}), associated with the corresponding relevant risk factors in the proportional hazard form as shown in the following equations:

$$\lambda_{12} = \lambda_{120} \times exp(\beta_1 \times (HP) + \beta_2 \times (Upper\ GI\ disease))$$

$$\lambda_{23} = \lambda_{230} \times exp(\beta_3 \times (IL1RN\ 2/2))$$

$$\lambda_{34} = \lambda_{340} \times exp(\beta_4 \times (Exercise) + \beta_5 \times (Fruit\ input)$$
$$+\beta_6 \times (Meat\ input) + \beta_7 \times (Picked\ food\ input)$$
$$+\beta_8 \times (Salty\ food\ input))$$

$$\lambda_{45} = \lambda_{450} \times exp(\beta_9 \times (p53) + \beta_{10} \times (\text{E-cadherin}\ 160\ AA, CA)$$
$$+\beta_{11} \times (MTHFR\ 677\ TT) + \beta_{12} \times (MSI)$$
$$+\beta_{13} \times (LOX) + \beta_{14} \times (p41ARC))$$

These four regression models are used for the development a personalized risk assessment model for deriving four transition risk scores for normal → CAG, CAG → AG, AG → IM, and IM → cancer, and also the composite score by combining four transition risk scores with the assignment of different weights to each transition risk score. The weights assigned to each transition (normal → CAG, CAG → AG, AG → IM, and IM → cancer) were based on

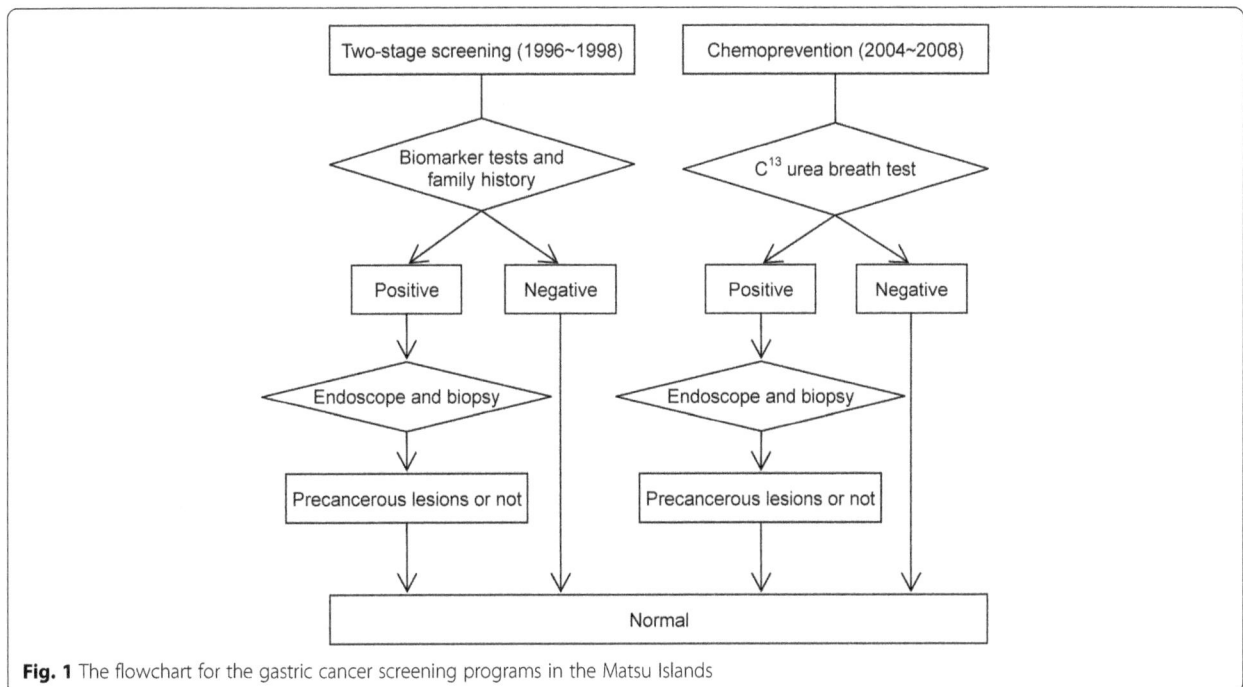

Fig. 1 The flowchart for the gastric cancer screening programs in the Matsu Islands

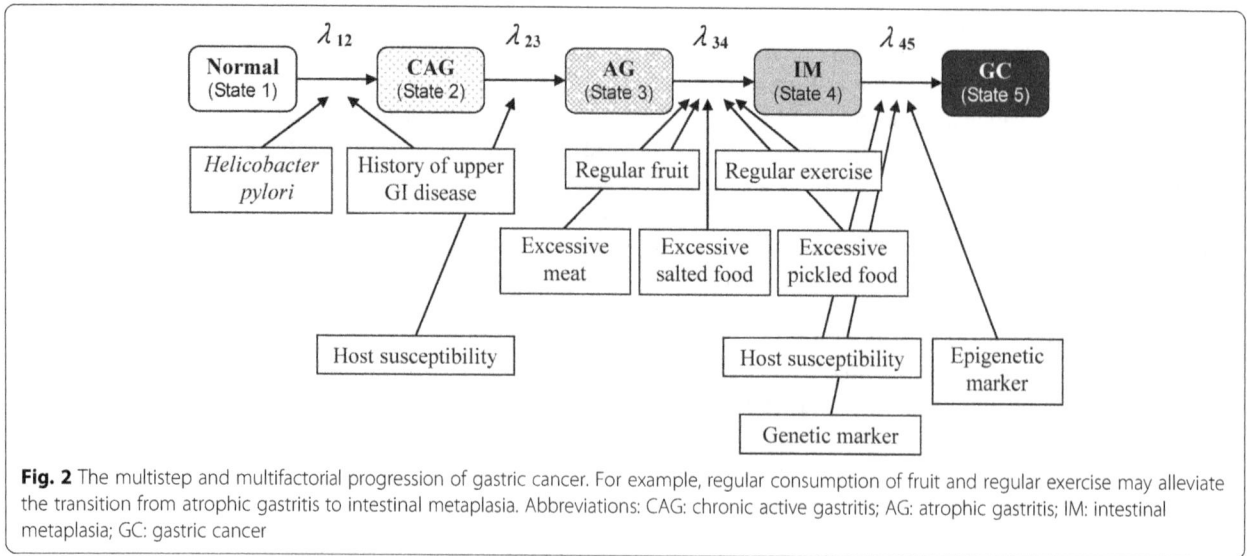

Fig. 2 The multistep and multifactorial progression of gastric cancer. For example, regular consumption of fruit and regular exercise may alleviate the transition from atrophic gastritis to intestinal metaplasia. Abbreviations: CAG: chronic active gastritis; AG: atrophic gastritis; IM: intestinal metaplasia; GC: gastric cancer

the relative value of taking the logarithm of baseline rate for the three transitions (normal → CAG, CAG → AG, and IM → cancer) in comparison with the reference group (AG → IM).

Computer simulation of the individual risk

We simulated a cohort of 100,000 subjects aged 30–79 years who were followed up for 10 years in order to generate the 10-year cumulative risk of developing gastric cancer. The infection with *H. pylori*, history of upper gastrointestinal disease, lifestyle, and dietary habits of this hypothetic cohort were determined by assigning the distributions of the cohort on the Matsu Islands. The rates of P53 codon 72 polymorphisms, E-cadherin-160A polymorphisms, microsatellite instability (MSI), and the methylation levels of LOX and p41ARC were also derived. The cohort was therefore classified into different risk groups according to deciles of the composite risk score as mentioned above.

Statistical analysis

A continuous-time five-state Markov process in the light of the Correa's model was developed by defining four transition rates as mentioned above into the intensity 5×5 matrix form. The transition probabilities during time t in terms of matrix for each transition were also derived by using the forward Kolmogorov equations. Given the Markov property that the disease status in each year for any individual was dependent on his/her disease status in the previous year but independent of the disease status previously, the log likelihood function was developed by using the available empirical data on each transition mode, respectively, including normal → CAG, CAG → AG, AG → IM, and

IM → cancer, to estimate four transition parameters and also the state-specific regression coefficients. The latter was formed as the basis for the development of transition risk score and composite risk score. All analyses were done using SAS software (version 9.4; SAS Institute, Cary, NC, USA).

Results

State-specific correlates associated with the Correa's multistate model

The state-by-state transition rates per year were 0.0053, 0.7523, 0.1750, and 0.0121 per year from normal to CAG, CAG to AG, AG to IM, and IM to gastric cancer, respectively. Table 1 shows the both effects of *H. pylori* infection and histories of upper gastrointestinal disease on the incidence of CAG; the effect of genetic susceptibility on the transition from CAG to AG; the effects of lifestyle and dietary habits on the transition from AG to IM; and the effects of genetic susceptibility, microsatellite instability, and DNA methylation level (epigenetic factor) on the transition from IM to gastric cancer. Accordingly, the transition rates between states before the development of invasive gastric cancer can be expressed as:

$$\lambda_{12} = 0.001232 \times exp(1.7733 \times (HP) + 1.0682 \times (Upper\ GI\ disease))$$

$$\lambda_{23} = 0.6838 \times exp(0.8198 \times (IL1RN\ 2/2))$$

$$\lambda_{34} = 0.1536 \times exp(-0.4463 \times (Exercise) - 0.5276 \times (Fruit\ input) + 0.7178 \times (Meat\ input) + 0.8629 \times (Intake\ of\ prickled\ food) + 1.1184 \times (Intake\ of\ salty\ food))$$

Table 1 The multifactorial effects of *H. pylori* infection, upper gastrointestinal disease, life style and dietary habit, genetic and epigenetic factors on the multistep progression of gastric cancer

Variables	Estimate	95% CI	References
Effect on transition from normal to CAG			
Transition rate (λ_{120})	0.0053	0.0051–0.0056	[10, 11]
RR of *H. pylori infection*	5.89	5.63–6.17	[10, 11]
RR of history of upper gastrointestinal disease	2.91	2.76–3.06	[10, 11]
Effect on transition from CAG to AG			
Transition rate (λ_{230})	0.7523	0.7071–0.7975	[10, 11]
RR of interleukin-1 RN VNTR polymorphism: 2/2 genotype	2.27	1.40–3.70	[14]
Effect on transition from AG to IM			
Transition rate (λ_{340})	0.1750	0.1640–0.1860	[10, 11]
RR of regular exercise	0.64	0.59–0.68	[10, 11]
RR of frequent fruit	0.59	0.53–0.65	[10, 11]
RR of frequent meat	2.05	1.82–2.30	[10, 11]
RR of frequent prickled food	2.37	1.86–3.02	[10, 11]
RR of frequent salty food	3.06	2.41–3.89	[10, 11]
Effect on transition from IM to GC			
Transition rate (λ_{450})	0.0121	0.0097–0.0145	[10, 11]
RR of p53 codon 72 polymorphism: Arg/Arg genotype	0.84	0.72–0.99	[15]
RR of E-cadherin (*CHD1*)-160A polymorphism: AA/CA genotype	0.81	0.67–0.99	[16]
RR of MTHFR 677 polymorphism: TT genotype	1.64	1.36–1.97	[17]
RR of microsatellite instability	3.09	2.79–3.42	[18]
RR of methylation level of *LOX*	2.37	2.17–2.59	[19]
RR of methylation level of *p41ARC*	3.72	3.29–4.21	[19]

Abbreviations: *RR* relative risk, *CI* confidence interval, *CAG* chronic active gastritis *AG* atrophic gastritis, *IM* intestinal metaplasia, *GC* gastric cancer, *RR* relative risk, *VNTR* variable number tandem repeat, *MTHFR* methylenetetrahydrofolate reductase

$$\begin{aligned}\lambda_{45} = 0.0005 \times\ &exp(-0.1744 \times (p53\ Arg, Arg) - 0.2107 \\ &\times (E\text{–cadherin } 160\ AA, CA) + 0.4947 \\ &\times (MTHFR\ 677\ TT) + 1.1282 \times (MSI) \\ &+ 0.8629 \times (LOX) + 1.3137 \times (p41ARC))\end{aligned}$$

According to these four transition rates, four corresponding transition risk scores for serial state transitions are developed by using their regression coefficients:

$$\begin{aligned}\text{Score (normal} \rightarrow \text{CAG}) = \{&1.7733 \times (HP) + 1.0682 \\ &\times (Upper\ GI\ disease)\}\end{aligned}$$

$$\text{Score (CAG} \rightarrow \text{AG}) = \{0.8198 \times (IL1RN\ 2/2)\}$$

$$\begin{aligned}\text{Score (AG} \rightarrow \text{IM}) = \{&-0.4463 \times (Exercise) - 0.5276 \\ &\times (Fruit\ input) + 0.7178 \times (Meat\ input) \\ &+ 0.8629 \times (Prikled\ food\ input) + 1.1184 \\ &\times (Salty\ food\ input)\}\end{aligned}$$

$$\begin{aligned}\text{Score (IM} \rightarrow \text{cancer}) = \{&(-0.1744 \times (p53\ Arg, Arg) - 0.2107 \\ &\times (E\text{–cadherin } 160\ AA, CA) \\ &+ 0.4947 \times (MTHFR\ 677\ TT) \\ &+ 1.1282 \times (MSI) + 0.8629 \\ &\times (LOX) + 1.3137 \times (p41ARC))\}\end{aligned}$$

The composite score in the light of four transition risk scores was also developed by assigning different weights to each transition risk score. The weights assigned to normal $\rightarrow$ CAG, CAG $\rightarrow$ AG, AG $\rightarrow$ IM, and IM $\rightarrow$ cancer were 15, 1, 5, and 20 based on the relative value of taking the logarithm of baseline rate for three baseline transitions in comparison with the reference group (AG $\rightarrow$ IM).

Kinetic epidemiological curves of the multistate outcomes
The kinetic epidemiological curves of multi-state outcomes (from normal to gastric cancer) for four hypothetical subjects at the low risk, intermediate risk, high risk, and extremely high risk are depicted in Fig. 3. For example, low risk could be defined as no *H. pylori* infection, with regular exercise and fruit intake, p53 codon 72

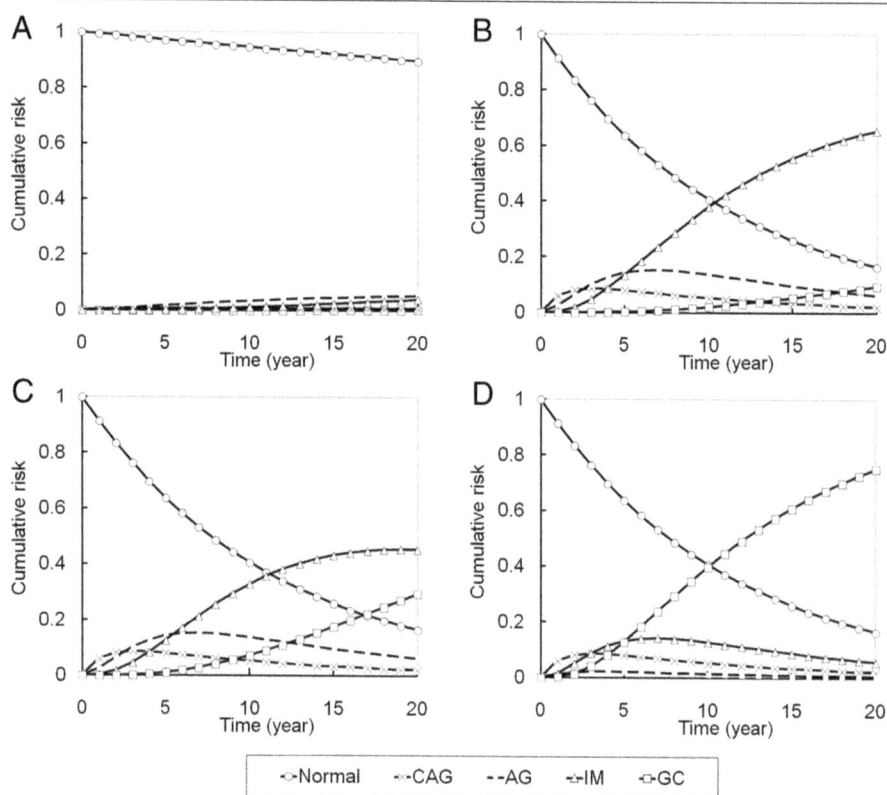

Fig. 3 The 20-year cumulative risk of multi-state outcomes of gastric neoplasms for four hypothetical subjects with: (a) low risk (without *H. pylori* infection, with regular exercise and fruit intake, p53 codon 72 Arg/Arg, E-cadherin C/C, MSI stable, and methylation levels LOX/p41 ARC: 7.2%/6.2%); (b) intermediate risk (with *H. pylori* infection/upper gastrointestinal disease history/large intake of meat, without regular exercise and fruit intake, p53 codon 72 Pro/Pro, E-cadherin A/A, MSI stable, and methylation LOX/p41 ARC: 7.2%/6.2%); (c) high risk (with *H. pylori* infection, upper gastrointestinal disease history, smoking, large intake of meat, without regular exercise or fruit intake, p53 codon 72 Pro/Pro, E-cadherin A/A, MSI stable, and methylation LOX/p41 ARC: 7.2%/11.2%); and (d) extremely high risk (with *H. pylori* infection, upper gastrointestinal disease history, smoking, large intake of meat, intake of salty fish and dry fish, without regular exercise or fruit intake, p53 codon 72 Pro/Pro, E-cadherin A/A, MSI instable, and with methylation levels: LOX/p41 ARC: 12.2%/11.2%). Abbreviations: CAG: chronic active gastritis; AG: atrophic gastritis; IM: intestinal metaplasia; GC: gastric cancer

Arg/Arg, E-cadherin C/C, MSI stable, and methylation levels LOX/p41 ARC: 7.2%/6.2%. Intermediate risk was defined as having *H. pylori* infection, a history of upper gastrointestinal disease, large intake of meat, no regular exercise or fruit intake, p53 codon 72 Pro/Pro, E-cadherin A/A, MSI stable, and methylation LOX/p41 ARC: 7.2%/6.2%. High risk was defined as having *H. pylori* infection, a history of upper gastrointestinal disease, smoking, large intake of meat, no regular exercise or fruit intake, p53 codon 72 Pro/Pro, E-cadherin A/A, MSI stable, and methylation LOX/p41 ARC: 7.2%/11.2%. Extremely high risk was defined as having *H. pylori* infection, a history of upper gastrointestinal disease, smoking, large intake of meat, intake of salty fish and dry fish, no regular exercise or fruit intake, p53 codon 72 Pro/Pro, E-cadherin A/A, MSI instable, and methylation levels: LOX/p41 ARC: 12.2%/11.2%.

For the intermediate risk condition relative to the low risk, the cumulative risk for intestinal metaplasia increased

significantly through time. For the high risk condition, although the cumulative risk for intestinal metaplasia increased less than for the intermediate risk condition, gastric cancer was more likely to develop. For the extremely high risk condition, the cumulative risk for gastric cancer development was up to 40% after 10 years.

Not only the different risk profile of an individual, Fig. 3 also demonstrates the pattern of dynamic transition from normal to the occurrence of gastric cancer. These curves provide a basis for the development of surrogate endpoint and primary endpoint for the evaluation of a personalized prevention program.

Personalized risk assessment for gastric cancer

We classified our cohort into four risk groups (low, intermediate, high, and extremely high) and deciles of risk and calculated the 10-year and lifetime risk of developing gastric cancer by using composite risk score (Table 2). Compared with the median risk group, the most risky

Table 2 The 10-year and lifetime risk of developing gastric cancer by using the composite risk score

Risk group	RR	10-year risk	Life-time risk
95–100	5.22	4.04%	21.04%
80–95	3.80	2.94%	16.50%
60–80	2.70	2.09%	13.01%
51–60	1.23	0.95%	7.30%
Median (50)	1.00	0.77%	5.43%
40–49	0.92	0.71%	4.64%
30–40	0.17	0.13%	0.98%
5–30	0.08	0.06%	0.53%
0–5	0.08	0.06%	0.42%

Abbreviations: *RR* relative risk

decile had a 5.22-fold risk of developing gastric cancer, and the least risky 5% around one-twelfth of the risk. The median 10-year risk for gastric cancer incidence and mortality were 0.77 and 0.53%, respectively. The median lifetime risk for gastric cancer incidence and mortality were 5.43 and 5.06%, respectively. By decile, the 10-year risk ranged from 0.06 to 4.04% and the lifetime risk ranged from 0.42 to 21.04%.

Discussion

Personalized dynamic risk assessment model for gastric cancer

Environmental risk factors and biological markers (including the genetic and epigenetic determinants) related to the progression from premalignant gastric lesions to gastric cancer provide an insight into the benefits of a prophylactic intervention and screening program. The development of an individually-tailored method to stratify the risk of multistate disease outcome for the underlying population plays an important role for the planning of personalized preventive strategies for gastric cancer. However, how to develop a systematic framework for such a purpose has been barely addressed before. In this article, we demonstrate how to develop a multistep and multifactorial risk assessment model, taking into account environmental, genetic, and epigenetic factors, and to produce a risk-score-based stratification upon which we can develop individualized prevention strategies to reduce the incidence and mortality of gastric cancer.

The personalized risk assessment model with the incorporation of personal characteristics and possible biological markers here provides a new insight into how to integrate genetic counseling, epidemiology, health information, and healthcare management into a unifying framework based on the risk of developing premalignant gastric lesion and gastric cancer, and throws light on how to develop an individual-tailored approach. For the risk assessment of gastric cancer, the currently available

blood tests mainly include the serum PG, which has long been considered a reliable biomarker of the functional and morphologic status of the gastric mucosa [22]. A meta-analysis of 1520 patients with gastric cancer and 27,723 controls showed a sensitivity of 70%, a specificity of 79%, and a positive likelihood ratio of 3.3 of the combination of PG-I level and the PG-I/II ratio to detect gastric cancer [23]. Also in our study population, a previous study has shown that a low serum PG-I level and/ or a low PG-I/II ratio were predictive of a higher risk of gastric cancer death following 16 years of follow-up [24]. Nonetheless, the subjects with abnormal PG level was found only associated with about 3–4 folds of gastric cancer risk; therefore, the predictability of using this serological marker remains limited as the phenotypes of gastric cancer may include the intestinal and the diffuse types, which may be in turn associated with different patterns of the genetic and epigenetic alternations. Also because PG testing only detects atrophic gastritis coexisting with cancer, about one third of gastric cancer cases (the diffuse type) may be missed by using the PG teste as a non-endoscopic biomarker for the detection of gastric cancer.

Comparison with the universal screening approaches

Several studies have indicated that the secondary prevention with endoscopic screening could decrease the mortality from gastric cancer. In the Korean Nationwide Screening Program, those who received endoscopic screening were associated with 47% reduction of death from gastric cancer [25]. A synthetic study that included 6 cohort studies and 4 case control studies in Asia (comprising 342,013 individuals) consistently showed a 40% reduction in gastric cancer mortality [26]. However, such a universal endoscopy approach greatly relied on the capacity of endoscopists and failed to decrease the incidence of gastric cancer. On the other way, the primary prevention through *H. pylori* eradication has greatly attracted attention as the strategy for gastric cancer prevention on a population-wide scale [1, 6, 27], which was supported by a consensus meeting that formally declared *H. pylori* gastritis as an infectious disease, which should be treated and cured [28]. In our previous meta-analysis that included 715 incident gastric cancers among a total of 48,064 individuals/340,255 person-years (also included the population on Matsu Islands), individuals with eradication of *H. pylori* infection had a reduction of 47% in gastric cancer risk than those who did not receive eradication therapy [8]. The magnitude of risk reduction related to *H. pylori* eradication would be greater in populations with the more aggressive *H. pylori* strains and the higher percentage of genetic trait that is more susceptible to carcinogens, which may lead to more intensive host-bacterial interaction, the more rapid carcinogenic process, and thus the higher risk of gastric cancer. Therefore, in high-risk populations, in addition to the intensive endoscopic surveillance, the combination of a mass eradication program is highly desirable.

The personalized preventive approach

In recent years, many genetic and epigenetic markers have been reported as promising biomarkers to predict and stratify gastric cancer risk [29–31]; however, none of them has been implemented on the population level. Our study highlights a method illustrating how to apply these novel biomarkers to a high-risk population that has initiated the mass eradication program, which has a significant implication for how to integrate the primary and secondary prevention strategies to maximize the benefit from a screening program and optimize the allocation of limited endoscopic resources. Such a personalized risk assessment model is very helpful for the development of personalized preventive strategies. According our proposed models, the median risk group might start screening in middle age with medium-range intervals, in late age with longer intervals for those at lower risk, and those at extremely high risk might start screening programs at younger ages with the shortest interval. The same logic can be applied to chemoprevention on age to commence.

It is noteworthy that such a personalized risk assessment model with multistep and multifactorial property also provides an opportunity of point-of-care for the dynamic transition of gastric cancer with personal viewpoint, which also makes major contribution to shared decision-making for personalized prevention for gastric cancer.

Short-term and long-term evaluations

Despite the advantage of using personalized strategies, evaluation of its effectiveness is intractable partly because of enormous costs and time in longitudinal follow-up study and partly because of the complex design of personalized strategy. The proposed dynamic multistate model with the underpinning of Correa's cascade may be a panacea. The Fig. 3 shows dynamic transition from normal to gastric cancer through the premalignant gastric lesions. Such a kinetic epidemiological curve provides an opportunity for the development of short-term indicators, such as AG and IM, and long-term indictors, such as incidence and mortality of gastric cancer.

Strengths and limitations of the study

Our strengths include the use of a cohort study design in a high-risk community with gastric cancer, which reduces the possibility of selection bias common in previous studies. A cohort with comprehensive demographic characteristics, baseline *H. pylori* infection status, and histological assessment presented a unique opportunity to estimate state-to-state transition rates accurately. We also simulated the clinical scenarios about how to implement such a risk-score-based stratification on the population level, which may be of great information for the healthcare policy makers to develop a policy that consists of individual risk profiles such that the incidence and mortality of gastric cancer can be efficiently reduced especially for the high-risk populations and the limited medical resources can be properly allocated.

However, there are several limitations in this study. First, gastric cancer is a heterogeneous disease. Molecular heterogeneity has been shown through the existence of subtypes that differ in histopathology and anatomic site, gene expression, DNA methylation, and oncogenic pathways [12]. Although the five-state Markov model and the resulting equations could not account for all potential genetic/epigenetic risk factors, the concept of risk-score-based stratification could provide a specific prevention strategy for high risk individuals to reduce their incidence and mortality rates of gastric cancer. Second, the development of dietary habits is highly dependent on the underlying culture and socioeconomic status of an individual. The present cohort was surveyed on dietary items in the 1990s. We found that most of the habits pertaining to the intake of salted foods were time-invariant, whereas the intake of meat, fruit, milk, and shrimp sauce were time-variant [13]. Therefore, whether our model based on the nutritional factors at the initial stage could be applied to the more modern population deserves further observation.

Conclusions

We demonstrate how to develop a personalized Correa gastric cancer model to stratify the risk of developing premalignant gastric lesions and gastric cancer using clinical and genomic factors. The proposed personalized risk assessment model provides a new insight into health planning for the development of preventive strategies regarding the eradication of *H. pylori* infection and early detection with endoscopy with short-term endpoints to reduce the premalignant gastric lesions and with long-term endpoints to reduce the incidence and mortality of gastric cancer.

Abbreviations
AG: Atrophic gastritis; CAG: Chronic active gastritis; IM: Intestinal metaplasia; MSI: Microsatellite instability; MTHFR: Methylenetetrahydrofolate reductase; PG: Pepsinogen; RR: relative risk; VNTR: Variable number tandem repeat

Acknowledgements
The authors would like to express their special thanks to the staff of the Eighth Core Lab, Department of Medical Research, National Taiwan University Hospital. The authors also thank the administrative support in Matsu Island from Dr. Cheng-Ying Liu of the Lienchiang County Government and Dr. Chun-Fu Hsieh of the Health Bureau of Lienchiang County.

Funding
This work was supported by the Innovation and Policy Center for Population Health and Sustainable Environment (Population Health Research Center, PHRC), College of Public Health, National Taiwan University from the Ministry of Science and Technology (MOST 107-3017-F-002-003) and Featured Areas Research Center Program within the framework of the Higher Education Sprout Project by the Ministry of Education (MOE) in Taiwan (NTU-107 L9003). This study was also supported by the National Taiwan University Hospital (107-T11).

Authors' contributions
AMY, YCL, and HHC have full access to the data and take responsibility for the integrity of the data and the accuracy of the data analysis. Conception and design of the study: All authors. Generation, collection, assembly, analysis and/or interpretation of data: All authors. Drafting or revision of the manuscript: All authors. Critical revision of the manuscript for important intellectual content: All authors. Administrative, technical, or material support: All authors. Approval of the final version of the manuscript: All authors. Study supervision: HHC. YCL, AMY, and HHC had the final responsibility for the decision to submit for publication.

Competing interests
The authors declare that they have no competing interests.

Author details
[1]Department of Health Industry Management, School of Healthcare Management, Kainan University, Taoyuan City, Taiwan. [2]Department of Internal Medicine, College of Medicine, National Taiwan University Hospital, No. 7, Chung-Shan South Road, Taipei 10002, Taiwan. [3]Department of Integrated Diagnostics and Therapeutics, National Taiwan University Hospital, Taipei, Taiwan. [4]Graduate Institute of Clinical Medicine, College of Medicine, National Taiwan University, Taipei, Taiwan. [5]School of Oral Hygiene, College of Oral Medicine, Taipei Medical University, No. 250, Wu-Hsing Street, Xinyi District, Taipei 110, Taiwan. [6]Institute of Epidemiology and Preventive Medicine, College of Public Health, National Taiwan University, Taipei, Taiwan. [7]Innovation and Policy Center for Population Health and Sustainable Environment, College of Public Health, National Taiwan University, Taipei, Taiwan.

References
1. IARC *Helicobacter pylori* Working Group. *Helicobacter pylori* Eradication as a Strategy for Gastric Cancer Prevention. Lyon: International Agency for Research on Cancer (IARC Working Group Reports, No. 8); 2014. Available at: http://publications.iarc.fr/Book-And-Report-Series/Iarc-Working-Group-Reports/-Em-Helicobacter-Pylori-Em-Eradication-As-A-Strategy-For-Preventing-Gastric-Cancer-2014. Accessed 14 July 2018.
2. Van Cutsem E, Sagaert X, Topal B, Haustermans K, Prenen H. Gastric cancer. Lancet. 2016;388:2654–64.
3. Correa P. Human gastric carcinogenesis: a multistep and multifactorial process--first American Cancer Society award lecture on Cancer epidemiology and prevention. Cancer Res. 1992;52:6735–40.
4. Plummer M, de Martel C, Vignat J, Ferlay J, Bray F, Franceschi S. Global burden of cancers attributable to infections in 2012: a synthetic analysis. Lancet Glob Health. 2016;4:e609–16.
5. Ferlay J, Soerjomataram I, Dikshit R, Eser S, Mathers C, Rebelo M, et al. Cancer incidence and mortality worldwide: sources, methods and major patterns in GLOBOCAN 2012. Int J Cancer. 2015;136:E359–86.
6. Lee YC, Chiang TH, Liou JM, Chen HH, Wu MS, Graham DY. Mass eradication of helicobacter pylori to prevent gastric cancer: theoretical and practical considerations. Gut Liver. 2016;10:12–26.
7. Graham DY, Shiotani A. The time to eradicate gastric cancer is now. Gut. 2005;54:735–8.
8. Lee YC, Chiang TH, Chou CK, Tu YK, Liao WC, Wu MS, et al. Association between helicobacter pylori eradication and gastric cancer incidence: a systematic review and meta-analysis. Gastroenterology. 2016;150:1113–24.
9. Lee YC, Wu HM, Chen TH, Liu TY, Chiu HM, Chang CC, et al. A community-based study of helicobacter pylori therapy using the strategy of test, treat, retest, and re-treat initial treatment failures. Helicobacter. 2006;11:418–24.
10. Liu CY, Wu CY, Lin JT, Lee YC, Yen AM, Chen TH. Multistate and multifactorial progression of gastric cancer: results from community-based mass screening for gastric cancer. J Med Screen. 2006;13(Suppl 1):S2–5.
11. Lee YC, Chen TH, Chiu HM, Shun CT, Chiang H, Liu TY, et al. The benefit of mass eradication of helicobacter pylori infection: a community-based study of gastric cancer prevention. Gut. 2013;62:676–82.
12. Cristescu R, Lee J, Nebozhyn M, Kim KM, Ting JC, Wong SS, et al. Molecular analysis of gastric cancer identifies subtypes associated with distinct clinical outcomes. Nat Med. 2015;21:449–56.
13. Hsiung HY, Fann JC, Yen AM, Chen SL, Chiu SY, Ku TH, et al. Stage-specific dietary factors associated with the Correa multistep and multifactorial process of human gastric carcinogenesis. Nutr Cancer. 2016;68:598–610.
14. Chen TH, Chiu YH, Luh DL, Yen MF, Wu HM, Chen LS, Taiwan Community-Based Integrated Screening Group, et al. Community-based multiple screening model: design, implementation, and analysis of 42,387 participants. Cancer. 2004;100:1734e43.
15. Dixon MF, Genta RM, Yardley JH, Correa P. Classification and grading of gastritis. The updated Sydney system. International workshop on the histopathology of gastritis, Houston 1994. Am J Surg Pathol. 1996;20:1161–81.
16. Peleteiro B, Lunet N, Carrilho C, Duraes C, Machado JC, La Vecchia C, et al. Association between cytokine gene polymorphisms and gastric precancerous lesions: systematic review and meta-analysis. Cancer Epidemiol Biomark Prev. 2010;19:762–76.
17. Zhou Y, Li N, Zhuang W, Liu GJ, Wu TX, Yao X, et al. P53 codon 72 polymorphism and gastric cancer: a meta-analysis of the literature. Int J Cancer. 2007;121:1481–6.
18. Wang GY, Lu CQ, Zhang RM, Hu XH, Luo ZW. The E-cadherin gene polymorphism 160C->A and cancer risk: a HuGE review and meta-analysis of 26 case-control studies. Am J Epidemiol. 2008;167:7–14.
19. Boccia S, Gianfagna F, Persiani R, La Greca A, Arzani D, Rausei S, et al. Methylenetetrahydrofolate reductase C677T and A1298C polymorphisms and susceptibility to gastric adenocarcinoma in an Italian population. Biomarkers. 2007;12:635–44.
20. Leung WK, Kim JJ, Kim JG, Graham DY, Sepulveda AR. Microsatellite instability in gastric intestinal metaplasia in patients with and without gastric cancer. Am J Pathol. 2000;156:537–43.
21. Maekita T, Nakazawa K, Mihara M, Nakajima T, Yanaoka K, Iguchi M, et al. High levels of aberrant DNA methylation in helicobacter pylori-infected gastric mucosae and its possible association with gastric cancer risk. Clin Cancer Res. 2006;12:989–95.
22. Samloff IM. Immunologic studies of human group I pepsinogens. J Immunol. 1971;106:962–8.
23. Huang YK, Yu JC, Kang WM, Ma ZQ, Ye X, Tian SB, et al. Significance of serum pepsinogens as a biomarker for gastric cancer and atrophic gastritis screening: a systematic review and meta-analysis. PLoS One. 2015;10: e0142080.
24. Chiang TH, Chiu SY, Chen SL, Yen AM, Fann JC, Liu CY, et al. Serum pepsinogen as a predictor for gastric cancer death: A 16-Year community-based cohort study. J Clin Gastroenterol. 2018. https://doi.org/10.1097/MCG.0000000000000992 [Epub ahead of print].
25. Jun JK, Choi KS, Lee HY, Suh M, Park B, Song SH, et al. Effectiveness of the Korean National Cancer Screening Program in reducing gastric cancer mortality. Gastroenterology. 2017;152:1319–28 e7.
26. Zhang X, Li M, Chen S, et al. Endoscopic screening in Asian countries is associated with reduced gastric cancer mortality: A meta-analysis and systematic review. Gastroenterology. 2018;155:347–54 e9.

27. Malfertheiner P, Megraud F, O'Morain CA, Gisbert JP, Kuipers EJ, Axon AT,
     European Helicobacter and Microbiota Study Group and Consensus panel,
     et al. Management of Helicobacter pylori infection--the Maastricht IV/
     Florence consensus report. Gut. 2012;61:646–64.

28. Sugano K, Tack J, Kuipers EJ, Graham DY, El-Omar EM, Miura S, faculty
     members of Kyoto Global Consensus Conference, et al. Kyoto global
     consensus report on helicobacter pylori gastritis. Gut. 2015;64:1353–67.

29. Asada K, Nakajima T, Shimazu T, Yamamichi N, Maekita T, Yokoi C, et al.
     Demonstration of the usefulness of epigenetic cancer risk prediction by a
     multicentre prospective cohort study. Gut. 2015;64:388–96.

30. Maeda M, Yamashita S, Shimazu T, Iida N, Takeshima H, Nakajima T, et al.
     Novel epigenetic markers for gastric cancer risk stratification in individuals
     after helicobacter pylori eradication. Gastric Cancer. 2018. https://doi.org/10.
     1007/s10120-018-0803-4 [Epub ahead of print].

31. Yamashita S, Kishino T, Takahashi T, Shimazu T, Charvat H, Kakugawa Y, et al.
     Genetic and epigenetic alterations in normal tissues have differential impacts
     on cancer risk among tissues. Proc Natl Acad Sci U S A. 2018;115:1328–33.

19

The monocyte-macrophage-mast cell axis in dengue pathogenesis

Shu-Wen Wan[1], Betty A. Wu-Hsieh[2], Yee-Shin Lin[3,4], Wen-Yu Chen[2], Yan Huang[5] and Robert Anderson[3,5,6*]

Abstract

Dengue virus, the causative agent of dengue disease which may have hemorrhagic complications, poses a global health threat. Among the numerous target cells for dengue virus in humans are monocytes, macrophages and mast cells which are important regulators of vascular integrity and which undergo dramatic cellular responses after infection by dengue virus. The strategic locations of these three cell types, inside blood vessels (monocytes) or outside blood vessels (macrophages and mast cells) allow them to respond to dengue virus infection with the production of both intracellular and secretory factors which affect virus replication, vascular permeability and/or leukocyte extravasation. Moreover, the expression of Fc receptors on the surface of monocytes, macrophages and mast cells makes them important target cells for antibody-enhanced dengue virus infection which is a major risk factor for severe dengue disease, involving hemorrhage. Collectively, these features of monocytes, macrophages and mast cells contribute to both beneficial and harmful responses of importance to understanding and controlling dengue infection and disease.

Keywords: Dengue pathogenesis, Mast cell, Monocyte, Macrophage, Vascular leakage

Introduction

Dengue is the most common mosquito-transmitted viral infectious disease, and therefore represents a major global health threat, especially in tropical and subtropical areas of the world. Over the past several decades, there has been an increase in dengue cases due to many factors, including increased air travel and climate change. It has been estimated that there are 390 million infections per year, of which 96 million cases show clinical manifestations [1]. Dengue virus (DENV) is a member of the Flavivirus genus of the Flaviviridae family and its genome is a single-stranded, positive-sense RNA, which encodes three structural proteins: envelope (E), premembrane/membrane (prM/M) and capsid (C) proteins, and seven nonstructural (NS) proteins [2]. There are at least four serotypes of DENV, all of which can cause disease. Most dengue patients present with dengue fever (DF) including fever, headache, bone pain and skin rash, but some may progress to life-threatening dengue hemorrhagic fever (DHF) or dengue shock syndrome (DSS) with major features of high levels of proinflammatory cytokines, vascular leakage, thrombocytopenia, hemorrhage, and hypotensive shock [3, 4]. There is still a demand for satisfactory vaccines and antiviral drugs. Although there is a licensed vaccine and several ongoing vaccine candidates in clinical trials, they confer only partial protection against DENV infection by some serotypes and may carry the risk of antibody-dependent enhancement (ADE) [5, 6]. The difficulty of eliciting balanced efficacy of neutralizing antibodies against all four DENV serotypes remains a major concern.

Both innate and adaptive immune responses to DENV play significant roles in protection against DENV, but can also elicit pathological responses which may worsen disease [2, 7]. Understanding the mechanisms that regulate immune-mediated protection versus pathogenesis is critical for the development of safe and effective dengue vaccines and therapeutic agents [4, 7]. DENV can perturb vascular endothelium by multiple mechanisms, including vasoactive factors from intravascular cells such as monocytes and lymphocytes, and from extravascular cells such as mast cells and tissue macrophages. Various factors produced by T cells, monocytes, macrophages, and mast cells have been proposed to increase vascular permeability, including tumor necrosis factor (TNF), IL-1β, IL-6, CXCL8 (IL-8), macrophage migration inhibitory factor (MIF), CCL2 (also known as monocyte chemoattractant protein-1,

* Correspondence: robert.anderson@dal.ca
[3]Department of Microbiology and Immunology, College of Medicine, National Cheng Kung University, Tainan, Taiwan
[5]Department of Microbiology & Immunology, Dalhousie University, Halifax, NS B3H 4R2, Canada
Full list of author information is available at the end of the article

MCP-1), high mobility group box-1 (HMGB-1) and matrix metalloproteinases [4, 8].

Although DENV infects several cell types, monocytes, macrophages and mast cells are major responders to DENV infection by producing potent immunological mediators, including cytokines, chemokines, lipid-derived mediators and more. By virtue of cell surface expressed Fc receptors they can also function as major amplifiers of DENV infection in the presence of subneutralizing levels of antibody by the mechanism of ADE. In this review, we will focus on cells and cellular networks encompassing monocytes, macrophages, and mast cells that can uniquely amplify DENV infection by ADE and modulate pathogenesis by release of cytokines, chemokines, proteases and other factors.

The monocyte-macrophage-mast cell axis

Monocytes (and monocyte-derived cells including macrophages) as well as mast cells originate from bone marrow common myeloid progenitors (CMPs) by two distinct pathways. Monocytes differentiate from CMP-derived granulocyte/monocyte progenitors (GMPs) while mast cells develop from CMP- or GMP-derived mast cell progenitors (MCPs) which home to peripheral tissues where they progress to mature mast cells [9]. Mature mast cells, like their precursor MCPs, express the stem cell factor receptor CD117 (c-kit) and the high affinity FcεR but differ from MCPs most notably by their high content of granules [10]. While monocytes remain largely in the circulation, monocyte-derived cells (including macrophages) as well as mast cells are resident in the tissues. All three cell types are potent producers of cytokines, chemokines and other factors some of which affect vascular integrity. Their locations either within or in close proximity to blood vessels as well as their potent innate immune responses to DENV infection allows them to function as an "axis" in regulating the fine balance between virus replication/suppression and disease.

Monocytes and DENV

Peripheral blood mononuclear cells, particularly monocytes have long been recognized as major targets of DENV infection and amplification [11–14], especially in the presence of low levels of dengue-specific antibody. The dramatic enhancement by dengue antibody of DENV replication in monocytes and certain other cells is known as ADE [15, 16]. DENV comprises four serotypes (designated 1–4) against each of which the respective homotypic antiserum is much more effective than heterotypic antiserum in virus neutralization. ADE is hypothesized to contribute to heightened dengue disease severity and is believed to arise upon sequential infection of an individual with two different DENV serotypes in which antibody produced against the first serotype enhances

infection of the second. The formation of virus-antibody complexes in such individuals gives rise to increased virus replication in cells bearing Fc receptors (eg. monocytes and a select number of other cells), triggering amplified virus- and immune-mediated pathogenic effects. In concordance with the ADE hypothesis is a study showing higher numbers of FcγRII bearing DENV-infected monocytes in DHF compared to DF patients [14]. Single nucleotide polymorphisms in the FcγRII gene are also associated with altered susceptibility to severe dengue disease [17].

ADE of DENV infection has been differentiated into intrinsic and extrinsic components, denoting intra- and extracellular events respectively [18, 19]. Extrinsic ADE is believed to result from increased virus binding and internalization via virus-antibody complex ligation of Fc receptors. Intrinsic ADE, which results from signaling through ligated FcRs, is postulated to suppress antiviral responses, selectively enhance cytokine production (particularly IL-10) and enhance virus replication [19]. Additional or alternative mechanisms may also be involved [20].

Infection of monocytes by DENV is dependent on monocyte phenotype, as defined by relative expression levels of certain protein markers which are associated with differentiation or activation status [14, 21, 22]. Human monocytes are in fact a heterogeneous population which can be grouped into at least three subsets [23, 24]. One study found DENV infection predominantly in one subset of monocytes expressing CD14, CD32, CD86 and CD11c [14]. Another study reported upregulation of CD14 and CD16 in DENV-infected blood monocytes which mediate B cell to plasmablast differentiation and production of IgM and IgG [22]. However, another study reported no increase in blood CD14+ CD16+ monocytes [25]. A correlation between DENV-induced monocyte activation and severity of disease has been reported [14].

DENV infection of monocytes triggers the release of numerous immunological factors, some of which modulate the function of other cells, particularly vascular endothelial cells. Endothelial cells are activated by TNF released by antibody-enhanced DENV-infected monocytes [26]. Circulating TNF levels are altered in severely afflicted dengue patients [27–29] and TNF is a crucial factor in DENV-induced hemorrhage in a mouse model [30]. Moreover, human genetic studies of cytokine gene polymorphisms highlight a strong role for TNF in the severity of dengue disease [17].

In addition to TNF, other monocyte-secreted factors can prime or trigger endothelial cell permeability leading to vascular leakage, a major hallmark of severe dengue disease. Other cells including lymphocytes and endothelial cells themselves can further contribute to vascular leakage via the secretion of similar or other vasoactive factors. Which of these factors predominate in triggering dengue-associated endothelial permeability is widely debated, but likely candidates include vascular endothelial growth factor (VEGF), platelet activating factor (PAF), leukotrienes, matrix metalloproteinase-9 (MMP-9), sphingosine-1-phosphate (S1P), DENV NS1 protein (reviewed in [8]) as well as MIF [31] and glycosaminoglycans such as hyaluronic acid and heparan sulfate [32]. The dominant source(s) of these factors awaits definitive identification, but likely includes monocytes, lymphocytes, endothelial cells and platelets. Platelets, which have been shown to undergo marked changes in protein expression during dengue infection [33], may also enhance cyto/chemokine production by DENV-infected monocytes through a contact-dependent mechanism [34].

A picture of complex cellular interplay during dengue infection is beginning to emerge. For example, dengue-infected monocyte-derived dendritic cells are able to activate natural killer (NK) cells which in turn may suppress DENV infection of monocytes by a mechanism involving interferon (IFN)-γ [35]. DENV replication in monocytes may also be suppressed by NK cell activation through a TRAIL-dependent mechanism augmented by type I IFNs [36]. On the other hand, monocyte-derived dermal macrophages bind and internalize DENV into early phagosomes but do not permit virus replication and may therefore have a role in sequestration and early control of the virus. Such DENV-exposed dermal macrophages apparently do not produce IFN-α [37] and therefore likely restrict virus replication in themselves without conferring antiviral resistance on other cells.

Monocyte-derived cells do not always have a protective role in DENV infection. In the mouse model, monocytes which migrate to the virus inoculation site in the dermis and differentiate into dendritic cells may become fresh targets for virus replication in the skin [38, 39].

It is important to note that DENV-induced cellular (including monocytic) infiltration into the skin is not generalized, but rather is restricted to the site of virus inoculation as indicated by studies on mice [38, 39] as well as cynomolgus macaques [25]. Although limited, studies on humans also indicate a lack of widespread cellular infiltration into skin even in patients showing severe dengue disease, i.e. DSS [25].

Monocytes and monocyte-derived cells therefore play seemingly synergistic as well as opposing roles in dengue disease. In addition to their important beneficial role in virus clearance by activating T cells in the draining lymph node [40], they may also contribute either negatively or positively to virus replication in the skin.

Role of apoptosis in DENV-monocyte interactions
Apoptosis of peripheral blood mononuclear cells (PBMCs), including lymphocytes and monocytes as well as phagocytic engulfment of apoptotic cells were noted in children with acute DENV infection [41]. Such apoptosis was proposed to represent a modulating mechanism for both virus replication as well as cell-mediated immune responses [41]. Apoptosis has also been observed in DENV-infected monocyte and/or macrophage cultures [42–46]. Multiple mechanisms of apoptosis induction have been proposed including components of both the intrinsic and extrinsic pathways. Caspase-8 activation and concomitant TNF production has been reported in DENV-infected monocyte-like U937 cells [43]. Caspase-1 has been implicated in both IL-1β production and pyroptosis in DENV-infected monocytes [47]. IL-1β is a known activator of endothelial cells and, along with monocyte-produced TNF [26], could contribute to vascular permeability in dengue disease.

Macrophages and DENV
Jessie et al. [48] identified DENV antigen and RNA in macrophages, multinucleated and reactive lymphoid cells in the spleen, Kupffer cells and sinusoid endothelial cells of liver, and macrophages and endothelial cells in the lungs of human autopsied and biopsied samples. Balsitis et al. [49] identified DENV NS3 protein in phagocytes of spleen and lymph nodes, in alveolar macrophages in the lungs, and in perivascular cells in the brains from dengue autopsy cases. An in vitro study also showed that primary human peripheral monocytes and splenic macrophages are permissive for DENV [50]. The mannose receptor on primary human macrophages that binds to the envelope protein of DENV through its carbohydrate-recognition domain may be responsible for recognition and uptake of the virus [51]. The observation that IL-4 treatment renders human dermal macrophages and dendritic cells isolated from healthy human abdominal skin permissive to DENV infection [52] could be the result of upregulation of the mannose receptor on macrophages by IL-4 [53].

In $Stat1^{-/-}$ mice infected with DENV, Chen et al. identified CLEC5A as a receptor for DENV [54]. Blocking CLEC5A protected mice from DENV-induced pathology and death [54]. CLEC5A has also been identified as the receptor that mediates DENV-induced IL-1β on GM-CSF-stimulated human monocyte-derived macrophages [55].

In AG129 mice infected subcutaneously with DENV2 (PL046 or mouse-adapted D2S10), viral E and NS1 proteins are detected in F4/80$^+$CD11b$^+$ macrophages and CD11c$^+$ dendritic cells in the spleen and other lymphoid tissues during the early phase of infection [56]. By inoculation of labeled DENV intravenously to AG129 mice, Prestwood et al. [57] found that macrophages, initially in lymphoid tissues, especially in the spleen, are the main virus targets. In the later phase of infection, however, macrophages in non-lymphoid tissues also become targets of DENV replication. In wild-type mice infected by DENV2 through the intradermal route, both macrophages and endothelial cells are targets of the virus [30].

Macrophages are recruited to the vicinity of endothelium during hemorrhage development [58]. Their recruitment and response to the virus has a profound impact on the pathogenesis of hemorrhage [30].

Cytokine production by macrophages in response to DENV

Human monocyte-derived macrophages infected with DENV in vitro produce TNF, IFN-α, IL-1β, CXCL8 (IL-8), IL-12, CCL3 (MIP-1α) and CCL5 (Regulated on Activation Normal T cell Expressed and Secreted, RANTES) [12]. Autopsy tissues from dengue patients showed elevated levels of IFN-γ and TNF expressing cells in livers, lungs and kidneys [59] and DENV RNA was detected in Kupffer cells producing these two cytokines [59]. The relationship between TNF and hemorrhage is worth noting. An early study in Thai children showed that plasma level of soluble TNF receptor (sTNFR) detected at < 72 h of fever is higher in children who developed DHF than those who had DF and TNF was detectable more often in children with DHF than with DF and children with fever from non-dengue-related illness [60]. TNF, which activates endothelial cells, is also produced by DENV-infected monocytes [26] and mast cells [61]. In a dengue hemorrhagic mouse model, skins obtained from hemorrhagic sites express higher levels of TNF transcripts and protein than that from non-hemorrhagic sites and TNF deficiency impedes DENV-induced hemorrhage development [30]. Immunofluorescence staining of hemorrhage tissues revealed that TNF co-localizes with macrophages and DENV infection of macrophages in vitro also induces TNF production [30]. These data demonstrate that TNF is important in severe dengue in humans as well as hemorrhage development in the mouse.

Role of apoptosis in DENV-macrophage interactions

Human liver Kupffer cells respond to DENV infection with cytokine production and apoptosis [62]. Although DENV replication is low or absent in cultured Kupffer cells [62], DENV antigen is detectable in Kupffer cells and hepatocytes in human autopsy studies [63]. Phagocytic Kupffer cells may also play a role in clearance of virus-induced apoptotic bodies in infected tissues [64].

Apoptosis is also observed in endothelial cells which are important targets of monocyte/macrophage action. Importantly, TNF and DENV-induced endothelial cell death resulted in alteration of endothelial permeability and pan-caspase treatment reversed its effect [58]. These results demonstrate that infection of endothelial cells by DENV in the presence of TNF changes endothelial permeability through caspase-dependent cell death. In the hemorrhage mouse model, hemorrhage development is accompanied by macrophage recruitment and endothelial cell death [58]. Macrophage production of TNF in the

vicinity of endothelium that is infected with DENV may enhance endothelial cell death which contributes to hemorrhage development.

It is of interest to note that DENV NS2B/3 protease enzymatic activity is critical to DENV-induced endothelial cell death [65]. DENV NS2B/3 protease cleaves host cell IκBα and IκBβ. By inducing IκBα and IκBβ cleavage and IκB kinase activation, enabling p50 and p65 translocation to the nucleus, DENV NS2B/3 protease activates NF-κB which results in endothelial cell death. Injecting DENV NS2B/3 protease packaged in adenovirus-associated virus-9 intradermally to mice induces macrophage infiltration, endothelial cell death and hemorrhage development [65]. Thus, the presence of TNF-producing macrophages near blood vessels contributes to DENV protease-induced endothelial cell death and hemorrhage development. A depiction of the possible events triggered by DENV infection that lead to hemorrhage development is shown in Fig. 1.

Mast cells and DENV

Mast cells are well known for their involvement in inflammation and allergy but recent studies indicate a broader role in immunological responses [66–69]. The abundance of mast cells at mucosal sites and skin confers on them a sentinel function for the early detection and disposition of invading pathogens. Upon appropriate stimulation, mast cells selectively produce and secrete a variety of mediators including chemokines, cytokines, lipid mediators and granule associated products. Mast cells reside mainly in the tissues and have been shown to associate closely with blood vessels [70] and nerves [71]. Human mast cells can express both FcεRI [72, 73] and some Fcγ receptors including FcγRI [74, 75] and FcγRII [76, 77] and contain FcγRIII mRNA [76].

Mast cells have aroused speculation for many years as to their possible involvement in dengue pathogenesis. Mast cells are located in the skin and mucosa which are the first line of defense against pathogens. In addition to dendritic cells (including Langerhans cells) and macrophages [78], mast cells also encounter DENV early in infection [79]. DHF patients exhibit increased levels of urinary and plasma histamine which is a major granule-associated mediator from mast cells [80, 81]. Levels of mast cell-derived VEGF and proteases are also increased in DSS patients [82]. Furthermore, mast cell-derived chymase also promotes vascular leakage in a DENV-infected mouse model [83]. In vitro studies indicated that antibody-enhanced DENV infection of mast cells selectively induces production of chemokines including CCL3, CCL4 and CCL5 [84, 85], as well as cytokines including IL-6, IL-1β and TNF [61, 86]. TNF produced from antibody-enhanced DENV infection of mast cells as well as of monocytes can trigger endothelial cell activation [26, 61]. These findings suggest that mast cells

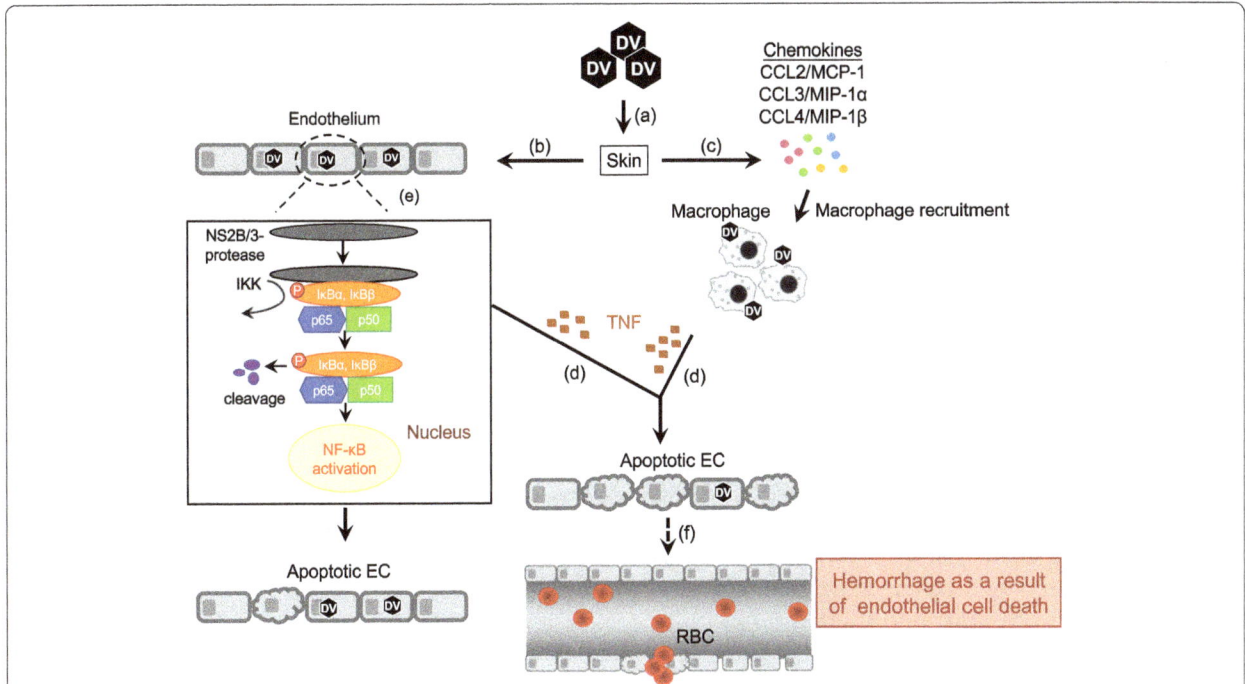

Fig. 1 Dengue virus interactions with macrophages and endothelial cells that lead to hemorrhage development. **a** Inoculation by mosquito bite of DENV (DV) into the skin. **b** The virus infects several cell types including endothelial cells (ECs). **c** DENV induces production of chemokines that attract macrophages. **d** DENV stimulates macrophages to produce TNF. **e** DENV NS2B/3 protease interacts with and cleaves cellular IκBα/IκBβ. DENV NS2B/3 protease also activates IKK, which phosphorylates IκBα and IκBβ. IκBα/IκBβ cleavage enables p50 and p65 translocation into the nucleus, thereby activating NF-κB which results in endothelial cell death. **f** The presence of TNF in the microenvironment enhances DENV-primed EC apoptosis. Endothelium damage/increased vascular permeability results in hemorrhage development. Solid arrows represent events that enhance endothelium damage. Dotted arrow indicates an event that is speculated to occur [30, 58, 65]

likely play a role in vascular function as well as leukocyte recruitment during DENV infection.

Most significantly, mast cells are susceptible to antibody-enhanced DENV infection via the mast cell FcγRII [87]. Mast cell responses to antibody-enhanced DENV infection have revealed potent immunoregulatory activities of these cells, including secretion of TNF [61] and the chemokines CCL3, CCL4 and CCL5 [84]. Together with other published reports [67, 68, 88, 89], these studies reinforce the role of mast cells as innate immune effectors in response to a variety of virus infections. Chemokines such as CCL3, CCL4 and CCL5 are important for the trafficking of leukocytes such as monocytes, T cells, and NK cells, all of which are suggested to play important roles in dengue infection. Serum levels of CCL3, CCL4 and CCL5 are altered [90–93] and tissue levels of chemokine-producing cells are elevated [59, 93] in dengue patients. In particular, serum levels of CCL4 are increased in mild dengue and may be of good prognostic value [93].

Induction of innate immune factors in DENV-infected mast cells

The cellular molecules by which DENV is detected by the innate immune system have been partly characterized. RIG-I or MDA5 have been implicated in the production of

CCL5 and CXCL8 by a number of viruses, including DENV as well as viral RNA homologs [85, 94, 95]. Upregulation of RIG-I and MDA5 mRNA has been demonstrated after DENV infection in a rodent mast cell line [79] as well as antibody-enhanced DENV infection of human mast cells [85]. Protein kinase dsRNA dependent (PKR) recognizes dsRNA and can mediate the inhibition of protein translation in response to type I IFNs and DENV dsRNA [96]. Together, all three RNA sensors provide a mechanism by which the innate immune system induces the antiviral response when the host is exposed to DENV.

In addition to the above-noted RNA sensors RIG-I, MDA5 and PKR, mast cells possess a battery of pattern recognition receptors the individual expression of which varies according to the host source and associated tissue or organ [97–100]. Human mast cells express the RNA sensor, Toll-like receptor (TLR)3 [89]. Recognition of viral dsRNA by mast cell TLR3 leads to signaling via TRIF to TBK1/IKKε to activate both IRF-3 and nuclear factor-κB (NF-κB) promoting the production of IFN stimulated genes, cytokines and chemokines. In the case of human mast cell lines HMC-1 and LAD-2 as well as primary peripheral CD34[+] mast cells, responses to extracellular polyinosinic·polycytidylic (polyI:C) were shown to involve upregulation of type I IFNs by RT-PCR [89].

Mast cells activated by polyI:C have also been reported to influence CD8[+] T cell recruitment [88]. Furthermore, polyI:C-exposed or reovirus-infected mast cells recruit NK cells in a CXCL8-dependent manner [101]. Along with other RNA sensors, TLR3 is also upregulated in antibody-enhanced DENV infection of mast cells [85].

Antibody-enhanced DENV-infected mast cells can produce sufficient amounts of type I IFNs to protect neighboring cells from infection [85]. The upregulation of RNA sensors such as RIG-I and MDA5 appears to be key for the suppression of DENV replication via establishment of the antiviral state [102–104]. The upregulation of PKR in mast cells upon antibody-enhanced DENV infection [85], is also consistent with induction of the antiviral state since protein translation inhibition during DENV infection is dependent on the PKR substrate, eIF2α [96]. The possibility that tissue-resident mast cells can initiate this vital response would therefore allow them to confer type I IFN-mediated protection upon neighboring cells at the tissue site early after virus inoculation.

Roles of mast cells in DENV clearance and vascular leakage

After DENV infection, mast cell-deficient mice showed increased viral burden within draining lymph nodes, compared with wild-type mice. In addition, the recruitment of NK and NKT cells into the DENV-infected skin was dependent on mast cell activation [79]. Such mast cell-dependent immune responses facilitate DENV clearance. Compared to wild-type mice, mast cell-deficient mice showed enhanced DENV infection, CCL2 production and macrophage infiltration at the skin inoculation site, suggesting other mechanisms for the interplay between mast cells and tissue macrophages to modulate DENV replication [105]. Therefore, during the initial stage, mast cells may play crucial roles in immune surveillance for DENV by promoting viral clearance and restricting viral replication (Fig. 2).

Several mast cell-derived mediators, such as tryptase, chymase and VEGF contribute to dengue disease severity [82]. Serum chymase levels could be a predictive biomarker of DHF in pediatric and adult patients [106]. DENV-infected mice show activated degranulated tissue mast cells. as well as elevated systemic levels of various vasoactive products, including chymase, histamine, and serotonin [83]. After DENV infection, mast cell-deficient mice showed significantly reduced vascular permeability compared to mast cell-sufficient controls [83]. Hence, at later stages of systemic infection, mast cells might play other important roles in DENV-induced vascular leakage (Fig. 2). Sub-neutralizing dengue-specific antibodies not only promote DENV infection but also enhance mast cell

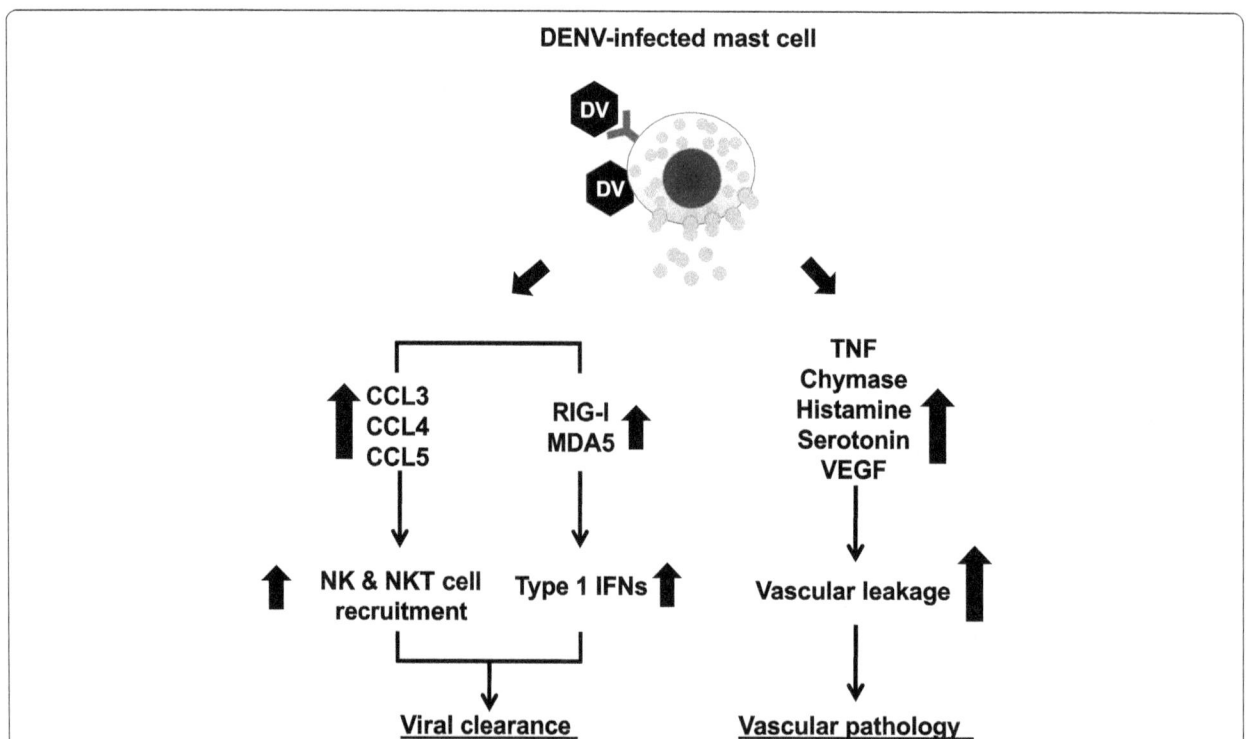

Fig. 2 The dual roles of mast cells in dengue infection. Mast cells respond to DENV (DV) infection via RNA sensors (RIG-I and MDA5) which are involved in type I IFN production to inhibit viral replication. DENV-infected mast cells also secrete chemokines including CCL3, CCL4 and CCL5, which recruit NK and NKT cells to help clear the virus. However, if initial control mechanisms fail, the virus may spread to other organs. DENV-infected mast cells in these organs secrete vasoactive products, including TNF, chymase, histamine, and serotonin and VEGF which contribute to vascular permeability

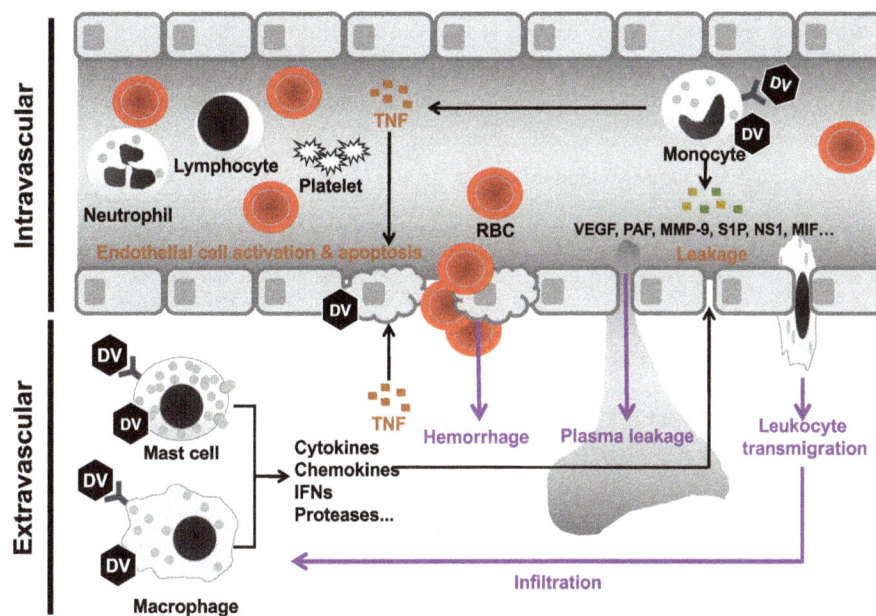

Fig. 3 Intra- and extravascular cells in the pathogenesis of dengue. DENV (DV) infection of monocytes triggers the intravascular release of numerous immunological factors to modulate the function of vascular endothelial cells. Besides TNF, other monocyte-secreted factors can prime or trigger endothelial cell permeability leading to vascular leakage and leukocyte transmigration to extravascular tissues. Extravascular mast cells and macrophages are target cells for DENV infection which elicits production of cytokines, chemokines, lipid-derived mediators and proteases which also contribute to endothelial cell permeability. In addition, macrophage production of TNF enhances DENV-infected endothelial cell death which leads to hemorrhage development

activation in an FcγR-dependent manner [87, 107]. During secondary DENV infection, antibody-mediated mast cell activation may therefore also contribute to the enhanced vascular pathology in severe dengue (Fig. 3).

The involvement of mast cells in dengue pathogenesis suggests they may be potential therapeutic targets. The mast cell-stabilizing drug, ketotifen, not only improves DENV-induced vasculopathy [83] but also reverses the DENV-induced host response without suppressing memory T cell formation [108]. Furthermore, antibodies against DENV NS1 provide protection in mice against DENV challenge and reduce mast cell degranulation and macrophage infiltration as well as the production of chemokines including CCL2, CCL5, and CXCL10 (IP-10) at local skin DENV infection sites [109].

Role of apoptosis in DENV-mast cell interactions

Antibody-enhanced DENV-infected mast cell-like KU812 cells show dramatic apoptosis [110]. Interestingly, apoptosis is observed mainly in DENV antigen-negative cells suggesting the involvement of apoptotic mediators produced by DENV-infected cells. Alternatively, apoptosis may be triggered very early in some DENV-infected cells so that cell death occurs prior to appreciable virus replication. Thus, as with monocytes and macrophages, apoptosis of mast cells

in DENV infection likely plays a role in regulating mast cell numbers and responses.

Conclusions

While differing in cellular developmental pathways, monocytes/macrophages and mast cells share intriguing features which come into play in vascular disease triggered by DENV infection. Their potent production of cytokines, chemokines and various vasoactive mediators in response to DENV makes them key orchestrators of some of the pathological vascular changes which occur in severe dengue disease. In particular, their expression of Fc receptors makes them powerful amplifiers of DENV replication as well as of virus-induced innate immune factors some of which act directly on vascular endothelium and others of which regulate the extent of virus replication.

Abbreviations

CCL: Chemokine (C-C motif) ligand; CMP: Common myeloid progenitor; CXCL: Chemokine (C-X-C motif) ligand; DENV: Dengue virus; DF: Dengue fever; DHF: Dengue hemorrhagic fever (DHF); dsRNA: double-stranded ribonucleic acid; DSS: Dengue shock syndrome; eIF: eukaryotic initiation factor; GMP: Granulocyte/monocyte progenitor; IFN: Interferon; IL: Interleukin; MIF: Macrophage migration inhibitory factor; MMP: Matrix metalloproteinase; NK: Natural killer; NS1: Non-structural protein 1; PKR: Protein kinase R; TLR: Toll-like receptor; TNF: Tumor necrosis factor

Acknowledgements
The authors gratefully acknowledge the contributions of numerous colleagues and collaborators, listed in previous publications.

Funding
Work performed in the authors' laboratories was supported by Grants from the Ministry of Science and Technology, Taiwan and the Canadian Institutes of Health Research.

Authors' contributions
All authors discussed and designed the concept. RA, SWW, BAWH, YSL, WYC and YH collected information, prepared and wrote the manuscript. All authors read and approved the final manuscript.

Competing interests
The authors declare that they have no competing interests.

Author details
[1]School of Medicine, College of Medicine, I-Shou University, Kaohsiung, Taiwan. [2]Graduate Institute of Immunology, College of Medicine, National Taiwan University, Taipei, Taiwan. [3]Department of Microbiology and Immunology, College of Medicine, National Cheng Kung University, Tainan, Taiwan. [4]Center of Infectious Disease and Signaling Research, National Cheng Kung University, Tainan, Taiwan. [5]Department of Microbiology & Immunology, Dalhousie University, Halifax, NS B3H 4R2, Canada. [6]Canadian Center for Vaccinology, Dalhousie University, Halifax, Canada.

References

1. Bhatt S, Gething PW, Brady OJ, Messina JP, Farlow AW, Moyes CL, et al. The global distribution and burden of dengue. Nature. 2013;496:504–7.
2. Rothman AL. Dengue: defining protective versus pathologic immunity. J Clin Invest. 2004;113:946–51.
3. Halstead SB. Dengue. Lancet. 2007;370:1644–52.
4. Guzman MG, Harris E. Dengue. Lancet. 2015;385:453–65.
5. Guy B, Lang J, Saville M, Jackson N. Vaccination against dengue: challenges and current developments. Annu Rev Med. 2016;67:387–404.
6. Vannice KS, Durbin A, Hombach J. Status of vaccine research and development of vaccines for dengue. Vaccine. 2016;34:2934–8.
7. Elong Ngono A, Shresta S. Immune response to dengue and zika. Annu Rev Immunol. 2018;36:279–308.
8. Malavige GN, Ogg GS. Pathogenesis of vascular leak in dengue virus infection. Immunology. 2017;151:261–9.
9. Voehringer D. Protective and pathological roles of mast cells and basophils. Nat Rev Immunol. 2013;13:362–75.
10. Dahlin JS, Hallgren J. Mast cell progenitors: origin, development and migration to tissues. Mol Immunol. 2015;63:9–17.
11. Halstead SB, O'Rourke EJ. Dengue viruses and mononuclear phagocytes. I. Infection enhancement by non-neutralizing antibody. J Exp Med. 1977;146:201–17.
12. Chen YC, Wang SY. Activation of terminally differentiated human monocytes/macrophages by dengue virus: productive infection, hierarchical production of innate cytokines and chemokines, and the synergistic effect of lipopolysaccharide. J Virol. 2002;76:9877–87.
13. Kou Z, Quinn M, Chen H, Rodrigo WW, Rose RC, Schlesinger JJ, et al. Monocytes, but not T or B cells, are the principal target cells for dengue

virus (DV) infection among human peripheral blood mononuclear cells. J Med Virol. 2008;80:134–46.
14. Durbin AP, Vargas MJ, Wanionek K, Hammond SN, Gordon A, Rocha C, et al. Phenotyping of peripheral blood mononuclear cells during acute dengue illness demonstrates infection and increased activation of monocytes in severe cases compared to classic dengue fever. Virology. 2008;376:429–35.
15. Halstead SB, Chow JS, Marchette NJ. Immunological enhancement of dengue virus replication. Nat New Biol. 1973;243:24–6.
16. Halstead SB, O'Rourke EJ. Antibody-enhanced dengue virus infection in primate leukocytes. Nature. 1977;265:739–41.
17. Xavier-Carvalho C, Cardoso CC, de Souza Kehdy F, Pacheco AG, Moraes MO. Host genetics and dengue fever. Infect Genet Evol. 2017;56:99–110.
18. Halstead SB. Dengue antibody-dependent enhancement: knowns and unknowns. Microbiol Spectr. 2014;2:AID-0022-2014.
19. Ubol S, Phuklia W, Kalayanarooj S, Modhiran N. Mechanisms of immune evasion induced by a complex of dengue virus and preexisting enhancing antibodies. J Infect Dis. 2010;201:923–35.
20. Kou Z, Lim JY, Beltramello M, Quinn M, Chen H, Liu S, et al. Human antibodies against dengue enhance dengue viral infectivity without suppressing type I interferon secretion in primary human monocytes. Virology. 2011;410:240–7.
21. O'Sullivan MA, Killen HM. The differentiation state of monocytic cells affects their susceptibility to infection and the effects of infection by dengue virus. J Gen Virol. 1994;75:2387–92.
22. Kwissa M, Nakaya HI, Onlamoon N, Wrammert J, Villinger F, Perng GC, et al. Dengue virus infection induces expansion of a CD14(+)CD16(+) monocyte population that stimulates plasmablast differentiation. Cell Host Microbe. 2014;16:115–27.
23. Saha P, Geissmann F. Toward a functional characterization of blood monocytes. Immunol Cell Biol. 2011;89:2–4.
24. Ziegler-Heitbrock L, Hofer TP. Toward a refined definition of monocyte subsets. Front Immunol. 2013;4:23.
25. Duyen HTL, Cerny D, Trung DT, Pang J, Velumani S, Toh YX, et al. Skin dendritic cell and T cell activation associated with dengue shock syndrome. Sci Rep. 2017;7:14224.
26. Anderson R, Wang S, Osiowy C, Issekutz AC. Activation of endothelial cells via antibody-enhanced dengue virus infection of peripheral blood monocytes. J Virol. 1997;71:4226–32.
27. Bethell DB, Flobbe K, Cao XT, Day NP, Pham TP, Buurman WA, et al. Pathophysiologic and prognostic role of cytokines in dengue hemorrhagic fever. J Infect Dis. 1998;177:778–82.
28. Hober D, Poli L, Roblin B, Gestas P, Chungue E, Granic G, et al. Serum levels of tumor necrosis factor-alpha (TNF-alpha), interleukin-6 (IL-6), and interleukin-1 beta (IL-1 beta) in dengue-infected patients. Am J Trop Med Hyg. 1993;48:324–31.
29. Yadav M, Kamath KR, Iyngkaran N, Sinniah M. Dengue haemorrhagic fever and dengue shock syndrome: are they tumour necrosis factor-mediated disorders? FEMS MicrobiolImmunol. 1991;89:45–50.
30. Chen HC, Hofman FM, Kung JT, Lin YD, Wu-Hsieh BA. Both virus and tumor necrosis factor alpha are critical for endothelium damage in a mouse model of dengue virus-induced hemorrhage. J Virol. 2007;81:5518–26.
31. Chen HR, Chuang YC, Lin YS, Liu HS, Liu CC, Perng GC, et al. Dengue virus nonstructural protein 1 induces vascular leakage through macrophage migration inhibitory factor and autophagy. PLoS Negl Trop Dis. 2016;10:e0004828.
32. Tang TH, Alonso S, Ng LF, Thein TL, Pang VJ, Leo YS, et al. Increased serum hyaluronic acid and heparan sulfate in dengue fever: association with plasma leakage and disease severity. Sci Rep. 2017;7:46191.
33. Trugilho MRO, Hottz ED, Brunoro GVF, Teixeira-Ferreira A, Carvalho PC, Salazar GA, et al. Platelet proteome reveals novel pathways of platelet activation and platelet-mediated immunoregulation in dengue. PLoS Pathog. 2017;13:e1006385.
34. Hottz ED, Medeiros-de-Moraes IM, Vieira-de-Abreu A, de Assis EF, Vals-de-Souza R, Castro-Faria-Neto HC, et al. Platelet activation and apoptosis modulate monocyte inflammatory responses in dengue. J Immunol. 2014;193:1864–72.
35. Costa VV, Ye W, Chen Q, Teixeira MM, Preiser P, Ooi EE, et al. Dengue virus-infected dendritic cells, but not monocytes, activate natural killer cells through a contact-dependent mechanism involving adhesion molecules. MBio. 2017;8:e00741.
36. Gandini M, Petitinga-Paiva F, Marinho CF, Correa G, De Oliveira-Pinto LM, de Souza LJ, et al. Dengue virus induces NK cell activation through TRAIL expression during infection. Mediat Inflamm. 2017;2017:5649214.

37. Kwan WH, Navarro-Sanchez E, Dumortier H, Decossas M, Vachon H, dos Santos FB, et al. Dermal-type macrophages expressing CD209/DC-SIGN show inherent resistance to dengue virus growth. PLoS Negl Trop Dis. 2008;2:e311.

38. Cerny D, Haniffa M, Shin A, Bigliardi P, Tan BK, Lee B, et al. Selective susceptibility of human skin antigen presenting cells to productive dengue virus infection. PLoS Pathog. 2014;10:e1004548.

39. Schmid MA, Harris E. Monocyte recruitment to the dermis and differentiation to dendritic cells increases the targets for dengue virus replication. PLoS Pathog. 2014;10:e1004541.

40. Tamoutounour S, Guilliams M, Montanana Sanchis F, Liu H, Terhorst D, Malosse C, et al. Origins and functional specialization of macrophages and of conventional and monocyte-derived dendritic cells in mouse skin. Immunity. 2013;39:925–38.

41. Myint KS, Endy TP, Mongkolsirichaikul D, Manomuth C, Kalayanarooj S, Vaughn DW, et al. Cellular immune activation in children with acute dengue virus infections is modulated by apoptosis. J Infect Dis. 2006;194:600–7.

42. Arias J, Valero N, Mosquera J, Montiel M, Reyes E, Larreal Y, et al. Increased expression of cytokines, soluble cytokine receptors, soluble apoptosis ligand and apoptosis in dengue. Virology. 2014;452-453:42–51.

43. Klomporn P, Panyasrivanit M, Wikan N, Smith DR. Dengue infection of monocytic cells activates ER stress pathways, but apoptosis is induced through both extrinsic and intrinsic pathways. Virology. 2011;409:189–97.

44. Levy A, Valero N, Espina LM, Anez G, Arias J, Mosquera J. Increment of interleukin 6, tumour necrosis factor alpha, nitric oxide, C-reactive protein and apoptosis in dengue. Trans R Soc Trop Med Hyg. 2010;104:16–23.

45. Espina LM, Valero NJ, Hernandez JM, Mosquera JA. Increased apoptosis and expression of tumor necrosis factor-alpha caused by infection of cultured human monocytes with dengue virus. Am J Trop Med Hyg. 2003;68:48–53.

46. Torrentes-Carvalho A, Azeredo EL, Reis SR, Miranda AS, Gandini M, Barbosa LS, et al. Dengue-2 infection and the induction of apoptosis in human primary monocytes. Mem Inst Oswaldo Cruz. 2009;104:1091–9.

47. Tan TY, Chu JJ. Dengue virus-infected human monocytes trigger late activation of caspase-1, which mediates pro-inflammatory IL-1beta secretion and pyroptosis. J Gen Virol. 2013;94:2215–20.

48. Jessie K, Fong MY, Devi S, Lam SK, Wong KT. Localization of dengue virus in naturally infected human tissues, by immunohistochemistry and in situ hybridization. J Infect Dis. 2004;189:1411–8.

49. Balsitis SJ, Coloma J, Castro G, Alava A, Flores D, McKerrow JH, et al. Tropism of dengue virus in mice and humans defined by viral nonstructural protein 3-specific immunostaining. Am J Trop Med Hyg. 2009;80:416–24.

50. Blackley S, Kou Z, Chen H, Quinn M, Rose RC, Schlesinger JJ, et al. Primary human splenic macrophages, but not T or B cells, are the principal target cells for dengue virus infection in vitro. J Virol. 2007;81:13325–34.

51. Miller JL, de Wet BJ, Martinez-Pomares L, Radcliffe CM, Dwek RA, Rudd PM, et al. The mannose receptor mediates dengue virus infection of macrophages. PLoS Pathog. 2008;4:e17.

52. Schaeffer E, Flacher V, Papageorgiou V, Decossas M, Fauny JD, Kramer M, et al. Dermal CD14(+) dendritic cell and macrophage infection by dengue virus is stimulated by Interleukin-4. J Invest Dermatol. 2015;135:1743–51.

53. Stein M, Keshav S, Harris N, Gordon S. Interleukin 4 potently enhances murine macrophage mannose receptor activity: a marker of alternative immunologic macrophage activation. J Exp Med. 1992;176:287–92.

54. Chen ST, Lin YL, Huang MT, Wu MF, Cheng SC, Lei HY, et al. CLEC5A is critical for dengue-virus-induced lethal disease. Nature. 2008;453:672–6.

55. Wu MF, Chen ST, Yang AH, Lin WW, Lin YL, Chen NJ, et al. CLEC5A is critical for dengue virus-induced inflammasome activation in human macrophages. Blood. 2013;121:95–106.

56. Kyle JL, Beatty PR, Harris E. Dengue virus infects macrophages and dendritic cells in a mouse model of infection. J Infect Dis. 2007;195:1808–17.

57. Prestwood TR, May MM, Plummer EM, Morar MM, Yauch LE, Shresta S. Trafficking and replication patterns reveal splenic macrophages as major targets of dengue virus in mice. J Virol. 2012;86:12138–47.

58. Yen YT, Chen HC, Lin YD, Shieh CC, Wu-Hsieh BA. Enhancement by tumor necrosis factor alpha of dengue virus-induced endothelial cell production of reactive nitrogen and oxygen species is key to hemorrhage development. J Virol. 2008;82:12312–24.

59. Povoa TF, Oliveira ER, Basilio-de-Oliveira CA, Nuovo GJ, Chagas VL, Salomao NG, et al. Peripheral organs of dengue fatal cases present strong pro-inflammatory response with participation of IFN-gamma-, TNF-alpha- and RANTES-producing cells. PLoS One. 2016;11:e0168973.

60. Hober D, Delannoy AS, Benyoucef S, De GD, Wattre P. High levels of sTNFR p75 and TNF alpha in dengue-infected patients. Microbiol Immunol. 1996;40:569–73.

61. Brown MG, Hermann LL, Issekutz AC, Marshall JS, Rowter D, Al-Afif A, et al. Dengue virus infection of mast cells triggers endothelial cell activation. J Virol. 2011;85:1145–50.

62. Marianneau P, Steffan AM, Royer C, Drouet MT, Jaeck D, Kirn A, et al. Infection of primary cultures of human Kupffer cells by dengue virus: no viral progeny synthesis, but cytokine production is evident. J Virol. 1999;73:5201–6.

63. Aye KS, Charngkaew K, Win N, Wai KZ, Moe K, Punyadee N, et al. Pathologic highlights of dengue hemorrhagic fever in 13 autopsy cases from Myanmar. Hum Pathol. 2014;45:1221–33.

64. Marianneau P, Flamand M, Deubel V, Despres P. Apoptotic cell death in response to dengue virus infection: the pathogenesis of dengue haemorrhagic fever revisited. Clin Diagn Virol. 1998;10:113–9.

65. Lin JC, Lin SC, Chen WY, Yen YT, Lai CW, Tao MH, et al. Dengue viral protease interaction with NF-kappaB inhibitor alpha/beta results in endothelial cell apoptosis and hemorrhage development. J Immunol. 2014;193:1258–67.

66. Marshall JS. Mast-cell responses to pathogens. Nat Rev Immunol. 2004;4:787–99.

67. Dawicki W, Marshall JS. New and emerging roles for mast cells in host defence. Curr Opin Immunol. 2007;19:31–8.

68. Metz M, Siebenhaar F, Maurer M. Mast cell functions in the innate skin immune system. Immunobiology. 2008;213:251–60.

69. Galli SJ, Tsai M. Mast cells: versatile regulators of inflammation, tissue remodeling, host defense and homeostasis. J Dermatol Sci. 2008;49:7–19.

70. Selye H. Mast cells and necrosis. Science. 1966;152:1371–2.

71. Wiesner-Menzel L, Schulz B, Vakilzadeh F, Czarnetzki BM. Electron microscopical evidence for a direct contact between nerve fibres and mast cells. Acta Derm Venereol. 1981;61:465–9.

72. Sperr WR, Bankl HC, Mundigler G, Klappacher G, Grossschmidt K, Agis H, et al. The human cardiac mast cell: localization, isolation, phenotype, and functional characterization. Blood. 1994;84:3876–84.

73. Guo CB, Kagey-Sobotka A, Lichtenstein LM, Bochner BS. Immunophenotyping and functional analysis of purified human uterine mast cells. Blood. 1992;79:708–12.

74. Okayama Y, Hagaman DD, Woolhiser M, Metcalfe DD. Further characterization of FcgammaRII and FcgammaRIII expression by cultured human mast cells. Int Arch Allergy Immunol. 2001;124:155–7.

75. Okayama Y, Kirshenbaum AS, Metcalfe DD. Expression of a functional high-affinity IgG receptor, fc gamma RI, on human mast cells: up-regulation by IFN-gamma. J Immunol. 2000;164:4332–9.

76. Okayama Y, Hagaman DD. Metcalfe DD. A comparison of mediators released or generated by IFN-gamma-treated human mast cells following aggregation of fc gamma RI or fc epsilon RI. J Immunol. 2001;166:4705–12.

77. Wedi B, Lewrick H, Butterfield JH, Kapp A. Human HMC-1 mast cells exclusively express the fc gamma RII subtype of IgG receptor. Arch Dermatol Res. 1996;289:21–7.

78. Wu SJ, Grouard-Vogel G, Sun W, Mascola JR, Brachtel E, Putvatana R, et al. Human skin Langerhans cells are targets of dengue virus infection. Nat Med. 2000;6:816–20.

79. St John AL, Rathore AP, Yap H, Ng ML, Metcalfe DD, Vasudevan SG, et al. Immune surveillance by mast cells during dengue infection promotes natural killer (NK) and NKT-cell recruitment and viral clearance. Proc Natl Acad Sci U S A. 2011;108:9190–5.

80. Tuchinda M, Dhorranintra B, Tuchinda P. Histamine content in 24-hour urine in patients with dengue haemorrhagic fever. Southeast Asian J Trop Med Public Health. 1977;8:80–3.

81. Phan DT, Ha NT, Thuc LT, Diet NH, Phu LV, Ninh LY, et al. Some changes in immunity and blood in relation to clinical states of dengue hemorrhagic fever patients in Vietnam. Haematologia (Budap). 1991;24:13–21.

82. Furuta T, Murao LA, Lan NT, Huy NT, Huong VT, Thuy TT, et al. Association of mast cell-derived VEGF and proteases in dengue shock syndrome. PLoS Negl Trop Dis. 2012;6:e1505.

83. St John AL, Rathore AP, Raghavan B, Ng ML, Abraham SN. Contributions of mast cells and vasoactive products, leukotrienes and chymase, to dengue virus-induced vascular leakage. elife. 2013;2:e00481.

84. King CA, Anderson R, Marshall JS. Dengue virus selectively induces human mast cell chemokine production. J Virol. 2002;76:8408–19.

85. Brown MG, McAlpine SM, Huang YY, Haidl ID, Al-Afif A, Marshall JS, et al. RNA sensors enable human mast cell anti-viral chemokine production and IFN-mediated protection in response to antibody-enhanced dengue virus infection. PLoS One. 2012;7:e34055.

86. King CA, Marshall JS, Alshurafa H, Anderson R. Release of vasoactive cytokines by antibody-enhanced dengue virus infection of a human mast cell/basophil line. J Virol. 2000;74:7146–50.

87. Brown MG, King CA, Sherren C, Marshall JS, Anderson R. A dominant role for FcgammaRII in antibody-enhanced dengue virus infection of human mast cells and associated CCL5 release. J Leukoc Biol. 2006;80:1242–50.

88. Orinska Z, Bulanova E, Budagian V, Metz M, Maurer M, Bulfone-Paus S. TLR3-induced activation of mast cells modulates CD8+ T-cell recruitment. Blood. 2005;106:978–87.

89. Kulka M, Alexopoulou L, Flavell RA, Metcalfe DD. Activation of mast cells by double-stranded RNA: evidence for activation through toll-like receptor 3. J Allergy Clin Immunol. 2004;114:174–82.

90. Perez AB, Garcia G, Sierra B, Alvarez M, Vazquez S, Cabrera MV, et al. IL-10 levels in dengue patients: some findings from the exceptional epidemiological conditions in Cuba. J Med Virol. 2004;73:230–4.

91. Cui L, Lee YH, Thein TL, Fang J, Pang J, Ooi EE, et al. Serum metabolomics reveals serotonin as a predictor of severe dengue in the early phase of dengue fever. PLoS Negl Trop Dis. 2016;10:e0004607.

92. van de Weg CA, Pannuti CS, de Araujo ES, van den Ham HJ, Andeweg AC, Boas LS, et al. Microbial translocation is associated with extensive immune activation in dengue virus infected patients with severe disease. PLoS Negl Trop Dis. 2013;7:e2236.

93. Bozza FA, Cruz OG, Zagne SM, Azeredo EL, Nogueira RM, Assis EF, et al. Multiplex cytokine profile from dengue patients: MIP-1beta and IFN-gamma as predictive factors for severity. BMC Infect Dis. 2008;8:86.

94. Wagoner J, Austin M, Green J, Imaizumi T, Casola A, Brasier A, et al. Regulation of CXCL-8 (interleukin-8) induction by double-stranded RNA signaling pathways during hepatitis C virus infection. J Virol. 2007;81:309–18.

95. Yoshida H, Imaizumi T, Lee SJ, Tanji K, Sakaki H, Matsumiya T, et al. Retinoic acid-inducible gene-I mediates RANTES/CCL5 expression in U373MG human astrocytoma cells stimulated with double-stranded RNA. Neurosci Res. 2007;58:199–206.

96. Diamond MS, Harris E. Interferon inhibits dengue virus infection by preventing translation of viral RNA through a PKR-independent mechanism. Virology. 2001;289:297–311.

97. Matsushima H, Yamada N, Matsue H, Shimada S. TLR3-, TLR7-, and TLR9-mediated production of proinflammatory cytokines and chemokines from murine connective tissue type skin-derived mast cells but not from bone marrow-derived mast cells. J Immunol. 2004;173:531–41.

98. McCurdy JD, Olynych TJ, Maher LH, Marshall JS. Cutting edge: distinct toll-like receptor 2 activators selectively induce different classes of mediator production from human mast cells. J Immunol. 2003;170:1625–9.

99. Kulka M, Metcalfe DD. TLR3 activation inhibits human mast cell attachment to fibronectin and vitronectin. Mol Immunol. 2006;43:1579–86.

100. Bonini S, Micera A, Iovieno A, Lambiase A, Bonini S. Expression of toll-like receptors in healthy and allergic conjunctiva. Ophthalmology. 2005;112:1528–34.

101. Burke SM, Issekutz TB, Mohan K, Lee PW, Shmulevitz M, Marshall JS. Human mast cell activation with virus-associated stimuli leads to the selective chemotaxis of natural killer cells by a CXCL8-dependent mechanism. Blood. 2008;111:5467–76.

102. Munoz-Jordan JL, Fredericksen BL. How flaviviruses activate and suppress the interferon response. Viruses. 2010;2:676–91.

103. Nasirudeen AM, Wong HH, Thien P, Xu S, Lam KP, Liu DX. RIG-I, MDA5 and TLR3 synergistically play an important role in restriction of dengue virus infection. PLoS Negl Trop Dis. 2011;5:e926.

104. Qin CF, Zhao H, Liu ZY, Jiang T, Deng YQ, Yu XD, et al. Retinoic acid inducible gene-I and melanoma differentiation-associated gene 5 are induced but not essential for dengue virus induced type I interferon response. Mol Biol Rep. 2011;38:3867–73.

105. Chu YT, Wan SW, Anderson R, Lin YS. Mast cell-macrophage dynamics in modulation of dengue virus infection in skin. Immunology. 2015;146:163–72.

106. Tissera H, Rathore APS, Leong WY, Pike BL, Warkentien TE, Farouk FS, et al. Chymase level is a predictive biomarker of dengue hemorrhagic fever in pediatric and adult patients. J Infect Dis. 2017;216:1112–21.

107. Syenina A, Jagaraj CJ, Aman SA, Sridharan A, St John AL. Dengue vascular leakage is augmented by mast cell degranulation mediated by immunoglobulin Fcgamma receptors. elife. 2015;4:e05291.

108. Morrison J, Rathore APS, Mantri CK, Aman SAB, Nishida A, St John AL. Transcriptional profiling confirms the therapeutic effects of mast cell stabilization in a dengue disease model. J Virol. 2017;91:e00617.

109. Chu YT, Wan SW, Chang YC, Lee CK, Wu-Hsieh BA, Anderson R, et al. Antibodies against nonstructural protein 1 protect mice from dengue virus-induced mast cell activation. Lab Investig. 2017;97:602–14.

110. Brown MG, Huang YY, Marshall JS, King CA, Hoskin DW, Anderson R. Dramatic caspase-dependent apoptosis in antibody-enhanced dengue virus infection of human mast cells. J Leukoc Biol. 2009;85:71–80.

20

Microbiota dysbiosis and barrier dysfunction in inflammatory bowel disease and colorectal cancers: exploring a common ground hypothesis

Linda Chia-Hui Yu (ID)

Abstract

Inflammatory bowel disease (IBD) is a multifactorial disease which arises as a result of the interaction of genetic, environmental, barrier and microbial factors leading to chronic inflammation in the intestine. Patients with IBD had a higher risk of developing colorectal carcinoma (CRC), of which the subset was classified as colitis-associated cancers. Genetic polymorphism of innate immune receptors had long been considered a major risk factor for IBD, and the mutations were also recently observed in CRC. Altered microbial composition (termed microbiota dybiosis) and dysfunctional gut barrier manifested by epithelial hyperpermeability and high amount of mucosa-associated bacteria were observed in IBD and CRC patients. The findings suggested that aberrant immune responses to penetrating commensal microbes may play key roles in fueling disease progression. Accumulative evidence demonstrated that mucosa-associated bacteria harbored colitogenic and protumoral properties in experimental models, supporting an active role of bacteria as pathobionts (commensal-derived opportunistic pathogens). Nevertheless, the host factors involved in bacterial dysbiosis and conversion mechanisms from lumen-dwelling commensals to mucosal pathobionts remain unclear. Based on the observation of gut leakiness in patients and the evidence of epithelial hyperpermeability prior to the onset of mucosal histopathology in colitic animals, it was postulated that the epithelial barrier dysfunction associated with mucosal enrichment of specific bacterial strains may predispose the shift to disease-associated microbiota. The speculation of leaky gut as an initiating factor for microbiota dysbiosis that eventually led to pathological consequences was proposed as the "common ground hypothesis", which will be highlighted in this review. Overall, the understanding of the core interplay between gut microbiota and epithelial barriers at early subclinical phases will shed light to novel therapeutic strategies to manage chronic inflammatory disorders and colitis-associated cancers.

Keywords: Colitis, colorectal cancers, intestinal dysbiosis, barrier function, epithelial permeability, bacterial internalization

Introduction

Human intestine harbors approximately 3.8×10^{13} bacteria, with over 1000 species found in a cohort [1]. Bacteria also habitat the skin, oral and nasal cavity, and vagina; however, the bacterial counts in extraintestinal organs are no more than 10^{12} [1, 2]. Along with the large amount of bacteria, other microorganisms including virus, archaea, and fungi inhabits the gastrointestinal tract and are collectively defined as the gut microbiota [3]. Keeping in mind that the number of gut bacteria is the same order as human cells and the bacterial genes outnumber human genes by 10- to 100- fold, a symbiotic relationship is maintained between the host and the lumen-confined microbes in a healthy state [4]. Recent evidence indicated that altered microbial communities (termed "microbiota dysbiosis") and intestinal barrier impairment are associated with the development of a number of chronic inflammatory disorders and systemic diseases [5–7]. These included

Correspondence: lchyu@ntu.edu.tw
Graduate Institute of Physiology, National Taiwan University College of Medicine, Suite 1020, #1 Jen-Ai Rd. Sec. 1, Taipei 100, Taiwan, Republic of China

inflammatory bowel disease (IBD), celiac disease, multiple sclerosis, rheumatoid arthritis, ankylosing spondylitis, psoriasis, type 2 diabetes, allergic diseases, cardiovascular and neurodegenerative diseases, and cancers [8–13]. An incoming speculation of common factors involved in the pathogenesis of chronic polygenic disorders has been proposed as the "common ground hypothesis", which placed microbiota dysbiosis and leaky gut in the core mechanisms of a wide array of diseases.

The breach of mucosal barrier may result in unlimited passages of microbes to lamina propria and systemic bloodstream, which could overturn immune tolerance to hyperactivation in the body. The epithelial barrier defects accompanied by an altered microbial community were observed in patients and experimental models of chronic and acute intestinal diseases, such as IBD (Crohn's disease (CD) and ulcerative colitis (UC)) [14–17], celiac disease[18–22], bowel obstruction [23–25], and gastrointestinal (GI) infection [26–29]. IBD is a multifactorial disease of unclear etiology, which arises as a result of the interaction of genetic, environmental, barrier and microbial factors leading to immunological responses and chronic inflammation in the intestine. Patients with IBD had a higher risk of developing colorectal carcinoma (CRC) in later life [30]. As genetic polymorphisms of innate immune receptors (such as nucleotide-binding oligomerization domain (NOD) 2/CARD15 and toll-like receptor (TLR) 4 [31–35]) are considered major risk factors for IBD development, aberrant immune response to host own commensal microbiota was considered to play key roles in fueling the progression of inflammatory diseases. Recent evidence demonstrated that immune-related gene mutations were also observed in CRC patients, including polymorphism in TLRs and ATG16L1 (an autophagy gene for control of immune responses to virus and bacteria) [36–38]. Experimental models provided evidence that aberrant epithelial innate immune responses were involved in the pathogenesis of colitis and tumor development [39–43], further supporting a link between microbe, inflammation and cancers.

The purpose of the review is to summarize the evidence of bacterial dysbiosis and barrier dysfunction in patients and experimental models of IBD and CRC, and to discuss the "common ground hypothesis" to explain abnormal host-microbe interactions underlying disease pathogenesis. Lastly, this review offers further speculation on the mechanisms of mucosal enrichment and conversion of commensal-derived pathobionts in the context of inflammation and cancers.

Microbiota dysbiosis and mucosa-associated bacteria in chronic inflammation

Microbiota dysbiosis is characterized by microbial population, diversity, spatial, or number change in the human body [9, 43]. Stool samples are often used as surrogates for the intestinal microbial contents because it is relatively easy to collect in clinical laboratories. Distinct fecal microbial communities were found between IBD patients and healthy control subjects [44–46]. An average of 25% less microbial richness was found in IBD patients compared to healthy individuals [47–49]. The reduction of microbial diversity with relative abundance or paucity of specific bacterial taxa was widely reported in IBD patients. However, a large variation of fecal bacterial composition in IBD patients was documented in the literatures [50, 51].

An inter-individual variability was readily noted in the fecal microbiota of healthy subjects. Although over one thousand bacterial species were identified in a cohort study with mainly four phyla (Bacteroidetes, Firmicutes, Proteobacteria and Actinobacteria), it should be emphasized that each person harbors around 160 species and that only 30-40 species as the bulk of microbiota are shared among individuals [48, 52, 53]. Studies with Crohn's patients have shown that *Enterobacteriaceae* family [54, 55], and *Fusobacterium* and *Enterococcus faecalis* [56] were significantly increased in the fecal samples compared to those of healthy subjects. Lower bifidobacterial populations and reduction of butyrate-producing bacteria (such as *Faecalibacterium*, *Eubacterium*, *Roseburia*, *Lachnospiraceae* and *Ruminococcaceae*) were found in fecal samples of patients with CD and UC [55, 57–59]. Despite variable results were documented, a reduction of fecal bacterial richness were commonly reported in patients with CD and UC [60–63]. This suggests that maybe fewer species could be making up the majority of a disease-associated microbial population.

While a general consensus exists that altered gut microbiota composition is associated with IBD, a direct causal relationship remains debatable in humans. The uncertainty of causation or correlation is partly due to the fact that stool samples are collected at one single time point in patients (after the diagnosis of IBD) and in healthy subjects without the disorder. Other confounding factors include the dietary habits and life style in individuals, and the use of antibiotics and immunotherapy in patients. Hence, the timing of bacteria dysbiosis relative to disease onset is hard to decipher in humans even by studies of pediatric cohorts [64–66]. The cause-effect relationship of microbiota dysbiosis and chronic inflammatory disorders relied mainly on data of experimental models.

Accumulating evidence indicated that mucosa-associated bacteria are different from fecal microbial population, and may better reflect regional changes in gut microbes at mucosal surfaces at sites of inflammation [50, 53]. In healthy states, indigenous symbiotic bacteria mostly reside in the intestinal lumen which are separated from the epithelial cells by inner firm mucus layers [67], and are not in direct contact with the epithelial cells in physiological conditions [68, 69]. Nevertheless, high densities of mucosa-associated bacteria were reported in IBD patients [64, 65, 70], and were suspected to play a more dominant role than fecal microbiota in promoting gut inflammation. A recent study demonstrated that microbiota obtained from IBD patients from a greater mass of biofilm containing bacteria and extracellular matrix compared to that of healthy controls [71]. Moreover, higher invasiveness of IBD biofilms in a model of human intestinal epithelia was observed compared to healthy control biofilms, demonstrating a more virulent phenotype of microbiota in IBD patients [71].

The enrichment of *Enterobacteriaceae, Bacteroides/ Prevotella, Veillonellaceae, and Fusobacteriaceae* were reported in ileal and colonic biopsies of new-onset treatment-naïve pediatric patients with CD and UC [64–66]. Other studies showed the abundance of the *Escherichia coli* in tissue biopsies of Crohn's patients [55, 60, 72–74]. In addition, adherent-invasive *E.coli* (AIEC) was found in the ileal lesions of Crohn's disease patients [72, 75]. Moreover, a high amount of adherent *Bacteroides fragilis* was found in the mucosal biofilm in patients with IBD [64]. Presence of *B. fragilis* and enterotoxigenic *B. fragilis* (ETBF) was found in the stool and biopsy specimens of healthy individuals, but significantly higher toxin genes were detected in UC patients [76–78]. Furthermore, *Enterococcus* strains with adherent and biofilm-forming ability were isolated from tissue biopsies of IBD patients [79]. Taken together, abundance of mucosa-associated bacteria is correlated to gut inflammation.

The role of gut microbiota in colitis development was confirmed by using animal models. Germ-free mice displayed minimal inflammation or delayed onset of chemically and genetically induced colitis (e.g. IL-2(-/-) and IL-10(-/-)) compared to the conventionally raised animals [80–84]. However, higher mortality was seen in germ-free than conventional mice after giving dextran sulfate sodium (DSS) due to massive gut epithelial injury [82, 83]. The seemingly paradoxical phenomenon could be explained by the lack of immune maturation and/or tolerance as well as the impairment of epithelial turnover (which is dependent on commensal colonization) in germ-free intestine [85–87]. With this said, germ-free models provided clear evidence that intestinal bacteria are crucial for the development of colitis. Other studies using co-housing and fecal transplantation experiments demonstrated the existence of "disease-predisposing microbiota" or "pathobionts" (an opportunistic bacteria derived from commensals) in the fecal microbiota [88, 89]. The animal experiments supported that intestinal bacteria played a disease-predisposing role in colitis development.

Recent studies by using monoassociation and inoculation experiments have helped teased out the roles of single strains of colitis-associated bacteria, and provided valuable information in addition to the overall dysbiotic microbiota. The gut bacterial species documented with pro-inflammatory roles are discussed in the following sections along with the underlying colitogenic mechanisms.

Escherichia coli

High levels of mucosa-associated bacteria with adherence and invasive ability were isolated from Crohn's disease patients [72, 75]. Oral inoculation of Crohn's associated AIEC (LF82 strain), but not the human laboratory *E.coli* K-12, resulted in severe colitis in transgenic mice overexpressing human carcinoemcryonic antigen adhesion molecule 6 (CEACAM6, a receptor to type 1 pili or fimbriae) [90]. In contrast, AIEC did not colonize nor induce colitis in wild type mice [90]. The colitogenic activity of AIEC was dependent on type 1 pili expression as bacteria deleted of the *fimH* gene failed to induce mucosal inflammation [90].

There are evidence indicated that virulence factors other than fimbriae may be crucial for the colitogenic effects. It is noteworthy that the fimH protein sequence of *E.coli* K-12 strain showed high degree of homology (97%) to the LF82, and it only differed from LF82 by variations at residues Ala-48, Ser-91, and Asn-99 [91]. Moreover, the adherence and invasive ability of fim-mutants of LF82 was restored to wild type levels by transforming a *fim* operon derived from *E. coli* K-12 to the mutant. The finding suggested that the fimbriae synthesized by K-12 also possess adherence properties despite of inability of promoting inflammation. In contrast, a non-invasive laboratory *E.coli* strain JM109 transformed with *fim* operons derived from LF82 or K-12 strains did not gain invasive properties, suggesting that although fimbriae-mediated adherence may facilitate bacterial invasion but is insufficient to cause translocation by itself [91]. Additional mechanisms of Crohn's associated AIEC related to its colitogenic ability included higher bacterial survival and replication inside macrophages and induction of proinflammatory cyclooxygenase (COX)-2 expression from macrophages [92, 93]. Recent data also showed that AIEC LF82 strain is capable of long term intracellular survival in gut epithelial cells by suppressing autophagy [94–96], which could contribute to long-term infection.

Other studies showed that monoassociation of non-pathogenic *E.coli* and *Enterococcus faecalis* to gnotobiotic IL-10(-/-) mice induced inflammation in the cecum and distal colon, respectively [81]. Dual-association of the two commensal bacteria in gnotobiotic IL-10(-/-) induces aggressive pancolitis and duodenal inflammation [97, 98].

The findings demonstrated that commensal bacteria isolated from healthy subjects could be colitogenic when monoassociated in mice with genetic deficiency but not in wild type mice, suggesting that opportunistic commensals may turn into pathobionts in genetically-predisposed hosts.

Bacteroides subspecies

Commensal *Bacteroides* spp., such as *B. fragils* and *B. vultagus,* have been reported to modulate colitis development. Abundance of enterotoxigenic *B. fragilis* (ETBF) was detected in the stool and biopsy specimens of UC patients [76–78]. ETBF but not its nontoxigenic strain causes persistent colitis after oral inoculation to wild type mice [99] and a more severe form of inflammation in models of chemically induced colitis [100]. Intestinal permeability was increased and epithelial E-cadherin was cleaved *in vivo* in the ETBF-colonized wild type mice [101]. The enterotoxin produced by *B. fragilis* (also known as fragilysin) acted as a metalloprotease for cleavage of junctional protein and induction of epithelial-derived IL-8 synthesis, which were suggested to be involved in the colitogenic ability [102, 103]. Moreover, gnotobiotic mice monoassociated with three strains of *B. vultagus* isolated from UC patients showed exacerbated cecal inflammation after DSS administration [104], suggesting potential pro-inflammatory ability of the bacteria.

Enterococcus species

Increased colonic inflammation was observed in IL-10(-/-) mice after inoculation or monoassociation with *Enterococcus faecalis* and *E. faecium* [105–107]. The colitogenic characteristics of *E. faecalis* was partly attributed to a bacterial gelatinase which was involved in intestinal barrier impairment and degradation of E-cadherin (a junctional protein) in mouse studies [106]. Moreover, bacterial adherence and penetration to mucosal layers and biofilm formation of *E. faecalis* were dependent on an enterococcal polysaccharide antigen [107]. A cell surface-associated lipoprotein on *E. faecalis* stimulated TLR2-mediated dendritic cell activation and contributes to inflammation [107].

In sum, animal models have provided clear evidence of a disease-predisposing role of certain gut bacteria, yet whether the altered bacterial population is involved in the initiation or perpetuation of intestinal inflammation remains debatable. Moreover, mucosa-associated adherent and invasive bacteria may play a more pathogenic role than fecal microbes in IBD progression. The conversion mechanisms and timing of specific commensal bacteria to turn into invasive or colitogenic pathobionts have yet to be determined. Overall, longitudinal investigation of mucosa-associated bacterial changes that represents a smaller pool of gut microbiota may help elucidate the driver or passenger roles of individual microbes for colitis development.

Microbiota dybiosis and mucosal biofilms in colon cancers

Colon carcinoma is the second most commonly diagnosed cancer. The majority (60-85%) of CRC is classified as sporadic cancers and around 10-30% is familial or hereditary, stressing the importance of environmental and microbial factors in tumorigenesis [108, 109]. IBD accounts for 1-2% of CRC cases, but the cancer risk in UC patients is 5 times higher than the general population and colitis-associated CRC is more aggressive [110]. The hereditary CRC which accounts for <5% of CRC cases have identifiable germline mutation, such as adenomatous polyposis coli (APC) tumor suppressor gene [109]. Patients with APC gene mutation develop hundreds to thousands of colorectal polyps at young age, of which the disease is termed familial adenomatous polyposis (FAP). The FAP patients had a 100% cumulative risk of progression to CRC by the age of 40 years, If the polyps were left untreated [111, 112]. To date, abundant studies have revealed altered fecal microbiota composition and enrichment of mucosa-associated bacteria in patients with CRC or FAP [113–116].

Recent evidence indicated that mucosa-associated bacterial population may play more dominant roles than fecal microbiota in colon carcinogenesis [116–118]. Overabundance of *E. coli* was noted in tumor biopsies in stage I to IV CRC samples, whereas *Fusobacterium nucleatum* was found in stage IV but not in earlier stages of cancers [119, 120]. A recent report showed that more than 50% of FAP patients harbor colonic biofilm with both *E. coli* and *Bacteroides fragilis* [113]. So far, these bacterial strains have been proposed as protumoral pathobionts based on experimental data of animal models.

The experimental models to investigate the roles of bacteria in colon carcinogenesis included conventionalized, germ-free, and gene-modified animals [121]. Studies of verifying an infectious carcinogen in conventionalized wild type situation would bear more resemblance to the heterogeneous population of human CRC. The benefits and caveats of each of these models are highlighted here. It is worth mentioning that commensal-derived pathobionts usually do not colonize well in a healthy gut with a diversified ecosystem. Many studies with bacterial inoculation experiments in conventionalized animals incorporated an antibiotic pretreatment protocol to overcome colonization resistance. However, the antibiotic regimen and the time frame of bacterial colonization varied in different reports [121]. The value of germ-free models is clearly seen as it would facilitate intestinal colonization or monoassociation of inoculated bacteria in a chronic setting of malignant transformation. Nevertheless, cautions were raised regarding the lack of intestinal and systemic immune maturation and/or tolerance in germ-free animals which might confound data interpretation [85–87]. Gene-modified mice that developed spontaneous colorectal cancers were also utilized to verify the hypothesis of protumoral bacteria, including APC(Min/+) mice [117, 122, 123] and mice deficient of NOD-like receptors [88, 89, 124, 125]. There are criticisms of using gene-modified or immune-deficient mice which already had a distinct gut microbiota as a result of altered host genetics, and the clinical implication may be limited to only subsets of patients. While the research values of germ-free and gene-modified animals are undoubtful, it is still difficult to tease out the temporal order of host abnormality versus bacterial dysbiosis in these models. The potential tumorigenic bacterial strains are discussed below.

Escherichia coli

Despite indication of Crohn's-associated AIEC triggering intestinal inflammation by using transgenic mice overexpressing human CEACAM6 [90], no direct evidence was shown for the involvement of AIEC in cancer development. The induction of local inflammation by AIEC has been implicated as a link for progression to intestinal malignancy. Another report demonstrated an increase in tumor susceptibility in CEACAM6-transgenic mice after AOM treatment [126], suggesting a role of fimbriae (without specifying the bacterial strains) in colon tumorigenesis.

Clinical studies showed that 40% of mucosa-associated E.coli from IBD patients, and 67-86% of mucosa-associated E. coli obtained from CRC or diverticulosis specimens harbored the pks pathogenicity island encoding genotoxic coilbactin [117, 127]. Inoculation of NC101 strain (a mouse isolate of pks-positive E.coli) increased colon inflammation and intestinal crypt proliferation in human CEACAM6-transgenic mice [127], and caused DNA damage in colonocytes and promoted tumor growth in AOM-treated IL-10(-/-) mouse models [117, 123]. Recent data demonstrated that monoassociation of pks-positivie E. coli increased the tumor burden in gnotobiotic APC(Min/+) mice and APC(Min/+); IL-10(-/-) mice [128]. Moreover, a clinical isolate CCR20 strain (a pks-positive E. coli obtained from human CRC samples) induced cellular senescence and increased tumor burden in AOM-treated IL-10(-/-) mouse models[129, 130]. Furthermore, the human CRC-associated E.coli triggered macrophage-derived COX-2 production in vitro in a pks-independent manner [93], suggesting a genotoxin-independent, immune-mediated mechanism for the protumoral activity of bacteria.

Enterotoxigenic Bacteroides fragilis

Presence of ETBF was identified in mucosal biopsies of 60% of FAP patients in contrast to 30% in control individuals [113]. Higher amount of ETBF and B. fragilis toxin were observed in late-stage CRC samples [77, 78, 131]. Previous studies demonstrated that colonization of ETBF but not its non-toxigenic counterparts induced chronic colitis and promoted colon tumorigenesis in APC(Min/+) mice [118, 122]. A number of tumorigenic mechanisms of B. fragilis toxin have been proposed. B. fragilis toxin triggered an inflammatory protumoral signaling caspase in colonic epithelial cells that caused the recruitment of polymorphonuclear immature myeloid cells to promote colon cancers [132]. Other studies indicated that B. fragilis toxin may cause oxidative DNA damage or induce epithelial E-cadherin cleavage for barrier disruption [99, 101, 118]. Moreover, ETBF drives Th17 inflammation and also promoted invasion of pks-positive E. coli by causing mucus degradation in AOM-treated wild type mice [113, 122]. The findings indicated that synergistic effects of various strains of bacteria in immunomodulation may be involved in promoting colon tumorigenesis.

Fusobacterium nucleatum

Abundance of Fusobacterium DNA was observed in tumor tissues positively associated with poor prognosis in cancer patients [133]. Higher tumor burden was demonstrated in APC(Min/+) mice following inoculation of clinical isolates of F. nucleatum, and was associated with activation of TLR4/MyD88/NFκB signaling and recruitment of tumor-infiltrating myeloid cells [116, 119]. One report showed that F. nucleatum did not induce colitis nor exacerbated colon inflammation in APC(Min/+) mice [116]. In addition, inoculation of F. nucleatum did not aggravate intestinal inflammation nor induce tumors in colitic models of IL-10(-/-) and T-bet(-/-)/Rag2(-/-) mice [116]. The findings indicated that inflammation was not involved in the pathogenesis of Fusobacteria-mediated tumor progression.

Virulence factors and invasiveness of F. nucleatum have been implicated in promoting colon tumorigenesis. Higher transcript levels of FadA (an adhesin of F. nucleatum) was identified in carcinoma samples compared to normal mucosal biopsies or adenoma tissues [134]. Xenograft studies in immunodeficient mice have shown that injection of purified FadA protein into the subcutaneously inoculated sites resulted in larger tumor size [134]. Moreover, the invasive characteristic of F. nucleatum has been linked to cancer growth. In vitro studies demonstrated that FadA-dependent adherence and invasion of F. nucleatum was involved in induction of cell hyperproliferation, and FadA binding to

E-cadherin induced nuclear translocation of β-catenin for oncogene transcription in human CRC cell lines [134]. Another study indicated that *F. nucleatum* invasion activated a TLR4/PAK-1 cascade for β-catenin signaling in CRC cell lines [135]. Lastly, FadA also enhanced the *E. coli* invasion in endothelial cell lines by using transwell assays [134, 136], further indicating that interaction between bacteria may be cause pathology to the hosts.

Gut barrier dysfunction in chronic inflammation
Gut leakiness manifested by epithelial hyperpermeability was long documented in CD [137–139] and UC patients [140–142]. Increased macromolecular flux in the intestine has been suggested as a predictor for inflammatory relapse in IBD patients in remission [143, 144]. Experimental models using chemical-induced colitis or genetic deficient mice which develop spontaneous enterocolitis with higher susceptibility to tumor formation have demonstrated that epithelial barrier dysfunction preceded the onset of mucosal inflammation [145–147]. An elegant study showed that mice expressing a dominant negative N-Cadherin mutant lacking an extracellular domain (loss of endogenous E-cadherin) developed histopathological features of Crohn's disease by 3 months of age [148], supporting that epithelial barrier disruption was a cause for intestinal inflammation. Other reports documented that inhibition of epithelial hyperpermeability attenuated the colitis severity in animal models, providing further evidence of the cause-and-effect relationship [149, 150]. In sum, the loss of gut barrier integrity is an early event which contributes to chronic inflammation.

The gut barrier is composed of a single layer of epithelial cells which display densely-packed microvilli (brush border, BB) rooted on terminal webs and are joined at their apical side by tight junctions (TJs) [151–153]. Among the epithelial ultrastructures, the apical BB formed by cytoskeletons separated bacteria from the cellular soma and acted as the transcellular barrier; the TJs formed the most marrow paracellular space and acted as the paracellular barrier. The TJ opening is regulated by activation of myosin light chain kinase (MLCK). In pathological conditions, bacteria may translocate across the epithelial layers through either transcellular or paracellular pathways (Fig. 1).

Both transcellular hyperpermeability (manifested by bacterial internalization to epithelia [154, 155]) and paracellular hyperpermeability (evidenced by abnormal TJ expression and upregulated MLCK activity [156–160]) were noted in mucosal biopsies of patients with CD and UC. While low to negligible amount of bacteria was detected in mucosal tissues of control subjects, presence of mucosal bacteria was found in 83% of colonic

specimens from the UC patients, in 56% of the ileal and in 25% of the colonic specimens from the CD patients [65]. Other reports showed 5- and 14-fold higher invasiveness of microbiota biofilms obtained from CD and UC patients, respectively, into a human model of intestinal epithelia, compared to those of healthy control biofilms [71]. Several strains of bacteria, including *E. coli, E. faecalis B. vultagus, Fusobacterium varium* isolated from CD or UC patients were found to invade epithelial cells *in vitro* [107, 155, 161]. Taken together, host barrier defects and microbial invasiveness were both documented in IBD patients.

Other than the transcytotic route, paracellular bacterial influx following TJ disruption was also observed in *in vitro* epithelial cultures [162–166]. However, the timing of two pathways (transcellular versus paracellular) was variable depending on the types of triggers in the context-specific models. To date, longitudinal studies that identify the time points of transcellular and paracellular barrier defects in animal models of colitis are still lacking. More studies are needed to decipher the timeline of epithelial barrier impairment and microbiota composition changes during the early course of colitis development.

Previous studies from our laboratory demonstrated that increased bacterial internalization to epithelial cells occurred prior to the onset of TJ damage using mouse models of bowel obstruction and superbug infection [24, 26, 67, 167]. It is believed that upon TJ destruction, luminal bacteria without strain specificity could flow freely through the paracellular space to underlying lamina propria and cause mucosal inflammation. On the other hand, only particular bacterial strains (such as *Escherichia, Staphylococcus, Bacteroides*) have been reported "inside" epithelial cells in our disease models of bowel obstruction and superbug infection [24, 26]. It is possible that the strain-specific bacterial internalization and intracellular survival may act as an initial trigger to evoke damage to paracellular junctional structures, leading to non-specific bacterial translocation and colitis development. The impact of bacterial internalization on epithelial cytoskeletal structures and perijunctional organization has yet to be explored. Furthermore, whether the mucosa-association of bacteria as an early event in transcellular barrier dysfunction may alter the fecal microbiota due to preferential "anchoring" advantage warrants further investigation.

Common ground hypothesis and further postulation
Disease-predisposing microbiota was found in a wide spectrum of chronic disorders, including IBD and CRC [8–12]. These findings have led to the speculation of a common factor in multigenic disease development. A

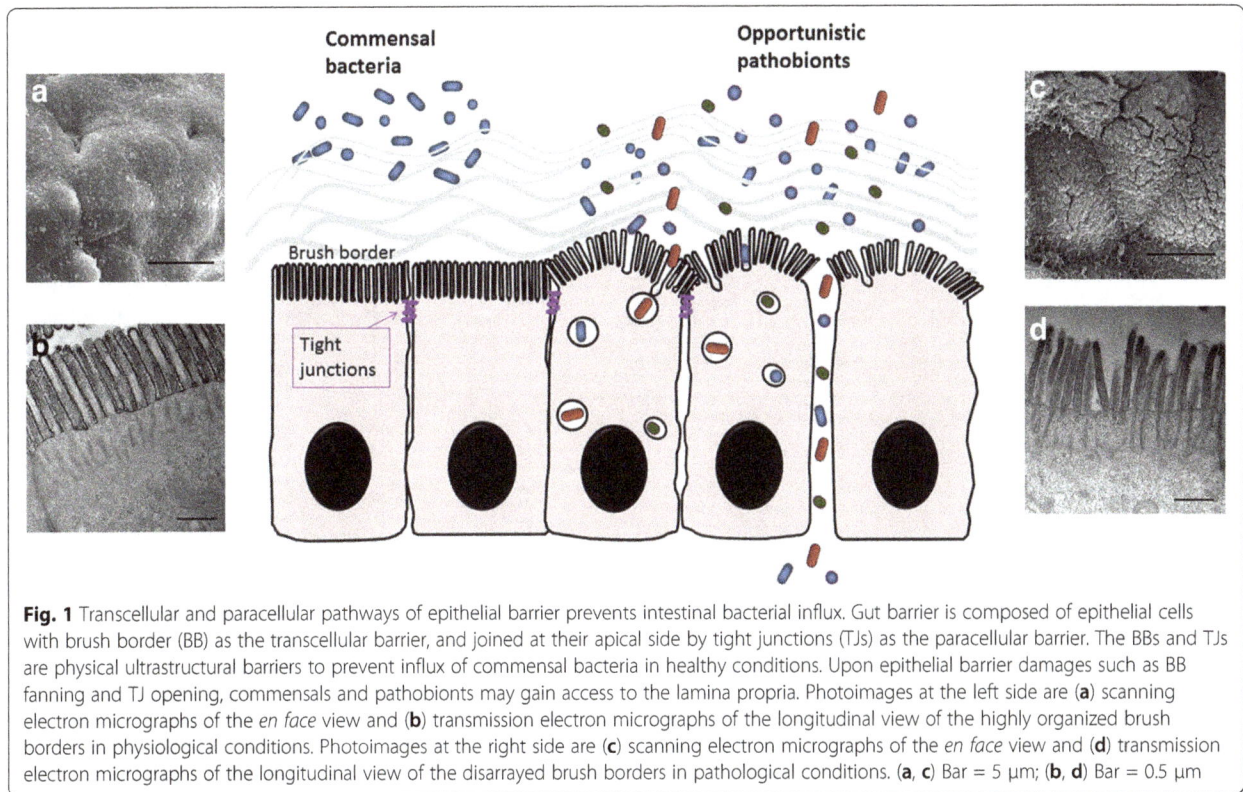

Fig. 1 Transcellular and paracellular pathways of epithelial barrier prevents intestinal bacterial influx. Gut barrier is composed of epithelial cells with brush border (BB) as the transcellular barrier, and joined at their apical side by tight junctions (TJs) as the paracellular barrier. The BBs and TJs are physical ultrastructural barriers to prevent influx of commensal bacteria in healthy conditions. Upon epithelial barrier damages such as BB fanning and TJ opening, commensals and pathobionts may gain access to the lamina propria. Photoimages at the left side are (**a**) scanning electron micrographs of the *en face* view and (**b**) transmission electron micrographs of the longitudinal view of the highly organized brush borders in physiological conditions. Photoimages at the right side are (**c**) scanning electron micrographs of the *en face* view and (**d**) transmission electron micrographs of the longitudinal view of the disarrayed brush borders in pathological conditions. (**a**, **c**) Bar = 5 μm; (**b**, **d**) Bar = 0.5 μm

"common ground hypothesis" was proposed to indicate the key roles of microbiota dysbiosis associated with a leaky gut in the pathogenesis of chronic polygenic diseases [9, 168, 169] (Fig. 2). The hypothesis, which still needs to be rigorously examined, first suggests that endogenous and exogenous factors which cause gut barrier impairment and low grade immune activation could impose selective pressure on the intestinal microbiota. The subclinical mucosal abnormalities that developed in individuals with genetic predisposition then favor the growth of opportunistic microbes with virulence emergence. The opportunistic microbes then aggravate the morphologic and functional changes with pathological consequences, and result in chronic inflammation and clinical symptoms in the host (Fig. 2).

Additional evidence also demonstrated that chronic inflammation may shape the gut microbiota and further contribute to dysbiosis [117, 170]. Several lines of evidence have shown that electron acceptors generated as by-products of the inflammatory responses promoted the outgrowth of facultative anaerobes, such as Enterobacteriaceae [171, 172]. Indeed, the mucosa-associated bacteria have higher oxygen tolerance and catalase expression relative to the fecal dominant species [173], which could be an advantage for microbial competition in the gut ecosystem. Alternatively, proinflammatory cytokines (e.g. IFNγ and TNFα) [24, 67, 164] and opportunistic pathobionts (e.g. AIEC and ETBF) [102, 103, 174] were

shown to disrupt epithelial integrity through both transcellular and paracellular pathways. Furthermore, chronic inflammation with high oxidative stress (such as superoxide and nitric oxide) caused epithelial death-dependent barrier loss, which may lead to a vicious cycle of aggravating barrier dysfunction and immune hyperactivation [175, 176].

Based on the current knowledge in intestinal barrier regulation (see review papers [67, 177]), we have reconstructed a more detailed hypothesis in attempt to explain the early interaction between epithelial barriers and microbial conversion. In accordance to the "common ground hypothesis", we speculated that an initial epithelial barrier dysfunction manifested by a low amount of passive bacterial internalization for enrichment of specific mucosa-associated bacteria was the first event causing an altered microbial community (Fig. 2). The internalized commensal bacteria inside epithelial cells with aerotolerance may acquire virulence factors to ensure survival, immune evasion, and anchoring advantage. The epithelia-associated driving of opportunistic commensals to pathobionts could be a point of no return leading to pathological consequences to the host. Bacterial internalization may also disturb the epithelial cytoskeletal contour and destabilize junctional structures, resulting in the passage of non-specific bacterial strains. The combination of host barrier defects and bacterial invasiveness may evoke a massive amount of

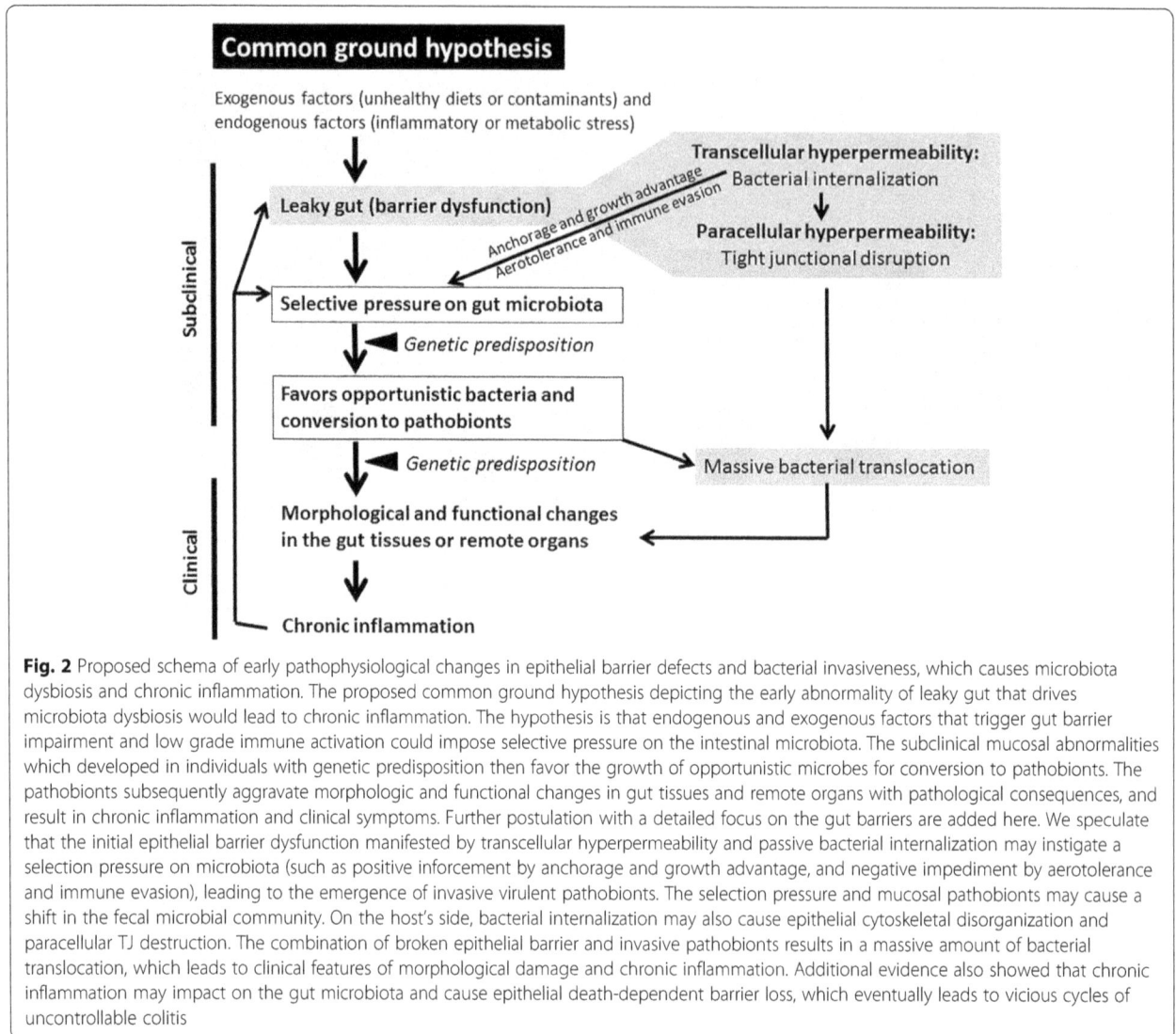

Fig. 2 Proposed schema of early pathophysiological changes in epithelial barrier defects and bacterial invasiveness, which causes microbiota dysbiosis and chronic inflammation. The proposed common ground hypothesis depicting the early abnormality of leaky gut that drives microbiota dysbiosis would lead to chronic inflammation. The hypothesis is that endogenous and exogenous factors that trigger gut barrier impairment and low grade immune activation could impose selective pressure on the intestinal microbiota. The subclinical mucosal abnormalities which developed in individuals with genetic predisposition then favor the growth of opportunistic microbes for conversion to pathobionts. The pathobionts subsequently aggravate morphologic and functional changes in gut tissues and remote organs with pathological consequences, and result in chronic inflammation and clinical symptoms. Further postulation with a detailed focus on the gut barriers are added here. We speculate that the initial epithelial barrier dysfunction manifested by transcellular hyperpermeability and passive bacterial internalization may instigate a selection pressure on microbiota (such as positive inforcement by anchorage and growth advantage, and negative impediment by aerotolerance and immune evasion), leading to the emergence of invasive virulent pathobionts. The selection pressure and mucosal pathobionts may cause a shift in the fecal microbial community. On the host's side, bacterial internalization may also cause epithelial cytoskeletal disorganization and paracellular TJ destruction. The combination of broken epithelial barrier and invasive pathobionts results in a massive amount of bacterial translocation, which leads to clinical features of morphological damage and chronic inflammation. Additional evidence also showed that chronic inflammation may impact on the gut microbiota and cause epithelial death-dependent barrier loss, which eventually leads to vicious cycles of uncontrollable colitis

bacterial translocation and immune hyperactivation in gut mucosa. The immune hyperactivation could impact on the microbiota and cause a further shift to a disease-promoting microbial composition in individuals with genetic predisposition, which eventually leads to chronic inflammation and malignant transformation (Fig. 2).

To date, our understanding of the role of gut microbiota in human health and disease has been fraught with challenges, partly due to the inability to elucidate this complex host-microbe interaction simply based on patient studies. Irrespective of the orders of host or microbial factors involved in disease progression, the co-existence of microbiota dysbiosis and barrier dysfunction (with reciprocal aggravation) appears to be a common instigator in chronic inflammation. Overall, experimental models evaluting subclinical pathophysiological abnormalities (i.e. microbiota dysbiosis and leaky

gut) based on the "common ground hypothesis" may serve as a roadmap to decipher the cause-and-effect relationship of disease mechanisms.

Unanswered questions and future directions
Despite a consensus exists for the presence of microbiota dysbiosis and barrier disruption, the order of the microbial and host factors in disease pathogenesis has not been established in chronic gut inflammation and colitis-associated CRC. Moreover, mucosa-associated pathobionts have been assumed to derive from unharmful gut commensals, yet without direct evidence. One of the proposed triggers for emergence of pathogenic commensals was the need for adaptation to oxidative stress [178, 179]. Other factors, such as mucosal enrichment and selective pressure, on pathobiont conversion remain to be tested. In addition, the virulence profiles to indicate the conversion of commensal to opportunistic

pathobionts still need to be determined. Alternatively, whether virulence factors found in opportunistic bacteria (mostly to confer microbial growth advantage) necessarily indicate pathogenic outcome in the hosts or only to those with genetic deficiency warrant further studies.

Furthermore, the majority of microbiome studies so far have focused on bacterial census, and the roles of virus and fungi are less well understood. Since bacteriophages are transferrable and are abundant in the human gut, their roles in modulating the bacterial ecosystems and conferring opportunistic virulence warrant thorough investigation [180, 181]. In addition, bacterial influx due to transcellular and paracellular hyperpermeability in intestinal epithelia was observed in IBD and CRC patients, yet the relative timing of each pathway remains unclear. Timeline studies in experimental models may answer this question, and will provide insights to the differential regulation of distinct transepithelial routes and their relationships to the shaping of gut microbiota.

Fecal microbiota transplantation (FMT) is now standard of care for recurrent *Clostridium difficile* infection, and emerging evidence also supports the use of FMT to treat IBD [182, 183]. A recent randomized double-blinded controlled trial had shown that FMT induced remission in patients with active UC, which was associated with increased microbial richness without adverse events following transplantation [184, 185]. Some studies reported worsening GI symptoms after FMT in IBD patients by lower GI delivery or in *Clostridium* infection[186], which may be due to variable donor microbial factors. The possible use of restoration of gut barrier as an indicator of colonization of a healthy microbiota following FMT warrant further studies.

Conclusions

Research for correction of abnormal microbe-host interaction by sealing the broken barrier and improvement of epithelial integrity is currently in progress to supplement anti-inflammatory and immunotherapies for IBD patients [187–189]. Moreover, novel microbe-focused intervention such as bacterial engineering, next-generation probiotics, microbe-specific bactericidal antibiotics, and fecal microbiota transplantation as a monotherapy or add-on therapy will be promising for IBD treatment [190, 191]. Based on the "common ground hypothesis", targeting the dysbiotic bacteria and intestinal barriers may be used as treatment for not only IBD but also extraintestinal inflammatory disorders and colitis-associated cancers. In addition, the use of microbial signatures in addition to genetic traits as diagnostic biomarkers to predict the prognosis and development of diseases have shown positive results in clinical studies and could be used for personalized medicine in

the future [192, 193]. Lastly, diet and prebiotics to affect microbe-microbe and microbe-host interaction would be another valuable approach beyond the known nutritive functions to restore intestinal homeostasis and barrier integrity [194]. In conclusion, the understanding of the core interplay between gut microbiota and host barriers at the early subclinical phase will shed light to novel therapeutic approaches to chronic inflammatory disorders and cancers.

Abbreviations
AIEC: adherent-invasive *Escherichia coli*; BB: brush border; CD: Crohn's disease; CEACAM: carcinoemcryonic antigen adhesion molecule; COX: cyclooxygenase; CRC: colorectal carcinoma; DSS: dextran sulfate sodium; ETBF: enterotoxigenic *Bacteroides fragilis*; FMT: fecal microbiota transplantation; IBD: inflammatory bowel disease; MLCK: myosin light chain kinase; NOD: nucleotide-binding oligomerization domain; TJ: tight junction; TLR: toll-like receptor; UC: ulcerative colitis

Acknowledgements
We thank the staff of the imaging core at the First Core Labs and the animal center in National Taiwan University College of Medicine, for technical assistance.

Funding
Ministry of Science and Technology (MoST 107-2320-B-002-041-MY3), and National Health Research Institute, Taiwan (NHRI-EX105-10520BI, NHRI-EX106-10520BI, NHRI-EX107-10520BI)

Authors' contributions
Guarantor of integrity of entire manuscript, LCY; manuscript drafting and revision for important intellectual content, literature research, and manuscript final version approval: LCY.

Competing interests
I declare that there is no competing interest.

References
1. Sender R, Fuchs S, Milo R. Are We Really Vastly Outnumbered? Revisiting the Ratio of Bacterial to Host Cells in Humans. Cell. 2016;164(3):337–40.
2. Nakamoto N, Schnabl B. Does the Intestinal Microbiota Explain Differences in the Epidemiology of Liver Disease between East and West? Inflamm Intest Dis. 2016;1(1):3–8.
3. Turnbaugh PJ, Ley RE, Hamady M, Fraser-Liggett CM, Knight R, Gordon JI. The human microbiome project. Nature. 2007;449(7164):804–10.
4. Yu LC, Wang JT, Wei SC, Ni YH. Host-microbial interactions and regulation of intestinal epithelial barrier function: From physiology to pathology. World J Gastrointest Pathophysiol. 2012;3(1):27–43.
5. Balzan S, de Almeida Quadros C, de Cleva R, Zilberstein B, Cecconello I. Bacterial translocation: overview of mechanisms and clinical impact. J GastroenterolHepatol. 2007;22(4):464–71.
6. Leaphart CL, Tepas JJ, III: The gut is a motor of organ system dysfunction. Surgery 2007, 141(5):563-569.
7. Ni J, Wu GD, Albenberg L, Tomov VT. Gut microbiota and IBD: causation or correlation? Nat Rev Gastroenterol Hepatol. 2017;14(10):573–84.

8. Bernstein CN, Forbes JD. Gut Microbiome in Inflammatory Bowel Disease and Other Chronic Immune-Mediated Inflammatory Diseases. Inflammatory Intestinal Diseases. 2017;2:116–23.

9. Lynch SV, Pedersen O. The Human Intestinal Microbiome in Health and Disease. N Engl J Med. 2016;375(24):2369–79.

10. Slyepchenko A, Maes M, Machado-Veira R, Anderson G, Solmi M, Sanz Y, Berk M, Kohler CA, Carvalho AF. Intestinal dysbiosis, gut hyperpermeability and bacterial translocation: missing links between depression, obesity and type 2 diabetes? Curr Pharm Des. 2016.

11. Rogler G, Rosano G. The heart and the gut. Eur Heart J. 2014;35(7):426–30.

12. Kohler CA, Maes M, Slyepchenko A, Berk M, Solmi M, Lanctot KL, Carvalho AF. The Gut-Brain Axis, Including the Microbiome, Leaky Gut and Bacterial Translocation: Mechanisms and Pathophysiological Role in Alzheimer's Disease. Curr Pharm Des. 2016;22(40):6152–66.

13. Chua HH, Chou HC, Tung YL, Chiang BL, Liao CC, Liu HH, Ni YH. Intestinal Dysbiosis Featuring Abundance of Ruminococcus gnavus Associates With Allergic Diseases in Infants. Gastroenterology. 2018; 154(1):154–67.

14. Prorok-Hamon M, Friswell MK, Alswied A, Roberts CL, Song F, Flanagan PK, Knight P, Codling C, Marchesi JR, Winstanley C, et al. Colonic mucosa-associated diffusely adherent afaC+ Escherichia coli expressing lpfA and pks are increased in inflammatory bowel disease and colon cancer. Gut. 2014;63(5):761–70.

15. Martin HM, Campbell BJ, Hart CA, Mpofu C, Nayar M, Singh R, Englyst H, Williams HF, Rhodes JM. Enhanced Escherichia coli adherence and invasion in Crohn's disease and colon cancer. Gastroenterology. 2004;127(1):80–93.

16. Kahrstrom CT. Bacterial pathogenesis: E. coli claims the driving seat for cancer. Nature Rev Microbiol. 2012;10(10):670.

17. Chassaing B, Gewirtz AT. Pathobiont hypnotises enterocytes to promote tumour development. Gut. 2014;63(12):1837–8.

18. Girbovan A, Sur G, Samasca G, Lupan I. Dysbiosis a risk factor for celiac disease. Med Microbiol Immunol. 2017;206(2):83–91.

19. Cinova J, De Palma G, Stepankova R, Kofronova O, Kverka M, Sanz Y, Tuckova L. Role of intestinal bacteria in gliadin-induced changes in intestinal mucosa: study in germ-free rats. PLoS One. 2011;6(1):e16169.

20. Silva MA, Jury J, Sanz Y, Wiepjes M, Huang X, Murray JA, David CS, Fasano A, Verdu EF. Increased bacterial translocation in gluten-sensitive mice is independent of small intestinal paracellular permeability defect. Dig Dis Sci. 2012;57(1):38–47.

21. Ludvigsson JF, Olen O, Bell M, Ekbom A, Montgomery SM. Coeliac disease and risk of sepsis. Gut. 2008;57(8):1074–80.

22. Caminero A, Galipeau HJ, McCarville JL, Johnston CW, Bernier SP, Russell AK, Jury J, Herran AR, Casqueiro J, Tye-Din JA, et al. Duodenal Bacteria From Patients With Celiac Disease and Healthy Subjects Distinctly Affect Gluten Breakdown and Immunogenicity. Gastroenterology. 2016;151(4):670–83.

23. Wu CC, Lu YZ, Wu LL, Yu LCH. Role of myosin light chain kinase in intestinal epithelial barrier defects in a rat model of bowel obstruction. BMC Gastroenterology. 2010;10:39–50.

24. Wu LL, Peng WH, Kuo WT, Huang CY, Ni YH, Lu KS, Turner JR, Yu LC. Commensal Bacterial Endocytosis in Epithelial Cells Is Dependent on Myosin Light Chain Kinase-Activated Brush Border Fanning by Interferon-gamma. Am J Pathol. 2014;184(8):2260–74.

25. Tian F, Gao X, Zhang L, Wang X, Wan X, Jiang T, Wu C, Bi J, Lei Q. Effects of n-3 PUFAs on Intestinal Mucosa Innate Immunity and Intestinal Microbiota in Mice after Hemorrhagic Shock Resuscitation. Nutrients. 2016;8(10).

26. Yu LC, Shih YA, Wu LL, Lin YD, Kuo WT, Peng WH, Lu KS, Wei SC, Turner JR, Ni YH. Enteric dysbiosis promotes antibiotic-resistant bacterial infection: systemic dissemination of resistant and commensal bacteria through epithelial transcytosis. Am J Physiol Gastrointest Liver Physiol. 2014;307(8):G824–35.

27. Ubeda C, Taur Y, Jenq RR, Equinda MJ, Son T, Samstein M, Viale A, Socci ND, van den Brink MR, Kamboj M, et al. Vancomycin-resistant Enterococcus domination of intestinal microbiota is enabled by antibiotic treatment in mice and precedes bloodstream invasion in humans. J Clin Invest. 2010;120(12):4332–41.

28. Beatty JK, Akierman SV, Motta JP, Muise S, Workentine ML, Harrison JJ, Bhargava A, Beck PL, Rioux KP, McKnight GW, et al. Giardia duodenalis induces pathogenic dysbiosis of human intestinal microbiota biofilms. Int J Parasitol. 2017;47(6):311–26.

29. Barash NR, Maloney JG, Singer SM, Dawson SC: Giardia Alters Commensal Microbial Diversity throughout the Murine Gut. Infect Immun. 2017;85(6): e00948-16.

30. Brackmann S, Andersen SN, Aamodt G, Langmark F, Clausen OP, Aadland E, Fausa O, Rydning A, Vatn MH. Relationship between clinical parameters and the colitis-colorectal cancer interval in a cohort of patients with colorectal cancer in inflammatory bowel disease. Scand J Gastroenterol. 2009;44(1):46–55.

31. Browning BL, Huebner C, Petermann I, Gearry RB, Barclay ML, Shelling AN, Ferguson LR. Has toll-like receptor 4 been prematurely dismissed as an inflammatory bowel disease gene? Association study combined with meta-analysis shows strong evidence for association. Am J Gastroenterol. 2007;102(11):2504–12.

32. De Jager PL, Franchimont D, Waliszewska A, Bitton A, Cohen A, Langelier D, Belaiche J, Vermeire S, Farwell L, Goris A, et al. The role of the Toll receptor pathway in susceptibility to inflammatory bowel diseases. Genes Immun. 2007;8(5):387–97.

33. Brand S, Staudinger T, Schnitzler F, Pfennig S, Hofbauer K, Dambacher J, Seiderer J, Tillack C, Konrad A, Crispin A, et al. The role of Toll-like receptor 4 Asp299Gly and Thr399Ile polymorphisms and CARD15/NOD2 mutations in the susceptibility and phenotype of Crohn's disease. Inflamm Bowel Dis. 2005;11(7):645–52.

34. Lakatos PL, Hitre E, Szalay F, Zinober K, Fuszek P, Lakatos L, Fischer S, Osztovits J, Gemela O, Veres G, et al. Common NOD2/CARD15 variants are not associated with susceptibility or the clinicopathologic characteristics of sporadic colorectal cancer in Hungarian patients. BMC Cancer. 2007;7:54.

35. Franchimont D, Vermeire S, El HH, Pierik M, Van SK, Gustot T, Quertinmont E, Abramowicz M, Van GA, Deviere J, et al. Deficient host-bacteria interactions in inflammatory bowel disease? The toll-like receptor (TLR)-4 Asp299gly polymorphism is associated with Crohn's disease and ulcerative colitis. Gut. 2004;53(7):987–92.

36. Slattery ML, Herrick JS, Bondurant KL, Wolff RK. Toll-like receptor genes and their association with colon and rectal cancer development and prognosis. Int J Cancer. 2012;130(12):2974–80.

37. Semlali A, Reddy Parine N, Arafah M, Mansour L, Azzi A, Al Shahrani O, Al Amri A, Shaik JP, Aljebreen AM, Alharbi O, et al. Expression and Polymorphism of Toll-Like Receptor 4 and Effect on NF-kappaB Mediated Inflammation in Colon Cancer Patients. PLoS One. 2016;11(1):e0146333.

38. Grimm WA, Messer JS, Murphy SF, Nero T, Lodolce JP, Weber CR, Logsdon MF, Bartulis S, Sylvester BE, Springer A, et al. The Thr300Ala variant in ATG16L1 is associated with improved survival in human colorectal cancer and enhanced production of type I interferon. Gut. 2016;65(3):456–64.

39. Kuo WT, Lee TC, Yang HY, Chen CY, Au YC, Lu YZ, Wu LL, Wei SC, Ni YH, Lin BR, et al. LPS receptor subunits have antagonistic roles in epithelial apoptosis and colonic carcinogenesis. Cell Death Differ. 2015;22(10):1590–604.

40. Rakoff-Nahoum S, Medzhitov R. Role of toll-like receptors in tissue repair and tumorigenesis. Biochemistry (Mosc). 2008;73(5):555–61.

41. Kuo WT, Lee TC, Yu LC. Eritoran Suppresses Colon Cancer by Altering a Functional Balance in Toll-like Receptors That Bind Lipopolysaccharide. Cancer Res. 2016;76(16):4684–95.

42. Fukata M, Hernandez Y, Conduah D, Cohen J, Chen A, Breglio K, Goo T, Hsu D, Xu R, Abreu MT. Innate immune signaling by Toll-like receptor-4 (TLR4) shapes the inflammatory microenvironment in colitis-associated tumors. Inflamm Bowel Dis. 2009;15(7):997–1006.

43. Yu LC, Wei SC, Ni YN. Interplay between the gut microbiota and epithelial innate signaling in colitis-associated colon carcinogenesis. Cancer Res Frontiers. 2017;3(1):1–28.

44. Nagalingam NA, Kao JY, Young VB. Microbial ecology of the murine gut associated with the development of dextran sodium sulfate-induced colitis. Inflamm Bowel Dis. 2011;17(4):917–26.

45. Samanta AK, Torok VA, Percy NJ, Abimosleh SM, Howarth GS. Microbial fingerprinting detects unique bacterial communities in the faecal microbiota of rats with experimentally-induced colitis. J Microbiol. 2012;50(2):218–25.

46. Brinkman BM, Becker A, Ayiseh RB, Hildebrand F, Raes J, Huys G, Vandenabeele P. Gut microbiota affects sensitivity to acute DSS-induced colitis independently of host genotype. Inflamm Bowel Dis. 2013;19(12): 2560–7.

47. Kolho KL, Korpela K, Jaakkola T, Pichai MV, Zoetendal EG, Salonen A, de Vos WM. Fecal Microbiota in Pediatric Inflammatory Bowel Disease and Its Relation to Inflammation. Am J Gastroenterol. 2015;110(6):921–30.

48. Qin J, Li R, Raes J, Arumugam M, Burgdorf KS, Manichanh C, Nielsen T, Pons N, Levenez F, Yamada T, et al. A human gut microbial gene catalogue established by metagenomic sequencing. Nature. 2010;464(7285):59–65.

49. Manichanh C, Rigottier-Gois L, Bonnaud E, Gloux K, Pelletier E, Frangeul L, Nalin R, Jarrin C, Chardon P, Marteau P, et al. Reduced diversity of faecal microbiota in Crohn's disease revealed by a metagenomic approach. Gut. 2006;55(2):205–11.

50. Miyoshi J, Chang EB. The gut microbiota and inflammatory bowel diseases. Transl Res. 2017;179:38–48.

51. Kostic AD, Xavier RJ, Gevers D. The microbiome in inflammatory bowel disease: current status and the future ahead. Gastroenterology. 2014;146(6):1489–99.

52. Ley RE, Turnbaugh PJ, Klein S, Gordon JI. Microbial ecology: human gut microbes associated with obesity. Nature. 2006;444(7122):1022–3.

53. Eckburg PB, Bik EM, Bernstein CN, Purdom E, Dethlefsen L, Sargent M, Gill SR, Nelson KE, Relman DA. Diversity of the human intestinal microbial flora. Science. 2005;308(5728):1635–8.

54. Seksik P, Rigottier-Gois L, Gramet G, Sutren M, Pochart P, Marteau P, Jian R, Dore J. Alterations of the dominant faecal bacterial groups in patients with Crohn's disease of the colon. Gut. 2003;52(2):237–42.

55. Chen L, Wang W, Zhou R, Ng SC, Li J, Huang M, Zhou F, Wang X, Shen B, AK M, et al. Characteristics of fecal and mucosa-associated microbiota in Chinese patients with inflammatory bowel disease. Medicine (Baltimore). 2014;93(8):e51.

56. Zhou Y, Chen H, He H, Du Y, Hu J, Li Y, Li Y, Zhou Y, Wang H, Chen Y, et al. Increased Enterococcus faecalis infection is associated with clinically active Crohn disease. Medicine (Baltimore). 2016;95(39):e5019.

57. Prosberg M, Bendtsen F, Vind I, Petersen AM, Gluud LL. The association between the gut microbiota and the inflammatory bowel disease activity: a systematic review and meta-analysis. Scand J Gastroenterol. 2016:1–9.

58. Maukonen J, Kolho KL, Paasela M, Honkanen J, Klemetti P, Vaarala O, Saarela M. Altered Fecal Microbiota in Paediatric Inflammatory Bowel Disease. J Crohns Colitis. 2015;9(12):1088–95.

59. Sokol H, Pigneur B, Watterlot L, Lakhdari O, Bermudez-Humaran LG, Gratadoux JJ, Blugeon S, Bridonneau C, Furet JP, Corthier G, et al. Faecalibacterium prausnitzii is an anti-inflammatory commensal bacterium identified by gut microbiota analysis of Crohn disease patients. Proc Natl Acad Sci U S A. 2008;105(43):16731–6.

60. Walker AW, Sanderson JD, Churcher C, Parkes GC, Hudspith BN, Rayment N, Brostoff J, Parkhill J, Dougan G, Petrovska L. High-throughput clone library analysis of the mucosa-associated microbiota reveals dysbiosis and differences between inflamed and non-inflamed regions of the intestine in inflammatory bowel disease. BMC Microbiol. 2011;7.

61. Hansen R, Russell RK, Reiff C, Louis P, McIntosh F, Berry SH, Mukhopadhya I, Bisset WM, Barclay AR, Bishop J, et al. Microbiota of de-novo pediatric IBD: increased Faecalibacterium prausnitzii and reduced bacterial diversity in Crohn's but not in ulcerative colitis. Am J Gastroenterol. 2012;107(12):1913–22.

62. Lepage P, Hasler R, Spehlmann ME, Rehman A, Zvirbliene A, Begun A, Ott S, Kupcinskas L, Dore J, Raedler A, et al. Twin study indicates loss of interaction between microbiota and mucosa of patients with ulcerative colitis. Gastroenterology. 2011;141(1):227–36.

63. Pascal V, Pozuelo M, Borruel N, Casellas F, Campos D, Santiago A, Martinez X, Varela E, Sarrabayrouse G, Machiels K, et al. A microbial signature for Crohn's disease. Gut. 2017;66(5):813–22.

64. Swidsinski A, Weber J, Loening-Baucke V, Hale LP, Lochs H. Spatial organization and composition of the mucosal flora in patients with inflammatory bowel disease. J Clin Microbiol. 2005;43(7):3380–9.

65. Kleessen B, Kroesen AJ, Buhr HJ, Blaut M. Mucosal and invading bacteria in patients with inflammatory bowel disease compared with controls. Scand J Gastroenterol. 2002;37(9):1034–41.

66. Gevers D, Kugathasan S, Denson LA, Vazquez-Baeza Y, Van Treuren W, Ren B, Schwager E, Knights D, Song SJ, Yassour M, et al. The treatment-naive microbiome in new-onset Crohn's disease. Cell Host & Microbe. 2014;15(3):382–92.

67. Yu LC. Commensal bacterial internalization by epithelial cells: An alternative portal for gut leakiness. Tissue Barriers. 2015;3(3):e1008895.

68. Johansson ME, Sjovall H, Hansson GC. The gastrointestinal mucus system in health and disease. Nat Rev Gastroenterol Hepatol. 2013;10(6):352–61.

69. Johansson ME, Gustafsson JK, Holmen-Larsson J, Jabbar KS, Xia L, Xu H, Ghishan FK, Carvalho FA, Gewirtz AT, Sjovall H, et al. Bacteria penetrate the normally impenetrable inner colon mucus layer in both murine colitis models and patients with ulcerative colitis. Gut. 2014;63(2):281–91.

70. Mylonaki M, Rayment NB, Rampton DS, Hudspith BN, Brostoff J. Molecular characterization of rectal mucosa-associated bacterial flora in inflammatory bowel disease. Inflamm Bowel Dis. 2005;11(5):481–7.

71. Motta JP, Allain T, Green-Harrison LE, Groves RA, Feener T, Ramay H, Beck PL, Lewis IA, Wallace JL, Buret AG. Iron Sequestration in Microbiota Biofilms As A Novel Strategy for Treating Inflammatory Bowel Disease. Inflamm Bowel Dis. 2018;24(7):1493–502.

72. Darfeuille-Michaud A, Boudeau J, Bulois P, Neut C, Glasser AL, Barnich N, Bringer MA, Swidsinski A, Beaugerie L, Colombel JF. High prevalence of adherent-invasive Escherichia coli associated with ileal mucosa in Crohn's disease. Gastroenterology. 2004;127(2):412–21.

73. Martinez-Medina M, Aldeguer X, Lopez-Siles M, Gonzalez-Huix F, Lopez-Oliu C, Dahbi G, Blanco JE, Blanco J, Garcia-Gil LJ, Darfeuille-Michaud A. Molecular diversity of Escherichia coli in the human gut: new ecological evidence supporting the role of adherent-invasive E. coli (AIEC) in Crohn's disease. Inflamm Bowel Dis. 2009;15(6):872–82.

74. Baumgart M, Dogan B, Rishniw M, Weitzman G, Bosworth B, Yantiss R, Orsi RH, Wiedmann M, McDonough P, Kim SG, et al. Culture independent analysis of ileal mucosa reveals a selective increase in invasive Escherichia coli of novel phylogeny relative to depletion of Clostridiales in Crohn's disease involving the ileum. ISME J. 2007;1(5):403–18.

75. Eaves-Pyles T, Allen CA, Taormina J, Swidsinski A, Tutt CB, Jezek GE, Islas-Islas M, Torres AG. Escherichia coli isolated from a Crohn's disease patient adheres, invades, and induces inflammatory responses in polarized intestinal epithelial cells. Int J Med Microbiol. 2008;298(5-6):397–409.

76. Sears CL, Islam S, Saha A, Arjumand M, Alam NH, Faruque AS, Salam MA, Shin J, Hecht D, Weintraub A, et al. Association of enterotoxigenic Bacteroides fragilis infection with inflammatory diarrhea. Clin Infect Dis. 2008;47(6):797–803.

77. Viljoen KS, Dakshinamurthy A, Goldberg P, Blackburn JM. Quantitative profiling of colorectal cancer-associated bacteria reveals associations between fusobacterium spp., enterotoxigenic Bacteroides fragilis (ETBF) and clinicopathological features of colorectal cancer. PLoS One. 2015;10(3):e0119462.

78. Boleij A, Hechenbleikner EM, Goodwin AC, Badani R, Stein EM, Lazarev MG, Ellis B, Carroll KC, Albesiano E, Wick EC, et al. The Bacteroides fragilis toxin gene is prevalent in the colon mucosa of colorectal cancer patients. Clin Infect Dis. 2015;60(2):208–15.

79. Golinska E, Tomusiak A, Gosiewski T, Wiecek G, Machul A, Mikolajczyk D, Bulanda M, Heczko PB, Strus M. Virulence factors of Enterococcus strains isolated from patients with inflammatory bowel disease. World J Gastroenterol. 2013;19(23):3562–72.

80. Hudcovic T, Stepankova R, Cebra J, Tlaskalova-Hogenova H. The role of microflora in the development of intestinal inflammation: acute and chronic colitis induced by dextran sulfate in germ-free and conventionally reared immunocompetent and immunodeficient mice. Folia Microbiol (Praha). 2001;46(5):565–72.

81. Kim SC, Tonkonogy SL, Albright CA, Tsang J, Balish EJ, Braun J, Huycke MM, Sartor RB. Variable phenotypes of enterocolitis in interleukin 10-deficient mice monoassociated with two different commensal bacteria. Gastroenterology. 2005;128(4):891–906.

82. Llewellyn SR, Britton GJ, Contijoch EJ, Vennaro OH, Mortha A, Colombel JF, Grinspan A, Clemente JC, Merad M, Faith JJ. Interactions between diet and the intestinal microbiota alter intestinal permeability and colitis severity in mice. Gastroenterology. 2017.

83. Hernandez-Chirlaque C, Aranda CJ, Ocon B, Capitan-Canadas F, Ortega-Gonzalez M, Carrero JJ, Suarez MD, Zarzuelo A, Sanchez de Medina F, Martinez-Augustin O. Germ-free and Antibiotic-treated Mice are Highly Susceptible to Epithelial Injury in DSS Colitis. J Crohns Colitis. 2016;10(11):1324–35.

84. Contractor NV, Bassiri H, Reya T, Park AY, Baumgart DC, Wasik MA, Emerson SG, Carding SR. Lymphoid hyperplasia, autoimmunity, and compromised intestinal intraepithelial lymphocyte development in colitis-free gnotobiotic IL-2-deficient mice. J Immunol. 1998;160(1):385–94.

85. Chung H, Pamp SJ, Hill JA, Surana NK, Edelman SM, Troy EB, Reading NC, Villablanca EJ, Wang S, Mora JR, et al. Gut immune maturation depends on colonization with a host-specific microbiota. Cell. 2012;149(7):1578–93.

86. Vannucci L, Stepankova R, Kozakova H, Fiserova A, Rossmann P, Tlaskalova-Hogenova H. Colorectal carcinogenesis in germ-free and conventionally reared rats: different intestinal environments affect the systemic immunity. Int J Oncol. 2008;32(3):609–17.

87. Rhee KJ, Sethupathi P, Driks A, Lanning DK, Knight KL. Role of commensal bacteria in development of gut-associated lymphoid tissues and preimmune antibody repertoire. J Immunol. 2004;172(2):1118–24.

88. Couturier-Maillard A, Secher T, Rehman A, Normand S, De Arcangelis A, Haesler R, Huot L, Grandjean T, Bressenot A, Delanoye-Crespin A et al: NOD2-mediated dysbiosis predisposes mice to transmissible colitis and colorectal cancer. J Clin Invest 2013, 123(2):700-711.

89. Hu B, Elinav E, Huber S, Strowig T, Hao L, Hafemann A, Jin C, Wunderlich C, Wunderlich T, Eisenbarth SC, et al. Microbiota-induced activation of epithelial IL-6 signaling links inflammasome-driven inflammation with transmissible cancer. Proc Natl Acad Sci U S A. 2013;110(24):9862–7.

90. Carvalho FA, Barnich N, Sivignon A, Darcha C, Chan CH, Stanners CP, Darfeuille-Michaud A. Crohn's disease adherent-invasive Escherichia coli colonize and induce strong gut inflammation in transgenic mice expressing human CEACAM. J Exp Med. 2009;206(10):2179–89.

91. Boudeau J, Barnich N, Darfeuille-Michaud A. Type 1 pili-mediated adherence of Escherichia coli strain LF82 isolated from Crohn's disease is involved in bacterial invasion of intestinal epithelial cells. Mol Microbiol. 2001;39(5):1272–84.

92. Glasser AL, Boudeau J, Barnich N, Perruchot MH, Colombel JF, Darfeuille-Michaud A. Adherent invasive Escherichia coli strains from patients with Crohn's disease survive and replicate within macrophages without inducing host cell death. Infect Immun. 2001;69(9):5529–37.

93. Raisch J, Rolhion N, Dubois A, Darfeuille-Michaud A, Bringer MA. Intracellular colon cancer-associated Escherichia coli promote protumoral activities of human macrophages by inducing sustained COX-2 expression. Lab Invest. 2015;95(3):296–307.

94. Lu C, Chen J, Xu HG, Zhou X, He Q, Li YL, Jiang G, Shan Y, Xue B, Zhao RX, et al. MIR106B and MIR93 prevent removal of bacteria from epithelial cells by disrupting ATG16L1-mediated autophagy. Gastroenterology. 2014;146(1):188–99.

95. Nguyen HT, Dalmasso G, Muller S, Carriere J, Seibold F, Darfeuille-Michaud A. Crohn's disease-associated adherent invasive Escherichia coli modulate levels of microRNAs in intestinal epithelial cells to reduce autophagy. Gastroenterology. 2014;146(2):508–19.

96. Sadaghian Sadabad M, Regeling A, de Goffau MC, Blokzijl T, Weersma RK, Penders J, Faber KN, Harmsen HJ, Dijkstra G: The ATG16L1-T300A allele impairs clearance of pathosymbionts in the inflamed ileal mucosa of Crohn's disease patients. Gut 2015, 64(10):1546-1552.

97. Kim SC, Tonkonogy SL, Karrasch T, Jobin C, Sartor RB. Dual-association of gnotobiotic IL-10-/- mice with 2 nonpathogenic commensal bacteria induces aggressive pancolitis. Inflamm Bowel Dis. 2007;13(12):1457–66.

98. Karrasch T, Kim JS, Muhlbauer M, Magness ST, Jobin C. Gnotobiotic IL-10-/-;NF-kappa B(EGFP) mice reveal the critical role of TLR/NF-kappa B signaling in commensal bacteria-induced colitis. J Immunol. 2007;178(10):6522–32.

99. Rhee KJ, Wu S, Wu X, Huso DL, Karim B, Franco AA, Rabizadeh S, Golub JE, Mathews LE, Shin J, et al. Induction of persistent colitis by a human commensal, enterotoxigenic Bacteroides fragilis, in wild-type C57BL/6 mice. Infect Immun. 2009;77(4):1708–18.

100. Rabizadeh S, Rhee KJ, Wu S, Huso D, Gan CM, Golub JE, Wu X, Zhang M, Sears CL. Enterotoxigenic bacteroides fragilis: a potential instigator of colitis. Inflamm Bowel Dis. 2007;13(12):1475–83.

101. Wick EC, Rabizadeh S, Albesiano E, Wu X, Wu S, Chan J, Rhee KJ, Ortega G, Huso DL, Pardoll D, et al. Stat3 activation in murine colitis induced by enterotoxigenic Bacteroides fragilis. Inflamm Bowel Dis. 2014;20(5):821–34.

102. Remacle AG, Shiryaev SA, Strongin AY. Distinct interactions with cellular E-cadherin of the two virulent metalloproteinases encoded by a Bacteroides fragilis pathogenicity island. PLoS One. 2014;9(11):e113896.

103. Hwang S, Gwon SY, Kim MS, Lee S, Rhee KJ. Bacteroides fragilis Toxin Induces IL-8 Secretion in HT29/C1 Cells through Disruption of E-cadherin Junctions. Immune Netw. 2013;13(5):213–7.

104. Setoyama H, Imaoka A, Ishikawa H, Umesaki Y. Prevention of gut inflammation by Bifidobacterium in dextran sulfate-treated gnotobiotic mice associated with Bacteroides strains isolated from ulcerative colitis patients. Microbes and infection / Institut Pasteur. 2003;5(2):115–22.

105. Barnett MP, McNabb WC, Cookson AL, Zhu S, Davy M, Knoch B, Nones K, Hodgkinson AJ, Roy NC. Changes in colon gene expression associated with increased colon inflammation in interleukin-10 gene-deficient mice inoculated with Enterococcus species. BMC Immunol. 2010;11:39.

106. Steck N, Hoffmann M, Sava IG, Kim SC, Hahne H, Tonkonogy SL, Mair K, Krueger D, Pruteanu M, Shanahan F, et al. Enterococcus faecalis metalloprotease compromises epithelial barrier and contributes to intestinal inflammation. Gastroenterology. 2011;141(3):959–71.

107. Ocvirk S, Sava IG, Lengfelder I, Lagkouvardos I, Steck N, Roh JH, Tchaptchet S, Bao Y, Hansen JJ, Huebner J, et al. Surface-Associated Lipoproteins Link Enterococcus faecalis Virulence to Colitogenic Activity in IL-10-Deficient Mice Independent of Their Expression Levels. PLoS Pathog. 2015;11(6):e1004911.

108. Pulusu SSR, Lawrance IC. Dysplasia and colorectal cancer surveillance in inflammatory bowel disease. Expert Rev Gastroenterol Hepatol. 2017;11(8):711–22.

109. Giglia MD, Chu DI. Familial Colorectal Cancer: Understanding the Alphabet Soup. Clin Colon Rectal Surg. 2016;29(3):185–95.

110. Fumery M, Dulai PS, Gupta S, Prokop LJ, Ramamoorthy S, Sandborn WJ, Singh S. Incidence, Risk Factors, and Outcomes of Colorectal Cancer in Patients With Ulcerative Colitis With Low-Grade Dysplasia: A Systematic Review and Meta-analysis. Clin Gastroenterol Hepatol. 2017;15(5):665–74 e665.

111. Giardiello FM, Krush AJ, Petersen GM, Booker SV, Kerr M, Tong LL, Hamilton SR. Phenotypic variability of familial adenomatous polyposis in 11 unrelated families with identical APC gene mutation. Gastroenterology. 1994;106(6): 1542–7.

112. Laurent S, Franchimont D, Coppens JP, Leunen K, Macken L, Peeters M, Plomteux O, Polus M, Poppe B, Sempoux C, et al. Familial adenomatous polyposis: clinical presentation, detection and surveillance. Acta Gastroenterol Belg. 2011;74(3):415–20.

113. Dejea CM, Fathi P, Craig JM, Boleij A, Taddese R, Geis AL, Wu X, DeStefano Shields CE, Hechenbleikner EM, Huso DL, et al. Patients with familial adenomatous polyposis harbor colonic biofilms containing tumorigenic bacteria. Science. 2018;359(6375):592–7.

114. Gao R, Kong C, Huang L, Li H, Qu X, Liu Z, Lan P, Wang J, Qin H. Mucosa-associated microbiota signature in colorectal cancer. Eur J Clin Microbiol Infect Dis. 2017.

115. Chen W, Liu F, Ling Z, Tong X, Xiang C. Human intestinal lumen and mucosa-associated microbiota in patients with colorectal cancer. PLoS One. 2012;7(6):e39743.

116. Kostic AD, Chun E, Robertson L, Glickman JN, Gallini CA, Michaud M, Clancy TE, Chung DC, Lochhead P, Hold GL, et al. Fusobacterium nucleatum potentiates intestinal tumorigenesis and modulates the tumor-immune microenvironment. Cell host & microbe. 2013;14(2):207–15.

117. Arthur JC, Perez-Chanona E, Muhlbauer M, Tomkovich S, Uronis JM, Fan TJ, Campbell BJ, Abujamel T, Dogan B, Rogers AB, et al. Intestinal inflammation targets cancer-inducing activity of the microbiota. Science. 2012;338(6103):120–3.

118. Goodwin AC, Destefano Shields CE, Wu S, Huso DL, Wu X, Murray-Stewart TR, Hacker-Prietz A, Rabizadeh S, Woster PM, Sears CL, et al. Polyamine catabolism contributes to enterotoxigenic Bacteroides fragilis-induced colon tumorigenesis. Proc Natl Acad Sci U S A. 2011;108(37):15354–9.

119. Yang Y, Weng W, Peng J, Hong L, Yang L, Toiyama Y, Gao R, Liu M, Yin M, Pan C, et al. Fusobacterium nucleatum Increases Proliferation of Colorectal Cancer Cells and Tumor Development in Mice by Activating Toll-Like Receptor 4 Signaling to Nuclear Factor-kappaB, and Up-regulating Expression of MicroRNA-21. Gastroenterology. 2017;152(4):851–66 e824.

120. Bonnet M, Buc E, Sauvanet P, Darcha C, Dubois D, Pereira B, Dechelotte P, Bonnet R, Pezet D, Darfeuille-Michaud A. Colonization of the human gut by E. coli and colorectal cancer risk. Clinical cancer research : an official journal of the American Association for Cancer Research. 2014; 20(4):859–67.

121. Yu LC, Wei SC, Ni YH. Impact of Microbiota in Colorectal Carcinogenesis: Lessons from Experimental Models. Intestinal Research. 2018.

122. Wu S, Rhee KJ, Albesiano E, Rabizadeh S, Wu X, Yen HR, Huso DL, Brancati FL, Wick E, McAllister F, et al. A human colonic commensal promotes colon tumorigenesis via activation of T helper type 17 T cell responses. Nat Med. 2009;15(9):1016–22.

123. Arthur JC, Gharaibeh RZ, Muhlbauer M, Perez-Chanona E, Uronis JM, McCafferty J, Fodor AA, Jobin C. Microbial genomic analysis reveals the

123. essential role of inflammation in bacteria-induced colorectal cancer. Nature Commun. 2014;5:4724.

124. Chen GY, Shaw MH, Redondo G, Nunez G. The innate immune receptor Nod1 protects the intestine from inflammation-induced tumorigenesis. Cancer Res. 2008;68(24):10060–7.

125. Normand S, Delanoye-Crespin A, Bressenot A, Huot L, Grandjean T, Peyrin-Biroulet L, Lemoine Y, Hot D, Chamaillard M. Nod-like receptor pyrin domain-containing protein 6 (NLRP6) controls epithelial self-renewal and colorectal carcinogenesis upon injury. Proc Natl Acad Sci U S A. 2011;108(23):9601–6.

126. Chan CH, Cook D, Stanners CP. Increased colon tumor susceptibility in azoxymethane treated CEABAC transgenic mice. Carcinogenesis. 2006;27(9):1909–16.

127. Raisch J, Buc E, Bonnet M, Sauvanet P, Vazeille E, de Vallee A, Dechelotte P, Darcha C, Pezet D, Bonnet R, et al. Colon cancer-associated B2 Escherichia coli colonize gut mucosa and promote cell proliferation. World J Gastroenterol. 2014;20(21):6560–72.

128. Tomkovich S, Yang Y, Winglee K, Gauthier J, Muhlbauer M, Sun X, Mohamadzadeh M, Liu X, Martin P, Wang GP, et al. Locoregional Effects of Microbiota in a Preclinical Model of Colon Carcinogenesis. Cancer Res. 2017;77(10):2620–32.

129. Cougnoux A, Dalmasso G, Martinez R, Buc E, Delmas J, Gibold L, Sauvanet P, Darcha C, Dechelotte P, Bonnet M, et al. Bacterial genotoxin colibactin promotes colon tumour growth by inducing a senescence-associated secretory phenotype. Gut. 2014;63(12):1932–42.

130. Dalmasso G, Cougnoux A, Delmas J, Darfeuille-Michaud A, Bonnet R. The bacterial genotoxin colibactin promotes colon tumor growth by modifying the tumor microenvironment. Gut Microbes. 2014;5(5):675–80.

131. Toprak NU, Yagci A, Gulluoglu BM, Akin ML, Demirkalem P, Celenk T, Soyletir G. A possible role of Bacteroides fragilis enterotoxin in the aetiology of colorectal cancer. Clin Microbiol Infect. 2006;12(8):782–6.

132. Chung L, Orberg ET, Geis AL, Chan JL, Fu K, DeStefano Shields CE, Dejea CM, Fathi P, Chen J, Finard BB, et al. Bacteroides fragilis Toxin Coordinates a Pro-carcinogenic Inflammatory Cascade via Targeting of Colonic Epithelial Cells. Cell Host & Microbe. 2018;23(3):421.

133. Mima K, Nishihara R, Qian ZR, Cao Y, Sukawa Y, Nowak JA, Yang J, Dou R, Masugi Y, Song M, et al. Fusobacterium nucleatum in colorectal carcinoma tissue and patient prognosis. Gut. 2016;65(12):1973–80.

134. Rubinstein MR, Wang X, Liu W, Hao Y, Cai G, Han YW. Fusobacterium nucleatum promotes colorectal carcinogenesis by modulating E-cadherin/beta-catenin signaling via its FadA adhesin. Cell host & microbe. 2013;14(2):195–206.

135. Chen Y, Peng Y, Yu J, Chen T, Wu Y, Shi L, Li Q, Wu J, Fu X. Invasive Fusobacterium nucleatum activates beta-catenin signaling in colorectal cancer via a TLR4/P-PAK1 cascade. Oncotarget. 2017;8(19):31802–14.

136. Fardini Y, Wang X, Temoin S, Nithianantham S, Lee D, Shoham M, Han YW. Fusobacterium nucleatum adhesin FadA binds vascular endothelial cadherin and alters endothelial integrity. Mol Microbiol. 2011;82(6):1468–80.

137. Hilsden RJ, Meddings JB, Sutherland LR. Intestinal permeability changes in response to acetylsalicylic acid in relatives of patients with Crohn's disease. Gastroenterology. 1996;110(5):1395–403.

138. D'Inca R, Annese V, di Leo V, Latiano A, Quaino V, Abazia C, Vettorato MG, Sturniolo GC. Increased intestinal permeability and NOD2 variants in familial and sporadic Crohn's disease. Aliment Pharmacol Ther. 2006;23(10):1455–61.

139. Peeters M, Geypens B, Claus D, Nevens H, Ghoos Y, Verbeke G, Baert F, Vermeire S, Vlietinck R, Rutgeerts P. Clustering of increased small intestinal permeability in families with Crohn's disease. Gastroenterology. 1997;113(3):802–7.

140. Schmitz H, Barmeyer C, Fromm M, Runkel N, Foss HD, Bentzel CJ, Riecken EO, Schulzke JD. Altered tight junction structure contributes to the impaired epithelial barrier function in ulcerative colitis. Gastroenterology. 1999;116(2):301–9.

141. Arslan G, Atasever T, Cindoruk M, Yildirim IS. (51)CrEDTA colonic permeability and therapy response in patients with ulcerative colitis. Nucl Med Commun. 2001;22(9):997–1001.

142. Buning C, Geissler N, Prager M, Sturm A, Baumgart DC, Buttner J, Buhner S, Haas V, Lochs H. Increased small intestinal permeability in ulcerative colitis: rather genetic than environmental and a risk factor for extensive disease? Inflamm Bowel Dis. 2012;18(10):1932–9.

143. Tibble JA, Sigthorsson G, Bridger S, Fagerhol MK, Bjarnason I. Surrogate markers of intestinal inflammation are predictive of relapse in patients with inflammatory bowel disease. Gastroenterology. 2000;119(1):15–22.

144. Jorgensen J, Ranlov PJ, Bjerrum PJ, Diemer H, Bisgaard K, Elsborg L. Is an increased intestinal permeability a valid predictor of relapse in Crohn disease? Scand J Gastroenterol. 2001;36(5):521–7.

145. Madsen KL, Malfair D, Gray D, Doyle JS, Jewell LD, Fedorak RN. Interleukin-10 gene-deficient mice develop a primary intestinal permeability defect in response to enteric microflora. Inflamm Bowel Dis. 1999;5(4):262–70.

146. Olson TS, Reuter BK, Scott KG, Morris MA, Wang XM, Hancock LN, Burcin TL, Cohn SM, Ernst PB, Cominelli F, et al. The primary defect in experimental ileitis originates from a nonhematopoietic source. J Exp Med. 2006;203(3):541–52.

147. Nenci A, Becker C, Wullaert A, Gareus R, van LG, Danese S, Huth M, Nikolaev A, Neufert C, Madison B, et al. Epithelial NEMO links innate immunity to chronic intestinal inflammation. Nature. 2007;446(7135):557–61.

148. Hermiston ML, Gordon JI. Inflammatory bowel disease and adenomas in mice expressing a dominant negative N-cadherin. Science. 1995;270(5239):1203–7.

149. Nighot P, Al-Sadi R, Rawat M, Guo S, Watterson DM, Ma T. Matrix metalloproteinase 9-induced increase in intestinal epithelial tight junction permeability contributes to the severity of experimental DSS colitis. Am J Physiol Gastrointest Liver Physiol. 2015;309(12):G988–97.

150. Liu X, Xu J, Mei Q, Han L, Huang J. Myosin light chain kinase inhibitor inhibits dextran sulfate sodium-induced colitis in mice. Dig Dis Sci. 2013;58(1):107–14.

151. Lee TC, Huang YC, Lu YZ, Yeh YC, Yu LC. Hypoxia-induced intestinal barrier changes in balloon-assisted enteroscopy. J Physiol. 2017;596(15):13.

152. Wei SC, Yang-Yen HF, Tsao PN, Weng MT, Tung CC, Yu LCH, Lai LC, Hsiao JH, Chuang EY, Shun CT, et al. SHANK3 Regulates Intestinal Barrier Function Through Modulating ZO-1 Expression Through the PKCepsilon-dependent Pathway. Inflamm Bowel Dis. 2017;23(10):1730–40.

153. Lu YZ, Huang CY, Huang YC, Lee TC, Kuo WT, Pai YC, Yu LC. Tumor Necrosis Factor alpha-Dependent Neutrophil Priming Prevents Intestinal Ischemia/Reperfusion-Induced Bacterial Translocation. Dig Dis Sci. 2017.

154. Swidsinski A, Ladhoff A, Pernthaler A, Swidsinski S, Loening-Baucke V, Ortner M, Weber J, Hoffmann U, Schreiber S, Dietel M, et al. Mucosal flora in inflammatory bowel disease. Gastroenterology. 2002;122(1):44–54.

155. Sobieszczanska BA, Duda-Madej AB, Turniak MB, Franiczek R, Kasprzykowska U, Duda AK, Rzeszutko M, Iwanczak B. Invasive properties, adhesion patterns and phylogroup profiles among Escherichia coli strains isolated from children with inflammatory bowel disease. Adv Clin Exp Med 2012; 21:591-9

156. Reuter BK, Pizarro TT. Mechanisms of tight junction dysregulation in the SAMP1/YitFc model of Crohn's disease-like ileitis. Ann N Y Acad Sci. 2009;1165:301–7.

157. Su L, Shen L, Clayburgh DR, Nalle SC, Sullivan EA, Meddings JB, Abraham C, Turner JR. Targeted Epithelial Tight Junction Dysfunction Causes Immune Activation and Contributes to Development of Experimental Colitis. Gastroenterology. 2009;136(2):551–63.

158. Zeissig S, Burgel N, Gunzel D, Richter J, Mankertz J, Wahnschaffe U, Kroesen AJ, Zeitz M, Fromm M, Schulzke JD. Changes in expression and distribution of claudin 2, 5 and 8 lead to discontinuous tight junctions and barrier dysfunction in active Crohn's disease. Gut. 2007;56(1):61–72.

159. Oshitani N, Watanabe K, Nakamura S, Fujiwara Y, Higuchi K, Arakawa T. Dislocation of tight junction proteins without F-actin disruption in inactive Crohn's disease. Int J Mol Med. 2005;15(3):407–10.

160. Blair SA, Kane SV, Clayburgh DR, Turner JR. Epithelial myosin light chain kinase expression and activity are upregulated in inflammatory bowel disease. Lab Invest. 2006;86(2):191–201.

161. Boudeau J, Glasser AL, Julien S, Colombel JF, Darfeuille-Michaud A. Inhibitory effect of probiotic Escherichia coli strain Nissle 1917 on adhesion to and invasion of intestinal epithelial cells by adherent-invasive E. coli strains isolated from patients with Crohn's disease. Aliment Pharmacol Ther. 2003;18(1):45–56.

162. Lewis K, Lutgendorff F, Phan V, Soderholm JD, Sherman PM, McKay DM. Enhanced translocation of bacteria across metabolically stressed epithelia is reduced by butyrate. Inflamm Bowel Dis. 2010;16(7):1138–48.

163. Wang A, Keita AV, Phan V, McKay CM, Schoultz I, Lee J, Murphy MP, Fernando M, Ronaghan N, Balce D, et al. Targeting mitochondria-derived reactive oxygen species to reduce epithelial barrier dysfunction and colitis. Am J Pathol. 2014;184(9):2516–27.

164. Clark E, Hoare C, Tanianis-Hughes J, Carlson GL, Warhurst G. Interferon gamma induces translocation of commensal Escherichia coli across gut epithelial cells via a lipid raft-mediated process. Gastroenterology. 2005;128(5):1258–67.

165. Smyth D, McKay CM, Gulbransen BD, Phan VC, Wang A, McKay DM. Interferon-gamma signals via an ERK1/2-ARF6 pathway to promote bacterial internalization by gut epithelia. Cell Microbiol. 2012;14(8):1257–70.

166. Wells CL, VandeWesterlo EM, Jechorek RP, Erlandsen SL. Effect of hypoxia on enterocyte endocytosis of enteric bacteria. Crit Care Med. 1996;24(6):985–91.

167. Wu LL, Chiu HD, Peng WH, Lin BR, Lu KS, Lu YZ, Yu LCH. Epithelial inducible nitric oxide synthase causes bacterial translocation by impairment of enterocytic tight junctions via intracellular signals of Rho-associated kinase and protein kinase C zeta. Critical Care Medicine. 2011;39:2087–98.

168. Saggioro A. Leaky gut, microbiota, and cancer: an incoming hypothesis. J Clin Gastroenterol. 2014;48(Suppl 1):S62–6.

169. Hansen TH, Gobel RJ, Hansen T, Pedersen O. The gut microbiome in cardio-metabolic health. Genome Med. 2015;7(1):33.

170. Lewis JD, Chen EZ, Baldassano RN, Otley AR, Griffiths AM, Lee D, Bittinger K, Bailey A, Friedman ES, Hoffmann C, et al. Inflammation, Antibiotics, and Diet as Environmental Stressors of the Gut Microbiome in Pediatric Crohn's Disease. Cell Host & Microbe. 2015;18(4):489–500.

171. Winter SE, Winter MG, Xavier MN, Thiennimitr P, Poon V, Keestra AM, Laughlin RC, Gomez G, Wu J, Lawhon SD, et al. Host-derived nitrate boosts growth of E. coli in the inflamed gut. Science. 2013;339(6120):708–11.

172. Winter SE, Lopez CA, Baumler AJ. The dynamics of gut-associated microbial communities during inflammation. EMBO Rep. 2013;14(4):319–27.

173. Albenberg L, Esipova TV, Judge CP, Bittinger K, Chen J, Laughlin A, Grunberg S, Baldassano RN, Lewis JD, Li H, et al. Correlation between intraluminal oxygen gradient and radial partitioning of intestinal microbiota. Gastroenterology. 2014;147(5):1055–63 e1058.

174. Denizot J, Sivignon A, Barreau F, Darcha C, Chan HF, Stanners CP, Hofman P, Darfeuille-Michaud A, Barnich N. Adherent-invasive Escherichia coli induce claudin-2 expression and barrier defect in CEABAC10 mice and Crohn's disease patients. Inflamm Bowel Dis. 2012;18(2):294–304.

175. Han X, Fink MP, Delude RL. Proinflammatory cytokines cause NO-dependent and -independent changes in expression and localization of tight junction proteins in intestinal epithelial cells. Shock. 2003;19(3):229–37.

176. Menconi MJ, Unno N, Smith M, Aguirre DE, Fink MP. Nitric oxide donor-induced hyperpermeability of cultured intestinal epithelial monolayers: role of superoxide radical, hydroxyl radical, and peroxynitrite. BiochimBiophysActa. 1998;1425(1):189–203.

177. Landy J, Ronde E, English N, Clark SK, Hart AL, Knight SC, Ciclitira PJ, Al-Hassi HO. Tight junctions in inflammatory bowel diseases and inflammatory bowel disease associated colorectal cancer. World J Gastroenterol. 2016;22(11):3117–26.

178. Marteyn B, Scorza FB, Sansonetti PJ, Tang C. Breathing life into pathogens: the influence of oxygen on bacterial virulence and host responses in the gastrointestinal tract. Cell Microbiol. 2011;13(2):171–6.

179. Green J, Rolfe MD, Smith LJ. Transcriptional regulation of bacterial virulence gene expression by molecular oxygen and nitric oxide. Virulence. 2014;5(8):794–809.

180. Mirzaei MK, Maurice CF. Menage a trois in the human gut: interactions between host, bacteria and phages. Nature Rev Microbiol. 2017;15(7):397–408.

181. De Sordi L, Lourenco M, Debarbieux L. "I will survive": A tale of bacteriophage-bacteria coevolution in the gut. Gut Microbes. 2018;1–18.

182. Allegretti J, Eysenbach LM, El-Nachef N, Fischer M, Kelly C, Kassam Z. The Current Landscape and Lessons from Fecal Microbiota Transplantation for Inflammatory Bowel Disease: Past, Present, and Future. Inflamm Bowel Dis. 2017;23(10):1710–7.

183. Costello SP, Soo W, Bryant RV, Jairath V, Hart AL, Andrews JM. Systematic review with meta-analysis: faecal microbiota transplantation for the induction of remission for active ulcerative colitis. Aliment Pharmacol Ther. 2017;46(3):213–24.

184. Moayyedi P, Surette MG, Kim PT, Libertucci J, Wolfe M, Onischi C, Armstrong D, Marshall JK, Kassam Z, Reinisch W, et al. Fecal Microbiota Transplantation Induces Remission in Patients With Active Ulcerative Colitis in a Randomized Controlled Trial. Gastroenterology. 2015;149(1):102–9 e106.

185. Vaughn BP, Vatanen T, Allegretti JR, Bai A, Xavier RJ, Korzenik J, Gevers D, Ting A, Robson SC, Moss AC. Increased Intestinal Microbial Diversity Following Fecal Microbiota Transplant for Active Crohn's Disease. Inflamm Bowel Dis. 2016;22(9):2182–90.

186. Qazi T, Amaratunga T, Barnes EL, Fischer M, Kassam Z, Allegretti JR. The risk of inflammatory bowel disease flares after fecal microbiota transplantation: Systematic review and meta-analysis. Gut Microbes. 2017;8(6):574–88.

187. Fries W, Belvedere A, Vetrano S. Sealing the broken barrier in IBD: intestinal permeability, epithelial cells and junctions. Curr Drug Targets. 2013;14(12):1460–70.

188. Bischoff SC, Barbara G, Buurman W, Ockhuizen T, Schulzke JD, Serino M, Tilg H, Watson A, Wells JM. Intestinal permeability--a new target for disease prevention and therapy. BMC Gastroenterol. 2014;14:189.

189. Lin KY, Peng SY, Chou CJ, Lee HS, Lin LC, Pan RY, Wu SC. Infusion of Porcine-Derived Amniotic Fluid Stem Cells for Treatment of Experimental Colitis in Mice. Chin J Physiol. 2017;60(6):345–52.

190. Motta JP, Bermudez-Humaran LG, Deraison C, Martin L, Rolland C, Rousset P, Boue J, Dietrich G, Chapman K, Kharrat P, et al. Food-grade bacteria expressing elafin protect against inflammation and restore colon homeostasis. Sci Transl Med. 2012;4(158):158ra144.

191. Carroll IM, Andrus JM, Bruno-Barcena JM, Klaenhammer TR, Hassan HM, Threadgill DS. Anti-inflammatory properties of Lactobacillus gasseri expressing manganese superoxide dismutase using the interleukin 10-deficient mouse model of colitis. Am J Physiol Gastrointest Liver Physiol. 2007;293(4):G729–38.

192. Kashyap PC, Chia N, Nelson H, Segal E, Elinav E. Microbiome at the Frontier of Personalized Medicine. Mayo Clin Proc. 2017;92(12):1855–64.

193. Zmora N, Zeevi D, Korem T, Segal E, Elinav E. Taking it Personally: Personalized Utilization of the Human Microbiome in Health and Disease. Cell Host & Microbe. 2016;19(1):12–20.

194. Nagpal R, Yadav H. Bacterial Translocation from the Gut to the Distant Organs: An Overview. Ann Nutr Metab. 2017;71(Suppl 1):11–6.

Permissions

List of Contributors

Sehrish Khan, Muhammad Shahid Mahmood, Sajjad ur Rahman and Hassan Zafar
Institute of Microbiology University of Agriculture, Faisalabad, Pakistan

Sultan Habibullah and Zulqarnain khan
Center of Agricultural Biochemistry and Biotechnology, University of Agriculture, Faisalabad, Pakistan

Aftab Ahmad
Department of Biochemistry/U.S.-Pakistan Center for Advanced Studies in Agriculture and Food Security (USPCAS-AFS), University of Agriculture Faisalabad (UAF), Faisalabad 38040, Pakistan

Shih-Han Kao and Kou-Juey Wu
Research Center for Tumor Medical Science, China Medical University, No. 91, Hseuh-Shih Rd, Taichung 40402, Taiwan
Drug Development Center, China Medical University, Taichung 40402, Taiwan

Kou-Juey Wu
Institute of New Drug Development, Taichung 40402, Taiwan
Graduate Institutes of Biomedical Sciences, China Medical University, Taichung 40402, Taiwan
Departmet of Medical Research, China Medical University Hospital, Taichung 40402, Taiwans

Han-Tsang Wu
Department of Cell and Tissue Engineering, Changhua Christian Hospital, Changhua City 500, Taiwan

Jianquan Zhao
Department of Cardiology, Bayannaoer City Hospital, 35 Xinhua District, Bayannaoer 015000, Inner Mongolia, China

Tiewei Lv, Junjun Quan and Weian Zhao
Department of Cardiology, Children's hospital, Chongqing Medical University, Chongqing, China

Jing Song and Longke Ran
Department of Bioinformatics, Chongqing Medical University, 1 Yixueyuan Road, Yuzhong District, Chongqing 400016, China

Zhuolin Li, Han Lei and Wei Huang
Department of Vascular Cardiology, the First Affiliated Hospital of Chongqing, Medical University, Chongqing, China

Victor Marinho, Thomaz Oliveira, Juliete Bandeira, Francisco Magalhães, Kaline Rocha, Carla Ayres, Valécia Carvalho and Silmar Teixeira
Neuro-innovation Technology & Brain Mapping Laboratory, Federal University of Piauí, Av. São Sebastião n° 2819 – Nossa Sra. de Fátima –, Parnaíba, PI CEP 64202-020, Brazil

Victor Marinho, Thomaz Oliveira, Giovanny R. Pinto, Anderson Gomes and Valéria Lima
Genetics and Molecular Biology Laboratory, Federal University of Piauí, Parnaíba, Brazil

Victor Marinho, Giovanny R. Pinto, Francisco Magalhães, Kaline Rocha, Valécia Carvalho and Silmar Teixeira
The Northeast Biotechnology Network (RENORBIO), Federal University of Piauí, Teresina, Brazil

Bruna Velasques and Pedro Ribeiro
Brain Mapping and Sensory Motor Integration Laboratory, Federal University of Rio de Janeiro, Rio de Janeiro, Brazil

Marco Orsini
Master's Program in Local Development Program, University Center Augusto Motta - UNISUAM, Rio de Janeiro, Brazil and Health Sciences Applied - Vassouras University, Rio de Janeiro, Brazil

Victor Hugo Bastos
Brain Mapping and Functionality Laboratory, Federal University of Piauí, Parnaíba, Brazil

Daya Gupta
Department of Biology, Camden County College, Blackwood, NJ, USA

Nikki P. Lee, Chung Man Chan, Lai Nar Tung, Hector K. Wang and Simon Law
Department of Surgery, The University of Hong Kong, Faculty of Medicine Building, 21 Sassoon Road, Pokfulam, Hong Kong

Mohamed El Amri and Gerhard Schlosser
Centre for Research in Medical Devices (CÚRAM), National University of Ireland, Galway, Biomedical Sciences Building, Newcastle Road, Galway, Ireland

Una Fitzgerald
Galway Neuroscience Centre, School of Natural Sciences, Biomedical Sciences Building, National University of Ireland, Newcastle Road, Galway, Ireland

Gerhard Schlosser
School of Natural Sciences and Regenerative Medicine Institute (REMEDI), National University of Ireland, Galway, Biomedical Sciences Building, Newcastle Road, Galway, Ireland

Jyh-Ming Liou, Yu-Ting Kuo and Ming-Shiang Wu
Division of Gastroenterology and Hepatology, Department of Internal Medicine, National Taiwan University Hospital, Taipei, Taiwan
Department of Internal Medicine, College of Medicine, National Taiwan University, No. 7, Chung-Shan S. Road, Taipei, Taiwan

Po-Yueh Chen
Division of Gastroenterology and Hepatology, Department of Internal medicine, Chia-Yi Christian Hospital, Chia-Yi, Taiwan

Kovit Pattanapanyasat, Premrutai Thitilertdecha and Nattawat Onlamoon
Biomedical Research Incubator Unit, Research Group and Research Network Division, Research Department, Faculty of Medicine Siriraj Hospital, Mahidol University, Bangkok, Thailand

Ladawan Khowawisetsut
Department of Parasitology, Faculty of Medicine Siriraj Hospital, Mahidol University, Bangkok, Thailand

Ampaiwan Chuansumrit, Kanchana Tangnararatchakit, Nopporn Apiwattanakul and Chonnamet Techasaensiri
Department of Pediatrics, Faculty of Medicine Ramathibodi Hospital, Mahidol University, Bangkok, Thailand

Kulkanya Chokephaibulkit
Department of Pediatrics, Faculty of Medicine Siriraj Hospital, Mahidol University, Bangkok, Thailand

Premrutai Thitilertdecha and Nattawat Onlamoon
Research group in Immunobiology and Therapeutic Sciences, Faculty of Medicine Siriraj Hospital, Mahidol University, 2 Wanglang Road, Bangkoknoi, Bangkok 10700, Thailand

Tipaporn Sae-Ung
Master of Science program in Immunology, Department of Immunology, Faculty of Medicine Siriraj Hospital, Mahidol University, Bangkok, Thailand

Matteo M Pusceddu and Melanie G Gareau
Department of Anatomy, Physiology and Cell Biology, School of Veterinary Medicine, University of California Davis, One Shield Avenue, Davis, CA, USA

Tsung-Yu Tsai
Ph.D. Program for Translational Medicine, China Medical University and Academia Sinica, Taichung and Taipei, Taiwan

Tsung-Yu Tsai, Cheng-Yuan Peng and Hsueh-Chou Lai
Division of Hepatogastroenterology, Department of Internal Medicine, China Medical University Hospital, 2, Yude St., North District, Taichung 404, Taiwan

Cheng-Yuan Peng
School of Medicine, China Medical University, Taichung, Taiwan

Hwai-I Yang, Ya-Lang Huang and Shie-Liang Hsieh
Genomics Research Center, Academia Sinica, 128, Academia Road, Sec. 2, Nankang District, Taipei 115, Taiwan

Mi-Hua Tao
Institute of Biomedical Sciences, Academia Sinica, 128, Academia Road, Sec. 2, Nankang District, Taipei 115, Taiwan

Shin-Sheng Yuan
Institute of Statistical Sciences, Academia Sinica, 128, Academia Road, Sec. 2, Nankang District, Taipei 115, Taiwan

Shie-Liang Hsieh
Institute of Clinical Medicine, National Yang-Ming University, Taipei, Taiwan

Department of Medical Research, Taipei Veterans General Hospital, Taipei, Taiwan

Tae Woo Jung
Research Administration Team, Seoul National University Bundang Hospital, 166 Gumi-ro, Bundang-gu, Seongnam 463-707, Korea

Tae Woo Jung, Hyung Sub Park, Geum Hee Choi, Daehwan Kim and Taeseung Lee
Department of Surgery, Seoul National University Bundang Hospital, Seoul National University College of Medicine, 166 Gumi-ro, Bundang-gu, Seongnam 463-707, Korea

Taeseung Lee
Department of Surgery, Seoul National University College of Medicine, Seoul, Korea

Ying-Qing Li, Na Liu, Qing-Mei He, Xin-Ran Tang, Xin Wen, Xiao-Jing Yang, Ying Sun, Jun Ma and Ling-Long Tang
Sun Yat-sen University Cancer Center; State Key Laboratory of Oncology in South China; Collaborative Innovation Center for Cancer Medicine; Guangdong Key Laboratory of Nasopharyngeal Carcinoma Diagnosis and Therapy, Guangzhou 510060, People's Republic of China

Ya-Fei Xu
Department of Cell Biology and Genetics, Shenzhen University Health Science Center, Shenzhen 518060, People's Republic of China

Hong-Ru Chen and Yen-Chung Lai
The Institute of Basic Medical Sciences, College of Medicine, National Cheng Kung University, Tainan, Taiwan

Trai-Ming Yeh
Department of Medical Laboratory Science and Biotechnology, College of Medicine, National Cheng Kung University, Tainan, Taiwan

Wei-Chen Hsin, Chan-Hua Chang, Chi-You Chang and Shin C. Chang
Institute of Microbiology, College of Medicine, National Taiwan University, No. 1, Jen-Ai Road, First Section, Taipei 100, Taiwan

Wei-Hao Peng and Chung-Liang Chien
Institute of Anatomy and Cell Biology, College of Medicine, National Taiwan University, No. 1, Jen-Ai Road, First Section, Taipei 100, Taiwan

Ming-Fu Chang
Institute of Biochemistry and Molecular Biology, College of Medicine, National Taiwan University, No. 1, Jen-Ai Road, First Section, Taipei 100, Taiwan

Feng-Woei Tsay and Ping-I Hsu
Division of Gastroenterology and Hepatology, Department of Internal Medicine, Kaohsiung Veterans General Hospital and National Yang-Ming University, 386 Ta Chung 1st Road, Kaohsiung 813, Taiwan, Republic of China

Feng-Woei Tsay
Cheng Shiu University, Kaohsiung, Taiwan, Republic of China

C. Sao Emani, M. J. Williams, I. J. Wiid and B. Baker
DST-NRF Centre of Excellence for Biomedical Tuberculosis Research; SAMRC Centre for Tuberculosis Research; Division of Molecular Biology and Human Genetics; Department of Biomedical Sciences, Faculty of Medicine and Health Sciences; Stellenbosch University, Francie van Zijl Drive, Tygerberg 8000, Cape Town, South Africa

Shu-Man Hsieh Li, Shu-Ting Liu, Yung-Lung Chang and Shih-Ming Huang
Department of Biochemistry, National Defense Medical Center, Taipei City 114, Taiwan, Republic of China

Ching-Liang Ho
Division of Hematology/Oncology, Department of Medicine, Tri-Service General Hospital, National Defense Medical Center, Taipei City 114, Taiwan, Republic of China

Jean Ching-Yuan Fann
Department of Health Industry Management, School of Healthcare Management, Kainan University, Taoyuan City, Taiwan

Tsung-Hsien Chiang, Yi-Chia Lee and Ming-Shiang Wu
Department of Internal Medicine, College of Medicine, National Taiwan University Hospital, No. 7, Chung-Shan South Road, Taipei 10002, Taiwan

Tsung-Hsien Chiang
Department of Integrated Diagnostics and Therapeutics, National Taiwan University Hospital, Taipei, Taiwan

Tsung-Hsien Chiang
Graduate Institute of Clinical Medicine, College of Medicine, National Taiwan University, Taipei, Taiwan

Amy Ming-Fang Yen
School of Oral Hygiene, College of Oral Medicine, Taipei Medical University, No. 250, Wu-Hsing Street, Xinyi District, Taipei 110, Taiwan

Yi-Chia Lee and Hsiu-Hsi Chen
Institute of Epidemiology and Preventive Medicine, College of Public Health, National Taiwan University, Taipei, Taiwan
Innovation and Policy Center for Population Health and Sustainable Environment, College of Public Health, National Taiwan University, Taipei, Taiwan

Shu-Wen Wan
School of Medicine, College of Medicine, I-Shou University, Kaohsiung, Taiwan

Betty A. Wu-Hsieh and Wen-Yu Chen
Graduate Institute of Immunology, College of Medicine, National Taiwan University, Taipei, Taiwan

Yee-Shin Lin and Robert Anderson
Department of Microbiology and Immunology, College of Medicine, National Cheng Kung University, Tainan, Taiwan

Yee-Shin Lin
Center of Infectious Disease and Signaling Research, National Cheng Kung University, Tainan, Taiwan

Yan Huang and Robert Anderson
Department of Microbiology & Immunology, Dalhousie University, Halifax, NS B3H 4R2, Canada
Canadian Center for Vaccinology, Dalhousie University, Halifax, Canada

Linda Chia-Hui Yu
Graduate Institute of Physiology, National Taiwan University College of Medicine, Suite 1020, #1 Jen-Ai Rd. Sec. 1, Taipei 100, Taiwan, Republic of China

Index

www.ingramcontent.com/pod-product-compliance
Lightning Source LLC
Chambersburg PA
CBHW061241190326
41458CB00011B/3546